**Pain Management
and
Regional Anesthesia
in
Trauma**

Commissioning Editor: Maria Khan
Project Manager: Emily Pillars
Typeset by Phoenix Photosetting, Chatham, Kent
Printed in China

Pain Management and Regional Anesthesia in Trauma

Edited by

Andrew D Rosenberg, MD
Vice Chairman Department of Anesthesiology
Hospital For Joint Diseases
Associate Professor of Clinical Anesthesiology
New York University School Of Medicine
New York City, New York

Christopher Grande, MD MPH
Executive Director
International Trauma Anesthesia and Critical Care Society
Baltimore, Maryland

Ralph L Bernstein, MD
Chairman Department Of Anesthesiology
Hospital For Joint Diseases
Professor of Clinical Anesthesiology
New York University School Of Medicine
New York City, New York

WB Saunders Company Ltd
London   Edinburgh   New York   Philadelphia   St Louis   Sydney   Toronto   2000

WB SAUNDERS
An imprint of Harcourt Publishers Limited

© Harcourt Publishers Limited 1999

 is a registered trademark of Harcourt Publishers Limited

The right of Dr Andrew Rosenberg, Dr Christopher Grande and
Dr Ralph Bernstein to be identified as editors of this work has been
asserted by them in accordance with the Copyright, Designs and
Patents Act 1988

First published 2000

ISBN 0-7020-2285-3

British Library Cataloguing in Publication Data
A catalogue record for this book is available from the British Library

Library of Congress Cataloging in Publication Data
A catalog record for this book is available from the Library of Congress

Note
Medical knowledge is constantly changing. As new information becomes
available, changes in treatment, procedures, equipment and the use of
drugs become necessary. The editors/authors/contributors and the
publishers have, as far as it is possible, taken care to ensure that the
information given in this text is accurate and up-to-date. However,
readers are strongly advised to confirm that the information, especially
with regard to drug usage, complies with the latest legislation and
standards of practice.

The
Publisher's
policy is to use
**paper manufactured
from sustainable forests**

Contents

Contributors   vii
Foreword   xi
Preface   xiii
Acknowledgements   xv
Dedication   xvii
Abbreviations   xix
Table of volume of local anesthetic suggested
for regional anesthesia   xxi

Section I. Basics: Interface of Trauma and Pain   1

1. General introduction on trauma   3
   KJ Gupta, MJA Parr and JP Nolan

2. Overview of pain mechanisms and
   neuroanatomy   29
   Maywin Liu and F Michael Ferrante

3. The effects of pain in the trauma patient   47
   Nileskumar Patel and Charles E Smith

4. Pharmacologic management of acute and
   chronic pain in trauma patients   55
   P Prithvi Raj and Craig Hartrick

5. Regional anesthesia and analgesia in
   trauma: advantages and disadvantages in
   specific medical and clinical situations   85
   Mitchell H Marshall

Section II. Location-Based Pain Management: Concepts and Considerations   107

6. Pain management in the pre-hospital
   EMS environment: on-site and
   transport   109
   Torben Wisborg and Hans Flaatten

7. Pain management in the ER: initial
   evaluation and interventions   119
   *Andreas R Thierbach, Markus DW Lipp
   and Monika Daubländer*

8. Pain management in the OR: regional
   anesthesia for operative intervention
   and to augment general anesthesia   131
   Noor M Gajraj and Adolph H Giesecke

9. Pain management and sedation in the
   ICU   137
   Laureen L Hill and Ronald G Pearl

10. Pain management in the rehabilitation
    centre   149
    *Frank JE Falco, P Prithvi Raj,
    Daniel Breitstein, Kenneth J Abrams
    and Christopher Grande*

Section III. Perioperative Pain Management in Trauma: Techniques and Applications   161

11. Patient-controlled analgesia   163
    *Andrew D Rosenberg, Burdett R Porter
    and Joel F Lupatkin*

12. Epidural and spinal techniques including
    patient-controlled epidural analgesia   175
    Sassan Hassassian and Hagop Tabakian

13. Continuous plexus blocks for
    the management of trauma to the
    extremities   209
    *Alon P Winnie, Kenneth D Candido
    and Maria L Torres*

14. Thoracic blocks   239
    Gilles Orliaguet and Pierre Carli

15. Non-pharmacologic techniques for pain
    management   253
    Barry R Snow and Paul Gusmorino

Section IV. Pain Management for Specific Trauma Patient Populations and Injured Organ Systems   263

16. Regional anesthesia for pediatric trauma 265
    Lynn M Broadman and Nancy L Glass

17. Pregnant trauma patient   287
    Patricia Dalby and Sivam Ramanathan

18. Burn patient   301
    Lauren J DeLoach and Judith L Stiff

19. Trauma patient with thoracic and
    abdominal injuries   311
    Raymond S Sinatra and Sean J Ennevor

20. Trauma patient with neurologic
    injuries   339
    *Irene P Osborne, Haroon F Choudhri and
    George Sandor*

21. Trauma patient with orthopedic injuries 351
    *Ralph L Bernstein, Andrew D Rosenberg
    and David B Albert*

22. Chronic pain after trauma: complex
    regional pain syndrome and phantom
    pain syndrome   369
    Pedro A Mendez-Tellez and Mark J Lema

23. Invasive pain management for the
    trauma patient   403
    Carol Harris, Miles Day and Gabor B Racz

Index   423

Contributors

Kenneth J Abrams, MD
Assistant Professor of Anesthesiology and Surgery
Mt Sinai School of Medicine
Regional Director
Department of Anesthesiology
Queens Health Network
New York City, New York
USA

David B Albert, MD
Attending Anesthesiologist
Department of Anesthesiology
Hospital for Joint Diseases
New York City, New York
USA

Ralph L Bernstein, MD
Chairman Department of Anesthesiology
Hospital for Joint Diseases
Professor of Clinical Anesthesiology
New York University School Of Medicine
New York City, New York
USA

Daniel Brietstein, MD
Assistant Professor of Anesthesiology
Mt Sinai School of Medicine
New York City, New York
USA

Lynn M Broadman, MD
Professor of Anesthesia and Pediatrics
West Virginia School of Medicine
Morgantown, West Virginia
USA

Kenneth D Candido, MD
Chief, Section of Trauma and Pain Management
Department of Anesthesiology and Pain Management
Cook County Hospital
Chicago, USA

Pierre Carli, MD
Chairman
Professor of Anesthesiology
Department of Anesthesiology and Critical Care
Hospital Necker – Enfants Malades
Paris, France

Haroon F Choudhri, MD
Resident
Department of Neurology
New York University School of Medicine
New York City, New York
USA

Patricia Dalby, MD
Assistant Professor of Anesthesiology and Critical Care Medicine
University of Pittsburgh
Staff Anesthesiologist
Magee Woman's Hospital
Pittsburgh, Pennsylvania
USA

Monika Daubländer, MD ES
Consultant Maxillofacial Surgeon
Clinic of Dental Surgery
Johannes Gutenberg-University
Mainz, Germany

Miles Day, MD
Assistant Professor Pain Services
Department of Anesthesiology
Texas Tech University Health Sciences Center
Lubbock, Texas
USA

Lauren J DeLoach, MD
Assistant Professor
Department of Anesthesiology
Johns Hopkins Bayview Medical Center
Baltimore, Maryland
USA

Sean J Ennevor, MD
Anesthesiology Fellow
Department of Anesthesiology
Yale University School of Medicine
New Haven, CT
USA

Frank JE Falco, MD
Clinical Assistant Professor
Department of Physical Medicine and Rehabilitation
Temple University Medical School
Philadelphia, Pennsylvania
USA

F Michael Ferrante, MD
Professor of Anesthesiology and
Director of Pain Medicine Program
University of Pennsylvania Medical Canter
Philadelphia, Pennsylvania
USA

H Flaatten, MD
Consultant Anesthesiologist
Department of Anesthesiology and Intensive Care
Hammerfest Hospital
Hammerfest, Norway

Noor M Gajraj, MD
Assistant Professor of Anesthesiology
Parkland Pain Clinic Director
University of Texas Southwestern Medical School
Dallas, Texas
USA

Adoph H Giesecke, MD
Professor of Anesthesiology
Department of Anesthesiology
University of Texas Southwestern Medical School
Dallas, Texas
USA

Nancy L Glass, MD
Associate Professor of Anesthesiology and Pediatrics
Department of Anesthesiology
Baylor College of Medicine
Texas Medical Center
Houston, Texas
USA

Christopher M Grande, MD MPH
Professor, Department of Anesthesiology
West Virginia University School of Medicine
Director of Trauma Anesthesia
Jon Michael Moore Trauma Center
Robert C Byrd Health Sciences Center
Morgantown, West Virginia
Executive Director
International Trauma Anesthesia and Critical Care Society (ITACCS)
ITACCS World Headquarters
Baltimore, Maryland
USA

KJ Gupta, FRCA
Specialist Registrar in Anesthesia and Intensive Care
Royal United Hospital
Combe Park, Bath
UK

Paul Gusmarino, MD
Clinical Assistant Professor of Psychiatry
New York University School of Medicine
Director Department of Behavioral Medicine
Hospital for Joint Diseases
New York City, New York
USA

Carol Harris, MD
Fellow, Department of Anesthesiology
Texas Tech University Health Sciences Center
Lubbock, Texas
USA

Craig Hartrick, MD
Director of Pain Medicine Section
Department of Anesthesia and Perioperative Medicine
Beaumont Hospital
Detroit, Michigan
USA

Sassan Hassassian, MD
Assistant Professor of Pain
Management/Anesthesiology
University of Maryland Pain Center
Baltimore, Maryland
USA

Laureen L Hill, MD
Assistant Professor of Anesthesiology
Department of Anesthesiology
Stanford University Medical Center
Stanford, California
USA

Mark J Lema, MD PhD
Professor and Chairman
Department of Anesthesiology
Roswell Park Cancer Institute
State University of New York at Buffalo School of
Medicine
Buffalo, New York
USA

Markus DW Lipp, MD PhD DDS
Consultant Anesthesiologist
Senior Lecturer
Clinic of Anesthesiology
Johannes Gutenberg-University
Mainz, Germany

Maywin Liu, MD
Director of Pain Management
Department of Anesthesia
St Joseph Medical Center
Baltimore, Maryland
USA

Joel F Lupatkin, MD
Anesthesiologist
Department of Anesthesiology
Hospital For Joint Diseases
New York City, New York
USA

Mitchell H Marshall, MD
Attending Anesthesiologist
Department of Anesthesiology
Hospital for Joint Diseases
New York City, New York
USA

Pedro Alejandro Mendez-Tellez, MD
Assistant Clinical Professor
Department of Anesthesiology
State University of New York at Buffalo School of
Medicine
Chief, Critical Care Medicine
Roswell Park Cancer Institute
Buffalo, New York
USA

JP Nolan, FRCA
Consultant in Anesthesia and Intensive Care
Royal United Hospital
Combe Park, Bath
UK

Gilles Orliaguet, MD
Assistant Professor of Anesthesiology
Department of Anesthesiology and Critical Care
Hôpital Necker-Enfants Malades
Paris
France

Irene P Osborne, MD
Assistant Professor of Clinical Anesthesiology
New York University School of Medicine
New York City, New York
USA

MJA Parr, MRCP FRCA FANZCA
Consultant in Anesthesia and Intensive Care
Liverpool Hospital
University of New South Wales
Sydney, Australia

Nileshkumar Patel, MD
Clinical Professor of Anesthesiology
Pikeville College School of Osteopathic Medicine
Advanced Pain Management
Wisconsin, USA

Ronald G Pearl, MD PhD
Associate Director
Intensive Care
Associate Professor and Vice-Chairman
Department of Anesthesiology
Stanford University Medical Center
Stanford, California
USA

Burdett R Porter, MD
Assistant Professor (Clinical Track)
Department of Anesthesiology
University of Iowa
Iowa City, Iowa
USA

Gabor B Racz, MD
Grover Murray Professor
Professor and Chairman Emeritus
Director of Pain Services
Texas Tech University Health Sciences Center
Lubbock, Texas
USA

P Prithvi Raj, MD
Professor and Co-Director
Pain Services
Texas Tech University Health Sciences Center
Lubbock, Texas
USA

Sivam Ramanathan, MD
Professor of Anesthesiology and Critical Care
Medicine
University of Pittsburgh
Chief of Anesthesia
Magee Woman's Hospital
Pittsburgh, Pennsylvania
USA

Andrew D Rosenberg, MD
Vice Chairman Department of Anesthesiology
Hospital for Joint Diseases
Associate Professor of Clinical Anesthesiology
New York University School Of Medicine
New York City, New York
USA

George Sandor, MD
Resident
Department of Anesthesiology
New York University School of Medicine
New York City, New York
USA

Raymond S Sinatra, MD PhD
Professor of Anesthesiology
Director of Acute Pain Management Services
Yale University School of Medicine
New Haven, Connecticut
USA

Charles E Smith, MD FRCPC
Associate Professor of Anesthesiology
Case Western Reserve University
MetroHealth Medical Center
Cleveland, Ohio
USA

Barry Snow, PhD
Clinical Psychologist and Director of Research
Pain Center
Hospital for Joint Diseases
New York City, New York
USA

Judith L Stiff, MD
Associate Professor
Department of Anesthesiology
Johns Hopkins Bayview Medical Center
Baltimore, Maryland
USA

Hagop Tabakian, MD
Assistant Professor of Pain
Management/Anesthesiology
St Louis University Health Sciences Center
Baltimore, Maryland
USA

Maria L Torres, MD
Chief, Section of Acute Pain Management
Department of Anesthesiology and Pain Management
Cook County Hospital
Chicago, USA

Andreas R Thierbach, MD
Consultant Anesthesiologist
Chief Emergency Physician
Clinic of Anesthesiology
Johannes Gutenberg-University
Mainz, Germany

Alon P Winnie, MD
Chairman
Department of Anesthesiology and Pain Management
Cook County Hospital
Chicago, USA

Torben Wisborg, MD DEAA
Consultant Anesthesiologist and Chairman
Department of Anesthesiology and Intensive Care
Hammerfest Hospital
Hammerfest, Norway

Foreword

Drs Rosenberg, Grande, and Bernstein have created a book *Pain Management and Regional Anesthesia in Trauma* that focuses on two areas of our medical practice often in need of additional attention – trauma and pain relief. I have had the distinct pleasure of reading an advance copy of this work. I believe the fundamental strength of their book is that it can be read as a complete work, or a specific chapter can be read alone to answer some narrower area of inquiry.

Dr René Leriche stated it well when he said:

"Physical pain is not a simple affair of an impulse, travelling at a fixed rate along a nerve. It is the resultant of a conflict between a stimulus and the whole individual."[1]

Leriche's comment necessarily emphasizes why the approach taken by many physicians in caring for patients needs to take the more comprehensive view of integrating traumatic pain states and our clinical practice. Rosenberg *et al.* have taken this comprehensive approach, and made every possible attempt to bind the "whole individual" to trauma and pain. There is necessarily some repetition between the four sections of this work;

1. Basics: Interface of Trauma and Pain
2. Location-Based Pain Management: Concepts and Considerations
3. Perioperative Pain Management in Trauma: Techniques and Applications
4. Pain Management for Specific Trauma Patient Populations and Injured Organ Systems;

though to me a wonderful balance has been maintained.

The contributors to this text come from a wide variety of institutions and backgrounds, which enlivens the coverage of topics.

During my review I was interested to see that continuous peripheral techniques for our trauma patients was covered by Winnie *et al.* in a way that really does help us focus on the future. The unique needs of our pregnant trauma patients were well covered by Drs Dalby and Ramanathan. This area of our practice often demands that physicians review the latest information prior to caring for "both" these patients. I think their chapter serves us and our patients well.

Finally, I enjoyed the "case studies" inserts found in the chapter by Bernstein, *et al.* on the orthopedic trauma patient. I have always found the case-based approach to education powerful and they have used it well.

Again, I would like to thank Drs Rosenberg, Grande and Bernstein for creating a needed work. I believe that this work helps us keep our focus on Leriche's quote about trauma and pain, and I know our patients will all be better served because of this text.

David L Brown, MD
Professor and Head
Department of Anesthesia
University of Iowa
USA

---

[1] Strauss MB. *Familiar Medical Quotations*. Little, Brown and Company, Boston, 1968.

Preface

We are pleased to present this new text, *Pain Management and Regional Anesthesia In Trauma*, on behalf of the International Trauma Anesthesia and Critical Care Society (ITACCS). Since 1987, ITACCS has served an important role worldwide, that of improving care for trauma patients. To that end, publications have stressed topics such as emergency resuscitation, airway management, and critical care, all crucial topics for management of critically ill trauma patients. However, one remaining area that needed to be addressed in a more comprehensive manner was pain management of the trauma patient.

Specifically, a book was lacking that would explain the pathophysiology of pain in the trauma patient, the modalities available to treat pain in specific trauma situations, and serve as a "how to" text for administering pain management. Our goal is to fill this void. The time is right for a text that addresses this topic. First, the field of pain management has grown exponentially in recent years. Secondly, physicians understand that treating the pathophysiologic stress response to pain can have a major beneficial impact on both the short and long term morbidity of trauma. Thirdly, multiple pain management modalities such as patient controlled analgesia (PCA), epidural analgesia in thoracic and lumbar regions (opiates and local anesthetics), plexus blocks and other regional pain management methods are now available. Fourthly, it is our observation that there has not been enough interaction between experts in the field of trauma care and experts in the field of pain management. This book then serves as the catalyst for a "fusion" between these two closely related areas of specialization.

From the moment of injury, pain can impose major physical and psychological barriers to successful rehabilitation and optimal restoration of "quality of life". During the 1990s, pain management developed into a subspecialty that has resulted in improved care of patients with both acute and chronic pain. The benefits of such advances should not be lost on the trauma patient,

but instead must be incorporated into perioperative management in order to maximize outcome. Thus, recent advances in knowledge and techniques of pain management and how they relate to the trauma patient, as well as those techniques that have stood the test of time, form the basis of this book.

The text is divided into four major sections. The first section, *Basics: Interface of Trauma and Pain*, is intended to create a foundation for the understanding of the basics of pain, pain pathways and pharmacological treatment. The section includes an introduction to trauma, including epidemiology, the basics of pain transmission and pain pathways, the effects of pain on the trauma patient, the pharmacolgic basis of medications utilized to treat pain, and appropriate use of pain techniques based on the pathophysiologic condition of the patient. *Section II. Location-Based Pain Management: Concepts and Considerations*, covers pain management of the trauma patient in various physical settings through which the seriously injured will typically pass; prehospital, emergency room, operating room, intensive care unit, and rehabilitation center. *Section III. Perioperative Pain Management in Trauma: Techniques and Applications*, describes how to perform and institute specific techniques and pain modalities such as PCA, plexus blocks, epidural and spinal techniques as well as non-pharmacologic techniques for pain management. These three sections set the stage for *Section IV. Pain Management for Specific Trauma Patient Populations and Injured Organ Systems*. In this section, management of the pediatric patient, the burn patient, the pregnant patient, the patient with thoracic and abdominal injuries, the patient with neurologic injuries, and the patient with orthopedic injuries are addressed. These patients represent the wide variety of concerns that frequently present to the traumatologist. In addition, this section contains two chapters dealing with chronic pain management, a rapidly expanding field with increasingly invasive management techniques.

Why publish a book with both pain management and regional anesthesia in the title? The field of pain management has grown to such an extent that it needs to be recognized as the major reason that this text is written. Naturally, a text on pain management in trauma should encompass care from the time of injury through the rehabilitation process, and this has been the focus of this work. However, the use of regional anesthetic techniques has become such an important component of pain management that we believe this also must be reflected in the title of the text.

As can be noted from the list of contributors, we have been fortunate to assemble leading experts from around the world in the field of pain management and trauma care. We are most grateful for the contributions of these authors. Gathering world experts in a given field is always interesting. Each person has developed the technique that works for him. This may be peculiar to the work environment (prehospital setting, emergency room, operating room, or clinic), the geographic area in which he practices, the culture of the patient and medical population, available equipment, or the skill of the practitioner. These differences result in varied approaches to management. It is the diverse approaches to the same problem that is particularly interesting to us, and therefore, when appropriate, we have included more than one author's management technique. For example, the chapter on *Thoracic Blocks* presents management modalities for thoracic pain, as does the chapter on *The Trauma Patient With Thoracic and Abdominal Injuries*. This allows the reader to choose which method might ultimately work best for him/her.

With these thoughts in mind we present this text to you the practitioner. We hope that you will utilize it in order to help improve pain management, and thus, the overall morbidity and mortality of the trauma patient.

Andrew D Rosenberg, MD
Christopher M Grande, MD MPH
Ralph L Bernstein, MD

Acknowledgements

To the various contributors to this text, who have given so much of themselves, and have shared their expertise and knowledge in this specialized area of trauma care. The important links between trauma and pain are just now beginning to become understood, and pain management in trauma care must become an area of increased focus in the treatment of the seriously injured.

To the various ITACCS Administrative Assistants who have helped to manage this literary project, most importantly, Stacey Zidi and Jewel Crum-Freeman.

To Ms Angelina Velez at the Hospital for Joint Diseases who contributed immeasurably to this project.

To Arrow International, Inc. and B.Braun Medical, Inc. for their financial support of the color reproduction in Chapter 13 – *Continuous plexus blocks for the management of trauma to the extremities*.

Dedication

This volume is dedicated to the continuing effort to alleviate the pain and suffering of trauma patients worldwide.

It is also dedicated to the improvement of educational, research and clinical efforts to those traumatologists in anesthesia, emergency medicine, surgery, critical care, and other disciplines involved in the perioperative management of the injured.

It is our hope that this work brings us one step closer to providing the injured the type of care that they deserve.

ADR, CMG, RLB

To my family, Maris, Gabe, Shira and Lexie; And to my teachers HT, Ram, and Butch.

ADR

To my lovely wife, Dr Lesley Wong, for being all that she has been to me. Next, to my co-editors, Drs Andy Rosenberg and Ralph Bernstein, who have provided me with mentorship and guidance since I first began to learn from them as a resident in anesthesiology in New York City.

CMG

To Trudy, Susan, Ken, Thomas, Marcy, Paul, Patty, Erica, Jamie, and David.

RLB

Abbreviations

ACh	acetylcholine	DKA	diabetic ketoacidosis
ACC	American College of Cardiology	DREZ	dorsal root entry zone
ACE	angiotensin-converting enzyme	DRG	dorsal root ganglion
ACP	American College of Physicians	DVT	deep vein thrombosis
ACS	acute compartment syndrome; American College of Surgeons	EAA	excitatory amino acid
ACTH	adrenocorticotropic hormone	EC	effective concentration
AHA	American Heart Association	ECG	electrocardiogram
AIS	Abbreviated Injury Scale	EEG	electroencephalogram
ALT	alanine aminotransferase	EMG	electromyogram
AMH	A-δ mechanoheat nociceptors	EMS	emergency medical service
aPTT	activated partial thromboplastin time	EP	evoked potentials
ARDS	adult respiratory distress syndrome	ER	emergency room
AROM	acute range of motion		
AS	aortic stenosis	FDA	United States Food and Drug Administration
ASA	American Society of Anesthesiologists	FDP	fibrin degradation product
ASHD	atherosclerotic cardiovascular disease	FEV_1	forced expiratory volume in 1 second
AST	aspartate aminotransferase	FRC	functional residual capacity
ATLS	advanced trauma life support	FVC	forced vital capacity
BTXA	botulinum toxin type A	GABA	gamma-aminobutyric acid
BUN	blood urea nitrogen	GCS	Glasgow Coma Scale
		GFR	glomerular filtration rate
CAT	comprehensive approach to trauma		
CBF	cerebral blood flow	5-HT	5-hydroxytryptamine (serotonin)
CCK	cholecystekinin		
CCS	chronic compartment syndrome	ICNB	intercostal nerves block
CGRP	calcitonin gene-related protein	ICD	International Classification of Diseases
CHF	congestive heart failure		
CNS	central nervous system	ICP	intracranial pressure
COPD	chronic obstructive pulmonary disease	ICU	intensive care unit
CPAP	continuous positive airway pressure		
CPM	continuous passive motion	IL	interleukin
C-PMN	C-polymodal nociceptors	IM	intramuscular
CPP	cerebral perfusion pressure	IMV	intermittent mandatory ventilation
CPT	chest percussive therapy	INR	International Normalized Ratio
CRPS	complex regional pain syndrome	IPA	intrapleural analgesia
CSF	cerebrospinal fluid	ISS	Injury Severity Score
CT	computed tomography	ITACCS	International Trauma Anesthesia and Critical Care Society
CTS	carpal tunnel syndrome		
CVS	cardiovascular	IVRB	intravenous regional blockade
		IV	intravenous
DIC	disseminated intravascular coagulation		

LDH	lactate dehydrogenase		PSA	power spectral analysis
LMWH	low molecular weight heparin		PT	prothrombin time
LVH	left ventricular hypertrophy		PTSD	post-traumatic stress disorder
			PTT	partial thromboplastin time
MAP	mean arterial pressure			
MI	myocardial infarction		q	every
MICI	mobile intensive care unit			
MLAC	minimum local analgesic concentration		ROM	range of motion
			RSD	reflex sympathetic dystrophy
MR	mitral regurgitation		RT	reptilase time
MRI	magnetic resonance imaging		RTS	Revised Trauma Score
MS	mitral stenosis			
MTOS	Major Trauma Outcome Study		SAMU	Service D'Aide Medicale Urgente
MVA	motor vehicle accident		SC	subcutaneous
			SCS	spinal cord stimulation
NGF	nerve growth factor		SIP	sympathetically-independent pain
NISS	New Injury Severity Score		SMP	sympathetically-maintained pain
NMBA	neuromuscular blocking agent			
NMDA	N-methyl-D-aspartic acid		TBSA	total body surface area
NSAID	nonsteroidal anti-inflammatory drug		TENS	transcutaneous electrical nerve stimulation
NS	nociceptive-specific			
NSC	National Safety Council (USA)		TRISS	Trauma Score – Injury Severity Score
			TS	Trauma Score
OPCS	Office of Population Censuses and Surveys (UK)		TSH	thyroid stimulating hormone
			TSO	thoracic outlet syndrome
OR	operating room		TT	thrombin time
			TV	tidal volume
PA	pulmonary artery			
PCA	patient-controlled analgesia		UMN	upper motor neuron
PCEA	patient-controlled epidural analgesia			
PDPH	post-dural puncture headache		VAS	Visual Analog Scale
PE	pulmonary embolism		VC	vital capacity
PEEP	positive end-expiratory pressure			
PEF	peak expiratory flow rate		WDR	wide dynamic range
PFT	pulmonary function testing		WHO	World Health Organization
PRN	pro re nata; as needed/as required			
PROM	passive range of motion		YPLL	years of potential life lost

BASICS: INTERFACE OF TRAUMA AND PAIN

General introduction on Trauma

K J Gupta, M J A Parr and J P Nolan

Introduction	**The role of the anesthesiologist in trauma care**
	Pre-hospital care
History of trauma anesthesia	In-hospital trauma resuscitation
	Advanced Trauma Life Support
Trauma epidemiology – the magnitude of the problem	Trauma team leader
Sources of data	The provision of analgesia
International trauma	Anesthesia in the operating room
Specific types of trauma	Pre- and postoperative critical care
	Attending physician for the transfer of a trauma patient
Costs of trauma care	
	Prevention of trauma
Outcome after trauma	
Scoring systems	**Conclusion**
Trauma outcome	

INTRODUCTION

Injury may be defined as physical harm or damage to the body resulting from an exchange of mechanical, chemical, thermal, or other environmental energy that exceeds the body's tolerance.[1] The terms 'injury' and 'trauma' are interchangeable, the former being used particularly by the lay public, while the latter may be more familiar to health care professionals. Commonly used major subdivisions of trauma deaths are homicide, suicide, and unintentional. The last term is preferred to accidental, which implies that injuries occur by chance and cannot be prevented.[2]

Trauma is the most serious public health problem facing developed societies and throughout the world is the leading cause of death during half of the human lifespan.[3] Developing nations are also blighted by trauma but in most of these countries there is very little hard data to quantify the problem. Humans have had to deal with the consequences of trauma since they first walked upon the Earth and this chapter includes a review of milestones in history that have helped shape current trauma management. The scale of the trauma epi-

demic is defined with a review of trauma data from across the world. This includes the causes of trauma, the outcome for its victims, and the costs it incurs. The anesthesiologist has a major role to play in the management of the trauma patient. The extent of this role is outlined, and an international comparison is made of the involvement of anesthesiologists in the management of trauma.

HISTORY OF TRAUMA ANESTHESIA

Trauma has been a major cause of death and injury throughout history.[4] Early civilizations made a variety of attempts at preventing and managing the effects of trauma. The Ebers Papyrus written close to 1500 BC was based on hundreds of years of practice in the Egyptian civilization, and describes many trauma therapies. The treatment of a human bite was described as follows:

Make thou for him a poultice of raw flesh on the first day. Afterwards treat him with oil and honey in order to do him good. Then put thou oil in wax in order to make him completely well at once.

Bryan's book on the Ebers Papyrus[5] describes the early use of a splint for a femoral fracture in a 14-year-old girl found in a cemetery near the modern village of Naga-ed Der on the east bank of the Nile. In some cases, therefore, the management of trauma in ancient Egypt was not so very different from today's.

The Bible frequently refers to wars, battles and domestic violence that were a constant feature of life in those times. The treatment of fractures is mentioned in Ezekiel (30:21):

Son of man, I have broken the arm of Pharaoh king of Egypt; and, lo, it shall not be bound up to be healed, to put a roller to bind it, to make it strong to hold the sword.

Chinese medicine has developed over many centuries. Tortoise shells with inscriptions dating from the Shang Dynasty (circa 1500 BC) are among the earliest medical texts from this civilization. Two classic acupuncture texts, the *Nei Ching SuWen* from many sources and *Classic of Acupuncture and Moxibustion* by Huang Fu Mi, date from the Warring States period about 300 BC and discuss the effects of pain relief and other ancillary measures for trauma care.

Analgesia was mentioned also in texts from the Greek and Roman civilizations. In Homer's *The Iliad*, written approximately 900 BC and set in the Mycenaean era, Patroclus was called to Eurypylus to treat a thigh injury. Part of his treatment involved the use of analgesia:

then he applied a bitter, pain assuaging root, rubbing it between his hands, which checked all his pain.

Gaius Plinius Secundus (Pliny the Elder) wrote about the importance of analgesia in the form of mandragora:

administered in doses proportional to the strength of the patient, the juice has a narcotic effect, a middling dose being one cyanthus. It is given too, for injuries inflicted by serpents and before incisions or punctures are made in the body, in order to ensure insensibility to the pain.[6]

The fall of the Roman Empire and the spread of the Barbarian hordes across Europe was followed by an abandonment of Greek and Roman medicine. Simple beliefs in magical or supernatural causes for disease became prevalent, and bloodletting became the main therapeutic intervention for

trauma. Islam, however, preserved much of the old Greek and Roman knowledge and subsequently returned it to Europe. Avicenna, the son of a Persian tax collector, began to write his *Canon of Medicine* in 1012. Influenced by the writings of Galen he described basic sound principles on the management of trauma. He wrote on the importance of analgesia:

When the pain is too intense, it may cause death, this resulting in the first place from coldness of the body, and secondly from tremor, with a small pulse, which finally fails thus bringing death.

He described opium as the most powerful of the stupefacients, and was also aware of the importance of careful positioning of the patient to lessen pain.[7]

During the Renaissance Paracelsus reintroduced opium for the relief of pain and refuted most of Galenic theory. Harvey's description of the circulation of the blood in the early 17th century had a profound influence on medicine in general.[8] This fundamental discovery paved the way for intravenous therapy. Wren, Boyle and Wilkins demonstrated the effects of intravenous opium on a dog in 1659. The first attempt at intravenous therapy in humans was probably by Major who documented his findings in two volumes.[9] Richard Lower performed animal to animal transfusion and demonstrated the technique in humans before the Royal Society of London in November 1667.[10] Blood transfusion, however, did not become truly successful or predictable for another 250 years.

A giant leap forward in the concept of patient care in the United Kingdom (UK) was made in 1774 when a society was founded to revive drowned people pulled from the River Thames in London. This became the Society for the Recovery of Persons Apparently Drowned, before changing its name to the Humane Society in 1776. The society offered money to people prepared to practice resuscitation and soon medical assistants were stationed along the Thames who could be called out when necessary. Prior to this, popular opinion stated that the best thing to do for a drowned man was to pick his pockets! Trying to restore life to a victim of sudden trauma was a new idea. On a similar note, Baron Larrey,[11] who was Napoleon's surgeon-in-chief, developed the idea of triage and rapid evacuation of casualties. In the same manner as the flying artillery, he created a 'flying ambulance' which was a mobile field hospital that followed the advanced guard. Urgent surgery within hours of the injury, before transport back to base hospitals, was a revolutionary concept.

Morton's successful public demonstration of ether anesthesia in Boston on 16 October 1846 started modern anesthesiology. Ether anesthesia was immediately accepted around the world and was employed with varying success in trauma patients.

Experience with anesthesia in civilian trauma was soon augmented by the traumas of war, and it is wars that have continued to exert a profound influence on the development of trauma anesthesia. By the First World War local anesthesia was firmly established and spinal anesthetics were becoming popular. Just before hostilities it was suggested that spinal anesthesia was the best choice for military service because of

increased safety and freedom from the toxaemia of general anaesthesia.

Also it was considered that

good relaxation was obtained, no anaesthetist was required, it was simple, portable and inexpensive, and lastly, it permitted single handed operations.[12]

The forthcoming war was to show how wrong this advice was. Nitrous oxide anesthesia was evolving in this period and was rapidly incorporated into an anesthetic machine by Gwathmey. This allowed a controlled concentration of nitrous oxide and oxygen to be delivered.[13] At St Bartholomew's Hospital in London, Boyle obtained two of Gwathmey's machines and was using them in his practice. The use of nitrous oxide became more popular during the war as its safety in severely injured patients was recognized.

The routine use of tracheal intubation was perfected soon after the First World War by Magill and Rowbotham.[14] This was a huge step forward in anesthetic care and the addition of cuffs to the tracheal tube by Guedel & Waters permitted reliable isolation of the airway for the first time.[15] Another major change occurring between the wars was the routine use of intravenous anesthesia after the introduction of barbiturates by Fischer & von Mering.[16] Thiopentone (sodium pentothal or STP) arrived just in time for the Second World War where its use in trauma patients was not without problems. Halford[17] reported how

when as small an amount as 0.5 gramme of pentothal sodium had been administered, there suddenly appeared a 'cyanosis decolletage' which was the inevitable and irremediable predecessor of death.

The same journal, however, carried another paper in the same issue describing the highly successful administration of STP to a shocked patient when given slowly in very small doses with 50% oxygen in nitrous oxide, and a blood transfusion. Information which has recently become available through US Freedom of Information legislation has revealed that the rumored death rate attributed to the use of STP at Pearl Harbor had been greatly exaggerated.[18]

During the Second World War the concept of the trauma anesthesiologist emerged. Crane & Sankey were enthusiastic about the involvement of anesthesiologists in resuscitation:

Recently medical anaesthetists have paid more attention to the application of restorative measures, including intravenous fluids and blood transfusion. Anesthetists should be prepared to supervise the administration of these valuable supportive measures both in the preoperative preparation of the seriously wounded and also during the operative procedure.[19]

This was strongly supported more than 10 years later when Egan, a Canadian physician writing in 1953 about his experiences during the Korean War,[20] said:

When a man has been wounded almost unto death his survival nowadays depends almost entirely on whether or not he can be kept alive and his vital processes restored to stand surgical repair, and, on whether or not he can be kept alive during the operation. Both of these, resuscitation on one hand, and anesthesia on the other, form the major portion of the practice and responsibilities of anesthesiology.

Huge advances in the drugs, techniques and apparatus used for anesthesia took place in the post-war years. In the UK, the structure of medicine changed with the introduction of the National Health Service and the recognition of anesthesiology as a specialty in its own right. Muscle relaxants were introduced in the 1940s and halothane in the 1950s.

Meanwhile in the Western world increasing traffic on the roads led to a massive increase in the number of motor vehicle accidents as a continuous source of trauma. Since then further advances in trauma management have included the development of pre-hospital care, trauma systems and trauma centers and the teaching and evaluation of trauma care. The role of the trauma anesthesiologist and critical care provider has become better defined and their role in establishing high standards of care for the victims of trauma is now well-established.[21]

TRAUMA EPIDEMIOLOGY – THE MAGNITUDE OF THE PROBLEM

Sources of data

Countries with reliable death registration systems produce mortality statistics which are published annually by the World Health Organization (WHO).[22,23] Such countries include all of western Europe, the United States of America (USA), Canada, Australia, New Zealand, Israel and Japan. Recently information has become available from several nations in Latin America and Asia (including selected areas of China). Also data are emerging from many of the former Soviet republics established around the period of the dissolution of the Warsaw Pact and the collapse of the United Soviet Socialist Republic (USSR).

Further information is also available from sources within specific countries. For example in the UK, the Office of Population Censuses and Surveys (OPCS) publish annual mortality statistics,[24] and in the USA the National Safety Council (NSC), a non-government public service organization, publishes data on the previous year's unintentional injuries in *Accident Facts*.[25] A global subsidiary of the NSC, the International Safety Council produces *International Accident Facts*[26] which provides international comparisons of accident data drawn from several sources. Data specific to individual groups or causes of trauma are also available. For example, data concerning motor vehicle accidents are available from American Automobile Manufacturers Association and the National Highway Traffic Safety Administration (NHTSA) in the USA and The Department of Transport in the UK.[27] Many of these organizations now also have web sites on the Internet.

International and national comparisons of trauma are possible because of a standardized coding system. The WHO provides a standard for the way in which causes of death are classified and coded. The underlying cause of death is defined as 'the disease or injury which initiated the train of morbid events leading directly to death, or the circumstances of the accident or violence which produced the fatal injury.'[28]

Deaths are classified and coded on the basis of the Manual of the International Classification of Diseases, Injuries, and Causes of Death, commonly known as the International Classification of Diseases or 'ICD'. The ICD has been revised ten times, almost on a decennial basis. The tenth revision (ICD-10) was published in 1992 and ICD-10 statistics will be available toward the end of the decade. The statistics used for this chapter adopt mainly the ninth revision which was instituted in 1979.[28] For deaths caused by injury and poisoning, ICD-9 provides a system of 'external cause' codes, or E-codes, to which the underlying cause of death is assigned. External causes of injury and poisoning are represented by codes E800 to E999 which permits precise information on the cause of injury to be recorded. The ICD system also includes a basic tabulation list of two-digit codes that cover all causes of death. The WHO tends to use this simpler system for displaying annual international health statistics. Codes E47 to E56 cover causes of trauma (Table 1.1).

Comparisons of data between countries can serve several different purposes. For example, the development of hypotheses to explain observed differences in trauma epidemiology can lead to the recommendation of programs, practices or environmental changes that may lower death and injury rates. It must be emphasized, however, that there are significant limitations to comparisons that must be understood before drawing conclusions from international accident data. Despite the existence of uniform coding systems for cause of death, such as ICD-9, differences still exist in definitions, recording systems and reporting practices that can significantly affect comparability of statistics. It is also necessary to consider the demographic, social, geographic, economic and cultural differences that exist between countries. Crude population death rates (usually expressed as death rate per 100 000 population) have been used for the international tables in this chapter. Crude death rates do not adjust for the age distribution differences that exist between countries; this requires the use of standardized population

Table 1.1   International Classification of Diseases, ninth revision. ICD-9 Basic tabulation list (E47 to E56) with equivalent codes in the supplementary classification – External causes of injury and poisoning (E800 to E999).

E47	**Transport accidents**	**E800–E848**
E470	Railway accidents	E800–E807
E471	Motor vehicle traffic accidents	E810–E819
E472	Other road vehicle accidents	E826–E829
E473	Water transport accidents	E830–E838
E474	Air and space transport accidents	E840–E845
E48	**Accidental poisoning**	**E850–E869**
E480	Accidental poisoning by drugs, medicaments and biologicals	E850–E858
E481	Accidental poisoning by other solid and liquid substances	E860–E866
E482	Accidental poisoning by gases and vapors	E867–E869
E49	**Misadventures during medical care, abnormal reactions, late complications**	**E870–E879**
E50	**Accidental falls**	**E880–E888**
E51	**Accidents caused by fire and flames**	**E890–E899**
E52	**Other accidents, including late effects**	**E900–E929**
E520	Accidents due to natural and environmental factors	E900–E909
E521	Accidental drowning and submersion	E910
E522	Foreign body accidentally entering orifice	E914, E915
E523	Accidents caused by machinery, and by cutting and piercing instruments	E919, E920
E524	Accidents caused by firearm missile	E922
E53	**Drugs, medicaments causing adverse effects in therapeutic use**	**E930–E949**
E54	**Suicide and self-inflicted injury**	**E950–E959**
E55	**Homicide and injury purposely inflicted by other persons**	**E960–E969**
E56	**Other violence**	**E970–E999**
E560	Injury undetermined whether accidentally or purposely inflicted	E980–E989
E561	Injury resulting from operation of war	E990–E999

death rates. The relationship between the two, however, is approximately linear.[26]

International trauma

More than 11 million people die in the world every year. Of these approximately 0.9 million (~8%) die as a result of trauma.[22] Table 1.2 lists the international death rates owing to trauma for each country ranked in descending order. Differences in reporting will have produced some anomalies but this table provides an overview. Recent information from some of the countries emerging from the breakdown of the USSR has had a significant influence on the ranking of international trauma data, since many of these emerging countries appear to have extremely high trauma rates. The range in trauma death rate is wide, with that in the Russian Federation being over four times that in the UK. The USA is often

regarded as having a relatively high level of trauma but actually falls towards the middle of the list with a rate less than half that of the top three countries. The very limited data available from developing countries make it impossible to make reliable comparisons with the developed world.

Trauma is amongst the top five leading causes of death in the world. In the vast majority of the countries submitting data to the WHO, heart disease and malignant neoplasms are the top two causes of death. Trauma ranks usually from third to fifth place along with cerebrovascular disease and respiratory diseases.[26]

In the USA, 2 268 553 people died in 1993.[25] Trauma accounted for 151 061 (6.7%) of these deaths (represented by codes E800 to E999 in the ICD-9 system). This ranks trauma as the third commonest cause of death in the USA, with fractionally more people dying from trauma than from strokes. Of those trauma deaths 90 523 were due

Table 1.2   International annual trauma fatality rates (per 100 000 population) ranked in order

Rank	Country	Year	Total trauma death rate	Rank	Country	Year	Total trauma death rate
1	Russian Federation	1991	129.5	25	Armenia	1990	54.4
2	Latvia	1990	129.1	26	Germany	1992	52.9
3	Hungary	1992	125.8	27	New Zealand	1991	52.8
4	Lithuania	1990	115	28	Sweden	1990	52.3
5	Belarus	1992	113	29	China (selected urban areas)	1990	51.4
6	Kazakhstan	1990	99.4	30	Italy	1990	50
7	China (selected rural areas)	1990	92.4	31	Trinidad and Tobago	1991	49.4
8	Kyrgyzstan	1990	87.9	32	Spain	1990	47.7
9	Finland	1992	85.9	33	Canada	1991	47.7
10	Czech Republic	1992	80.1	34	Japan	1992	46.3
11	France	1992	76.3	35	Mauritius	1992	45.5
12	Switzerland	1992	75.1	36	Argentina	1990	43.7
13	Romania	1992	74	37	Greece	1991	40.9
14	Poland	1992	72.8	38	Ireland	1991	39.4
15	Denmark	1992	72	39	Iceland	1992	39
16	Bulgaria	1992	66.6	40	Australia	1992	38.5
17	Mexico	1991	65	41	Costa Rica	1991	37.2
18	Puerto Rico	1991	65	42	Netherlands	1991	35.7
19	Luxembourg	1992	64.3	43	Israel	1990	34.8
20	Austria	1992	64	44	Malta	1992	33.8
21	Belgium	1989	61.6	45	Singapore	1991	31
22	Norway	1991	59.1	46	UK	1992	30.3
23	USA	1991	58	47	Hong Kong	1991	29.9
24	Portugal	1992	55.7				

Table constructed from calculations based on data from WHO *World Health Statistics Annual, 1993.*

to unintentional injuries, and this group alone ranks as the fifth commonest cause of death in the USA. Table 1.3 lists the leading causes of death in 1993 based on figures from the National Center for Health Statistics published by the NSC.[25] This table shows that the precise order of ranking of any particular cause of death depends on how the other causes of death are grouped. For example, if pneumonia and chronic obstructive pulmonary disease are combined, then deaths from respiratory disease far outnumber those due to trauma. Deaths from the human immunodeficiency virus (HIV) have more than doubled between 1988 and 1993.[29]

In the UK, trauma accounts for 3.1% of total deaths which is less than half the equivalent proportion in the USA. Consequently, in comparison with the USA, it does not rank as highly in the causes of death table[30] (Table 1.4). In 1994, there were 627 636 deaths in the UK. Of these, 19 151 died of trauma. 63% (12 062) of these were due to unintentional injuries. This ranks trauma as the sixth commonest cause of death in the UK.

Table 1.3   Leading causes of death – USA, 1993

Cause of death (ICD-9 code)	Total no. of deaths
All causes	**2 268 553**
Heart disease	743 460
Cancer	529 904
All trauma (E800–E999)	151 061
Stroke	150 108
COPD	101 077
Unintentional injuries (E800–E949)	90 523
Pneumonia	82 820
Diabetes mellitus	53 894
HIV infection	37 267
Suicide	31 102
Homicide	26 009
Chronic liver disease	25 209
Nephritis and nephrosis	23 317

COPD, chronic obstructive pulmonary disease.
HIV, human immunodeficiency virus.
Compiled from NSC data, *Accident Facts 1996.*

Table 1.4   Leading causes of death – UK, 1994

Causes of death (ICD-9 code)	Total no. of deaths
All causes	**627 636**
Neoplasms	160 806
Ischemic heart disease	154 842
Respiratory system	90 864
Cerebrovascular disease	68 190
Pneumonia	54 269
Digestive system	21 251
All trauma (E800–E999)	19 151
Unintentional deaths (E800–E929)	12 062
Genito-urinary system	7878
Diabetes mellitus	6486
Suicide	4381

Table constructed from OPCS data, *Annual Abstract of Statistics, 1997.*

Unfortunately, non-adjusted crude death rates have significant limitations. For example, they do not give any impression of the changing risk of death with age. It is well recognized that trauma tends to affect a younger population and this is clearly demonstrated in Figure 1.1 which separates the principal causes of death in different age groups in the USA in 1993. Unintentional injuries are the leading cause of death among all persons aged 1 to 38 years in the USA, and trauma is responsible for 76% of all deaths in the 15 to 24 age group.[25] This is similar in the UK where trauma is the leading cause of death among all persons aged 1 to 34 years.[31] In the USA, HIV is the leading cause of death in the 25 to 44 age group.

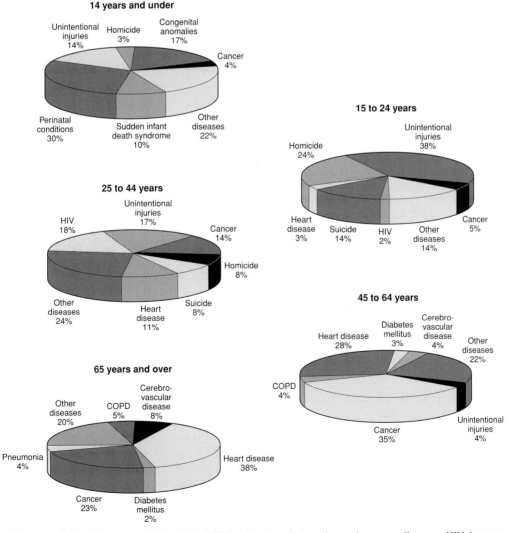

Fig. 1.1   Causes of death by age – USA, 1993. COPD, chronic obstructive pulmonary disease; HIV, human immunodeficiency virus. (Charts reproduced with permission from National Safety Council 1996 *Accident Facts*.)

Years of potential life lost

Trauma affects young people and therefore removes from the community men and women who would otherwise have had many years of productive life. This has great social and economic consequences to a country. Calculation of these 'years of potential life lost' (YPLL) is an effective method of highlighting the significance of deaths. Crude mortality rates give equal weight to all deaths. However YPLL before the age of 65 years (YPLL-65) emphasizes the significance of deaths among younger people by not counting deaths occurring after the age of 65 years and by positively weighting deaths that occur at younger ages. Ranked in this way unintentional injuries are the most significant cause of death accounting for over 1.9 million such years lost in 1992. This represents about 25% of a total estimated 7.5 million years lost.[25] Table 1.5 shows the top six causes of death according to their estimated YPLL-65 for the USA in 1992. If suicide and homicide are added to unintentional injuries, then trauma accounts for a staggering 3.4 million years of life lost, almost 50% of the total derived from the top six leading causes.

This calculation emphasizes the huge importance of deaths from trauma in the USA in a way that crude mortality rates, or even age-adjusted rates do not show. We have seen that trauma is the leading cause of death in the first four decades of life in both the USA and the UK. In the UK the impact of trauma on YPLL, although still significant, is less than in the USA. UK YPLL data from 1994 and 1995 show that unintentional injury ranks as the third leading cause of death but malignant neoplasms and ischemic heart disease are still the conditions that take 'most life' away from the population.[31]

Table 1.5 Estimated years of potential life lost (YPLL) from selected causes – USA, 1992

Cause of death	YPLL (millon years)
Unintentional injury	1.9
Malignant neoplasms	1.8
Heart disease	1.4
Human immunodeficiency virus	0.9
Homicide and legal intervention	0.8
Suicide	0.7

Table constructed from NSC data, *Accident Facts, 1996.*

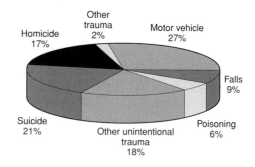

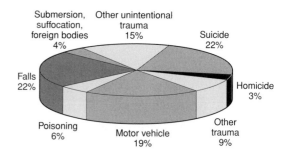

Fig. 1.2   Trauma fatalities by cause – USA and England & Wales, 1993. (USA data from National Safety Council 1996 *Accident Facts*; English and Welsh data from OPCS, 1993.)

Specific types of trauma

Of roughly 0.9 million trauma deaths in the world, approximately 600 000 are due to unintentional injury, 190 000 due to suicide and 80 000 due to homicide.[22] The single biggest killer amongst all trauma is motor vehicle accidents (MVA) which account for approximately 210 000 deaths in the world each year. In Table 1.6 the trauma fatalities for each nation are subdivided into separate categories: all accidents, MVA (the major sub-group of accidents), suicide and homicide. Figure 1.2 shows the cause of all the trauma deaths in the USA and England & Wales for 1993.

Motor vehicle accidents

In most countries MVAs are the most frequent cause of death from unintentional injury. From Table 1.6 it appears that Latvia and Lithuania have the highest mortality rate from MVAs at

Table 1.6   International death rates per 100 000 population by types of trauma

Country	Year	Accidents and adverse effects (E47–E53)	Motor vehicle traffic accidents (E471)	Homicide and injury purposely inflicted by others (E55)	Suicide (E54)
Argentina	1990	32	9.1	5	6.7
Armenia	1990	45.5	18.9	6.1	2.8
Australia	1992	24.9	10.8	1.6	12
Austria	1992	40.2	14.9	1.5	22.3
Belarus	1992	80.7	21.3	8.7	23.6
Belgium	1989	40.9	18.4	1.4	19.3
Bulgaria	1992	44.1	12.5	4.7	17.8
Canada	1991	32.2	12.7	2.3	13.2
China (selected rural areas)	1990	68.5	8.8	1.5	22.4
China (selected urban areas)	1990	40.4	8.5	2.4	8.6
Costa Rica	1991	28.9	13.3	4.1	4.2
Czech Republic	1992	58.9	14.4	1.9	19.3
Denmark	1992	n/a	11.1	1.3	22
Finland	1992	53.7	11.3	3.4	28.8
France	1992	55	15.3	1	20.3
Germany	1992	35	12.7	1.2	16.7
Greece	1991	35.7	22	1.5	3.7
Hong Kong	1991	15.1	5.8	1.8	13
Hungary	1992	83.1	22.7	4	38.7
Iceland	1992	27.2	7.7	1.1	10.7
Ireland	1991	29	12.1	0.6	9.8
Israel	1990	26.6	7.9	1.7	6.5
Italy	1990	39.7	15.8	2.7	7.6
Japan	1992	28.5	12	0.6	17.2
Kazakhstan	1990	68.5	21.8	11.8	19.1
Kyrgyzstan	1990	61.4	23.1	14	12.5
Latvia	1990	93.9	39.1	9.2	26
Lithuania	1990	81.3	30.9	7.6	26.1
Luxembourg	1992	47.3	19.3	2	15
Malta	1992	27.1	6.6	1.7	5
Mauritius	1992	28.6	15.1	3	13.9
Mexico	1991	45.1	16.4	17.5	2.4
Netherlands	1991	23.8	8.2	1.2	10.7
New Zealand	1991	36.8	19.5	2	14
Norway	1991	41.8	7.5	1.5	15.8
Poland	1992	55	19.2	2.9	14.9
Portugal	1992	45.4	28.1	1.5	8.8
Puerto Rico	1991	32.5	16.3	22.5	10
Romania	1992	57.5	15	4.9	11.6
Russian Federation	1991	87.6	26	15.3	26.6
Singapore	1991	17.6	9.3	1.8	11.6
Spain	1990	39.2	20.5	1	7.5
Sweden	1990	33.8	8.7	1.3	17.2
Switzerland	1992	n/a	10.9	1.5	20.8
Trinidad and Tobago	1991	30	11.8	7.6	11.8
UK	1992	21.4	8.1	0.9	8
USA	1991	35.4	16.9	10.4	12.2

n/a, ICD-9 data not available: Denmark ICD-8 (72); Switzerland ICD-8 (75.1). Table constructed from WHO data, *World Health Statistics Annual 1993/94*.

39.1 and 30.9 deaths per 100 000 population respectively. Third in the table is Portugal at 28.1 per 100 000 population, although this represents a much higher proportion of unintentional injuries than it does in the first two countries.

The range across western Europe is very large with Portugal and Greece at one extreme and the UK and Norway at the other with a death rate approximately three times lower. The USA lies 16th out of the 46 countries listed in the table with a rate of 16.9 per 100 000 population in 1991.

Factors affecting the mortality rate from MVAs include the volume of traffic, number of vehicles, population density, distance traveled in vehicles and definitions of death. A fatality rate together with a ratio of population to vehicles is more meaningful, since the ratio gives some indication of the dependence of the population on the motor vehicle as a means of transport. Better still is information derived by comparing the figures for deaths on the basis of distance travelled (the mileage death rate). This information is not fully available from many countries but Table 1.7 shows information from several developed countries that do produce this data.[27]

In accordance with the commonly agreed international definition, most countries define a MVA fatality as being due to a road accident where death occurs within 30 days of the accident. The official road accident statistics of some countries limit the reported fatalities to those occurring within shorter periods after the accident. For these countries numbers of deaths and death rates have been adjusted in the table, according to the factors used by the Economic Commission for Europe and the European Conference of Ministers of Transport, to represent standardized 30-day deaths. The mileage death rates in the table are for car users only and therefore differ from other quoted rates that include trucks and pedestrians. For example, other USA sources quote the 1994 death rate per 100 million miles, for all vehicles, as 1.81[25] which is higher than the 1.4 car-user deaths per 100 million car miles displayed in this table. Examination of this data shows how crude mortality data for MVAs can be misleading. Mileage

Table 1.7   International comparisons of road deaths: number and rates for different road users – 1994

Country	Total number of road deaths*	Road deaths per 100 000 population	Motor vehicles per 1000 population	Road deaths per 10 000 vehicles	Car-user deaths per 100 million car miles	Pedestrian deaths per 100 000 population
Australia[1]	1952	11.1	591	1.9	n/a**	1.9
Austria	1338	16.7	578	2.9	n/a	2.8
Belgium	1692	16.8	500[2]	3.2	n/a	2
Canada[1]	3615	12.6	617	2	n/a	1.7
Denmark	546	10.5	408[2]	2.4	1.3	1.8
Finland	480	9.5	456	2.1	1.1	1.7
France	9019	15.6	518	3	n/a	2.1
Germany	9814	12.1	572[2]	2.1	1.9	1.8
Greece[1]	2104	20.3	324[2]	5.6	n/a	4.7
Hungary	1562	15.2	248[2]	5.9	n/a	4.6
Irish Republic	404	11.4	339	3.4	1.4	3.4
Italy[1]	7177	12.6	666	1.9	n/a	1.8
Japan	12768	10.2	657	1.6	2.1	2.8
Luxembourg	74	18.5	n/a	2.4	n/a	2.5
Netherlands	1298	8.5	470	1.8	1.1	0.8
New Zealand	580	16.5	649[2]	2.5	n/a	1.5
Norway	281	6.5	552	1.2	n/a	1.1
Portugal	2700	28.7	530[2]	4.4	n/a	7.4
Spain	5615	14.4	519	2.8	n/a	2.6
Sweden	589	6.7	509	1.3	n/a	1
Switzerland	679	9.7	629	1.5	n/a	1.8
UK	3807	6.5	442	1.6	0.8	2
USA	40676	15.6	746[2]	2.1	1.4	2.2

* Adjusted to represent standardized 30-day deaths. Actual definition in parenthesis with adjustment: Italy (7 days) = 8%; France (6 days) = 5.7%; Greece (3 days) = 15%; Portugal (1 day) = 30%.
[1] 1993 data.
[2] All motor vehicles other than motorcycles < 50 cc per 1000 population.
** n/a, not available.
Modified from The Department of Transport. Road Accidents Great Britain: 1995. The Casualty Report.

death rates are only available from a few countries, so comparisons should be made with caution.

In 1995, 43 900 people were killed in MVAs in the USA, giving a death rate of 16.7 per 100 000 population, 2.15 per 10 000 vehicles and 1.83 per 100 million vehicle miles.[25] Figure 1.3 shows that MVAs account for approximately half of all the deaths from unintentional injury in the USA. Although these figures represent a slight rise on 1994 figures, the general trend is downward. Compared with 1985, motor vehicle deaths 10 years later were down by approximately 4%. To put these figures into perspective, in 1912 there were 3100 fatalities representing a death rate of 33 per 10 000 registered vehicles, a figure way above today's value of under 2.

MVAs also account for a huge number of non-fatal injuries every year. Figures from the National Health Interview Survey in the USA (see Non-fatal injuries, p. 16) show that in 1994 over 3 million people were injured as a result of a moving motor vehicle.[25] Approximately 2 300 000 of these had disabling injuries (defined as one which results in death, some degree of permanent impairment or renders the injured person unable to perform their regular duties or activities for a full day beyond the day of the injury). This represents an enormous workload not only on medical services but on the entire economy of the country (see Costs of trauma care, p. 17). The implication is that for every person killed in a MVA, 73 people are injured, and 52 of these will suffer disabling injuries. In the USA motor vehicles account for a death every 12 minutes and an injury every 14 seconds.[25]

In the UK, in contrast to the USA, deaths from falls outnumber those from MVAs (Fig. 1.3). Nevertheless MVAs still place a large demand on trauma services. In the UK in 1995 there were 230 376 road accidents,[30] causing a total of 310 506 casualties (i.e. any person killed or injured in a MVA). Of these casualties 3621 were fatal. Table 1.8 displays the distribution of these deaths by type of road user. This table reveals the excess risk associated with riding motorcycles.

USA – Total: 90 523

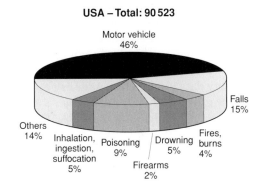

England & Wales – Total: 10 342

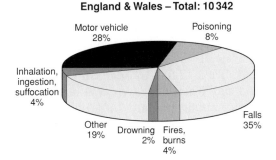

Fig. 1.3   Deaths from unintentional injury by type – USA and England & Wales, 1993. (USA data from National Safety Council 1996 *Accident Facts*; UK data from OPCS, 1993.)

Table 1.8   Road accidents in Great Britain by road user – 1995

	All road accidents	Car users	Motor cycles	Pedal cycles	Pedestrians
Fatalities	3621	1749	445	213	1038
All casualties	310506	193992	23480	24913	47029
Traffic volume[1]	2724	2208	26	28	
Casualty rate[2]	114	87.9	903.1	889.8	83[3]
Death rate[2]	1.3	0.8	17.4	7.6	

[1] 100 million vehicle miles.

[2] Per 100 million vehicle miles.

[3] Per 100 000 population.

Produced from Department of Transport data.

The calculated death rate for motorcycles from this table is 17.4 deaths per 100 million motorcycle miles, which is some **twenty times** higher than the equivalent rate of 0.8 for cars. Motorcycles are also associated with a higher mortality in the USA where the death rate has been calculated to be 24 per 100 million miles of motorcycle travel, some 17 times higher than for other types of vehicle.[25] It may be that this rate is higher than in the UK because of the lack of compulsory helmet laws in some states; in 1993 only 25 states plus the District of Columbia had legislation requiring compulsory helmet use for riders of all ages.[25] It is interesting to note from Table 1.8 that the risks of injury on a pedal cycle are almost as high as on motorcycles on the basis of risk per mile traveled. The calculation of deaths per 100 million vehicle miles, however, is less relevant for pedal cyclists because on the whole cyclists travel very small distances. The comparative risk to the individual riding a pedal cycle is therefore much lower than for a motorcyclist.

Falls

Over 90% of countries report falls as being amongst the top three causes of death from unintentional injury.[25] International comparison shows a wide range of death rates between countries; Hungary, Denmark, Switzerland, Norway and France all report death rates over 20 per 100 000 population, and Brazil, Jamaica, Spain, Hong Kong and Singapore report death rates less than 3.0.[26] The rate in the USA was 5.1 per 100 000 population in 1993[25] and was 7.4 in the UK in 1991.[26] Whilst these figures are interesting they are of limited value for international comparison because they take no account of the age distribution within each country. The vast majority of deaths from falls occur in elderly people. In the USA, for example, 13 141 people died from falls in 1993. Of these, 8760 (67%) occurred in those over 75 years. In this age group falls are the commonest cause of death from unintentional injuries, with a death rate of 62 per 100 000 population, some twelve times higher than for the nation as a whole. If an international comparison is made for death rates in the elderly population more meaningful results can be obtained. For example, analysis of data from 1981 to 1991 in the over 75 age group show that in Hungary, Denmark, France, Italy, Norway and Switzerland the death

rate from falls is over 200. In Japan, Korea, Hong Kong, Iceland, Spain and Singapore (as well as several developing countries) the death rate is less than 50 per 100 000 population.

Homicide

International crude homicide rates vary widely, ranging from 22.5 per 100 000 population in Puerto Rico to 0.6 in the Republic of Ireland and Japan (Table 1.6).[22] In 1987/88 the USA had the dubious honor of being 'top' of the international league table made up from WHO information[29] with a homicide rate of 8.6 per 100 000 population. In 1990/91 the US lay sixth on this international table. This is because of the emergence of mortality data from many countries not previously reporting to the WHO, rather than a decreasing incidence of homicide in the USA. On the contrary, the reported homicide rate had increased during this period to 10.4 per 100 000 population.

In 1993 the death rate from homicide (E960 to E969, E55) in the USA was 10.1 per 100 000 population, representing 26 009 cases of intentional killing (of which 356 were due to legal intervention). Homicide therefore accounted for 17.2% of all trauma related deaths and 1.1% of deaths from all causes in the USA that year (Fig. 1.2 and Table 1.3). In marked contrast, in England and Wales there were 434 homicides in 1993, accounting for only 2.8% of the 15 728 trauma related fatalities[24] and less than 0.1% of the deaths from all causes.

As with MVAs and falls, homicide rates are significantly influenced by the age of the population being studied. For example within the 15 to 24 year age group in the USA, homicides account for 23.7% of all deaths (Fig. 1.1). It is not surprising therefore that the homicide ranks as the fifth leading cause of years of potential life lost in the USA (Table 1.5). Intentional violence amongst this age group is showing an increasing trend in several countries and is the subject of extensive epidemiological studies.[32] There are many different factors influencing the amount and type of intentional violence occurring within a country, or even within a community. Violence is the common end-point of many quite different behavioral pathways. Each of these pathways, and each type of violence, are associated with a unique set of causes or risk factors.[33]

Homicide represents only the tip of the iceberg

of interpersonal violence, but given that mortality is generally more accurately documented than morbidity, it is an extremely important epidemiological tool. Homicide rates are influenced by many factors. The influence of race and ethnicity is profoundly demonstrated by the fact that the lifetime chance of becoming a homicide victim in the USA is approximately 1 in 240 for whites as compared to 1 in 45 for blacks and other ethnic minorities.[34] Socio-economic status[35] and intrafamily factors[36] are amongst several other well-described influential factors. The role of firearms, however, requires particular attention because of its profound and unique influence on homicide and trauma in the USA.

Firearms are a major public health problem in the USA. Deaths from firearms occur 90 times more frequently in the USA than in any other industrialized nation.[37] In 1993 firearms were used in the homicide of 18 253 people (more than 70% of all homicides in the USA, Fig. 1.4) and in the suicide of 18 940 people in that country. In total, firearms alone killed 39 277 people in the USA in 1993, accounting for 26% of all trauma deaths, rivaling the number killed in MVAs. In 1991, deaths from firearms exceeded those from MVAs in seven states and the District of Columbia.[38] The trend is one of a rapid rise and it is estimated that if these trends continue, firearms will become the leading cause of trauma deaths in the whole of the USA by the year 2003.[38,39] What makes this increase even more serious is that it is affecting mainly the younger population. In fact, the increase in total homicide rate for the whole of the US population has been entirely attributable to the increase in firearm homicide in the 15- to 24-year-old age group.[40] Firearms also account for a large number of non-fatal injuries. In 1992 in the USA, it is estimated that the rate of non-fatal firearm-related injuries treated in hospital emergency departments was 2.6 times the national rate of fatal firearm-related injuries.[41]

Undoubtedly there are many variables that may explain the international differences in firearm-related trauma and homicide rates, including cultural values, judicial systems and law enforcement practices. However, the existence of strict gun control laws in most other industrialized nations stands out as the main factor contributing to these major differences. Guns are highly lethal. It has been shown that 60% of gun assaults are fatal, compared to only 4% of knife assaults and <1% of assaults with blunt weapons.[42] Similarly, only 8% of victims survive suicide attempts with a firearm, compared with 33% surviving drowning attempts, 73% surviving poisoning attempts, and 96% surviving knife wounds.[43] It is perhaps not surprising, therefore, that the presence of a gun in the home increases the risk of homicide by a factor of 2.7 and the risk of successful suicide by a factor of 4.8.[44,45] The risk of suicide in the 15- to 24-year-old age group increases ten times if there is a gun in the home, yet 49% of USA households have one or more firearm.[46]

Suicide

In many European countries, in the Americas, and in Asia, suicide rates have been recorded for extended periods of time. The reported rates vary immensely; between 1990 and 1992, the countries with the highest rates were Hungary (38.7 deaths per 100 000 population), Finland (28.8 per 100 000 population) and the Russian Federation (26.6 per 100 000 population). The lowest rates

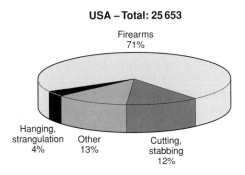
USA – Total: 25 653

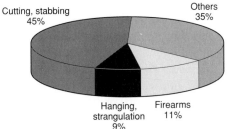
England & Wales – Total: 434

Fig. 1.4 Methods of homicide – USA and England & Wales, 1993. (USA data from National Safety Council 1996 *Accident Facts*; UK data from OPCS, 1993.)

recorded in the same years were Mexico (2.4), Armenia (2.8) and Greece (3.7) (Table 1.6). The same data source[22] records the suicide rates for the USA and the UK during these years as 12.2 and 8.0 per 100 000 population respectively, representing just over 20% of the trauma deaths occurring in each country (Fig. 1.2).

There is some debate on whether national suicide mortality statistics can be assumed to be a reliable source of data on which to base comparative epidemiological studies. Methods and criteria used in identifying suicides vary so much between different countries that they may account for the differences in rates. In 1982 a World Health Organization Working Group examined all the empirical evidence available on the matter.[47] This review indicated clearly that differences in ascertainment procedures do not explain differences in suicide rates between populations. The most likely alternative categories for suicide deaths (E54, E950 to E959) is likely to be either 'undetermined cause of death (E980 to E989) or 'accidental deaths' (E800 to E949). Studies looking at the effects of this however have shown that these are insufficient to affect the ranking of countries or to explain the differences in rates between them.[48,49] Overall, it seems that the effects of under-reporting, and the errors encountered in reporting mortality figures generally, appear to be a random effect that permits cautious epidemiological comparisons of rates within countries, between countries and over time.[50]

Assessment of international data shows that men are at considerably higher risk of suicide than women. For most countries (including the USA and UK) the male to female ratio is above three. This phenomenon is well known and not restricted to any continent or geographic area.[50] It also holds true across the age groups. Suicides account for a high proportion of the deaths occurring in the younger population. For example in the USA suicide accounts for almost 14% of all deaths in the 15 to 24 year age group (Fig. 1.1) with a death rate of 13.5 per 100 000 population of this age.[25] Other countries with high adolescent and young adult suicide rates are Canada (15 per 100 000 in 1990), Finland (25.1 in 1991), Austria and Switzerland (both with rates of 16.2 in 1991).[50] In many countries the rate of adolescent suicide has shown a marked increase over the last 35 years. This has been particularly high in Ireland, Norway and the Netherlands whilst countries such as Canada, Colombia and the USA have shown less dramatic increases. Japan is one of the few countries where a clear decrease in adolescent suicide can be established.[50]

It is difficult to know which specific sociocultural or other relevant aspects explain the similarities and differences between suicide rates in different countries. There are clear correlations between suicide and unemployment rates,[51] divorce and crime rates[52] and wars.[47] Many other complex factors are likely to be involved, such as religious affiliation. Suicide rates in Islamic countries are considerably lower than in Buddhist countries, and rates in Protestant northern Europe and North America are higher than in Roman Catholic southern Europe and Latin America.[50] Psychological risk factors also exist such as mental illness, alcoholism and financial problems. Two factors strongly and directly related to the frequency of suicidal acts are easy access to a killing agent or method, and publicity about suicidal acts. Examples of the former have been demonstrated in Western Samoa with the easy availability of the herbicide paraquat,[53] and also, as has been mentioned earlier, in the USA with widespread firearms' availability. The effect of publicity on suicide rates is sometimes described as the 'Werther effect' after its description by the 18th century German writer Goethe in his novel 'Die Leiden des jungen Werther'. This has been demonstrated in relation to television and press coverage in Germany and Austria.[54,55] Both of these factors are important in the epidemiology of suicide because they have wide implications when considering strategies for prevention.

Non-fatal injuries

There is no national injury surveillance system in the USA that provides reliable estimates of non-fatal injury. Estimates of the number of disabling injuries are made from the National Health Interview Survey, conducted by the US Public Health Service. This is a continuous personal interview of households to obtain information about the health status of household members, including injuries experienced during the 2 weeks prior to the interview. For 1994's figures 45 705 out of the 97 100 000 households were interviewed.[25] From this, an estimated 60 452 000 people were injured in 1994 in the USA (23.3 per

100 persons per year). This survey defines an injury for inclusion if it is medically attended or if it causes one half-day or more of restricted activity.

This data is not published until about 12 months after the reference year. For this reason the NSC uses injury to death ratios to estimate non-fatal disabling injury rate in the current year. The NSC defines a 'disabling injury' as one which results in death, some degree of permanent impairment, or renders the injured person unable to effectively perform their regular duties or activities for a full day beyond the day of injury. Using this system the estimated number of patients suffering disabling injuries in 1995 was 19 300 000 in the USA. This approximates to roughly 400 traumatic injuries and 130 disabling injuries for every death owing to trauma.

Table 1.9 Injury-related hospital emergency department visits – USA 1993

Cause of injury (ICD-9 code)	No. of visits (000)	%
All injury-related visits	**36492**	**100**
Other accidents (E916–E928)	11350	31.1
Accidental falls (E880–E888)	7616	20.9
Motor vehicle accidents, Traffic and non-traffic (E810–E825)	3987	10.9
Homicide and injury purposely inflicted by other persons (E960–E969)	1406	3.9
Accidents due to natural and environmental factors (E900–E909)	1228	3.4
Accidents due to submersion, suffocation, and foreign bodies (E910–E915)	936	2.6
Accidental poisoning by drugs, medicinal substances, and biologicals (E850–E858)	551	1.5
Other road vehicle accidents (E826–E829)	522	1.4
Adverse effects of drugs in therapeutic use (E930–E949)	495	1.4
Accidental poisoning by other solid and liquid substances, gases and vapors (E860–E869)	348	1
Accidents caused by fire and flames (E890–E899)	171	0.5
Suicide and self-inflicted injury (E950–E959)	167	0.5
Complications, misadventures of surgical, medical care (E878–E879)	35	0.1
Other	317	0.9
Unknown	7363	20

From NSC data, *Accident Facts 1996.*

This number of injured people makes huge demands on medical services at substantial expense. According to the National Hospital Ambulatory Medical Care Survey conducted for the National Center for Health Statistics, about 40% of all hospital emergency department visits in the USA are injury related. In 1993 there were approximately 90.3 million visits made to emergency departments, of which about 36.5 million were injury related (Table 1.9). More than one-third of all injuries resulting in emergency department visits occurred at home, the most common place of injury. The street or highway was the place of injury for about 14% of the total, while work accounted for 12% and school 4%.

COSTS OF TRAUMA CARE

Many factors must be taken into consideration when estimating the financial burden trauma represents to a country's economy. These are listed in Table 1.10. Estimated in this way, the financial impact of trauma is found to be immense. For example in the USA in 1995, the costs arising from unintentional injuries alone were estimated to be $434.8 billion.[25] Figure 1.5 shows the distribution of the components of this figure. The chart shows that the largest slice of the costs arises from wage and productivity losses. This represents a person's contribution to the wealth of the nation and is usually measured in terms of wages and household production. The total of wages and fringe benefits together with an estimate of the replacement cost value of household services provide an estimate of this lost productivity.[25] These costs include the differential effects of fatalities, permanent partial disabilities and temporary disabilities.

Table 1.10 Factors contributing to the financial burden imposed on a country's economy by trauma

- Medical expenses including emergency medical service costs
- Wage and productivity losses
- Administrative expenses, which include the administrative costs of private and public insurance plus police and legal costs
- Damage to property and goods
- Employer costs, representing the financial value incurred by remaining or newly-trained workers
- Costs arising from both fatal and non-fatal injuries

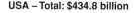

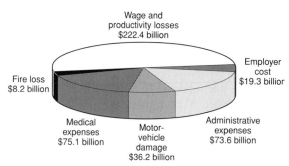

USA – Total: $434.8 billion

Wage and productivity losses $222.4 billion

Employer cost $19.3 billion

Fire loss $8.2 billion

Medical expenses $75.1 billion

Motor-vehicle damage $36.2 billion

Administrative expenses $73.6 billion

Fig. 1.5 Cost of unintentional injuries by component – USA, 1995. (Data from National Safety Council 1996 *Accident Facts*, with permission.)

In order to put these figures into perspective, the estimated total cost ($434.8 billion) is equivalent to 58 cents of every dollar spent on food in the USA in 1995. If the same costing mechanism is applied to injuries arising from MVAs alone, the resultant costs are estimated to be $170.6 billion.[25] This is the equivalent of purchasing 730 gallons of gasoline for every registered vehicle in the USA.

Such economic costs provide a measure of productivity lost and expenses incurred because of unintentional injuries. Economic costs, however, should not be used for cost benefit analysis because they do not reflect what society is willing to pay to prevent a fatality or injury. Comprehensive costs include not only the economic cost components, but also a measure of the value of lost quality of life associated with the deaths and injuries, that is, what society is willing to pay to prevent them. The values of lost quality of life can be estimated through empirical studies of what people actually pay to reduce their health and safety risks, such as through the purchase of air-bags or smoke detectors. In 1995 in the USA, such lost quality of life was estimated to have a value of $775.8 billion,[25] making the comprehensive cost of unintentional injury in the USA $1210.6 billion.

As dramatic as the financial costs may seem, the ultimate tragedy is not financial but personal. The loss experienced by victims and their families is, of course, incalculable. It is clear, therefore, that the main answer to reducing the costs of trauma lies not in improved diagnostic and therapeutic efficiency, nor in financial wizardry or major overhauls in the organization of trauma care systems, but in the prevention of trauma (see p. 24).

OUTCOME AFTER TRAUMA

Scoring systems

It is difficult to compare the outcome of trauma victims managed in different centers, particularly on an international scale. Meaningful comparisons of mortality and morbidity require a demonstration of equivalence in the type, severity, etiology and demography of the trauma load. Classification systems are therefore necessary to measure and classify the severity of injuries. Since the establishment of the first civilian trauma unit at Cook County Hospital in Chicago in 1966, we have seen the introduction of the concept and utilization of many such trauma scoring systems.[56]

Trauma scoring systems have the potential for many different uses. They were initially introduced to allow comparison between patient populations and to aid triage, but they also allow predictions of outcome, evaluation of current and new methods of treatment, and provide information that is useful in quality assurance and resource allocation. Any evolving trauma system must have the facility to measure and document injury severity.

Many scoring systems are based on the anatomy and severity of a patient's injuries. As anatomic scoring systems rely to an extent on retrospective data, they are of limited use in initial assessment and triage in the field. Scores that are based on physiology are of more practical use at this stage in the management of the trauma patient.

Physiologic-based scoring systems assign values depending on the extent of deviation from normal. They may include an assessment of blood pressure, heart rate, peripheral perfusion, ventilatory status, and level of consciousness. The data obtained may then be used to grade severity of injury, aid patient triage, assess response to therapy, and predict outcome.

At present no individual scoring system is applicable to all age-groups in all settings, while taking account of prior disease states and the mechanism of injury. However, the most commonly used scoring systems in current use are the Abbreviated Injury Scale (AIS), the Injury Severity Score (ISS), Glasgow Coma Scale

(GCS), and the Revised Trauma Score (RTS). Recently an adaptation of the ISS, the New Injury Severity Score (NISS) has been described.

Abbreviated Injury Scale

The AIS is an anatomical scoring system and was published in 1971 by the American Medical Association, the American Association for Automotive Medicine, and the Society of Automotive Engineers.[57] The AIS aimed to provide a uniform grading for persons injured in MVAs, but has undergone many revisions and now also includes penetrating trauma and other causes of blunt trauma. In its present form, the AIS assigns a score from 1 (minor) to 6 (fatal) to injuries that are coded based on their anatomic site, nature, and severity.

Injury Severity Score

ISS is an anatomical scoring system developed from the AIS, and was published originally in 1974.[58] It provides a severity score for patients with multiple injuries. Each injury is given an AIS code and classified into one of six body regions. The ISS is calculated by adding the squares of the highest AIS scores from the three most severely injured body regions. Any injury coded as 6 automatically converts the ISS to 75 (range 1–75), which is the maximum score ($5^2 + 5^2 + 5^2$). An ISS of 16 or more is taken as defining major trauma and corresponds with an average mortality rate of 10%.

The scale has been validated for road traffic casualties in relation to mortality, time of death, hospital treatment time, and disability. It shows good correlation with length of hospital stay, time of death, disability, the need for surgery, and plasma cortisol concentrations.[59–63]

The ISS remains virtually the only anatomic scoring system currently in use, but it may be criticized on several points:

1. Any error in scoring the AIS will increase the ISS error.
2. A wide diversity of injuries yield the same ISS score.
3. There is no weighting of values for injuries to different body regions, whereas, in practice, the same severity scores to different regions may have greatly differing mortalities.

4. The ISS will not differentiate a severe injury from a milder one which is poorly managed.[64]

Because it is complex and time-consuming, the ISS is not a useful triage tool. However, the combination of ISS (anatomic score) and trauma score (TS) (physiologic score) improves their predictive power (see TRISS).

New Injury Severity Score

This was created in an effort to improve the ISS by making it simpler to calculate.[65] The NISS dispenses with the question of body region and is simply the sum of the squares of the three highest AIS scores wherever they are.

Surprisingly, NISS not only makes the calculation a lot simpler but it also predicts survival better than ISS, as found in an analysis of 3136 consecutive admissions to the Level 1 trauma center in Albuquerque, New Mexico. It has been claimed that if further validation repeats these results, NISS will replace the use of ISS.[66]

Glasgow Coma Scale

The Glasgow Coma Scale was introduced in 1974 by Teasdale & Jennett.[67] It is the most frequently used neurologic scoring system and is also a component of several other scoring systems. This scale allows the grading of impairment of consciousness in both trauma and non-trauma situations. It is simple to use and learn, consistent for different observers,[68] and provides an accurate indication of neurologic status, outcome, and prognosis.[69–72] The scale assesses eye opening, motor response, and verbal response. Scores range from 3 to 15, the higher scores indicating increased level of consciousness. A non-verbal pediatric coma scale has been advocated for use in small children.[71]

Revised Trauma Score

In 1980, Champion and others derived indices from physiological variables known to correlate with mortality following blunt trauma. Taking weighted values for the five strongest variables (eye opening, verbal response, motor response, respiratory expansion, and capillary refill), the Triage Index was created.[73] Evaluation of the index showed it had high inter-rater reliability, demonstrated accuracy in ranking for possibility of death, and was easy to use.

In 1981 the Triage Index was modified by the addition of respiratory rate and systolic blood pressure to create the Trauma Score (TS).[74] The TS had shortcomings because capillary refill and respiratory effort (shallow or retractive) are very difficult to assess in the field under adverse conditions and in poor lighting, and the TS underestimated the severity of some head injuries. The RTS eliminates these assessments and requires only three of the five parameters of the TS (GCS, systolic blood pressure, and respiratory rate).[75] A range for each parameter is allocated a value that is multiplied by an assigned weight. The sum of the resulting values (the RTS) ranges from 0 (dead) to 7.8408 (normal). The RTS is superior to the original TS in that predictions of outcome and severe head injury are more reliable.[76] The GCS component carries most of the weight in the RTS, which allows identification of severe head injury in the absence of multi-system injury or major physiologic changes. A cut-off value of less than 4 has been suggested as identifying those individuals requiring care in a trauma center.[77]

Trauma Score – Injury Severity Score method

Physiological derangement and anatomical injury are the most important determinants of the threat to life, but age and the method of wounding are also relevant; a blunt assault produces different injury characteristics than does a penetrating object. The 'TRISS (Trauma Score – Injury Severity Score) methodology' described by Boyd[77] combines these four elements (in the form of RTS and ISS weighted by a coefficient based on age and mechanism of injury) to provide a measure of the probability of survival (Ps). The Ps is merely a mathematical calculation; it is not an absolute measure of mortality but only of the probability of death. It should not, therefore, be used as a predictive tool for death in an individual patient. It does, however, allow comparison of the effectiveness of trauma management on a local basis, as well as comparison of different populations and the identification of an unexpected outcome.

Trauma outcome
The Major Trauma Outcome Study

The Major Trauma Outcome Study (MTOS)[78] was initiated by the American College of Surgeons Committee on Trauma and began in 1982. Its aim is to improve injury severity scoring systems, to establish national outcome data, and to provide objective evaluation of quality assurance and outcome. Up to 1989, data had been recorded on over 170 000 seriously injured patients, from over 150 institutions. This included information on ISS, TS/RTS, age, management, outcome, and length of hospital stay. It is upon this empirical set of information that normative values can be set.

An equivalent multi-center prospective cohort study of trauma victims was set up as an independent UK MTOS in 1988. A Royal College of Surgeons Working Party reported on the management of patients with major injuries in November 1988 and highlighted several deficiencies in the care of the seriously injured in the UK.[79] A preliminary report from the MTOS (UK) data confirmed many of these deficiencies.[80] This reported on 14 648 trauma patients admitted to 33 hospitals across the UK. They found that 21% of seriously injured patients took over 1 hour to reach hospital, and that when they arrived in the emergency room, more than half were attended by relatively inexperienced junior doctors. Less than half the patients judged to require early operation arrived in the operating room within 2 hours. Mortality for more than 6000 patients sustaining blunt injury was substantially higher than in a comparable North American data set. The MTOS (UK) now encompasses 117 hospitals and there are approximately 86 000 patients on the database. Data analysis up to 1996 shows that there has been some improvement in the outcome of major trauma in the UK with the overall mortality ratio (the observed number of deaths divided by the expected number of deaths × 100) decreasing from 124 to 97.[81] Also over the 7-year period 1989–95, after severity of injury is controlled for, the odds of death in children and young adults (<24 years), after severe injury, declined by 16% a year.[82] In 1997 MTOS (UK) changed its name to the UK Trauma Audit & Research Network.

Trimodal distribution

The timing of death after trauma can be described as following a trimodal distribution (Fig. 1.6).[83] In this trimodal distribution, the first peak of death is within seconds to minutes of injury and accounts for 50% of the total. These deaths are the result of catastrophic injuries such as lacerations of the brain, brainstem or upper spinal cord, heart, aorta or other large blood vessels. Very few of these patients can be saved and only measures to prevent trauma will reduce it.

The second peak accounts for 30% of deaths and occurs up to 4 hours after injury. These deaths are usually caused by intracranial hematomas, hemopneumothorax, or significant blood loss from lacerated intra-abdominal organs or multiple musculoskeletal injuries. Most injuries in this group are considered treatable. These patients should benefit from a well-organized trauma care system that reduces the time interval between injury and expert definitive treatment and this period is often referred to as the 'Golden Hour' to emphasize the time following injury when resuscitation and stabilization are critical.[84]

The remaining trauma fatalities from the third peak of 'late deaths' occur after 4 hours. This is usually days to weeks after injury and is often the result of sepsis and multiple organ dysfunction. Appropriate, timely management and aggressive restoration of cellular oxygenation in the resuscitation phase should help reduce this third peak of deaths. This philosophy has molded trauma care

services in both the USA and the UK, and resulted in the development of paramedic services and trauma centers.

Trunkey's original work describing this distribution of deaths was based on an analysis, over 2 years, of trauma deaths in San Francisco nearly two decades ago. Whether or not those figures are still valid today has recently been questioned,[85,86] particularly in the UK where the causes of trauma and the systems for dealing with it differ considerably from those in the USA. An analysis of trauma deaths occurring over a 2-year period in the Lothian and Borders region of Scotland, for example, revealed a different distribution of the timing of death (Fig. 1.6). Similar results were found when the same group analyzed data for trauma in children in the same region.[87] The distribution of time of deaths is probably a reflection of the type of trauma seen and also due to improvements in early trauma care. If these figures are mirrored throughout the UK, they will fuel the debate on the role of pre-hospital trauma resuscitation. These figures imply that earlier definitive care at the scene will make little difference to early mortality since 98% of the deaths occurring within 1 hour occurred instantaneously in patients with unsurvivable injuries (AIS 6, ISS 75).

This conflicts with a recent retrospective study of pre-hospital trauma deaths in North Staffordshire in the UK[88] which reported that, on the basis of post-mortem evidence, airway obstruction had been present in two-thirds of those patients in whom death was judged not to have been inevitable. These authors concluded that more bystanders should be trained in simple first aid and the interval between the time of injury and arrival of the emergency services must be reduced. Whatever the outcome of these continuing debates the philosophy of rapid, systematic and appropriate management will remain.

THE ROLE OF THE ANESTHESIOLOGIST IN TRAUMA CARE

The anesthesiologist is one of the few specialists who can potentially provide continuity of care for the severely injured patient from the pre-hospital phase, to the emergency room, the operating room and through to intensive care (i.e. 'the Continuum of Acute Trauma Care'). The roles

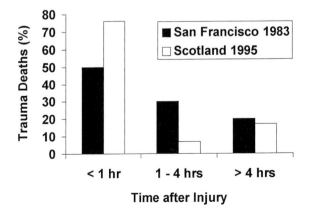

Fig. 1.6 Timing of death after trauma in San Francisco compared with south-east Scotland, 1995. Data derived from reference 85.

Table 1.11   Role of anesthesiologists in management of trauma patient resuscitation in different countries

	Pre-hospital EMS	Team leader	IV access	Inv. procedure	Airway	Lab data interp.	Diagnosis
Austria	+	+	+	+	+	+	+
Chile	−	−	+	+	+	−	−
England	±	±	+	+	+	±	±
France	+	+	+	+	+	+	+
Germany	+	+	+	+	+	+	+
Italy	±	±	+	+	+	±	±
Japan	−	−	±	±	±	−	−
Mexico	−	−	−	−	−	−	−
Netherlands	±	−	±	±	±	−	−
Norway	+	−	+	+	+	±	−
Switzerland	+	−	+	+	+	±	−
USA[1]	−	−	±	±	±	±	−

+ Anesthesiologists play a major role.

− Anesthesiologists play a minimal role.

± Anesthesiologists have a variable role.

EMS, Emergency Medical Service; IV, Intravenous; Inv, Invasive procedures such as inserting chest tubes, urinary catheters, arterial lines; Lab. data interp, laboratory data interpretation – leading role for anesthesiologist.

[1] Among 83 Level 1 trauma centers.

Table devised by C F Mackenzie based on data from Grande EM, ed. Textbook of trauma anesthesia and critical care. St Louis: Mosby-Yearbook, 1993.

undertaken by anesthesiologists managing trauma patients vary between institutions and between countries (Table 1.11). They may be summarized as follows:

1. Pre-hospital care
2. In-hospital trauma patient resuscitation as a member of the trauma team
3. Trauma team leader
4. The provision of analgesia
5. Anesthesia in the operating room
6. Pre- and postoperative critical care.
7. Attending physician for the transfer of a trauma patient.

Pre-hospital care

An effective pre-hospital emergency medical service (EMS) system requires short response times, adequate training of individuals who carry appropriate equipment, and the full support of communications and hospital facilities.

Controversies in pre-hospital trauma management concern the type of pre-hospital provider and the interventions they perform. Like the EMS in the USA, the UK utilizes a paramedic-based system. In other parts of Europe (in particular, France, Germany, and Belgium) ambulance technicians are supported by physicians, usually anesthesiologists, in mobile intensive care units (MICU). In the UK, ambulance technicians are trained in basic airway management, cervical spine control, and shock advisory defibrillation. Paramedics have the additional skills of tracheal intubation, intravenous cannulation, fluid therapy, and use of intravenous analgesia.[89] Supplemental skills provided by physicians in general, and anesthesiologists in particular, include the use of neuromuscular blocking drugs and a broader range of analgesia and fluids, insertion of chest drains, cricothyroidotomy, and the ability to triage the patient to the most appropriate hospital. In some states in the USA, paramedics are trained to use neuromuscular blocking drugs and to perform cricothyroidotomies. In theory, the doctor's ability to provide a more sophisticated and individualized continuum of patient care (not necessarily protocol driven) in the initial hospital phase may expedite definitive care. Certainly, the French anesthesiologists working within the Service D'Aide Medicale Urgente (SAMU) strongly support this hypothesis.[90]

Unfortunately, there are no good randomized controlled trials proving that the outcome for trauma patients is influenced by the type of pre-hospital provider or even the procedures performed. There are only small, retrospective, observational studies which have produced conflicting results.[91–96] Some studies have suggested that advanced life support procedures improve physiological variables but not outcome.[97] Except where patients are trapped, it would seem logical to limit interventions at the scene to establishing an open airway and effective ventilation, controlling external hemorrhage with pressure and expediting transport to a trauma center. For penetrating cardiac injuries delays of just 15 minutes in transportation increase morbidity and mortality so rapid transport with basic life support may give the best chance of survival.[98]

One of the problems with pre-hospital trauma studies is the lack of a uniform system or set of definitions for reporting results. An ITACCS-led working group has been convened to develop 'Guidelines for Uniform Recording and Reporting of Performance and Outcome Following Trauma' very much along the lines of the Utstein template for the reporting of pre-hospital cardiac arrest.[99] It is hoped that this will enhance the ability to compare data derived from different EMS systems.

In-hospital trauma resuscitation

The anesthesiologist has particular skills in airway and ventilatory management and in obtaining intravenous access. In most countries this individual plays a vital role within the trauma team (Table 1.11). However, a recent survey of Level 1 trauma centers in the USA showed that an anesthesiologist was included routinely on the trauma team in only 30% of cases.[100] In many institutions airway management during trauma patient resuscitation is performed primarily by emergency physicians.[101] Yet, as anesthesiologists in the USA begin to embrace the concept of the 'perioperative physician' their involvement in the 'pre-OR' phase of acute trauma care is likely to increase.

Advanced Trauma Life Support

A considerable advance in trauma patient resuscitation has been made by the Advanced Trauma Life Support (ATLS) Course.[102] Unfortunately, any benefit is very difficult to prove and only one group has documented a reduction in trauma mortality after the introduction of ATLS.[103,104]

The ATLS course manual and slides are produced by the Committee on Trauma of the American College of Surgeons (ACS). The course focuses on the initial management of patients with major injuries during the 'Golden Hour'. By its very nature, the course is didactic and an identical core content is taught to all doctors on ATLS courses across the world. Inevitably there are some controversial areas, particularly in airway management,[105] but many of these issues have been, and are being, resolved in later editions of the manual. Anesthesiologists make an important contribution to ATLS courses. In the UK, the current Chairman of the ATLS Committee is an anesthesiologist and more ATLS instructors are from anesthesia than from any other specialty (1997).

There are now plans for a trauma course which goes 'one step beyond' the skills and knowledge provided by ATLS. A number of ITACCS members are now designing the 'Comprehensive Approach to Trauma (CAT)' course. It is likely that an ATLS-provider certificate will be a mandatory prerequisite for admission to the CAT course.

Trauma team leader

The team leader plays a vital role in coordinating the activities of the rest of the trauma team. This person must be experienced in trauma patient resuscitation and must be capable of liaising with all the relevant specialists. In many European countries this role is often taken by an appropriately experienced anesthesiologist, although this is rarely the case in the USA.[100] In the future, the CAT course will provide essential elements for 'trauma team leader' training.

The provision of analgesia

The anesthesiologist obviously has particular skills in the provision of pain relief and anesthesia, both of vital importance in the early management of the severely injured patient. As a theme promulgated throughout this text, analgesia should be regarded as part of the resuscitation process for it brings with it not only compassionate relief but also cardiovascular stability and subsequently improved organ and tissue perfusion.[106] Effective relief of severe pain in the compromised patient requires not only knowledge and experience of the wide variety of analgesic agents but also the skill to support the vital functions involved in respiration and the circulation which may be depressed by effective analgesic doses. The postoperative trauma patient may benefit from more advanced analgesic techniques such as epidural analgesia or patient-controlled analgesia. These techniques, and many others, are discussed throughout this book.

Anesthesia in the operating room

The anesthetic management of severe trauma patients in the operating room can be challenging, even for the very experienced anesthesiologist. This is one area where the requirement for an appropriately trained anesthesiologist is undisputed. The patient requires ongoing resuscitation and correction or prevention of hypothermia and coagulopathy.

Pre- and postoperative critical care

In many countries anesthesiologists have primary responsibility for the management of trauma patients in the critical care unit. The management of trauma patients in the critical care unit demands extensive knowledge and experience in multiple organ support which is relevant to any critically ill patient. This might include advanced modes of ventilation, inotropic therapy, and renal replacement therapy. Facets of care that are specific to the trauma patient include the management of head injuries, burns, and spinal trauma, which are the subjects of other ITACCS-sponsored specialized texts.

Attending physician for the transfer of a trauma patient

Severely-injured patients frequently require intra-hospital or inter-hospital transport. The regionalization of trauma services will necessitate an increase in the number of long distance trauma patient transfers. Irrespective of the distance the patient needs to be transported, there is the potential for complications unless attended by suitably experienced personnel. The accompanying doctor must be skilled in airway management and have thorough knowledge of the benefits and limitations of portable ventilators and monitors. There is little doubt that an experienced anesthesiologist is ideally suited to this task. The Association of Anaesthetists of Great Britain and Ireland has recently published recommendations for the transfer of head-injured patients.[107]

PREVENTION OF TRAUMA

Trauma is a major cause of death, disability and injury across the world. Its impact on society is enormous. It rids a population of its young men and women and accounts for vast numbers of years of potential life lost. It has huge financial implications on a country with respect to both the acute medical costs, and to the loss of life of young people who would otherwise have been productive members of society.

Much attention in recent years has been focused on establishing systems of management that allow faster, more efficient and higher quality care for the trauma victim so that deaths from trauma can be reduced. While these systems have improved the chances of survival of the injured patient it is clear that the most effective means of reducing trauma morbidity and mortality lies in prevention.

Thirty years ago injuries were virtually ignored by the public health community. Their epidemiology was a mystery and few were advocating their prevention through research. At that time, injuries from trauma were labeled 'accidents,' a word associated with connotations of chance and inevitability.

Today, the word 'unintentional' is preferred to 'accidental' because it is now recognized that many types of trauma are not just chance occurrences, and therefore inevitable, but are in fact quite predictable and therefore preventable. This has resulted, in recent years, in several legislative changes that have led to a reduction in injuries from certain types of trauma. Motor vehicle-related trauma, for example, has come under intense scrutiny. Legislation concerning alcohol consumption, laminated windshields, energy-absorbing steering wheels, crash-resistant fuel systems, front and rear seat belts, and most recently, driver and passenger airbags have all had a major impact on deaths and injury in motor vehicles.

Lately, passenger airbags have received some adverse publicity after a series of case reports of children being killed during airbag deployment.[108] A total of 32 fatal injuries occurred during January 1993 to November 1996. Most of these occurred in children who were either unrestrained or incorrectly restrained by seat belts or who were in rear-facing child safety seats. To reduce the problems associated with children in front passenger seats automotive safety engineers are designing 'smart' airbags that will be appropriate for different ages and sizes of occupants. In the meantime clearer guidelines have been issued by the NHTSA, National Transport Safety Board, the American Academy of Pediatrics, and the Centers for Disease Control and Prevention.[108]

The scope for trauma prevention is enormous and its discussion is well beyond the remit of this chapter. Susan Baker, whilst giving the William T. Fitts Oration at the 56th Annual Meeting of the American Association for the Surgery of Trauma in 1996,[66] highlighted three particular areas that demand urgent changes in order to further reduce injury in the USA. These were:

- firearm legislation
- speed limit controls
- correct child occupant restraint in cars.

It is clear that these are just a few examples of many potential areas where there is a need for the introduction of measures to prevent injuries and deaths from trauma.

Whilst trauma prevention is a priority, it is important that appropriate resources are invested into the acute care of the trauma victim in order to maximize the chance of quality survival. Every link in the 'trauma chain of survival' (Fig. 1.7) is essential to the patient's survival.

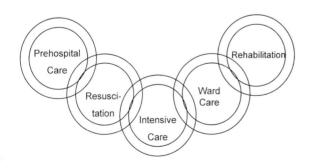

Fig. 1.7 The trauma chain of survival.

CONCLUSION

Trauma is a major cause of morbidity and mortality world-wide. It is clear that maximizing survival in trauma victims requires definitive care as soon as possible after injury and a continuing high quality of care to improve long-term survival. The anesthesiologist has many skills essential to this process and has an important role to play in most phases of the 'trauma chain of survival'. Whilst the 'biggest bang for the buck' lies with trauma prevention the onus is on us to maximize the quality of acute care for the trauma patient. We must make every effort to attract the funding and resources that this critically important specialty deserves.

REFERENCES

1. National Safety Council. Accident Facts Chicago: The Council; 1990.
2. Baker SP, O'Neill B, Karpf RS. Motor vehicle crashes. In: Baker SP, O'Neill B, Karpf RS, eds. The Injury Fact Book. Lexington: Lexington Books; 1984.
3. Baker SP, O'Neill B, Ginsburg M, Guohua L. Introduction. In: Baker SP, O'Neill B, Ginsburg M, Guohua L, eds. The Injury Fact Book. New York: Oxford University Press; 1992.
4. Wilkinson DJ. The history of trauma anesthesia. In: Grande C, ed. Textbook of Trauma Anesthesia and Critical Care. St Louis: Mosby–Yearbook; 1993: 199–204.
5. Bryan CP. The Papyrus Ebers. London: Geoffrey Bles; 1930.
6. Gaius Plinius Secundus (translated by Bostock J, Riley HT). Natural History. London: Henry J Bohn; 1861: 139–140.
7. Gruner OC. A treatise on the cannon of medicine of Avicenna. London: Luzac; 1930.
8. Harvey W. Exercitatio anatomica de motu cordis et sanguinis in animali. Frankfurt: William Fitzer; 1628.
9. Major JD. Chirurgia infusoria. Keil: 1662 and 1667.
10. Lower R. A method of transfusing blood. Philosophical Transactions 1667; 9.
11. Larrey DJ (translated by Hall RW). Memoirs of military surgery and campaigns of the French Army. Baltimore: Joseph Cushing; 1814.
12. Haughton JW. Spinal analgesia in military service; with a note on 600 cases BMJ 1913; 2: 305–306.
13. Gwathmey JT. Anesthesia. New York: Appleton; 1914.

14. Rowbotham S. Intra-tracheal anaesthesia by the nasal route for operations on the mouth and lips. BMJ 1920; 2: 590–591.

15. Guedel AE, Waters RM. A new intra-tracheal catheter. Anesth Analg 1928; 7: 238–239.

16. Fischer E, von Mering J. Ueber eine neue Klasse von Schlafmittein. Ther Gegenwart 1903; 5: 97–101.

17. Halford FJ. A critique of intravenous anesthesia in war surgery. Anesthesiology 1943; 4: 67–69.

18. Bennetts FE. Thiopentone anaesthesia at Pearl Harbor. Br J Anaesth 1995; 75: 366–368.

19. Crane RM, Sankey BB. Recent developments in anesthesia of significance to the military surgeon. Anesth Analg 1941; 20: 151–155.

20. Egan CF. Resuscitation and anesthesia at the Korean front. Curr Anesth Analg 1953; 32: 90–101.

21. Grande C. The trauma anaesthesia/critical care specialist. In: Grande C, ed. Textbook of trauma anesthesia and critical care. St Louis: Mosby–Yearbook; 1993.

22. World Health Organization. World health statistics annual, 1993. Geneva: WHO; 1994.

23. World Health Organization. World health statistics annual, 1994. Geneva: WHO; 1995.

24. Office of Population Censuses and Surveys. Mortality statistics, cause. Review of the Registrar General on deaths by cause, sex and age in England and Wales 1993; Series DH2 No 20; 1995.

25. National Safety Council. Accident facts. Itasca: National Safety Council; 1996.

26. National Safety Council. International Accident Facts. Itasca: National Safety Council; 1995.

27. The Department of Transport. Road Accidents Great Britain: 1995. The casualty report. London: HMSO; 1996: July.

28. World Health Organization. Manual of the international statistical classification of diseases, injuries and causes of death. Ninth Revision. Geneva: WHO; 1977; 1: 763.

29. Nolan J. Trauma statistics and demographics. In: Grande C, ed. Textbook of trauma anesthesia and critical care. St Louis: Mosby–Yearbook; 1993.

30. Office for National Statistics. Annual abstract of statistics. London: The Stationery Office; 1997: No. 133.

31. Department of Health. On the state of the public health, 1995. A report from the Chief Medical Officer. London: HMSO; 1996.

32. Jeanneret O, Sand EA. Intentional violence among adolescents and young adults: an epidemiological perspective. World Health Stat Q 1993; 46: 1.

33. Rosenberg ML, Mercy JA. Assaultive violence. In: Rosenberg ML, Fenley MA, eds. Violence in America: A public health approach. New York: Oxford University Press; 1991.

34. Rosenberg ML, Mercy JA. Homicide: Epidemiologic analysis at the national level. Bull N Y Acad Med 1986; 62(5): 376–399.

35. Hodgins S. Mental disorder, intellectual deficiency and crime. Evidence from a birth cohort. Arch Gen Psychiatry 1992; 49(6): 476–483.

36. Schellenbach CJ, Guernez LF. Identification of adolescent abuse and future intervention prospects. J Adolesc 1987; 10(1): 1–12.

37. The Violence Prevention Task Force of the Eastern Association for the Surgery of Trauma. Violence in America: A public health crisis–the role of firearms. J Trauma 1995; 38: 163–168.

38. Centers for Disease Control and Prevention. Deaths resulting from firearm and motor-vehicle related injuries–United States 1968–1991. MMWR Morb Mortal Wkly Rep 1994; 43: 37–42.

39. Fingerhut LA, Jones C, Makuo D. Firearm and motor-vehicle injury mortality–variation by state and race and ethnicity: United States 1990–1991. Advance Data from Vital and Health Statistics: No. 242. Hyattsville, Maryland: National Center for Health Statistics; 1994.

40. Trends in rates of homicide: United States, 1985–1994. MMWR Morb Mortal Wkly Rep 1996; 45: 460.

41. Annest J, Mercy J, Gibson D, et al. National estimates of nonfatal firearm-related injuries. Beyond the tip of the iceberg. JAMA 1995; 273: 1749.

42. Hedboe J, Charles AV, Neilson J, et al. Interpersonal violence: Patterns in a Danish community. Am J Public Health 1985; 75: 651.

43. Webster DW, Chaulk CP, Teret SP, et al. Reducing firearm injuries. Issues Sci Technol 1991: 73.

44. Kellermann AL, Rivara FP, Rushforth NB, et al. Gun ownership as a risk factor for homicide in the home. N Engl J Med 1993; 329: 1084.

45. Kellermann AL, Rivara FP, Somes G, et al. Suicide in the home in relation to gun ownership. N Engl J Med 1992; 327: 467.

46. Fontanarosa PB. The unrelenting epidemic of violence in America. Truths and consequences. JAMA 1995; 273: 1792–1793.

47. World Health Organization. Changing patterns in suicide behaviour. Report of a WHO working group (Athens, 29 September–2 October 1981) EURO Reports and Studies no. 74 (E,F,G,R) 1982. Copenhagen, Regional Office for Europe: WHO; 1982.

48. Barraclough B. Differences between national suicide rates. Br J Psychiatry 1973; 122: 95–96.

49. Sainsbury P, Barraclough B. Differences between suicide rates. Nature 1968; 2202: 1252.

50. Diekstra RFW, Gulbinat W. The epidemiology of suicidal behaviour: a review of three continents. World Health Stat Q 1993; 46(1): 52–68.

51. Platt S. Suicidal behaviour and unemployment: a literature review. In: Westcott G, Svensson PG, et al, eds. Health policy implications of unemployment. Copenhagen: WHO; 1985: 87–132.

52. Diekstra RFW. Suicide and parasuicide: a global perspective. In: Diekstra RFW, Gulbinat WH, eds. Preventive strategies on suicide. Leiden: EJ Brill; 1993.

53. Bowles JR. Suicide in Western Samoa: an example of a suicide prevention program in a developing country. In: Diekstra RFW, Gulbinat WH, eds. Preventive strategies on suicide. Leiden: EJ Brill; 1993: 126–156.

54. Schmidtke A, Hafner H. The Werther effect after television films: new evidence for an old hypothesis. Psychol Med 1988; 18: 665–675.

55. Sonneck G. Subway suicide in Vienna (1980–1990): a contribution to the imitation effect in suicidal behaviour. In: Diekstra RFW, Gulbinat WH, eds. Preventive strategies on suicide. Leiden: EJ Brill; 1993: 215–223.

56. Parr MJA, Grande CM. Concepts of trauma: In: Grande C, ed. Textbook of trauma anesthesia and critical care. St Louis: Mosby–Yearbook; 1993.

57. Committee on Medical Aspects of Automotive Safety. Rating the severity of tissue damage: I. The abbreviated scale. JAMA 1971; 215: 277–280.

58. Baker SP, O'Neill B, Haddon W, Long WB. The injury severity score: a method for describing patients with multiple injuries and evaluating emergency care. J Trauma 1974; 14: 187–196.

59. Stoner HB, Barton RN, Little RA, Yates DW. Measuring the severity of injury. BMJ 1977; 2: 1247–1249.

60. Semmlow JL, Cone R. Utility of the injury severity score: a confirmation. Health Serv Res 1976; 11: 45–52.

61. Copes WS, Champion HR, Sacco WJ, et al. The injury severity score revisited. J Trauma 1988; 28: 69–77.

62. Teasdale G, Knill-Jones R, van der Sande J. Observer variability in assessing impaired consciousness and coma. J Neurol Neurosurg Psychiatry 1978; 41: 603–610.

63. Langfitt TW. Measuring the outcome from head injuries. J Neurosurg 1978; 148: 673–678.

64. Rutledge R. The injury severity score is unable to differentiate between poor care and severe injury. J Trauma 1996; 40: 944–950.

65. Osler TM, Baker SP, Long WB. NISS: The new injury severity score. The Eastern Association for the Surgery of Trauma: Sanibel, Fla; 1997: January 16 (abstract).

66. Baker SP. Advances and adventures in trauma prevention. J Trauma 1997; 42: 369–373.

67. Teasdale G, Jennett B. Assessment of coma and impaired consciousness: a practical scale. Lancet 1974; 2: 81–83.

68. Jane JA, Rimel RW. Prognosis in head injury. Clin Neurosurg 1982; 29: 346–352.

69. Jennett B, Teasdale G, Braakman R, et al. Predicting outcome in individual patients after severe head injury. Lancet 1976; 1: 1031–1034.

70. Lanza DC, Koltai PJ, Parnes SM. Predictive value of the Glasgow Coma Scale for tracheostomy in head-injured patients. Ann Otol Rhinol Laryngol 1990; 99: 38–41.

71. Morray JP, Tyler DC, Jones TK, et al. Coma scale for use in brain-injured children. Crit Care Med 1984; 12: 1018–1020.

72. Champion HR, Gainer PS, Yackee E. A progress report on the trauma score in predicting a fatal outcome. J Trauma 1986; 26: 927–931.

73. Champion HR, Sacco WJ, Hannan DS, et al. Assessment of injury severity: the triage index. Crit Care Med 1980; 8: 201–208.

74. Champion HR, Sacco WJ, Carnazzo AJ, et al. Trauma score. Crit Care Med 1981; 9: 672–676.

75. Champion HR, Sacco WJ, Copes WS, et al. A revision of the trauma score. J Trauma 1989; 29: 623–629.

76. Ornato J, Mlinek EJ Jr, Craren EJ, et al. Ineffectiveness of the trauma score and the CRAMS scale for accurately triaging patients to trauma centers. Ann Emerg Med 1985; 14: 1061–1064.

77. Boyd CR, Tolson MA, Copes WS. Evaluating trauma care: the TRISS method. J Trauma 1987; 27: 370–378.

78. Champion HR, Copes WS, Sacco WJ, Lawnick MM, et al. The Major Trauma Outcome Study: establishing national norms for trauma care. J Trauma 1990; 30: 1356–1365.

79. Royal College of Surgeons of England. Report of the working party on the management of patients with major injuries. London: RCSE; 1988.

80. Yates DW, Woodford M, Hollis S. Preliminary analysis of the care of injured patients in 33 British hospitals: first report of the United Kingdom major trauma outcome study. BMJ 1992; 305: 737–740.

81. The UK Trauma Audit & Research Network. A guide for clinicians. Manchester: The University of Manchester; 1996.

82. Roberts I, Campbell F, Hollis S, Yates D. On behalf of the Steering Committee of the Major Trauma Outcome Study Group. Reducing acci-

dent death rates in children and young adults: the contribution of hospital care. BMJ 1996; 313: 1239–1241.

83. Trunkey DD. Trauma. Sci Am 1983; 249: 28–35.

84. Cowley R. The resuscitation and stabilization of major multiple trauma patients in a trauma center environment. Clin Med 1976; 83: 14.

85. Wyatt J, Beard D, Gray A, et al. The time of death after trauma. BMJ 1995; 310: 1502.

86. Sauaia A, Moore FA, Moore EE, et al. Epidemiology of trauma deaths. J Trauma 1995; 38: 185–193.

87. Wyatt JP, McLeod D, Beard D, et al. Timing of paediatric deaths after trauma. BMJ 1997; 314: 868.

88. Hussain LM, Redmond AD. Are pre-hospital deaths from accidental injury preventable? BMJ 1994; 308: 1077–1080.

89. Simpson HK, Smith GB. Survey of paramedic skills in the United Kingdom and Channel Islands. BMJ 1996; 313: 1052–1053.

90. Carli PA, Riou B, Barriot P. France. In: Grande C, ed. Textbook of trauma anesthesia and critical care. St Louis: Mosby–Yearbook; 1993: 199–204.

91. Kaweski SM, Sise MJ, Virgilio RW. The effect of pre-hospital fluids on survival in trauma patients. J Trauma 1990; 30: 1215–1219.

92. Potter D, Goldstein G, Fung SC, Selig M. A controlled trial of prehospital advanced life support in trauma. Ann Emerg Med 1988; 17: 582–588.

93. Sampalis JS, Lavoie A, Williams JI, et al. Impact of on-site care, prehospital time, and level of in-hospital care on survival in severely injured patients. J Trauma 1993; 34: 252–261.

94. Sampalis JS, Boukas S, Lavoie A, et al. Preventable death; evaluation of the appropriateness of the onsite trauma care provided by Urgences-Sante physicians. J Trauma 1995; 39: 1029–1035.

95. Schmidt U, Frame SB, Nerlich ML, et al. On-scene helicopter transport of patients with multiple injuries–comparison of a German and an American system. J Trauma 1992; 33: 548–555.

96. Smith JP, Bodai BL, Hill AS, Frey CF. Prehospital stabilization of critically injured patients: a failed concept. J Trauma 1985; 25: 65–70.

97. Cayten CG, Murphy JG, Stahl WM. Basic life support versus advanced life support for injured patients with an injury severity score of 10 or more. J Trauma 1993; 35: 460–467.

98. Gervin AS, Fischer RP. The importance of prompt transport in salvage of patients with penetrating heart wounds. J Trauma 1982; 22: 443–446.

99. Task Force of the American Heart Association, the European Resuscitation Council, the Heart and Stroke Foundation of Canada, and the Australian Resuscitation Council. Recommended guidelines for uniform reporting of data from out of hospital cardiac arrest: The Utstein Style. Circulation 1991; 84: 960–975.

100. Mackenzie CF, Nolan J, Kahn R, Delaney PA, Grande C. Trauma anesthesia practices, training and facilities. Anesthesiology 1996; 85: A252.

101. Cheng EY, Nimphius N, Kampine JP. Anesthetic drugs and emergency departments. Anesth Analg 1992; 74: 272–275.

102. Committee on Trauma of the American College of Surgeons. Advanced Trauma Life Support Manual. Chicago: American College of Surgeons; 1989/1997.

103. Ali J, Adam R, Butler AK, et al. Trauma outcome improves following the advanced trauma life support program in a developing country. J Trauma 1993; 34: 890–898.

104. Ali J, Adam R, Stedman M, Howard M, Williams JI. Advanced Trauma Life Support program increases emergency room application of trauma resuscitative procedures in a developing country. J Trauma 1994; 36: 391–394.

105. Bennett JR, Bodenham AR, Berridge JC. Advanced Trauma Life Support. A time for reappraisal. Anaesthesia 1992; 47: 798–800.

106. Rady MY. Possible mechanisms for the interaction of peripheral somatic nerve stimulation, tissue injury, and hemorrhage in the pathophysiology of traumatic shock. Anesth Analg 1994; 78: 761–765.

107. Working Party of the Neuroanaesthesia Society of Great Britain and Ireland and the Association of Anaesthetists of Great Britain and Ireland. Recommendations for the transfer of patients with acute head injuries to neurosurgical units. London: The Association of Anaesthetists of Great Britain and Ireland; 1996.

108. From the Centers for Disease Control and Prevention. Leads from the Morbidity and Mortality Weekly Report. Update: Fatal air bag-related injuries to children–United States, 1993–1996. JAMA 1997; 277(1): 11–12.

2

Overview of pain mechanisms and neuroanatomy

Maywin Liu and F Michael Ferrante

Introduction

Peripheral components of nociception
    Peripheral neuroanatomy of nociception
    Peripheral neurochemistry

Central components of nociception and pain
    Central nervous system anatomy
    Central sensory neurochemistry

    Ascending sensory pathways
    Descending inhibitory controls

Classification of pain
    Somatic pain
    Visceral pain
    Neuropathic pain

Summary

INTRODUCTION

Pain is a sensory modality by which the body can recognize actual or potential damage. The aversive nature of this sensation contributes to its protective function. Acutely, pain serves to allow healing to occur by preventing further damage to the injured area, e.g. by preventing weight-bearing on a broken leg. Trauma can result in many types of pain, including somatic, visceral, and neuropathic pain. Pain may also be classified as acute or chronic pain.

Noxious stimuli are transmitted from the injured areas (skin, bone, viscera) by sensory fibers called *nociceptors*. Nociceptors terminate peripherally as free sensory nerve endings. Nociceptors are classified according to their myelination, activating stimuli, and speed of conduction. The nerve fibers identified as nociceptors are the C and A-δ fibers.[1] Any injury to somatic or visceral structures necessarily activates nociceptors.

Pain perception requires noxious stimuli to be *transduced, transmitted, modulated*, and *perceived*. When a noxious stimulus is encountered, it is transformed from its native form (mechanical, chemical, thermal energy) by the activated nociceptor into electrical signals which are then trans-mitted along the corresponding nociceptive nerve fiber. These fibers in turn synapse onto second order neurons, in the spinal cord. These interneurons are located in the dorsal horn. (Nociception of the face is mediated via the trigeminal nerve which synapses onto interneurons in the brainstem. The nociceptive pathway of the face will not be detailed here.) It is at the level of the interneurons where the initial modulation of nociceptive input occurs. Here, the afferent nociceptive input may be modified or decreased by intraspinal or supraspinal sources. From the spinal cord, nociceptive signals can be transmitted to the brainstem, thalamus, and subsequently the cortex. The suprathalamic aspects of the pain pathway are responsible for the affective component (perception) of pain.

PERIPHERAL COMPONENTS OF NOCICEPTION

Peripheral neuroanatomy of nociception

Nociceptive transmission begins with the activation of the free nerve endings of the nociceptors of the skin, muscle, and joints. Nociceptors may be activated by thermal, chemical, or mechanical stimuli.[2] C and A-δ fibers have been identified as nociceptors. The skin, joints, and periosteum are richly innervated with C and A-δ nociceptors as well as the non-nociceptive A-β sensory fibers.

Nociceptors are classified according to their activating stimuli, speed of transmission, and whether they are unmyelinated or myelinated (Table 2.1).[1,3] A-δ fibers are lightly myelinated and responsible for the sensation of *first pain*, the initial sharp pain experienced following an injury.[4,5] These fibers are activated by noxious mechanical and heat stimuli.[1,6] C fibers are unmyelinated, slowly conducting, and responsible for the sensation of *second pain*, the slowly-building, throbbing, burning pain experienced following an injury.[4,5] C fibers are activated by noxious chemical, heat, and mechanical stimuli.

Using electromyography, several subtypes of nociceptors have been identified (Table 2.2). Not all C and A-δ fibers participate in pain transmission. C fibers can be silent, heat-sensitive, mechanically sensitive, or mechanoheat sensitive.[7-12] Silent C fibers under normal physiologic circumstances do not respond to stimuli. However, under extreme conditions, e.g. severe chemical burn, these fibers may be activated.[12] These 'silent' fibers represent only a small portion of the C fibers. Other C fibers have been found to be solely activated by heat or mechanical stimuli. The majority of C fibers respond to both heat and

mechanical stimuli.[11,12] These C fibers are called C-polymodal nociceptors (C-PMNs).

Several subtypes of A-δ fibers have been identified, including high threshold mechanoheat, low threshold mechanoheat, and high threshold mechanical receptors.[13] A-δ fibers are classified according to their thresholds for activation. Type I A-δ fibers are low threshold mechanoheat (AMH) receptors; Type II have high thresholds. Type I AMHs respond quickly to noxious stimuli but also adapt quickly, i.e. they will stop firing despite continued stimulation. Type II AMHs respond only to intense noxious stimuli and are slowly adapting. These receptors have a delayed response to stimuli but will continue to fire in the presence of continued noxious stimulation.[1,6]

When nociceptors are activated, the thresholds for subsequent activation decrease and magnitude of response increases, e.g. a touch on burned skin will cause pain. This is known as nociceptive *sensitization*. Nociceptor activation can also lead to temporal summation and central sensitization (decreasing the threshold and increasing magnitude of responses of the secondary neurons in the spinal cord).[14] When central sensitization has occurred, repetitive C fiber activation will result in a larger response. This is known as temporal summation or *wind-up*.[15-17] For wind-up to occur, the series of noxious stimuli must be delivered within

Table 2.1   Classification of sensory fibers

Sensory receptor	Speed of transmission	Sensory function	Myelination
C- fibers	0.5–2 m/sec	Noxious chemical, mechanical, thermal activation Slow, burning, second pain	Unmyelinated
A-δ fibers	2–20 m/sec	Noxious chemical, thermal, mechanical stimuli Sharp, fast, first pain	Lightly myelinated
A-β fibers	20–50 m/sec	Non-painful, light touch, pressure, vibration, proprioception	Heavily myelinated

Table 2.2   Classification of nociceptor subtypes

Nociceptor subtypes	Stimulus intensity	Stimulus	
C-Polymodal	High threshold	Chemical, thermal, mechanical	Quickly adapting
Type I A-δ mechanoheat	Low threshold	Mechanical, thermal, chemical	Quickly adapting
Type II A-δ mechanoheat	High threshold	Mechanical, thermal	Slowly adapting

a certain amount of time (3 to 10 seconds). Wind-up occurs only with substance P-containing C fibers.[15] With central sensitization, spatial summation is also seen.[18]

Peripheral neurochemistry

Following injury, local inflammatory mediators are released by the traumatized cells resulting in inflammation, vasodilatation, erythema, and swelling in the area of injury. Commonly released inflammatory mediators implicated in pain and hyperalgesia include bradykinins, potassium, substance P, cytokines, calcitonin-gene-related protein (CGRP), histamine, hydrogen ions, and arachidonic acid derivatives (leukotrienes, prostacyclins, prostaglandins) (Table 2.3).[1,19]

Bradykinin is derived from plasma kininogen as part of the clotting cascade. Bradykinin when applied locally (intradermally or intra-arterially) can cause or increase pain. When given in an area of injury, bradykinins can cause hyperalgesia and allodynia.[19] However, bradykinin alone is not sufficient to account for the pain associated with inflammation. Only low concentrations of bradykinin are found at the site of injury, and the amounts present do not correlate with severity of symptoms, i.e. higher amounts are not seen in patients with severe pain. Bradykinin activates phospholipase A_2. So, the algogenic effects of bradykinin may be potentiated or augmented by prostaglandins.[20]

Prostaglandins, prostacyclins, and leukotrienes (derivatives of arachidonic acid) are formed at the site of inflammation in significant quantities.[21,22]

Table 2.3 Peripheral neurochemistry: algogenic agents

Algogenic agent	Derived/released from	Action on nociceptors
Bradykinin	Plasma kininogen	Activates
Substance P	C-fiber terminals	Sensitizes
Potassium	Injured cells	Activates
Hydrogen ions	Injured cells	Activates
Arachidonic acid derivatives	Injured cells	Sensitizes
Cytokines	White blood cells	Sensitizes
Serotonin	Platelets, mast cells	Sensitizes
Norepinephrine	Adrenals, sympathetic efferents	Activates (high conc.), sensitizes after injury

These agents do not cause pain when administered,[23] but contribute to hyperalgesia and can potentiate pain.[24,25] Prostaglandins sensitize activated C and A-δ cutaneous nociceptors.[26] Prostaglandin levels can increase with C nociceptor stimulation and in response to bradykinin and acetylcholine.[27] They may also play a role in joint hyperalgesia through an interaction with substance P.

Substance P is released from activated C fiber terminals. Substance P itself is weakly algogenic but its nociceptive effect is increased when combined with bradykinin. Substance P causes vasodilatation and plasma extravasation, producing a wheal and flare reaction in the area. Following activation of one portion of the C fiber, an antidromic response will be propagated to all aspects of that C fiber, i.e. all distal terminals, causing a flare reaction and release of substance P from all terminals. This is termed the *axonal reflex*.[28] Substance P can also cause histamine release from local mast cells. Histamine can sensitize nociceptors and contributes to the substance P-induced vasodilatory response. The effects of substance P are also potentiated by CGRP, a peptide released locally by nociceptors.[29]

Cytokines (IL-1β, IL-8, IL-6, TNF_α) have also been found to contribute to nociception. These cytokines do not directly cause pain but cause the release of algogenic neuropeptides and augment the inflammatory response by increasing the concentration of nerve growth factor (NGF) in the area. Increased NGF, in turn, increases the amount of substance P and CGRP, causing hypersensitivity of the injured area.[28]

Another locally released agent involved in nociception is serotonin. Serotonin is released from nearby platelets and mast cells. Serotonin causes mild pain upon injection. Its main action appears to be sensitization of nociceptors and potentiation of the effects of bradykinin.[29]

Two protons important in nociception are potassium and hydrogen. Both can cause pain by directly activating nociceptors. Potassium and hydrogen are released locally from injured cells.[29,30] Hydrogen ions can cause prolonged activation of nociceptors and local mechanosensitivity. The mechanism of this is unknown.[29]

In addition to the algogenic agents, peripheral inhibitory agents have also been identified (Table 2.4). Recently, there has been evidence that opioid receptors may exist in the periphery.[31] All

Table 2.4 Peripheral neurochemistry: inhibitory agents

Agent	Derived from	Action
Opioids	Adrenal medulla, CNS	Inhibits
Somatostatin	Pancreas, CNS	Inhibits

three types of opioid receptors (μ, δ, and κ) have been identified peripherally on both myelinated and unmyelinated nociceptors.[32] These peripheral opioid receptors appear to be inactive until the area is traumatized or inflamed.[33] This has been shown to be of some clinical utility in the post-operative setting, as demonstrated by the greater analgesia obtained using a small amount of morphine injected directly into the wound following knee arthroscopy compared to the same amount administered systemically.[34] Administration of opioids peripherally, directly in the area of pain may decrease the amount of opioids required overall and thus, opioid-related side effects.[35]

Somatostatin has also been identified as a peripheral and central nociceptive inhibitory agent. It can decrease afferent excitability and algogenic neuropeptide release.[29]

CENTRAL COMPONENTS OF NOCICEPTION AND PAIN

Central nervous system anatomy

Signals from noxious stimuli are transmitted along the axons of the primary afferent to their cell bodies in the dorsal root ganglion (DRG), and then centrally by synapsing onto secondary neurons in the dorsal horns of the spinal cord. The DRG serves mainly as a relay station. Little modulation of the signal occurs in the DRG.

The spinal cord is divided into white and gray matter. Descending and ascending axons are located in the white matter.[36,37] Cell bodies of secondary neurons and interneurons are located in the gray matter. The gray matter of the spinal cord is classified into ten layers (Rexed layers I–X) (Fig. 2.1) with layers I–VI representing the dorsal horn of the cord[38] (Table 2.5). The dorsal horn is capped by the Lissauer's tract which consists of branches of cutaneous A-δ and C fibers and a few visceral afferents.[39,40] As the nociceptive fibers enter the spinal canal, they may send fibers, which travel in Lissauer's tract, a short distance rostrally and caudally from their entry site.[40]

Nociceptive fibers (A-δ and C fibers) terminate in the more superficial layers of the dorsal horns (laminas I and II) while the non-painful, myelinated fibers terminate in the deeper layers (laminas III–VI).[41] However, both nociceptive and non-nociceptive sensory fibers and interneurons

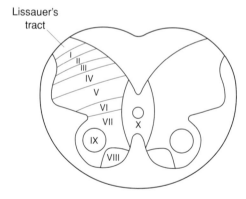

Lissauer's tract

Fig. 2.1 Schematic representation of the Rexed classification of the laminas of the gray matter of the spinal cord.

Table 2.5 Rexed classification of the spinal cord

Layer	Afferent input
I (nociceptive-specific)	Somatic C, few A-δ nociceptors, visceral
II (nociceptive-specific)	C nociceptors, few A-δ, few visceral
III (low-threshold mechanoreceptors)	A-β fibers
IV (low-threshold mechanoreceptors)	A-β fibers, some visceral
V (wide-dynamic range)	Somatic A-β and A-δ nociceptors, visceral
VI (lumbar and cervical only)	Proprioception, some visceral
VII	Wide-receptive fields
VIII	Wide-receptive fields
IX (autonomic cells)	
X (central area)	Some visceral, wide-receptive fields

synapse on the cells of lamina V.[42] These second-order neurons are labeled *wide-dynamic range (WDR) neurons* because of their varied primary input. Laminas I and II interneurons are nociceptive-specific (NS). Nociceptive fibers from somatic and visceral structures can terminate in these laminas.[41,42]

Lamina II has the highest concentration of opioid receptors in the spinal cord. This lamina contains interneurons which project to other laminas and to spinal segments. Modulation and inhibition of nociception may occur at this level through the use of opioids (systemic and/or neuraxial). Lamina II also contains a large number of γ-aminobutyric acid (GABA) receptors, another neurotransmitter involved in inhibition of sensory transmission. Laminas III–IV (nucleus propulsus) interneurons receive input from nociceptive and non-nociceptive fibers (NS and WDR interneurons located in these laminas) (Fig. 2.3).

Visceral afferents synapse in laminas I and V, and to a lesser extent, IV, VI, VII. Unlike the somatic afferents, visceral afferents have few synapses, i.e. their synapses are simple.[43,44] The neurons of laminas I, V, VII, and VIII contain the majority of the cell bodies of spinothalamic tract neurons.

The spinal cord is extremely plastic, i.e. changes in transmission and pain processing can occur in the dorsal horns in response to various stimuli. Constant, brief C-fiber nociceptive input to the dorsal horn could result in a more exaggerated response to subsequent C-fiber stimuli or peripheral tissue injury.[15,46–50] This phenomenon is termed temporal summation, central hypersensitization, or 'wind-up'.[15–17] A certain threshold frequency of stimulation (3 to 10 seconds) is required to induce wind-up.[50] Once wind-up is achieved, an exaggerated or prolonged response to the stimulus can be obtained even following cessation of the inciting stimulus. Wind-up occurs only in the C fibers terminating in lamina I. Some of the central changes associated with pain can possibly be pre-empted by blocking the afferent barrage to the dorsal horn.[51]

Processing of nociceptive information can occur at the level of the spinal cord. Nociceptive signals may be transmitted rostrally, or to other laminas, or inhibited. Nociceptive information can also be processed entirely in the spinal cord as in the case of spinal reflexes. With spinal reflexes, nociceptive input enters the spinal cord, and synapses onto its interneuron at the same level of entry. The interneuron, in turn, synapses onto an anterior horn cell or preganglionic autonomic cell, producing the efferent response. An example of this is pulling the hand away from a hot stove. Another example would be the production of a muscle spasm in response to a cutaneous stimulus or sympathetic stimulation with subsequent release of algogenic mediators. Spinal reflexes can be blocked at the level of the spinal cord, e.g. with local anesthetics.

Nociceptive information is transmitted from the spinal cord to the thalamus via the spinothalamic tracts (pain and temperature) and the dorsal columns (visceral sensation, including pain, and touch and proprioception). The spinothalamic tracts travel in the anterolateral portion of the spinal cord. From the thalamus, nociceptive information can be transmitted to the cortex, resulting in a subjective response to the noxious stimulus. It is not entirely clear which areas of the brain participate in processing of nociceptive input. The thalamus, hypothalamus, and brainstem nuclei have all been described as part of the pain pathway.[52–54] Using positron electron spectroscopy, areas of increased blood flow and thus, neuronal activity, in the thalamus, primary somatosensory cortex, anterior cingulate cortex, posterior insular cortex, and posterior parietal cortex indicate these structures are involved in pain processing.[55–57] The basal ganglia may also play a role[58,59] by modulating nociceptive information to higher motor areas.[59] Pain perception may also be modulated by the cingulate gyrus and frontal lobe, which may suppress the affective component of noxious stimuli.[60]

Central sensory neurochemistry

Centrally, a variety of neurotransmitters have been identified as being possibly involved in nociceptive transmission.[61,62] The major classes of neurotransmitters identified in the central nervous system thus far are the peptides, including substance P, opioids, monoamines, and the excitatory amino acids, glutamate and aspartate (Table 2.6).

The endogenous opioids serve as inhibitory transmitters of nociceptive transmission. Opioids are produced in the hypothalamus and in the adrenal medulla. Opioid receptors are located both spinally and supraspinally.[62,63] Spinally, opioid receptors are concentrated in lamina II (sub-

Table 2.6   Classification of central neurotransmitters

Peptides	Excitatory amino acids
Tachykinins	Aspartate
neuropeptide Y	Glutamate
substance P	Glycine
neurokinin A	
Calcitonin gene-related protein	**Monoamines**
(CGRP)	Norepinephrine
Vasoactive intestinal peptide	Serotonin
Somatostatin	Dopamine
Cholecystokinin (CCK)	
Opioid	
leu-enkephalin	
met-enkephalin	
β-endorphin	
γ-aminobutyric acid (GABA)	
Galanin	

stantia gelatinosa)[64,65] and on primary afferent fibers.[31] Opioids modulate pain transmission spinally by acting on the neurons of the spinothalamic tract. (Lamina II neurons have multiple connections to other laminas.) Supraspinally, opioid receptors are located in the periaqueductal gray area and rostroventral medulla.[63]

Three major opioid receptors have been identified: μ, κ, δ.[66] (The sigma (σ) receptor, responsible for the dysphoric effects, is not considered an opioid receptor.[67])

The μ receptors are located intraspinal and supraspinal. Two different subtypes of μ receptors have been identified: μ_1 and μ_2. The μ_1 subtype is responsible for the analgesic effects of opioids; the μ_2 subtype is responsible for the opioid-related side effects of sedation, respiratory depression, and constipation. There is no ceiling to the analgesia from μ receptor stimulation. Currently, there are no opioids that are selective for the μ_1 subtype.

The κ and δ opioid receptors are predominantly located in the spinal cord. Subtypes of these receptors have also been identified, though they are not yet well characterized.[68] An analgesic ceiling effect is seen with these receptors; however, a concomitant ceiling to respiratory depression is also seen.

Four endogenous opioids have been identified: leu-enkephalin, met-enkephalin, dynorphin, and β-endorphin. Of these, β-endorphin is the most potent. Dynorphin, though found in many areas

of the central nervous system (CNS), is analgesic only in the spinal cord (no effect supraspinally). Met- and leu-enkephalin are distributed widely throughout the CNS. However, they are primarily spinal opioid receptor agonists. β-endorphin is localized in the basal hypothalamus neurons. These neurons project to the limbic system and to the midbrain, periaqueductal gray, and locus ceruleus.

Another neurotransmitter involved in nociceptive transmission is substance P, a neuropeptide released from C-fiber terminals proximally in the dorsal horn of the spinal cord and peripherally distally with nociceptor activation and inflammation. Substance P is also found in nociceptive secondary neurons and in ascending nociceptive fibers.[69] In the dorsal horn, it binds to receptors in laminas I, II and V.[70,71] Substance P centrally is not an algogenic agent. It increases the perception of noxious stimuli but does not cause pain when injected intrathecally. The action of substance P may be dependent on nitric oxide synthesis.[72,73]

A second class of neurotransmitters has recently been found to play a significant role in central nociceptive modulation. These neurotransmitters are the excitatory amino acids (EAAs) which include glutamate, aspartate, and glycine. All bind to the N-methyl-D-aspartate (NMDA) receptors. They appear to play a role in allodynia, hyperalgesia, second pain, and wind-up.[43,74–77] Nitric oxide appears to mediate NMDA-induced hyperalgesia.[73,78] NMDA receptors are located post-synaptically on the interneurons and ascending neurons.[79] Blockade of the NMDA receptors can lead to a decrease in wind-up and hyperalgesia in both experimentally-induced pain[80] and in phantom limb pain.[81]

The EAAs are released by both myelinated and unmyelinated fibers.[82,83] Receptors for the EAAs are located post-synaptically. Glutamate can activate nociceptors and appears to have a role in hyperalgesia and second pain.[83] Currently available NMDA receptor antagonists (ketamine, dextromethorphan) have shown some efficacy in treating neuropathic pain.[81,84] However, their therapeutic index is small. CNS side effects were seen at the doses at which some degree of analgesia was achieved.[84] NMDA receptors may also play a role in modulating opioid tolerance, with opioid tolerance decreasing when a NMDA receptor antagonist is co-administered.[85]

A third excitatory amino acid, glycine, has a

binding site on the NMDA receptor that is different from that of aspartate and glutamate. Its role appears to be in potentiating aspartate or glutamate NMDA receptor activation.[86,87]

Monoamines are important as neurotransmitters of some of the descending inhibitory tracts. Increased central levels of norepinephrine and serotonin can increase the inhibition of nociceptive transmission.[88–90]

Cholecystekinin (CCK) is another peptide that also appears to play a role in central nociceptive transmission. However, its exact role is unknown. It is widely distributed throughout cortical gray matter, periaqueductal gray matter, ventromedial thalamus and spinal dorsal horn. CCK may act as an endogenous opiate antagonist[91] and function as a regulator of the endogenous opioid systems in the control of pain.[92]

Ascending sensory pathways

The peripheral sensory neurons synapse onto secondary interneurons of the dorsal horn. The axons of the non-nociceptive secondary neurons travel ipsilaterally in the dorsal columns of the spinal cord as the fasciculus cuneatus (upper body through T6) and fasciculus gracilis (lower body below T6), and synapse in the thalamus. The axons of the nociceptive secondary neurons, after synapsing, travel contralaterally in the anterolateral aspects of the spinal cord as the neospinothalamic and paleospinothalamic tracts. The neospinothalamic tract carries fine discriminations of pain, e.g. location, duration, intensity, and *first pain*. The paleospinothalamic fibers are responsible for *second pain* and the stress response to noxious stimuli (tachycardia, hypertension, increased catecholamines, etc.). The paleospinothalamic tract synapses in the thalamus, hypothalamus, and the limbic system. It appears to play a role in the emotional aspects of pain via the limbic system. The thalamus has multiple connections to the cortex and limbic system.[93]

Descending inhibitory controls

The descending controls of pain project specifically onto laminas I, II, and V of the dorsal horn from the mesencephalon, raphe nuclei, and the reticular tract. The mesencephalon is rich in opioid receptors. This area sends excitatory transmissions to the rostroventral medulla which sends

norepinephrine and serotonin inhibitory tracts via the dorsolateral funiculus to laminas I, II, and V.[94] The locus ceruleus may also contribute to the norepinephrine fibers. The norepinephrine and serotonin fibers modulate transmission between the primary afferents and the secondary neurons of the dorsal horn.[88,89] Increased activity of these fibers leads to increased inhibition of pain transmission. Tricyclic antidepressants, e.g. amitriptylline, desipramine, which have efficacy in treating neuropathic pain, inhibit the re-uptake of these inhibitory transmitters by affecting the catecholamine pump.[95,96]

A second area that contributes to the descending control of nociceptive transmission is the subnucleus reticularis dorsalis. This area may be involved in spinoreticular loops.[97] Nociception and pain perception may be modified by stimulating these areas of the brain.

CLASSIFICATION OF PAIN

Pain may be classified as somatic, visceral, or neuropathic. It is not unusual for an injury to involve more than one of these pain types. Each type of pain has typical characteristics (Table 2.7).

Table 2.7 Pain subtypes

	Pain descriptors	Examples
Somatic	Well-localized, sharp	Knife wound to thigh
Visceral	Diffuse, dull, deep, poorly localized	Bowel perforation
Neuropathic	Burning, radiating	Partial avulsion of the brachial plexus

Somatic pain

Somatic pain includes pain arising from cutaneous, muscular, osseous, and articular structures and is most commonly associated with acute or postoperative pain. Somatic pain is often described as an initial, sharp pain (*first pain*) followed by a second, slower, throbbing component (*second pain*). Cutaneous pain is often well-localized. Deeper structures, e.g. muscle, are often poorly localized. Cutaneous pain results from direct activation of nociceptors.

Muscular pain

Muscular pain is commonly encountered following almost all trauma. Muscular pain is transmitted by both unmyelinated (Group IV) and thin, lightly myelinated (Group III) sensory fibers that correspond to the cutaneous C and A-δ nociceptors (Table 2.8). Muscle nociceptors are located in the connective tissue between muscle fibers, in the tendons, and in the blood vessels of the muscle.[98] These nociceptors are sensitive to chemical, temperature, and mechanical activation.[99–101] The Group III fibers respond to noxious mechanical stimuli (pressure) to the muscle or its tendon but not to stretch or contraction. These nociceptors can be activated by bradykinin.[101]

The unmyelinated Group IV muscle nociceptors correspond to the cutaneous C-PMNs and respond to noxious thermal, chemical, and mechanical stimuli.[100,101] Like the C-PMNs, there are several subtypes of unmyelinated fibers, including mechanically-sensitive, chemically-sensitive, thermal-sensitive, and mechanoheat-chemo-sensitive.[1,101]

Muscle pain is often described as a dull, achy pain that may not be well-localized. It can result from stimulation of the muscle, tendon, or fascia. In addition to direct damage to the muscle or surrounding connective tissue, nociceptive fibers may be activated by ischemia.[102] Muscular pain can radiate beyond the area of injury and can mimic neuropathic pain, but the muscular radicular pattern is often limited to areas of similar innervation. Hyperalgesia of overlying cutaneous areas may also be seen. Radiating muscular pain and hyperalgesia may result from a combination of peripheral and central nervous system components. Peripherally, local mediators are released at the site of injury (e.g. arachidonic acid derivatives, bradykinin) and may sensitize or activate nociceptors of nearby somatic structures. Centrally, the radiation and hyperalgesia may be due to convergence of cutaneous and muscular afferents onto the same secondary neurons in the dorsal horn.

Joint pain

Joints are innervated by both C and A-δ nociceptors as well as non-nociceptive A-β and unmyelinated post-ganglionic sympathetic fibers.[103–105] The majority of nerve fibers are unmyelinated (C fibers and sympathetic fibers).[106] Joint pain is often described as dull and poorly localized. The most common etiologies of joint pain are inflammation and trauma. Hyperalgesia of the joint, defined as pain with movement or weight-bearing, can accompany joint pain and may be due to local release of inflammatory mediators. Substance P appears to play a role in sensitizing the affected joints.[1,2,107,108] C fibers innervating an inflamed joint have been found to have increased substance P in their terminals.[109] Substance P can increase the number of synoviocytes.[108]

Visceral pain

Trauma may also involve injury to viscera. Viscera are innervated by nociceptors (A-δ and C fibers) which are located in or on the surfaces of the viscera. Not all viscera will produce pain when injured. It is not clear if visceral pain results from activation of nociceptors or because of excessive activity in receptors normally involved in regulatory function of the affected viscera. The visceral afferents travel with the sympathetic and parasympathetic nerves. The origin of the thoracic visceral innervation is in the upper thoracic spinal cord (T1–4). The abdominal viscera (lower esophagus to the transverse colon) are innervated by the lower thoracic spinal cord nuclei (T5–9). The lower abdominal viscera and the pelvic visceral afferent innervation originate in the lower thoracic and upper lumbar neurons. The parasympathetic innervation travel with the vagus and the sacral cord (S2–4).

The viscera are not as well innervated as somatic structures. Perception of pain from viscera differs from pain from cutaneous or muscular nociceptors. Visceral pain is usually described as a deep, dull, crampy sensation that is poorly localized and often accompanied by motor and autonomic reflex activation. Visceral nociceptors do not respond to cutting or burning stimuli but are activated by stretching, ischemia, and pressure

Table 2.8 Classification of muscle sensory receptors

Muscle sensory fiber	Stimulus	Corresponding cutaneous fiber
Group I	Stretch	No equivalent
Group II	Touch	A-β fiber
Group III	Noxious pressure	A-δ fiber
Group IV	Thermal, chemical, mechanical	C fiber

pain. The high threshold nociceptors appear to respond to acute pain of short duration. The longer-lasting pain, e.g. hypoxia, inflammation, appears to be due to sensitization of previously inactive high threshold receptors.[110]

Visceral pain can be *referred* to cutaneous areas. However, pain from superficial structures does not refer to the viscera. Several theories have been proposed regarding the patterns of referral. Afferents from the viscera and skin converge on the same secondary neurons (viscerosomatic neurons) (Fig. 2.2). It is this somatic and visceral convergence that may in turn lead to referral of the pain.[110] An example of this is primary afferents mediating anginal pain which synapse on the same secondary neurons as the primary afferents innervating the arm. As a result, pain which be perceived in the arm sharing the secondary neuron. Viscerosomatic convergence may occur at the level of the spinal cord, thalamus, hypothalamus, ventrolateral orbital cortex[110–114] and in the autonomic regulatory areas of the brainstem.[114] In the spinal cord, the majority of the viscerosomatic cells are located in laminas I and V (a few visceral afferents also synapse in laminas II, IV, VI, and X). Fewer sensory afferents emanate from the viscera than from somatic structures. However, these visceral afferents synapse on secondary neurons at many more levels and laminas in the spinal cord than somatic structures. Somatic nociceptive afferents enter the spinal canal and send branches

to one or two spinal segments; visceral afferents send collaterals to multiple spinal segments (Fig. 2.3). Within each spinal segment level, somatic sensory input tends to 'cluster' in the superficial layers (laminas I and II) of the dorsal horn, whereas the visceral afferents may travel several laminas prior to synapsing (Fig. 2.4). Visceral afferents synapse ipsilaterally and contralaterally;[110] somatic nociceptive input synapses ipsilaterally.[93] The diffuse synapsing of the visceral

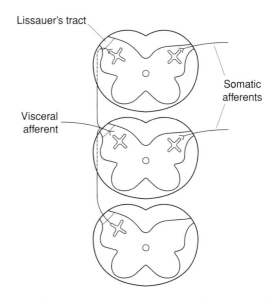

Fig. 2.3 Visceral afferents synapse onto secondary neurons over several spinal segments. Somatic nociceptive afferents essentially synapse at level of entry into the spinal canal.

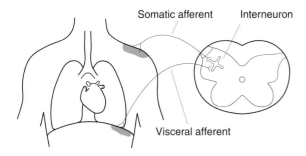

Fig. 2.2 Possible theory of referred pain: visceral afferents and somatic afferents synapse onto the same secondary neurons in the spinal cord. Pain in the viscera (diaphragm) activates the secondary neurons which then causes perception of pain in the area (shoulder) innervated by the somatic neuron sharing the secondary spinal neuron.

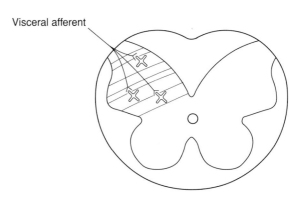

Fig. 2.4 Intrasegmental synapses of visceral afferents. Visceral afferents synapse at many different laminas.

afferents may account for the difficulty in localizing visceral pain. Despite the shared visceral and somatic input to the secondary neurons, it is unclear why pain does not refer from cutaneous structures to the viscera.

Hyperalgesia may be experienced in viscera.[115] This, as in the cutaneous structures, may be due to sensitized nociceptors. Excitation and wind-up can be seen in the viscerosomatic cells with prolonged noxious stimulation.[116]

Neuropathic pain

Neuropathic pain is defined as pain initiated by injury to a nerve, e.g. gunshot wound through the ulnar nerve, or owing to nerve dysfunction, e.g. reflex sympathetic dystrophy. It is commonly characterized as a sharp, shooting, burning pain. Mechanical allodynia (pain owing to a normally innocuous stimulus such as a light touch) and hyperalgesia (a decreased pain threshold and a greater pain response than would be expected from a painful stimulus) are often seen with neuropathic pain. Common examples of neuropathic pain include avulsion of the brachial plexus, sciatica, and postsurgical scar entrapment of nerves.

Several possible mechanisms for neuropathic pain exist. Spontaneous neuronal excitatory activity may be seen following nerve injury.[117–119] Following axonal injury, neuronal sprouting commonly occurs at the site of injury. Most of these sprouts will die. However, some of the sprouts will grow distally into the pathway created (and preserved) by the intact Schwann cells and result in regeneration of the nerve. Some of the sprouts will invade the proximal portion of the injured nerve and create a neuroma (Fig. 2.5). Peripheral nerves are composed of many types of sensory nerve fibers (C, A-δ, A-β). Because nociceptive fibers are involved, neuromas, which are often spontaneously active, can produce pain. Neuromas often become mechanically sensitive, as indicated by the presence of Tinel's sign over the neuroma[2,118] and can be stimulated by sympathetic stimulation.[119]

Neuroma formation can also indicate the normal regeneration of an injured nerve. With regeneration, the location of the neuroma can be used to follow the progression of regrowth. As the neuroma is mechanically sensitive, a Tinel's sign will be present over the neuroma. Regeneration can be tracked by following the distal progression of the Tinel's sign over time (usual growth rate is 1 cm

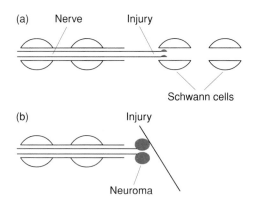

Fig. 2.5 Formation of neuromas. (A) In normal regeneration, nerve fibers grow into the pathway lined by the Schwann cells. (B) With abnormal nerve growth/neuroma formation, nerve fibers grow back onto the proximal end of the injured nerve.

per month). Regeneration is more common following a crush injury (close to 100%) than a nerve transection injury (less than 20%). Spontaneous activity in the injured nerves may also result from spontaneous firing in the DRG.[120,121] Evidence of increased electrical activity has been found at the proximal nerve synapses of the injured nerve. The DRGs and the proximal central terminals are found to have markedly less peptidergic neurotransmitters than surrounding neurons with normal axons, indicating increased discharges and release of neurotransmitters.[122]

Injured nerves (C fibers) may develop adrenergic sensitivity.[118,123–125] Spontaneous activity of the C fiber may result from continued adrenergic activation.

Direct nerve injury can result in areas of hypesthesia (decreased sensation) as well as allodynia (pain due to an innocuous stimulus) and hyperalgesia (decreased pain threshold). These areas can extend to areas beyond those innervated by the injured nerve. Both muscular and cutaneous sensory deficits can be observed in areas outside the nerve territory.[126–129] Interestingly, relief of the pain can lead to a decrease in the areas of sensory and motor deficit.[127]

Reflex sympathetic dystrophy and causalgia

Two forms of neuropathic pain that may be encountered following orthopedic injuries or any trauma involving major nerve damage are reflex sympathetic dystrophy (RSD) and causalgia. (It should be noted that both RSD and causalgia have been reclassified as complex regional pain syndromes (CRPS). RSD is now known as CRPS I; causalgia, CRPS II.[130])

RSD and causalgia may be seen a few days to a few weeks following trauma, e.g. orthopedic injury or surgery, or a gunshot wound through a nerve. RSD and causalgia pain is often characteristic (Table 2.9). Pain is constant and mechanical allodynia and cold hyperalgesia are often present. With RSD, the pain distribution is often non-anatomical, e.g. glove- or stocking-like; with causalgia, the pain, allodynia, and hyperalgesia are often in the distribution of the affected nerve. In the early phase, the affected limb may be warm and erythematous with increased hair growth. In later stages, the limb may become edematous (non-pitting), the skin hairless and shiny, and the nails dry and brittle. With RSD, osteoporosis and altered bone metabolism may be seen on bone scan.[130]

Causalgia and RSD are differentiated by the inciting injury. Causalgia is due to a known partial nerve injury, e.g. gunshot wound to the femoral nerve. RSD is usually associated with a minor or deep tissue injury. In some cases, patients may not recall any injury to the limb.

The mechanisms of RSD and causalgia are not known. However, an interaction between the peripheral and central nervous systems may be required initially. The interaction may be due to adrenergic sensitivity of the nociceptors at the injured site, resulting in increased nociceptive input centrally. Early in the course of the disease process, the treatment of choice is a series of sympathetic blocks. It is not known, however, if use of regional blockade shortly after injury, i.e. with surgery to repair damage, can prevent these pain syndromes from occurring. As part of the work-up for patients presenting with RSD-like symptoms, it is important to check to ensure that no occult, underlying cause for the pain, e.g. stress fracture, unhealed fracture, scar entrapment of a nerve, exists. The pain from the associated allodynia and hyperalgesia may mask the pain of the inciting injury.[131]

Allodynia/hyperalgesia/sensitization

With injury, a sensitized state in the affected area may be seen. The increased sensitivity can be to both painful and innocuous stimuli. This increased sensitivity at the site of injury is known as *primary hyperalgesia*. If pain owing to normally non-painful stimuli, e.g. a light touch, is present, this is known as *mechanical allodynia* (MA). A decreased threshold to pain or an increased

Table 2.9 Clinical symptoms in reflex sympathetic dystrophy (CRPS I) and causalgia (CRPS II)

Causalgia (CRPS II)	RSD (CRPS I)
Pain mainly along injured nerve's distribution	Non-anatomical pain distribution
Rarely spreads to other limbs	Can spread to other limbs
Constant pain always present	Usually has constant pain
Mechanical allodynia in nerve distribution	Non-anatomical mechanical allodynia
Cold hyperalgesia	Cold hyperalgesia
Skin and blood flow changes related to injured nerve distribution	Non-anatomical skin and blood flow changes (mottled skin)
	Non-pitting edema
Motor deficits related to injured nerve	Generalized decreased active motor strength of affected limb
Stages of causalgia and RSD	
Early stage	*Late stage*
Warmth of affected area	Cool, moist, shiny skin
Erythema	Trophic changes, e.g. brittle, dry nails
Hairy skin	Hairless skin
	Non-pitting edema
	Osteoporosis on radiographs (RSD)
	Abnormal bone metabolism on three-phase bone scan (RSD)

response to a normally painful stimulus is termed *hyperalgesia*. Decreased sensation can be seen following nerve injury. This is called *hypesthesia*. Hyperalgesia and allodynia may occur in areas surrounding the primary site of injury. This is called *secondary hyperalgesia* (Fig. 2.6).

There are several forms of hyperalgesia, including pinprick, thermal, and cold hyperalgesia. *Pinprick hyperalgesia* is defined as a greater pain response than usually associated with a painful, punctate stimulus. *Thermal hyperalgesia*, commonly seen following an injury involving somatic structures, is pain at a temperature below the usual thermal pain threshold (42–46°C). *Cold hyperalgesia* is pain at temperatures above the temperature usually associated with the production of pain. Cold hyperalgesia can be seen in patients with certain types of neuropathic pain, e.g. RSD.

Hyperalgesia may be found in both the injured area and the uninjured area surrounding the original insult site. Pinprick and thermal hyperalgesia and MA are present in the area of primary injury, whereas, only pinprick hyperalgesia and MA are found in the secondary, uninjured zones. Primary heat hyperalgesia appears to be mediated peripherally by the Type I AMHs and the C-PMNs.[13,132–135] Type I AMHs become sensitized following severe heat damage and C-PMNs with mild heat damage. The mechanism of pinprick hyperalgesia is unclear. Secondary hyperalgesia is thought to be mainly a central effect.[136] Following an injury, the central nervous system also can be sensitized. A stimulus in the area of injury will activate more nociceptors (C-PMNs and AMHs) than in the uninjured state, e.g. larger receptor field size.[137]

Central sensitization results in expansion of receptor field size, reduction in the threshold, and prolongation of afterdischarges.[46,138,139] MA may be a manifestation of central sensitization. MA may be classified as dynamic or static allodynia. Dynamic allodynia is pain due to a normally innocuous moving stimulus, e.g. light brush moving across the skin. Static allodynia is pain due to static pressure at thresholds which normally do not cause pain.[138,139]

Following trauma, primary MA is often seen in the injured area. Primary MA is thought to be due to sensitization of local nociceptors by chemical mediators, e.g. bradykinin, serotonin, prostaglandins.[1] However, MA may also be seen outside the area of the original injury or beyond the area innervated by the injured nerve (secondary hyperalgesia). Possible explanations for this phenomenon include a peripheral and/or a central mechanism. Much of the evidence indicates that an interaction between peripheral and central elements may be necessary. Through use of differential nerve blocks and through electromyography, MA in the secondary areas appears to be mediated by the A-β fibers, fibers which are not nociceptive fibers.[138,140,141] MA and hyperalgesia have been shown to cross peripheral nerve territories, supporting a central mechanism for these phenomena.[142] Centrally, 'misinterpretation' of the non-nociceptive signal as nociceptive may occur.[136] One theory is through shared peripheral input to the spinal interneurons. In the spinal cord, the WDR interneurons of layer V receive both nociceptive and non-nociceptive input (Fig. 2.7). The barrage of nociceptive input to the WDR interneurons may cause the input from the A-β fibers to be interpreted as painful.[143] As further evidence of a central mechanism, MA, but not ongoing pain, was seen when capsaicin, a C fiber-specific activator, was injected into a C fiber-insensate area. However, in areas where all sensation was intact, both ongoing pain and MA were perceived.[144]

The central misinterpretation of the innocuous stimuli alone is not enough to explain MA production. A peripheral 'trigger' may also be required to sustain the central changes.[137,146] In several patients with chronic pain and MA, an area of maximal pain was identified. Following

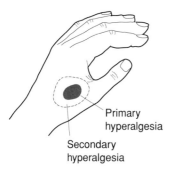

Primary
hyperalgesia

Secondary
hyperalgesia

Fig. 2.6 Sensory changes following heat injury to the skin. The area of injury (■) has primary hyperalgesia to heat and mechanical allodynia. In the area surrounding the burn (---), only mechanical allodynia and hyperalgesia are seen. No heat hyperalgesia is present in the secondary zone.

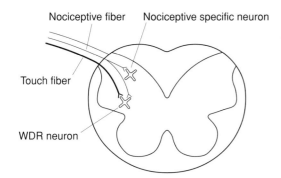

Fig. 2.7 Illustration of one theory of secondary hyperalgesia and allodynia production. In the spinal cord, the wide-dynamic range (WDR) neurons receive afferent input from both the touch fibers and the nociceptive fibers. The nociceptive fibers have multiple branches which may synapse on more than one cell. In this case, the nociceptive fiber synapses on both the WDR and the nociceptive-specific (NS) neuron.

local anesthetic blockade of that area, the surrounding MA resolved.[146] Continuously stimulated C-nociceptors may be responsible for this peripheral 'trigger'. Following nerve injury, C fibers are found to become adrenergically sensitive.[123–125,147] Adrenergic stimulation may cause continued C fiber activity with continued central stimulation. This adrenergic sensitivity may be blocked with the use of post-ganglionic blockade[129] or with the use of α-adrenergic blockers.[148] Using phentolamine, a mixed α_1 and α_2 antagonist, secondary MA produced by intradermal capsaicin could be decreased, suggesting the possible role of adrenergic receptors in MA production.[149] Adrenergic sensitivity appears to be solely an unmyelinated fiber phenomenon as adrenergic sensitivity has never been identified on the myelinated fibers.[150]

SUMMARY

Pain perception is a process involving a complex interaction between the peripheral and central components of the nervous system. Though many aspects of the peripheral and central components of nociception have been characterized, there are additional neurotransmitters and central pain pathways whose roles in nociceptive transmission are not yet well understood. Greater understand-

ing of the nociceptive transmission and modulation may lead to future developments of more effective pain therapies.

REFERENCES

1. Raja SN, Meyer RA, Campbell JN. Peripheral mechanisms of somatic pain. Anesthesiology 1988; 68: 571–590.
2. Wall PD. Mechanisms of acute and chronic pain. In: Kruger L, Liebeskind JC, eds. Advances in Pain Research and Therapy, vol 6. New York: Raven Press; 1984: 95–104.
3. Collins WF, Nulsen FE, Randt CT. Relation of peripheral nerve fiber size and sensation in man. Arch Neurol 1960; 3: 381–385.
4. Price DD, Dubner R. Mechanisms of first and second pain in the peripheral and central nervous systems. J Invest Dermatol 1977; 69: 167–171.
5. Melzack R, Wall PD, Ty TC. Acute pain in an emergency clinic: latency of onset and descriptor patterns related to different injuries. Pain 1982; 14: 33–43.
6. Treede RD, Meyer RA, Raja SN, Campbell JN. Evidence for two different heat transduction mechanisms in nociceptive primary afferents innervating monkey skin. J Physiol 1995; 483: 747–758.
7. Iggo A. Cutaneous mechanoreceptors with afferent C fibers. J Physiol (London) 1960; 152: 337–353.
8. Bessou P, Perl ER. Responses of cutaneous sensory units with unmyelinated fibers to noxious stimuli. J Neurophysiol 1969; 32: 1025–1043.
9. Torebjörk HE. Afferent C units responding to mechanical, thermal and chemical stimuli in human non-glabrous skin. Acta Physiol Scand 1974; 92: 374–390.
10. Meyer RA, Davis KD, Cohen RH, Treede RD, Campbell JN. Mechanically insensitive afferents (MIAs) in cutaneous nerve of monkey. Brain Res 1991; 561: 252–261.
11. Davis KD, Meyer RA, Campbell JN. Chemosensitivity and sensitization of nociceptive afferents that innervate the hairy skin of monkey. J Neurophysiol 1993; 69: 1071–1081.
12. Schmidt R, Schmelz M, Forster C, Ringkamp M, Torebjörk E, Handwerker H. Novel classes of responsive and unresponsive C nociceptors in human skin. J Neurosci 1995; 15: 333–341.
13. Burgess PR, Perl ER. Myelinated afferent fibres responding specifically to noxious stimulation of the skin. J Physiol (London) 1967; 190: 541–562.
14. Beitel RE, Dubner R. Response of unmyelinated (C) polymodal nociceptors to thermal stimuli

applied to monkey's face. J Neurophysiol 1976; 39: 1160–1175.

15. Mendell LM. Physiological properties of unmyelinated fiber projection to the spinal cord. Exp Neurol 1966; 16: 316–332.

16. Mendell LM, Wall PD. Responses of single dorsal cord cells to peripheral cutaneous unmyelinated fibers. Nature 1965; 206: 97–99.

17. Woolf CJ, King AE. Physiology and morphology of multireceptive neurons with C-afferent fiber inputs in the deep dorsal horn of the rat lumbar spinal cord. J Neurophysiol 1987; 58: 460–479.

18. Thalhammer JG, LaMotte RH. Spatial properties of nociceptor sensitization following heat injury of the skin. Brain Res 1982; 231: 257–265.

19. Treede RD, Meyer RA, Raja SN, Campbell JN. Peripheral and central mechanisms of cutaneous hyperalgesia. Progr Neurobiol 1992; 38: 397–421.

20. Vane JR. Pain of inflammation. In: Bonica JJ, Lindblom U, Iggo A, eds. Advances in pain research and therapy, vol 5. New York: Raven Press; 1983: 597–603.

21. Moncada S. Biological importance of prostacyclin. Br J Pharmacol 1982; 76: 3–31.

22. Greaves MW, Sondergaard J, McDonald-Gibson W. Recovery of prostaglandins in human cutaneous inflammation. BMJ 1971; 2: 258–260.

23. Lewis P. Prostaglandins in inflammation. J Reticulendothel Soc 1977; 22: 389–402.

24. Collier JG, Karin SMM, Robinson B, Somers K. Action of prostaglandins A2, B1, E2, F2a on superficial hand veins of man. Br J Pharmacol 1972; 44: 374–375.

25. Collier HOJ, Schneider C. Nociceptive response to prostaglandins. Nature 1972; 236: 141–143.

26. Chahl LA, Iggo A. The effects of bradykinin and prostaglandin E1 on rat cutaneous afferent nerve activity. Br J Pharmacol 1977; 59: 343–347.

27. Juan H, Lembeck F. Release of prostaglandins from the isolated perfused rabbit ear by bradykinin and acetylcholine. Agents Actions 1976; 6: 642–645.

28. LaMotte RH, Shain CN, Simone DA, Tsai EFP. Neurogenic hyperalgesia: psychophysical studies of underlying mechanisms. J Neurophysiol 1991; 66: 190–211.

29. Dray A. Neurogenic mechanisms and neuropeptides in chronic pain. Progr Brain Res 1996; 110: 85–94.

30. Lembeck F. Pharmacology of the primary nociceptive neuron. Recent Results Cancer Res 1984; 89: 59–63.

31. Stein C. Peripheral mechanisms of opioid analgesia. Anesth Anal 1993; 76: 182–191.

32. Stein C. The control of pain in peripheral tissues by opioids. N Engl J Med 1995; 332: 1685–1690.

33. Schaefer M, Imai Y, Uhl GR, Stein C. Inflammation enhances peripheral mu-opioid receptor-mediated analgesia but not mu-opioid receptor transcription in dorsal root ganglion. Eur J Pharmacol 1995; 279: 165–169.

34. Stein C, Comisel K, Haimerl E, Yassouridis A, Lehrberger K, Herz A, Peter K. Analgesic efficacy of intraarticular morphine after arthroscopic knee surgery. N Engl J Med 1991; 325: 1123–1126.

35. Stein C, Schaefer M, Hassan AH. Peripheral opioid receptors. Ann Med 1995; 27: 219–221.

36. Briner RP, Carlton SM, Coggeshall RE, Chung K. Evidence for unmyelinated sensory fibers in the posterior columns in man. Brain 1988; 111: 999–1007.

37. Patterson JT, Coggeshall RE, Lee WT, Chung K. Long ascending unmyelinated primary afferent axons in the rat dorsal column: immunohistochemical localizations. Neurosci Lett 1990; 108: 6–10.

38. Rexed B. The cytoarchitectonic organization of the spinal cord in the cat. J Comp Neurol 1952; 96: 415–495.

39. Coggeshall RE, Chung K, Chung JM, Langford LA. Primary afferent axons in the tract of Lissauer in the monkey. J Comp Neurol 1981; 196: 431–442.

40. LaMotte C. Distribution of the tract of Lissauer and the dorsal root fibers in the primate spinal cord. J Comp Neurol 1977; 172: 529–561.

41. Fitzgerald M, Wall PD. The laminar organization of dorsal horn cells responding to peripheral C fibre stimulation. Exp Brain Res 1980; 41: 36–44.

42. Foreman RD, Hancock MB, Willis WD. Responses of spinothalamic tract cells in the thoracic spinal cord of the monkey to cutaneous and visceral inputs. Pain 1981; 11: 149–162.

43. Price DD, Hull CD, Buchwald NA: Intracellular responses of dorsal horn cells to cutaneous and sural nerve A and C fiber stimuli. Exp Neurol 1971; 33: 291–309.

44. Cervero F. Mechanisms of visceral pain: past and present. In: Gebhart GF (ed) Visceral Pain, Progress in Pain Research and Management, Vol 5, Seattle, IASP Press; 1995: 25–40.

45. Suguira Y, Tonosaki Y. Spinal organization of unmyelinated visceral afferent fibers in comparison with somatic afferents. In: Gebhart GF (ed) Visceral Pain, Progress in Pain Research and Management, Vol 5, Seattle, IASP Press; 1995: 41–59.

46. Price DD, Browe AC. Responses of spinal cord neurons to graded noxious and non-noxious stimuli. Brain Res 1973; 64: 425–429.

47. Price DD, Hayes RL, Ruda MA, Dubner R. Spatial and temporal transformations of input to

spinothalamic tract neurons and their relation to somatic sensation. J Neurophysiol 1978; 41: 933-947.

48. Woolf CJ. Evidence for a central component of post-injury pain hypersensitivity. Nature 1983; 306: 686-68.

49. Koltzenburg M, Handwerker HO. Differential ability of human cutaneous nociceptors to signal mechanical pain and to produce vasodilatation. J Neurosci 1994; 14: 1756-1765.

50. Dubner R, Sharav Y, Gracely RH, Price DD. Idiopathic trigeminal neuralgia: sensory features and pain mechanisms. Pain 1987; 31: 23–33.

51. Bach S, Noreng MF, Tjellden NU. Phantom limb pain in amputees during the first 12 months following limb amputation after preoperative lumbar epidural blockade. Pain 1988; 33: 297–301.

52. Craig AD, Bushnell MC, Zhang ET, Blomqvist A. A thalamic nucleus specific for pain and temperature sensation. Nature 1994; 372: 770–773.

53. Fuchs PN, Melzack R. Analgesia induced by morphine microinjection into the lateral hypothalamus of the rat. Exp Neurol 1995; 134: 277–280.

54. Villanueva L, Bouhassira D, Bing Z, LeBars D. Convergence of heterotopic nociceptive information onto subnucleus reticularis dorsalis neurons in the rat medulla. J Neurophys 1988; 60: 980–1009.

55. Coghill RC, Talbot JD, Evans AC, et al. Distributed processing of pain and vibration by the human brain. J Neurosci 1994; 14: 4095–4108.

56. Coghill RC, Sang CN, Nelson KA, Bennett GJ, Max MB, Iadarola MJ. Regional brain activation in patients with post-herpetic neuralgia. VIIIth World Congress on Pain, Seattle: IASP Press; 1996: 443.

57. Duncan GH, Bushnell MC, Talbot JD, Evans AC, Meyer E, Marrett S. Pain and activation in the thalamus. Trends Neurosci 1992; 15: 252–253.

58. Chudler EH, Dong WK. The role of the basal ganglia in nociception and pain. Pain 1995; 60: 3–38.

59. Hu ZT, Wang QP, Huang DK, Li KY, He LF. Changes of central glucose metabolism following caudate stimulation produced analgesia in the rat-an autoradiographic deoxyglucose study. Sheng Li Hseuh Pao-Acta Physiologica Sinica 1992; 44: 355–361.

60. Davis KD, Hutchison WD, Lozano AM, Dostrovsky JO. Altered pain and temperature perception following cingulotomy and capsulotomy in a patient with schizoaffective disorder. Pain 1994; 59: 189–199.

61. Mayer DJ, Price DD. Central nervous system mechanisms of analgesia. Pain 1976; 2: 379–404.

62. Yaksh TL, Hammond DL. Peripheral and central substrates in rostral transmission of nociceptive information. Pain 1982; 13: 1–85.

63. Basbaum AI, Fields HL. Endogenous pain control systems: brainstem spinal pathways and endorphin circuitry. Annu Rev Neurosci 1984; 7: 309–338.

64. Kanjhan R. Opioids and pain. Clin Exp Pharmacol Physiol 1995; 22: 397–403.

65. Glazer EJ, Basbaum AI. Opioid neurons and pain modulation: an ultrastructural analysis of enkephalin in cat superficial dorsal horn. Neuroscience 1983; 10: 357–376.

66. Dhawan BN, Cesselin F, Raghubir R, et al. International Union of Pharmacology. XII. Classification of opioid receptors. Pharmacological Rev 1996; 48: 567–592.

67. Chavkin C. The sigma enigma: biochemical and functional correlates emerge for the haloperidol-sensitive sigma binding site. Trends Pharmacol Sci 1990; 11: 213–215.

68. Pasternak GW. Pharmacological mechanisms of opioid analgesics. Clin Neuropharmacol 1993; 16: 1–18.

69. Hokfelt T, Kellerth J-O, Nilsson G, Pernow B. Substance P: Localization in the central nervous system and in some primary sensory neurons. Science 1975; 190: 889–891.

70. Henry JL. Effects of substance P on functionally identified units in cat spinal cord. Brain Res 1976; 114: 439–451.

71. Ribeira-da-Silva A, Claudio-Cuello A. Organization of peptidergic neurons in the dorsal horn of the spinal cord: anatomical and functional correlates. In: Nyberg F, Sharm HS, Wiesenfeld-Hallin Z, eds. Progress in Brain Research, vol 104, Amsterdam: Elsevier Science; 1995: 41–57.

72. Wilcox GL. Spinal mediators of nociceptive neurotransmission and hyperalgesia. Relationships among synaptic plasticity analgesics, tolerance, and blood flow. APS J 1993; 2: 265–275.

73. Radhakrishnan V, Henry JL. L-NAME blocks responses to NMDA, substance P, and noxious cutaneous stimuli in cat dorsal horn. Neuroreport 1993; 4: 323–326.

74. Aanonsen LM, Lei S, Wilcox GL. Excitatory amino acid receptors and nociceptive neurotransmission in rat spinal cord. Pain 1990; 41: 309–321.

75. Price DD, Mao J, Frenk H, Mayer DJ. The N-methyl-D-aspartate receptor antagonist dextromethorphan selectively reduces temporal summation of second pain in man. Pain 1994; 59: 165–174.

76. Woolf CJ, Thompson SW. The induction and maintenance of central sensitization is dependent on N-methyl-D-aspartic acid receptor activation: implications for the treatment of post-injury pain hypersensitivity states. Pain 1991; 44: 293–299.

77. Dickenson AH, Sullivan AF. Evidence for a role of the NMDA receptor in the frequency dependent potentiation of deep rat dorsal horn nociceptive neurons following C fibre stimulation. Neuropharmacol 1987; 26: 1235–1238.

78. Kitto KF, Haley JE, Wilcox GL. Involvement of nitric oxide in spinally mediated hyperalgesia in the mouse. Neurosci Lett 1992; 148: 1–5.

79. Dickenson AH. Spinal cord pharmacology of pain. Br J Anaesth 1995; 75: 193–200.

80. Andersen OK, Felsby S, Nicolaisen L, Bjerring P, Jensen TS, Arendt-Nielsen L. The effect of ketamine on stimulation of primary and secondary hyperalgesic areas induced by capsaicin–a double-blind, placebo-controlled, human experimental study. Pain 1996; 66: 51–62.

81. Felsby S, Nielsen J, Arendt-Nielsen L, Jensen TS. NMDA receptor blockade in chronic neuropathic pain: a comparison of ketamine and magnesium chloride. Pain 1996; 64: 283–291.

82. Battaglia G, Rustioni A. Coexistence of glutamate and substance P in dorsal root ganglion neurons of rat and monkey. J Comp Neurol 1988; 277: 302–312.

83. DiBiasi S, Rustioni A. Glutamate and substance P coexist in primary afferent terminals in the superficial laminae of spinal cord. Proc Natl Acad Sci USA 1988; 85: 7820–7824.

84. Nelson KA, Park KM, Robinovitz E, Tsigos C, Max MB. High-dose oral dextromethorphan in diabetic neuropathy pain and post-herpetic neuralgia: a double-blind, placebo controlled study. Neurology 1997; in press.

85. Mao J, Price DD, Mayer DJ. Mechanisms of hyperalgesia and morphine tolerance: a current view of their possible interactions. Pain 1995; 62: 259–274.

86. Lester RA, Tong G, Jahr CE. Interactions between the glycine and glutamate binding sites of the NMDA receptor. J Neurosci 1993; 13: 1088–1096.

87. Budai D, Wilcox GL, Larson AA. Enhancement of NMDA-evoked neuronal activity by glycine in the rat spinal cord in vivo. Neurosci Lett 1992; 135: 265–268.

88. Roberts MH. Involvement of serotonin in nociceptive pathways. Drug Design Delivery 1989; 4: 77–83.

89. Proudfit HK. Pharmacologic evidence for the modulation of nociception by noradrenergic neurons. Progr Brain Res 1988; 77: 357–370.

90. Carstens E, Gilly H, Schreiber H, Zimmermann M. Effects of midbrain stimulation and iontophoretic application of serotonin, noradrenaline, morphine and GABA on electrical thresholds of afferent C- and A-fibre terminals in cat spinal cord. Neuroscience 1987; 21: 395–406.

91. Baber NS, Dolerish CT, Hill Dr. The role of CCK caerulein and CCK antagonists in nociception. Pain 1989; 39: 307–328.

92. Noble F, Derrien M, Roques BP. Modulation of opioid antinociception by CCK at the supraspinal level: evidence of regulatory mechanisms between CCK and enkephalin systems in the control of pain. Br J Pharmacol 1993; 109: 1064–1070.

93. Katz N, Ferrante FM. Nociception. In: Ferrante FM, VandeBoncouer TR, eds. Postoperative pain management. New York; Churchill Livingstone; 1993: 17–67.

94. Bonica JJ. Anatomic and physiologic basis of nociception and pain. In: Bonica JJ, ed. The management of pain. 2nd edn. 1990: 28–94.

95. Max MB, Kishore-Kumar R, Schafer SC, et al. Efficacy of desipramine in painful diabetic neuropathy: a placebo-controlled trial. Pain 1991; 45: 69.

96. Max MB, Lynch SA, Muir J, Shoaf SE, Smoller B, Dubner R. Effects of desipramine, amitriptylline, and fluoxetine on pain in diabetic neuropathy. New Engl J Med 1992; 326: 1250–1256.

97. Villanueva L, Bouhassira D, LeBars D. The medullary subnucleus reticularis dorsalis (SRD) as a key link in both the transmission and modulation of pain signals. Pain 1996; 67: 231–240.

98. Stacey MJ. Free nerve endings in skeletal muscle of the cat. J Anat 1969; 105: 231–254.

99. Iggo A. Non-myelinated afferent fibres from mammalian skeletal muscle. J Physiol 1961; 155: 52–53.

100. Kumazawa T, Mizumura K. The polymodal C-fiber receptor in the muscle of the dog. Brain Res 1976; 101: 589–593.

101. Kumazawa T, Mizumura K. Thin-fibre receptors responding to mechanical, chemical, and thermal stimulation in the skeletal muscle of the dog. J Physiol 1977; 273: 179–194.

102. Mense S, Stahnke M. Response in muscle afferent fibers of slow conduction velocity to contractions and ischemia in the cat. J Physiol 1983; 342: 383–397.

103. Freeman MAR, Wyke B. The innervation of the knee joint. An anatomical and histological study in the cat. J Anat 1967; 101: 505–532.

104. Kidd BL, Morris VH, Urban L. Pathophysiology of joint pain. Ann Rheum Dis 1996; 55: 276–283.

105. Schaible HG, Grubb BD. Afferent and spinal mechanisms of joint pain. Pain 1993; 55: 5–54.

106. Langford LA, Schmidt RF. Afferent and efferent axons in the medial and posterior articular nerves of the cat. Anat Rec 1983; 206: 71–78.

107. Levine JD, Clark R, Devor M, Helms C, Moskowitz MA, Basbaum AI. Intraneuronal substance P contributes to the severity of experimental arthritis. Science 1984; 226: 547–549.

108. Lotz M, Carson DA, Vaughn JH. Substance P activation of rheumatoid synoviocytes: Neural pathway in pathogenesis of arthritis. Science 1987; 235: 893–895.

109. Lembeck F, Donnerer FC, Colpaert FC. Increase in substance P in primary afferent nerves during chronic pain. Neuropeptides 1981; 1: 175–180.

110. Cervero F. Mechanisms of visceral pain: past and present. In: Gebhart GF, ed. Visceral pain, progress in pain research and management, vol 5. Seattle; IASP Press; 1995: 25–40.

111. Cervero F, Tattersall JEH. Somatic and visceral sensory integration in the thoracic spinal cord in visceral sensation. In: Cervero F, Morrison JFB, eds. Progress in brain research, vol 67. Amsterdam: Elsevier; 1980: 189–205.

112. Apkarian AV, Brüggemann J, Shi T, Airapetian LR. A thalamic model for true and referred visceral pain. In: Gebhart GF, ed. Visceral pain, progress in pain research and management, vol 5. Seattle: IASP Press; 1995: 217–259.

113. Snow PJ, Lumb BM, Cervero F. The representation of prolonged and intense, noxious somatic and visceral stimuli in the ventrolateral orbital cortex of the cat. Pain 1992; 48: 89–99.

114. Cechetto DF. Supraspinal mechanisms of visceral representation. In: Gebhart GB, ed. Visceral pain, progress in pain research and management, vol 5. Seattle: IASP Press; 1995: 261–290.

115. Ness TJ, Metcalf AM, Gebhart GF. A psychophysical study using phasic colonic distention as a noxious visceral stimulus. Pain 1990; 43: 377–386.

116. Cervero F, Laird JM, Pozo MA. Selective changes of receptive field properties of spinal nociceptive neurons induced by visceral noxious stimulation in the cat. Pain 1992; 51: 335–342.

117. Kajander KC, Bennett GJ. Onset of a painful peripheral neuropathy in rat: a partial and differential deafferentation and spontaneous discharge in A beta and A delta primary afferent neurons. J Neurophysiol 1992; 68: 734–744.

118. Devor M. The pathophysiology of damaged peripheral nerves. In: Wall PD, Melzack R, eds. Textbook of pain. 3rd ed. Edinburgh: Churchill Livingstone; 1994: 79–100.

119. Jänig W. Activation of afferent fibers ending in an old neuroma by sympathetic stimulation in the rat. Neurosci Lett 1990; 111: 309–314.

120. Wall PD, Devor M. Sensory afferent impulses originate from dorsal root ganglia as well as from the periphery in normal and nerve-injured rats. Pain 1983; 17: 321–339.

121. Study RE, Kral MG. Spontaneous action potential in isolated dorsal root ganglion neurons from rats with painful neuropathy. Pain 1996; 65: 235–242.

122. Barbut D, Polak JM, Wall PD. Substance P in spinal cord dorsal horn decreases following nerve peripheral injury. Brain Res 1981; 205: 289–298.

123. Sato J, Perl ER. Adrenergic excitation of cutaneous pain receptors induced by peripheral nerve injury. Science 1991; 251: 1608–1610.

124. Sato J, Suzuki S, Iseki T, Kumazawa T. Adrenergic excitation of cutaneous nociceptors in chronically inflamed rats. Neurosci Lett 1993; 164: 225–228.

125. Korenman EMD, Devor M. Ectopic adrenergic sensitivity in damaged peripheral nerve axons in the rat. Exp Neurol 1981; 72: 63–81.

126. Kelly M. Spread of sensory and motor loss after nerve injury. Neurol 1952; 2: 36–45.

127. Nathan PW. Improvement in cutaneous sensibility associated with relief of pain. J Neurol Neurosurg Psychiat 1960; 23: 202–206.

128. Lindblom U, Verrillo RT. Sensory functions in chronic neuralgia. J Neurol Neurosurg Psychiat 1979; 42: 422–435.

129. Loh L, Nathan PW. Painful peripheral states and sympathetic blocks. J Neurol Neurosurg Psychiat 1978; 41: 664–671.

130. Boas RA. Complex regional pain syndrome: a reappraisal. In: Jänig W, Stanton-Hicks M, eds. Reflex sympathetic dystrophy; A reappraisal, progress in pain research and management, vol 6. Seattle: IASP Press; 1996: 79–92.

131. Bennett GJ, Roberts WJ. Animal models and their contribution to our understanding of complex regional pain syndrome I and II. In: Jänig W, Stanton-Hicks M, eds. Reflex sympathetic dystrophy: A reappraisal, progress in pain research and management, vol 6. Seattle: IASP Press; 1996: 107–122.

132. Fitzgerald M, Lynn B. The sensitization of high threshold mechanoreceptors with myelinated axons by repeated heating. J Physiol 1977; 265: 549–563.

133. Meyer RA, Campbell JN. Myelinated nociceptive afferents account for the hyperalgesia that follows a burn to the hand. Science 1981; 213: 1527–1529.

134. LaMotte RH, Thalhammer JG, Torebjörk HE, Robinson CJ. Peripheral neural mechanisms of cutaneous hyperalgesia following mild injury by heat. J Neurosci 1982; 2: 765–781.

135. LaMotte RH, Thalhammer JG, Robinson CJ.

Peripheral neural correlates of magnitude of cutaneous pain and hyperalgesia: a comparison of neural events in monkey with sensory judgements in humans. J Neurophysiol 1983; 50: 1–26.

136. LaMotte RH, Shain CN, Simone DA, Tsai EFP. Neurogenic hyperalgesia psychophysical studies of underlying mechanisms. J Neurophysiol 1991; 66: 190–211.

137. Dickenson AH, Sullivan AF. Peripheral origins and central modulation of subcutaneous formalin-induced activity of rat dorsal horn neurons. Neurosci Lett 1987; 83: 207–211.

138. Koltzenburg M, Lundberg LER, Torebjörk HE. Dynamic and static components of mechanical hyperalgesia in human hairy skin. Pain 1992; 51: 207–219.

139. Ochoa JL, Yarnitsky D. Mechanical hyperalgesias in neuropathic pain patients: dynamic and static subtypes. Ann Neurol 1993; 33: 465–472.

140. Campbell JN, Raja SN, Meyer RA, MacKinnon SE. Myelinated afferents signal the hyperalgesia associated with nerve injury. Pain 1988; 32: 89–94.

141. Raja SN, Campbell JN, Meyer RA. Evidence for different mechanisms of primary and secondary hyperalgesia following heat injury to the glabrous skin. Brain 1984; 107: 1179-1188.

142. Sang CN, Gracely RH, Max MB, Bennett GJ. Capsaicin-evoked mechanical allodynia and hyperalgesia cross nerve territories. Evidence for a central mechanism. Anesthesiology 1996; 85: 491-496.

143. Cervero F, Laird JMA. Mechanisms of touch-evoked pain (allodynia): a new model. Pain 1996; 68: 13-23.

144. Treede RD, Cole JD. Dissociated secondary hyperalgesia in a subject with a large-fibre sensory neuropathy. Pain 1993; 53: 169-174.

145. Levine JD, Dardick SJ, Basbaum AI, Scipio E. Reflex neurogenic inflammation. I. Contribution of the peripheral nervous system to spatially remote inflammatory responses that follow injury. J Neurosci 1985; 5: 1380-1386.

146. Gracely RH, Lynch SA, Bennett GJ: Painful neuropathy: altered central processing maintained dynamically by peripheral input. Pain 1992; 5: 175-194.

147. Häbler H-J, Jänig W, Koltzenburg M. Activation of unmyelinated afferents in chronically lesioned nerves by adrenaline and excitation of sympathetic efferents in the cat. Neurosci Lett 1987; 82: 35-40.

148. Raja SN, Treede RD, Davis KD, Campbell JN. Systemic alpha-adrenergic blockade with phentolamine: a diagnostic test for sympathetically-maintained pain. Anesthesiol 1991; 74: 691-698.

149. Liu M, Max MB, Parada S, Rowan JS, Bennett GJ: The sympathetic nervous system contributes to capsaicin-evoked mechanical allodynia but not pinprick hyperalgesia in humans. J Neurosci 1996; 16: 7331-7335.

151. Liu M, Max MB, Parada S, Rowan JS, Bennett GJ. The sympathetic nervous system contributes to capsaicin-evoked mechanical allodynia but not pinprick hyperalgesia in humans. J Neurosci 1996; 16: 7331–7335.

152. Bossut DF, Perl ER. Effects of nerve injury on sympathetic excitation of A delta mechanical nociceptors. J Neurophysiol 1995; 73: 1721-1723.

3

The effects of pain in the trauma patient

Nileshkumar Patel and Charles E Smith

Introduction

Mechanisms of pain – the axes
 Hypothalamic–pituitary–adrenal axis
 Sympathomedullary–adrenal axis
 Lympho–adrenal axis

Mechanisms of pain – the biochemical response
 Endocrine response to stress
 Metabolic response to pain

Clinical effects of pain – ebb and flow phases
 Central hypersensitization and 'wind-up'

Organ system responses to pain
 Cardiovascular responses
 Pulmonary dysfunction
 Gastrointestinal complications
 Hematologic and immune consequences of pain

Preventing the stress response to pain

Pre-emptive analgesia

Conclusion

INTRODUCTION

The confluence of hormonal, immunologic, cardiovascular, metabolic, and inflammatory responses that occur after major trauma results in the surgical stress response, the primary purpose of which is to restore and maintain cellular homeostasis. These biologic responses after injury occur in several phases, the magnitude and duration of which vary considerably and are related to severity of injury. The 'ebb phase' occurs immediately after trauma and is manifested by decreased energy expenditure, decreased oxygen consumption, hyperglycemia, vasoconstriction, and decreased body temperature. The 'flow phase' occurs after resuscitation and is characterized by a hyperdynamic state. This consists of increased cardiac output and minute ventilation, accelerated lipolysis and skeletal muscle proteolysis, and increased synthesis of acute phase proteins and glucose. In addition to these responses, there is activation of clotting mechanisms, major fluid shifts, blood flow redistribution, leukocyte immo-

bilization, and macrophage and specialized T cell production.

Much of the data concerning the effects of pain in the trauma population has been extrapolated from the 'controlled' situation of elective surgery. Although these data can equally apply to 'uncontrolled' tissue injury sustained by victims of major trauma, important differences exist such as the emergent nature of the surgery, shock, fluid resuscitation, blood transfusion, electrolyte imbalance, infections, airway compromise, and ventilatory instability.

The purpose of this chapter is to review the effects of pain in the trauma setting, with particular reference to the mechanisms and neuroendocrine response to pain, and to develop a clinical approach to effectively modulating the stress response to pain, to the benefit of the patient. Current data indicate that reduction of the stress response is associated with improved physiology and outcome. This knowledge can be utilized in the clinical care of the trauma population.

MECHANISMS OF PAIN – THE AXES

Hypothalamic–pituitary–adrenal axis

Afferent sensory nerve fibers provide a direct and rapid route for signals to arrive at the central nervous system. There is evidence that pain is the initial afferent signal after tissue trauma, and that these pain signals are essential to stimulate the hypothalamic–pituitary–adrenal axis.[1] Transection of the spinal cord above the level of injury, section of the medulla oblongata, or section of peripheral nerves to the area of injury prevents the adrenocortical response.[2] The efferent response prompts the release of hypothalamus-releasing factors, which in turn stimulate the release of pituitary and adrenal hormones, and hepatic release of glucagon and insulin (Table 3.1).

The hypothalamus secretes a number of substances including corticotropin-releasing hormone into the adenohypophysis, which in turn release propiomelanocortin. This latter substance breaks down into endorphins including beta-endorphin and adrenocorticotropic hormone (ACTH). The adrenal cortex responds to ACTH by releasing cortisol and other hormones (Table 3.1). Acute traumatic injury engenders production of endogenous endorphins. There is a positive correlation between injury severity score and serum beta endorphin levels.[3] Glucocorticoids and other steroids released by the adrenal cortex have potent effects on substrate and mineral metabolism. Cortisol mobilizes amino acids from skeletal muscle and increases gluconeogenesis and insulin resistance.

Sympathomedullary–adrenal axis

The chief mediators secreted from this system in response to stress are the catecholamines, epinephrine and norepinephrine (Table 3.1). These catecholamines, in turn, exert regulatory effects on cardiac output, regional circulation, serum glucose, and oxidative metabolism, which result in glycogenolysis, increased lactate production from skeletal muscle, and insulin resistance.

Lympho–adrenal axis

This axis is most notably responsible for the release of ACTH by lymphocytes. In the 1950s, the falling eosinophil count was used as weak index of adrenocortical response to trauma.[4]

MECHANISMS OF PAIN – THE BIOCHEMICAL RESPONSE

Endocrine response to stress

The clinical consequences of the stress response include hypertension, tachycardia, cardiac arrhythmias, protein catabolism, immune system suppression, hypercoagulable state, and elevated oxygen consumption.[5] It is of interest that the clinical effects of mild to moderate hypothermia in the trauma patient, such as impaired immunologic function, elevated catecholamines, and compensatory increased oxygen consumption during rewarming[6] are similar to the neuroendocrine effects of pain. Furthermore, it is likely that shock, thermal injury, and sepsis all activate various components of the stress response, such as cytokines and other peptide regulatory factors.

Increased catabolism is mediated by the counter-regulatory hormones, ACTH, cortisol, antidiuretic hormone, growth hormone and catecholamines, and the inflammatory mediators, specifically interleukin-2. Concurrently, there is a decrease in anabolism mediated chiefly by insulin. The combination of the increased catabolism and decreased anabolism leads to a hyperglycemic state in an effort to lead the body into preparedness for the increased energy requirements of the stressful situation. Vasopressin and aldosterone contribute to water and salt retention. The catecholamines also are responsible for hypertension, tachycardia, arrhythmias, gluconeogenesis, and glycogenolysis. Glucagon further promotes gluconeogenesis and ketogenesis.

Table 3.1 Hormones released after major trauma

Corticotropin-releasing hormone	Cortisol
Propriomelanocortin	Anti-diuretic hormone (ADH)
Beta-endorphins	Growth hormone
Adrenocorticotropic hormone (ACTH)	Vasopressin
Epinephrine	Aldosterone
Norepinephrine	Glucagon

Table 3.2 Hypermetabolic response to trauma

Increased lipolysis and ketogenesis
Increased muscle proteolysis
Increased acute phase proteins
Increased gluconeogenesis and glycogenolysis
Insulin resistance
Increased lactate production in skeletal muscle

Metabolic response to pain (Table 3.2)

The hyperglycemic response is due to the combined effect of the counter-regulatory hormones glucagon, cortisol, and catecholamines, as well as protein breakdown that, in part, fuels the formation of glucose and facilitates amino acid and fat mobilization. The acute phase reactive proteins, including C-reactive protein, are elevated. Ketone levels are typically elevated during the stress response because of accelerated lipolysis and oxidation of free fatty acids.

CLINICAL EFFECTS OF PAIN

Ebb and flow phases

The clinical features of injury are graded responses. In general, the greater the injury, the greater the response until a maximal response occurs. The 'ebb phase' occurs immediately after trauma and typically lasts the first 24 hours (Fig. 3.1). This early low-flow ebb phase is characterized by alpha-receptor mediated vasoconstriction, and decreased urine flow and oxygen utilization. Cardiac output is increased or decreased, and stress hormone levels are elevated. There is also a transient hypometabolic state characterized by decreased temperature and insulin levels. Many of these early changes are related to hypovolemia and reduced tissue perfusion.

With restoration of perfusion and time, the ebb phase is followed by the 'flow phase'. This flow phase, or chronic hyperdynamic phase, typically lasts 2 to 5 days and involves an increased cardiac output, elevation of oxygen consumption, beta adrenoreceptor mediated increases in regional blood flow, and a hypermetabolic state (Fig. 3.1). The components of this phase include protein catabolism, lipolysis, gluconeogenesis, glycogenolysis, and an increased core temperature. This hyperdynamic phase may explain the increased

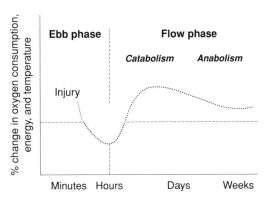

Fig. 3.1 The 'ebb' and 'flow' phases following trauma.

incidence of myocardial infarctions observed 2 to 3 days following surgery. Inadequate control of nociception during this phase may contribute to higher mortality and morbidity because of immunosuppression, increased myocardial oxygen demand, increased thrombogenicity, a hypercoagulable state, reduced body mass and tissue reserve as well as impaired pulmonary function (see Table 3.4).[7,8]

Tissue trauma causes the release of certain algesic agents including serotonin, bradykinin, hydrogen ions, potassium, and prostaglandins, into the local region (see Ch. 2). These substances excite the primary afferent fibers to heighten responsiveness such that a stimulus that would not normally cause firing in the affected neuron does so in an unexpected manner.[9] The primary injury phase is followed by a subsequent inflammatory phase associated with the release of the traditional inflammatory mediators as well as cytokines, purines, leukotrienes, neuropeptides, nitric oxide and nerve growth factors in the region of the tissue injury. This 'inflammatory soup' may cause sensitization of nociceptors, provide persistent input to the spinal cord beyond the initial insult, and maintain the pain patterns in the post-injury phase.[10]

Central hypersensitization and 'wind-up'

With any continuous afferent nociceptive central nervous system barrage, there is progressive 'wind-up' of the dorsal horn neurons such that the receptive fields widen and expand.[11,12] Associated with this are the morphological changes in the neurons of the dorsal horn of the spinal cord. The noxious stimulus thereby imparts changes in the physiology and anatomy of the dorsal horn such that nociceptive stimuli can force the spinal cord into a new state of excitability which is then sustained by mechanisms within the spinal cord.[13] Further noxious stimulus from the peripheral tissue damage produces prolonged changes in the processing of afferent information in the central nervous system including decreased pain threshold, pain to normal stimulation (allodynia), and increased duration of response to brief stimulation. This is the phenomenon of central sensitization.[14]

ORGAN SYSTEM RESPONSES TO PAIN (Tables 3.3, 3.4)

Cardiovascular responses (Table 3.3)

Evidence from the elective surgery population indicates that the magnitude of the surgical stress response correlates with the 'invasiveness' and severity of the surgery. Peripheral surgeries are associated with minimal stress response, lower abdominal and pelvic surgeries with mild to moderate stress response, whereas abdominal surgery and thoracic surgery are associated with maximal stress response. The trauma patient with thermal and head injuries is likely to have a severe stress response.

Much of the data available for surgical stress (i.e. a controlled trauma) can be applied to the trauma population. The cardiovascular responses to stress include increase in heart rate, systemic vascular resistance, cardiac output and coronary vascular resistance (see Table 3.1), all of which place the susceptible patient at an increased risk of myocardial ischemia. These hemodynamic responses are partially due to segmental spinal cord reflex

Table 3.3 Cardiovascular responses to major trauma (note that these responses may vary depending on the phase, type, and severity of injury, volume status, and tissue perfusion)

Increased sympathetic nerve activity
Increased heart rate
Peripheral vasoconstriction
Increased cardiac output
Altered interstitial fluid matrix configuration
Increased oxygen consumption

Table 3.4 Other organ system responses to major trauma (note that these responses may vary depending on the phase, type, and severity of injury)

Impaired pulmonary function (e.g. thoracic trauma)
Impaired gastrointestinal tone and ileus
Decreased urinary output
Release of inflammatory mediators (e.g. tumor necrosis factor, leukotrienes)
Hypercoagulable state
Increased platelet reactivity
Decreased fibrinolysis
Activation of coagulation cascade
Activation of cytokine cascade and release of interleukins (e.g. IL-1, IL-2, IL-6, IL-8)
Activation of complement cascade
Activation of neutrophils
Stimulation of lymphocytes
Immune dysfunction
Immunosuppression (e.g. prostaglandin E2)

responses; nociceptive impulses that initiate positive feedback loops that stimulate segmental sympathetic neurons. Moreover, pain impulses that reach the hypothalamus and the limbic system cause a general increase in the sympathetic tone that further increase cardiac output, blood pressure, and cardiac workload as well as increase body metabolism and oxygen consumption.[15] Additionally, sympathetic stimulation results in decrements in coronary blood flow,[16] and sympathectomy improves coronary circulation.[17]

Pulmonary dysfunction

As a result of acute pain, especially following trauma to the thorax and abdomen, there is significant impairment of pulmonary function (see Chs 14 and 19).[18,19] A combination of factors including diaphragmatic muscle inhibition via phrenic nerve dysfunction and reflex muscle spasm, and involuntary splinting of thoracic and abdominal muscles produces ventilation perfusion (V/Q) abnormalities.

In addition, direct injury to muscle tissue produces reductions in inspiratory capacity, vital capacity, and functional residual capacity resulting in negative transpulmonary pressure in the gravity dependent areas of the lung. This leads to narrowing and collapse of the small airways and further loss of functional residual capacity. Failure of the airway to re-open leads to the total collapse of the lung unit served by that airway, producing atelectasis. Consequently, low V/Q relationship results in impaired gas exchange and hypoxemia. Multiple rib fractures, flail chest, and pulmonary contusion cause further pain and impaired gas exchange.

Gastrointestinal complications

The sympathetic innervation to the gut arises from the thoracolumbar sympathetic chain (T5–L2), the parasympathetics from the vagus and the sacral outflow (S1–S4). Stress-mediated increases in sympathetic nerve activity result in a decrease in the gastrointestinal tone, producing distension, ileus, and decreased bowel motility, as well as nausea and vomiting.[20,21] Additionally, abdominal pain per se activates reflex arcs which inhibit intestinal motility.[22] Surgical sympathectomy prevents ileus following abdominal surgery, further supporting the proposal that the ileus is a result of sympathetic hyperactivity.[23] Delayed return of bowel function and prolonged nausea and vomiting in the trauma patient may translate into prolonged hospitalization, higher costs, and added morbidity.

Hematologic and immune consequences of pain

Hypercoagulability leads to thrombosis and pulmonary embolism, and is a function of the activation of the coagulation cascade, increased platelet reactivity, decreased level of endogenous anticoagulants and a decreased fibrinolytic activity.[24,25] Thrombus formation occurs with greater frequency in the postoperative patient whose pain is inadequately relieved, especially if fear of pain leads to immobility.[26] Immune dysfunction from surgical stress leading to a higher incidence of infection is a well-known phenomenon,[27] and is particularly related to suppression of the natural killer cell cytotoxic function.[28] Additional stress-related factors, including alterations in the hormonal milieu, also contribute to impaired host defenses.[29,30]

PREVENTING THE STRESS RESPONSE TO PAIN

Effective acute pain management can improve postoperative outcome by altering many of the pathophysiological responses to acute pain. Blockade of surgical stress-related sympathetic activation can lead to lower postoperative cortisol levels,[31] serum glucose,[32] and protein catabolism.[33] Attenuating the sympathetic nervous system hyperactivity with epidural opioids leads to lower norepinephrine levels.[34] In the study, neuraxial blockade attenuated the sympathetic response to a greater degree than the pituitary adrenal cortical response.[34] Randomized, prospective studies have shown that epidural anesthesia and analgesia attenuate the postoperative stress response, reduce the postsurgical hypercoagulable state, and decrease morbidity from cardiovascular aberrations, major infections, and vascular graft re-occlusion.[31,35,36]

In the trauma patient, adequate analgesia improves oxygenation, ventilation, and comfort.[37] In a review of pulmonary-related mortality, it was shown that epidural analgesia was associated with lower mortality when compared with a group of patients receiving general anesthesia.[38] Effective pain control with neuraxial analgesia has also been shown to reduce postoperative intubation time, intensive care unit stay, and hospital costs.[31,39] More recently, epidural analgesia has been shown to allow earlier return of bowel function and earlier achievement of objective discharge criteria compared with intravenous patient-controlled analgesia (IV-PCA).

While it is evident that neuraxial blockade provides excellent pain relief, blunts the stress response, and is associated with beneficial clinical effects such as improved oxygenation, intrapleural analgesia improves pain scores but does not result in any significant improvement in oxygenation in patients who have suffered blunt traumatic chest wall injuries.[40] Kehlet has surmised that pain relief per se is not adequate for improved surgical outcome in that the neuroendocrine stress response must also be blunted for improved outcome.[41–43] These views are supported by animal studies that suggest that neuraxial blockade blunts the catecholamine surge and improves survival in experimental hemorrhagic shock.[44,45]

The need for adequate pain relief and blunting of the stress response in trauma has been well documented and advocated.[5,46,47] Despite the documented beneficial effects of pain relief, it is evident that peripheral nerve blocks and neuraxial techniques are underutilized in the trauma population.[48]

PRE-EMPTIVE ANALGESIA

The concept of pre-emptive analgesia can easily be applied to the surgical patient where operative trauma is anticipated and pre-emptive analgesia is feasible. However, in the acute trauma population, such interventions are not usually possible. Nonetheless, long-term effects of pain can probably be blunted in many individuals by adequate pain control at the earliest opportunity. This is because pronounced neuroplastic changes occur in the dorsal horn of the spinal cord and at higher centers in response to chronic pain. These neuroplastic changes are deemed significant in the pathophysiology of chronic pain syndromes. Sympathetic-mediated pain syndromes and phantom limb pain are examples of neuropathic pains (see Ch. 22). For example, if the pre-operative pain is experienced at the time of amputation, there is a higher probability that pain will persist in the phantom limb.[49] Although controversial, epidural analgesia with local anesthetics and opioids before undergoing limb amputation decreased the frequency of post-amputation phantom limb pain.[50,51] Similarly, symptoms of sympathetic mediated pain may be prevented by prior neural blockade.[52]

CONCLUSION

The effect of pain in the trauma patient is evident at the biochemical, histological, and clinical levels. While the effect of pain may transiently improve the survival potential of the patient in the immediate time frame, its consequences in the medium- to long-term range is rarely beneficial. All attempts should be made to blunt pain and more importantly, its neuroendocrine stress response in an attempt to alleviate suffering and improve outcome. A clear understanding of the pathophysiology of the stress response should aid the traumatologist in achieving this goal.

REFERENCES

1. Hume DM, Egdahl RH. The importance of the brain in the endocrine response to injury. Ann Surg 1958; 150: 697.
2. Wilmore DW. Homeostasis. In: Sabiston DC, Lyerly HK, eds. Textbook of surgery. The biological basis of modern surgical practice. 15th ed. Philadelphia: WB Saunders; 1997.
3. Bernstein L, Garzone PD, Rudy T, Kramer B, Stiff D, Peitzman A. Pain perception and serum beta endorphin in trauma patient. Psychosomatics 1995; 36: 276–284.
4. Roche M, Thorn GW, Hills AG. The levels of circulating eosinophils and their responses to ACTH in surgery. N Engl J Med 1950; 242: 307–314.
5. Kehlet H. The surgical stress response: should it be prevented? Can J Surgery 1991; 34: 565–567.
6. Smith T, Patel N. Hypothermia in the trauma patient. Am J Anesthesiology 1996.
7. Kehlet H. Br J Anaesth 1982; 63: 189.
8. Kehlet H. Acta Chir Scand Suppl 1989; 550: 22.
9. Raja SN, Meyer RA, Campbell JN. Peripheral mechanisms of somatic pain. Anesthesiology 1988; 68: 571–590.
10. Raja SN. Editorial: Is an ounce of preoperative local anesthesia better than a pound of postoperative analgesic? Reg Anesth 1996; 21: 277–280.
11. Woolf CJ. Evidence for a central component of post injury hypersensitivity. Nature 1983; 306: 686–688.
12. Cook AJ, Woolf CJ, Wall PD, McMohan SB. Dynamic receptive field plasticity in the rat spinal cord dorsal horn following C-primary afferent input. Nature 1987; 325: 151–153.
13. Wall PD. The prevention of postoperative pain. Pain 1988; 33: 289–290.
14. Coderra TJ, Melzack R. Cutaneous hyperalgesia: Contributions of the peripheral and central nervous system to the increase in pain sensitivity after injury.
15. Bonica JJ. Management of post operative pain. In: Bonica JJ, ed. The management of pain, 2nd ed. Philadelphia: Lea & Febiger 1990; 461–480.
16. Uchida Y, Murao S. Sustained decrease in coronary blood flow and excitation of cardiac sensory fibers following sympathetic stimulation. Jpn Heart J 1975; 16: 265–279.
17. Klassen GA, Bramwell RS, Bromage PR, Zaborowska-Sluis DT. Effect of acute sympathectomy by epidural anesthesia on the canine coronary circulation. Anesthesiology 1980; 52: 8–15.
18. Craig DB. Post operative recovery of pulmonary function. Anesth Analg 1981; 60: 46–52.
19. Spence AA. In: Gray TC, Nunn JF, Utting F, eds. Post operative pulmonary complications in general anesthesia, vol. 1. London: Butterworths; 1981; 591–608.
20. Kehlet H. Modifications of response to surgery and anesthesia by neural blockade. In: Cousins MJ, Bridenbaugh PO, eds. Neural blockade in clinical anesthesia and management of pain. Philadelphia: JB Lippincott; 1987; 145.
21. Livingston EH, Passero EP. Post operative ileus. Dig Dis Sci 1990; 35: 121–132.

22. Furness JB, Costa M. Adynamic ileus, its patho-genesis and treatment. Med Biol Eng Compat 1974; 82–89.

23. Bayliss W, Starling E. The movements and inner-vation of the small intestine. J Physiol (Lond) 1899; 24: 8–143.

24. Collins GJ, Barker JA, Zajtchuk E, Vanek D, Malogne LA. The effects of operative stress on coagulation profile. Am J Surg 1977; 133: 612–616.

25. Rosenfeld BA, Faraday N, Campbell D, Dise K, Bell W, Goldschmidt F. Hemostatic effects of stress hormone infusion. Anesthesiology 1994; 81: 1116–1126.

26. Modig JP. Respiration and circulation after total hip replacement surgery. Acta Anaesthesiol Scand 1976; 20: 225.

27. Slade MS, Simmons RC, Yunis E, Greenberg LS. Immunodepression after major surgery in normal patients. Surgery 1975; 78: 363.

28. Ucheida A, Kolb R, Micksche M. Generation of suppressor cells for natural killer activity in cancer patients after surgery. J Natl Cancer Inst 1982; 68: 735–741.

29. Faist E, Ertel W, Mewes A, et al. Trauma induced alteration of the lymphokine cascade. In: Faist E, Ninneman J, Green D, eds. Immune conse-quences of trauma, shock and sepsis: Mechanisms and therapeutic approaches. Berlin: Springer Verlag; 1989; 79–94.

30. Alexander JW. Mechanism of immunologic sup-pression in burn injury. J Trauma 1990; 30: 570.

31. Yeager MP, Glass DD, Neff RK, Brink-Johnsosen T. Epidural anesthesia and analgesia in high-risk surgical patients. Anesthesiology 1987; 66: 729–736.

32. Wattwill M, Thorea T, Heunerdel S, Garvill JE. Epidural anesthesia with bupivacaine reduces post-operative paralytic ileus after hysterectomy. Anesth Analg 1989; 68: 353–358.

33. Vedrinne C, Vedrinne JM, Guiraud M, et al. Nitrogen sparing effect of local anesthesia in colon surgery. Anesth Analg 1989; 69: 354–359.

34. Breslow MJ, Jordan DA, Christopherson K, et al. Epidural morphine decreases post operative hyper-tension by attenuating sympathetic nervous hyper-activity. JAMA 1989; 261: 3577–3581.

35. Tuman KJ, McCarthy RJ, March RJ, et al. Effects of epidural anesthesia and analgesia on complica-tion and outcome after major vascular surgery. Anesth Analg 1991; 73: 693–704.

36. Christopherson R, Beatie C, Frank SM, Morris EJ, et al. Perioperative morbidity in patients random-ized to epidural and general anesthesia for lower extremity vascular surgery. Anesthesiology 1993; 79: 422–434.

37. O'Kelly E, Gary B. Continuous pain relief for mul-tiple fractured ribs. Br J Anaesth 1981; 53: 988–999.

38. Sharrock, et al. Anesth Analg 1995; 80: 242–248.

39. deLeone Casasola, et al. Reg Anesth 1994; 19: 307–315.

40. Short K, Scheers D, Mlakar J, Dean R. Evaluation of intrapleural anesthesia in the management of blunt traumatic chest wall pain: a clinical trial. Am Surg 1996; 62: 488–493.

41. Kehlet H. Modification of responses to surgery and anesthesia by neural blockade: clinical impli-cations. In: Cousins MJ, Bridenbaugh PO, eds. Neural blockade in clinical anesthesia and man-agement of pain. 3rd ed. Philadelphia: JB Lippincott; 1996.

42. Kehlet H. Postoperative pain relief: A look from the other side. Reg Anesth 1994; 72: 369–377.

43. Kehlet H. General outcome improvement overview. Reg Anesth 1986; 21: 5–8.

44. Shibata K, Yamamoto Y, Murakami S. Effects of epidural anesthesia in cardiovascular response and survival in hemorrhagic shock in dogs. Anesthesiology 1989; 71: 953–959.

45. Shibata K, Yamamoto Y, Kobayashi T, Murakami S. Beneficial effects of upper thoracic epidural anesthesia in experimental hemorrhagic shock: Influence of circulating catecholamines. Anesthesiology 1991; 74: 303–308.

46. Mackersie RL, Karagianes TG. Pain management following trauma. Crit Care Clin 1990; 6: 433–449.

47. Cohen SS, Alagesan R, Jain S. Acute and chronic post traumatic pain. Probe in Anesth 1994; 8: 487–517.

48. Brown DL. Special situations for regional anesthe-sia: trauma. Reg Anesth 1996; 2: 122–125.

49. Katz J, Melzack R. Pain 'memories' in phantom limbs: review and critical observation. Pain 1990; 43: 319–336.

50. Bach S, Noreng MF, Tjellden NU. Phantom limb pain in amputees during the first 12 months following limb amputation after perioperative lumbar epidural blockade. Pain 1988; 33: 297–301.

51. Jahangir M, Bradley JWP, Jayatunga AP. Prevention of phantom limb pain after major lower limb amputation by epidural infusion of diamor-phine, clonidine and bupivacaine. Ann R Coll Surg Engl 1994; 76: 324–326.

52. Pedeson JL, Crawford ME, Dahl JB, Brennen J, Kehlet H. Effect of pre-emptive nerve block on inflammation and hyperalgesia after human thermal injury. Anesthesiology 1996; 84: 1020–1026.

Pharmacologic management of acute and chronic pain in trauma patients

P Prithvi Raj and Craig Hartrick

Introduction

Pain caused by acute injury
    Rationale for pain management
    General principles
    Concerns of hypovolemia and hypotension

The development of chronic post-traumatic pain
    Psychological factors

Acute post-traumatic pain management
    Systemic analgesia

Regional anesthesia

Chronic pain management
    General principles of management

Drugs used in acute and chronic trauma patients
    Narcotics

Nonsteroidal anti-inflammatory analgesics
    Mechanism of action
    Specific drugs

Anti-depressants
    Guidelines for using anti-depressants

Neuroleptics
    Guidelines for using neuroleptics

Anticonvulsants

Sedative-hypnotics and anxiolytics

Antihistamines and muscle relaxants

Local anesthetics
    Physical and chemical properties
    Mechanisms of local anesthetic function
    Factors that affect blockade
    Addition of vasoconstrictor agents
    Specific local anesthetics
    Toxicity of local anesthetics

Summary

INTRODUCTION

Each year tens of millions of Americans suffer accidental injuries that result in persistent pain. These injuries account for a large percentage of the chronic pain seen in the USA. Bonica, reviewing cases in which pain was the predominant symptom,[1] found that more than one-third of all Americans experience persistent or recurrent pain requiring medical therapy. For these patients, it is the pain and not the underlying pathology that is the primary reason for their being nonproductive. In addition to the obvious personal and social impact post-traumatic pain and its resultant disabilities project onto patients and their families, the economic impact on the USA secondary to lost productivity and health care expenses for all chronic pain is conservatively estimated in excess of $85 billion annually.[2]

Heightened awareness of the importance of early intervention with effective pain management measures is reflected in both public policy[3] and medical professional guidelines.[4,5] In recent years, organized acute and chronic pain management services, previously available only in large tertiary care centers, have become common in communities remote from major medical centers. This chapter highlights the pharmacologic approaches to post-traumatic pain, emphasizes the importance of early effective intervention, and suggests some strategies for selection of appropriate systemic pain management modalities.

PAIN CAUSED BY ACUTE INJURY

When the trauma patient arrives in the emergency room, attention is at once directed toward initial resuscitation and stabilization. Priority is given to establishing ventilatory and cardiovascular stability, control of external hemorrhage, and restoration of fluid and blood volume. Depending on the sites of injury, attention may then shift to intra-abdominal or intrathoracic bleeding and the repair of hollow viscus injury, followed by urological, neurosurgical, and orthopedic intervention.

Following the institution of therapeutic intervention, pain relief often continues to have low priority. Analgesics should not be delayed once the initial assessment is complete. In fact, far from confusing diagnosis, Zoltie & Cust demonstrated in a prospective double-blind trial that narcotic administration in the emergency department can facilitate correct diagnosis.[6] The choice of analgesic and route of administration, however, must be carefully selected with due consideration of the prevailing hemodynamic, respiratory, and neurological circumstances, as well as the possibility of aspiration of gastric contents.

Although most preliminary diagnostic and therapeutic procedures (e.g. tracheal intubation, paracentesis, chest tube insertion) can be performed with local or topical anesthetics, *systemic* or *regional* techniques may be required for optimal performance of certain imaging studies and painful procedures such as fracture splinting or reduction. Aside from facilitating specific diagnostic and therapeutic interventions, there is ample evidence that pain relief can minimize both patient anxiety and stress response.[7]

Rationale for pain management

An important goal in post-traumatic pain management is the early restoration of function. Cellular function depends on blood flow for delivery of nutrients to the tissues. Vasoconstriction, whether secondary to pain or direct vascular injury resulting from trauma or surgical manipulation, interferes with nutrient supply. *Sympathetic blockade* can be used to decrease vascular resistance and improve skin and vascular graft flow, while decreasing pain-mediated vasoconstriction.[8] Regional block for relief of pain can permit improved mobilization of the injured part.[9–11] Early mobilization helps to preserve normal myofascial and gastrointestinal function. Improved nutrient supply, as measured by gastric emptying time, is significantly better with epidural analgesia than with systemic narcotic administration.[12]

A second goal in post-traumatic pain management is the modulation of both early and delayed sequelae following injury. Reduced postoperative morbidity has been associated with the use of epidural analgesia in high-risk surgical patients.[13,14] Additionally, myofascial pain syndromes resulting from injury to musculoskeletal structures and disuse secondary to pain and muscle spasm are minimized with early ambulation and mobilization of injured extremities. The development of late post-traumatic pain syndromes may also partially depend upon initial pain management.

General principles

The treatment selected must be compatible with the pathophysiology of the injured patient

Both hemorrhage and reduced cardiac output in the severely traumatized patient alter the pharmacokinetic and pharmacodynamic effects of administered drugs. Organ perfusion may also be altered, affecting the clearance and terminal elimination rates of analgesics. Extremely high plasma levels of analgesics or their metabolites may result in undesirable side effects. Similarly, muscle blood flow may be impaired, limiting usefulness of intramuscular analgesic administration.

Care should be taken to ensure that the analgesic regime does not further interfere with the mechanics of respiration (e.g. chest muscle function, airway patency) or with central control when chest injury or pre-existing pulmonary compromise is present. A rise in $PaCO_2$ caused by hypoventilation may result in cerebral vasodilation, thus potentially aggravating increased intracranial pressure in closed head injuries.

The patient may be intoxicated with alcohol or other drugs. Further, the state of consciousness may be altered following closed head injuries. Drugs that mask or imitate the signs of raised intracranial pressure should be administered with caution. The stomach may be full and gastric emptying delayed. Drugs should not be given by the oral route. This is particularly inappropriate if a general anesthetic will be needed for surgical intervention or imaging studies.

The analgesic approach should consider the possibility of pain from either multiple sites or multiple simultaneous causative factors

If more than one strategy needs to be employed to cover pain emanating from noncontiguous sites, interactions must be considered. Additionally, traumatized patients concomitantly suffer varying degrees of anxiety and emotional stress.[15] Consideration should be given to anxiety reduction, not only to minimize side effects precipitated by analgesics,[16] but also to attempt to reduce the subsequent incidence of chronic pain related to post-traumatic stress disorder.[17]

Although behavioral changes are most frequently associated with chronic pain syndromes, acute pain may also be accompanied by psychiatric disturbances that can confound and conceal underlying pathology.[18,19] Neurologic injury following closed head injury may give rise to altered behavior. Movement disorders such as kinisophobia[20] and, rarely, acute dystonia[21] may follow even minor peripheral trauma.

Early return to normal physiologic function is an important goal with any acute injury. Attention to not only the injured site, but to the surrounding musculature should be directed towards mobilization. The return of function prevents painful contracture and allows normal physiologic stresses to aid remodeling of tendon and bone.[22] Some form of anesthesia should be used during reduction of dislocations. The resultant analgesia and muscle relaxation protect the joint from excessive stress and prevent damage to articular surfaces.[23]

The extent of tissue damage, functional impairment, and joint instability must be assessed early in the evaluation process. Ligamentous laxity, once developed, tends not to improve spontaneously. Repair of unstable joints is better undertaken before the onset of fibrosis and contracture.[23] Corticosteroids reduce the inflammatory response, and hence interfere with the first stage of healing; they should be used with caution in acute strains and only when the joint is to be placed at rest.[22,23]

Continued tissue swelling following crushing or blunt traumatic extremity injury may predispose the patient to subsequent development of a compartment syndrome. Analgesic selection should consider potential masking of evolving neurologic sequelae of both peripheral and central origins.

Concerns of hypovolemia and hypotension

In the trauma patient hypovolemia and hypotension play a large part in the appropriate selection of analgesic agents. The choice of analgesic drugs and techniques is largely influenced by the severity of hemorrhage and the adequacy of the resuscitation.[24] The patient should be carefully observed for signs of hypovolemia such as pallor, tachycardia, hypotension, cold extremities, collapsed veins with low venous pressure, and reduced urine output. Hypovolemia resulting from a loss of more than 40% of blood volume will cause confusion, restlessness, air hunger, and coma. Signs of hypovolemic shock appear earlier in geriatric patients. Patients with injury to the cervical portion of the spinal cord, cardiac tamponade, or pneumothorax may mimic the signs of hypovolemic shock even though their blood volume is not reduced.

Patients with minor injuries and minimal blood loss can be anesthetized in the same way as elective cases for similar surgical procedures. Either regional analgesia or general anesthesia is appropriate. The trachea should be intubated when a full stomach is suspected, when field avoidance is required, when controlled ventilation is planned, or when the integrity of the airway is questioned. The following are commonly used agents and techniques for patients with minor injuries and minimal blood loss:

1. Ketamine, 5 mg/kg IM or 0.5 mg/kg IV, is suitable in infants and children for reduction of fractures, suturing of lacerations, minor

debridement, or application of dressings. Ketamine anesthesia alone does not preserve airway reflexes. The tracheas of patients with full stomachs should be intubated.

2. Diazepam, 0.3–0.5 mg/kg IV, is suitable for closed reduction and casting of fractures.

3. An intravenous regional block is useful for brief procedures on the forearm or hand. A double cuff is applied to the arm proximal to the site of an intravenous puncture which is placed near the injury. The arm is then elevated to exsanguinate the limb and the proximal cuff inflated to 200 mmHg. 40 mL of 0.5% lidocaine is introduced intravenously and, as the block takes effect, the distal cuff is inflated and the proximal one released. Obviously care must be taken to avoid accidental escape of local anesthetic solution from the limb as this will result in convulsions or cardiac arrest.

Patients with moderate trauma or loss of 10 to 30% of blood volume will be tachycardic, hypotensive, vasoconstricted, and oliguric and will exhibit respiratory distress and mental confusion. Because of partial resuscitation during transport and in the emergency room, such a patient may arrive in the operating room with nearly normal vital signs only to become hypotensive secondary to abolition of compensatory vasoconstriction by IV narcotics and/or anesthetic induction with potent cardiovascular depressants. If the blood volume has been completely restored, the patient may respond to potent analgesics without serious changes in vital signs.

Patients with major trauma and loss of 50% of blood volume or greater will be severely hypotensive and tachycardic. Low venous pressure, severe respiratory distress, marked vasoconstriction, anuria, advanced hypoxia, and metabolic acidosis will be observed. The patients are usually semiconscious and may become comatose. Immediate surgery is a necessity. Anesthesiologists must accept the responsibility for the care of these patients even though preoperative data may not exist. They usually need no anesthetics. Even small doses of intravenous narcotics may precipitate complete and irreversible cardiovascular collapse. Pain appreciation is usually abolished in this state, and patients offer little resistance to endotracheal intubation, controlled ventilation, and, for that matter, the surgical procedure. Oxygen

only should be given or, at the most, very small doses of anesthetic (i.e. 0.25 MAC isoflurane).

THE DEVELOPMENT OF CHRONIC POST-TRAUMATIC PAIN

Pain persisting beyond the normal recovery period, often greatly exceeding that which might be anticipated relative to the residual pathology, can be considered chronic post-traumatic pain. Although it is widely assumed that psychological factors become increasingly important as acute pain progresses to become chronic, it is perhaps less well appreciated that a number of pathophysiological changes also occur in both central and peripheral pain pathways. Consequently, the response of chronic pain patients to various therapeutic interventions, including the response to local anesthetic blockade, often varies from what one might expect in the acute pain setting.[25,26] Modification of the approach to treatment is required.

It is poorly understood why some patients suffer traumatic injuries that result in chronic-pain states while other patients with similar injuries escape this fate. Genetic predisposition to chronic neuropathic pain has been suggested by both experimental,[27–29] and clinical studies.[30] Premorbid psychological factors have also been implicated in the subsequent development of chronic low back pain[31,32] and chronic regional pain syndrome (CRPS) I reflex sympathetic dystrophy (RSD).[33] High levels of anxiety,[34] personality disorder,[35,36] passive coping strategies,[37] and job dissatisfaction[38] all predict the progression of acute low back pain to chronic pain and disability. Yet the persistence and intensity of acute pain may be crucial to the initiation of processes leading to chronic pain in susceptible individuals.[39] This impression is based upon clinical studies involving phantom limb pain[40–43] and low back pain.[34–36] The intensity of acute pain predicted the severity and persistence of pain in these conditions. An overwhelming afferent barrage owing to severe pain may then lead to the pathophysiologic alterations associated with chronic pain in a manner consistent with the central neuroplasticity previously discussed.[44]

Site of injury is certainly one important factor in the development of persistent pain. Sports-related injuries that seem more likely to become chronic pain problems include injuries involving the spine and spinal cord, brachial plexus injuries including thoracic outlet syndrome and other syndromes of neurovascular compression, and certain extremity injuries. Mechanical shoulder and knee injuries producing recurrent joint dislocation, bursitis, post-traumatic arthritis or tendinitis, and myofascial dysfunction involving muscle groups about the joint are particularly common. The risk factors predicting overuse musculoskeletal injuries, however, relate to poor conditioning,[45–48] predisposing anatomic characteristics,[48–50] and intensity of activity,[51] but not to accident-prone psychological factors.[52] Extremity injuries are also most prone to the development of CRPS I (RSD). The sympathetic dysfunction seen in the upper extremity following shoulder injury has long been referred to as shoulder hand syndrome.[53] RSD of the knee has been more recently recognized to be a fairly common ailment.[54]

Similarly, chronic pain conditions seem to more commonly occur following surgical trauma involving the extremities, especially the hands and feet. Spinal surgery, thoracotomy, extensive facial and scalp surgery, cholecystectomy, and radical mastectomy also seem particularly vulnerable to persistent pain problems.[55] Chronic post-traumatic pain in the lower abdomen and groin is frequently seen following appendectomy, inguinal herniorrhaphy, varicocele ligation, obstetrical/gynecological procedures with Pfannenstiel incisions, nephrectomy, femoral thrombectomy, femoral–popliteal bypass grafting, vein stripping, lumbar sympathectomy, and uterine suspension procedures.[56,57] Visceral, myofascial, neuropathic, and psychogenic etiologies contribute.[57] Hitchcock & Alvarez[58] reported a 2% incidence of chronic postincisional scar pain. They found the most common sites to be (in decreasing order) the lower abdomen, thorax, lumbosacral area, head and neck, flank, and palm. Neuroma formation was diagnosed in 43.3% of cases, whereas 23.3% had deafferentation pain. Psychological factors were thought to be important in 33.3% of cases.

Psychological factors

Psychological factors play important roles in the outward expression and adjustment to both acute and chronic pain; they may also play a role in the eventual evolution of acute pain into chronic pain states. Anxiety states, depression, organic brain dysfunction, and post-traumatic stress disorder

can all lead to expression of pain seemingly out of proportion to what would be typically expected based strictly on the overt physical damage.[17,59] The afferent neural traffic, however, clearly can be altered by psychological factors.[60] Human volunteers have been taught to control the amount of afferent activity measured by somatosensory evoked potentials with extremity stimulation.[61] Other primates have been conditioned so that discharge of pain-transmitting neurons has been observed in anticipation of a noxious stimulus.[62] Psychological factors may not only alter the outward expression of pain, but may actually increase the afferent barrage following a given traumatic insult. Early identification of warning signs in the acute pain stage facilitates aggressive intervention and thus aids in the prevention of chronic-pain states.[59] Denial, anxiety, depression, irritability, family problems, sleep disorders, and increasing narcotic use or dependence on alcohol or tranquilizers are frequent indicators[59] and should be actively searched for in trauma victims.

Post-traumatic stress disorder (PTSD) is a state characterized by high levels of anxiety following a traumatic incident. Pain attacks, phobic reactions related to stimuli involving the original traumatic event, and pain symptomatology predominate.[17,59] Certain types of injuries (e.g. burns and electrical shock) seem particularly prone to PTSD-related pain.[63,64] Furthermore, PTSD following electrical burns is more resistant to treatment than PTSD following nonelectrical burns.[65] Symptoms consistent with PTSD in chronic-pain patients are associated with affective distress[66] and depression.[67] The Post-traumatic Chronic Pain Test has been developed as a screening instrument to aid in early detection of PTSD.[68] The Minnesota Multiphasic Personality Inventory has also been used with trauma victims to help distinguish between PTSD and functional disorders.[69]

ACUTE POST-TRAUMATIC PAIN MANAGEMENT

Systemic analgesia

Narcotic analgesics are the mainstay of the analgesic armamentarium for the trauma victim. Intravenous administration is the route of choice. The IV route gives immediate access to the circulation and therefore allows rapid onset of drug action. The use of a continuous IV infusion makes short-acting narcotic administration practical. Thus the infusion rate can be altered to rapidly produce the desired change in plasma level or clinical effect. A steady state can be rapidly achieved with either a bolus dose or a two-rate infusion. In conscious patients patient-controlled analgesia is effective.

Patient-controlled analgesia (PCA) pumps allow the patient to self-administer predetermined aliquots of IV narcotic without the assistance of hospital personnel and the attendant delay in analgesia (see Ch. 11). Appropriate drug, dosage, and lock-out interval selection should permit maintenance of a plasma level with peaks below the toxic level and troughs above the therapeutic level in a manner similar to that of the ideal intravenous infusion. Just as inappropriately low or high infusion rates can lead to either subtherapeutic or toxic plasma drug levels, respectively. Therapeutic failure can also occur with PCA at either extreme. Subtherapeutic levels result when bolus dosages are set too low or lock-out intervals are too long. Toxic levels often result when less lipophilic drugs are selected in an attempt to increase the duration of action from each aliquot injected. The lag between peak levels in the plasma and the central nervous system (CNS) may be significant, and if inappropriately short lock-out intervals are selected, the patient may inject a second or even third dose before the first dose has achieved maximal effect. The addition of a basal infusion along with the PCA mode is a further refinement that is especially beneficial as it reduces sleep disturbance owing to pain.

Wide variation in post-traumatic analgesic requirements can be expected because of pre-existing variations in coping styles,[70] psychological factors,[71] and possibly physiological factors such as individual adenosine, endorphin and substance P levels.[72] Pediatric use of the PCA apparatus is appropriate for children capable of quantifying pain, generally 4 years of age or older. Parent- or nurse-assisted use bypasses the intrinsic safety of this technique.

Systemic analgesia with narcotics can be supplemented with adjunctive intravenous analgesics. Two adjunctive agents that are, in certain circumstances, sufficiently powerful to replace opioids are ketamine and ketorolac. Ketamine produces a profound analgesia and may be used in high doses as the sole agent for emergency and trauma surgery. At lower dosages, it can be used as an analgesic.[73,74] The efficacy of ketamine in the treatment of pain following burn injuries is well known. This may be in part due to ketamine's ability to inhibit central temporal summation.[75] This agent also possesses sympathomimetic action, which may be beneficial in injured patients with a depressed cardiovascular system or shock. Ketamine, however, increases intracranial pressure and is contraindicated in head injuries. Ketorolac is an intravenous nonsteroidal anti-inflammatory agent that can be administered as a bolus or by continuous infusion.[76] The ability to inhibit prostaglandin synthesis makes this drug particularly effective following injury to bone.

In less severe trauma, where alterations in skin and subcutaneous blood flow, gastrointestinal function, and hemodynamic perturbations are less profound, alternative routes of systemic analgesic administration can be considered. Transdermal delivery systems for narcotics take hours to achieve steady state and are not appropriate for acute titration.

REGIONAL ANESTHESIA

Before the application of neural blockade, assess the patient's present physical condition and take a complete history to assure appropriateness of the procedure. It is important to ascertain if the patient has had any past reactions to local anesthetics. Patients scheduled for nerve blocks should refrain from eating 8 hours before the procedure because vomiting may occur either as a psychogenic response or secondary to a systemic reaction. Ambulatory patients need to be transported home; they should not be permitted to drive. Obtain consent only after full disclosure as to the purposes of the blockade, the procedural steps, effect and duration of the medications, and possible side effects and complications. Assure IV access and monitor vital signs. Sedation with a benzodiazepine will allay apprehension and protect the patient from possible systemic reaction by increasing the level for CNS seizure threshold. Calculate in advance the appropriate amount of the drug needed to avoid toxic dose potentials by understanding the anatomic considerations and knowing the optimal site for injection to attain the desired effects with the least amount of local anesthetic solution.

Injection should be unhurried with frequent

Table 4.1   Differential diagnosis of local anesthetic reactions

Etiology	Major clinical features	Comments
Local anesthetic toxicity		
Intravascular injection	Immediate convulsion and/or cardiac toxicity	Injection into vertebral or a carotid artery may cause convulsion after administration of small dose
Relative overdose	Onset in 5–15 min of irritability, progressing to convulsions	
Reaction to vasoconstrictor	Tachycardia, hypertension, headache, apprehension	May vary with vasopressor used
Vasovagal reaction	Rapid onset Bradycardia Hypotension Pallor, faintness	Rapidly reversible with elevation of legs
Allergy		
Immediate	Anaphylaxis ($\downarrow$ BP, bronchospasm, edema)	Allergy to amides extremely rare
Delayed	Urticaria	Cross-allergy possible, e.g. with preservatives in local anesthetics and food
High spinal or epidural block	Gradual onset Bradycardia* Hypotension Possible respiratory agent	May lose consciousness with total spinal block and onset of cardiorespiratory effects more rapid than with high epidural or with subdural block
Concurrent medical episode†	May mimic local anesthetic reaction	Medical history important

*Sympathetic block above T4 adds cardioaccelerator nerve blockade to the vasodilatation seen with blockade below T4, total spinal block may have rapid onset.
†Asthma attack, myocardial infarction.
$\downarrow$ BP, decreased blood pressure.
From Covino BG. Clinical pharmacology of local anesthetic agents. In: Cousins MJ, Bridenbaugh PO, eds. Clinical anesthesia and management of pain. Philadelphia: JB Lippincott; 1988.

aspirations for blood or cerebrospinal fluid (CSF), and multiple test doses are encouraged. Continuous conversation with the patient assures the patient and it also alerts the physician to possible adverse reactions secondary to the drug misplacement. Monitor for adverse reactions or delayed complications; Table 4.1 lists possible reactions. Record a complete summary of the procedure, drug dosages, effects, and adverse reactions. At the end of the procedure debrief the patient about the experience and inform the patient what to do if an untoward reaction occurs.

CHRONIC PAIN MANAGEMENT

General principles of management

The treatment of post-traumatic pain that persists because of deranged patterns of healing, the development of altered pain pathways, chronic ischemia, or the misuse or disuse of myofascial structures is far more complex than the treatment of acute pain syndromes. As previously discussed, the contribution of psychological factors to the interpretation and outward expression of pain must always be considered in chronic pain patients; resultant behavioral changes often contribute to the perpetuation of pain. Furthermore, the group of patients suffering from chronic pain is far from homogeneous. Instead, these patients represent a complex clinical syndrome manifesting varying degrees of psychosocial, physical, and vocational dysfunction. Obviously, no one approach can be expected to achieve the desired goals of reducing pain, improving the quality of life, and reducing dependency on the health care system. Consequently, a goal-oriented, multidisciplinary approach to chronic pain continues to be accepted as essential to proper and cost-effective management of chronic pain.

Such an approach requires not only accurate medical diagnosis, but also behavioral and functional considerations utilized in concert with medical and physical therapeutic modalities. No single mode of treatment can be expected to consistently provide satisfactory results. Protocols using outcome predictors to assign patients into various therapeutic regimes have been developed to aid in structuring treatment plans.

Brena and Chapman[77] provide a conceptually useful template. They classified patients into four clusters and recommended differing approaches to treatment for each group. Patients with low pathology and high behavioral scores (Cluster I) are directed into structured rehabilitation-oriented tracks. Those with low behavioral and low pathology scores (Cluster II) should be offered activities of daily living instruction, relaxation, and self-control and pacing educational tracks. Patients in Clusters III and IV are potential candidates for medically-related intervention. Patients with both high pathology and high behavioral scores (Cluster III) require matched and psychological rehabilitation-directed programs. Patients with low behavioral scores with high pathology scores (Cluster IV) require medically-oriented intervention structured with restraint so as to preserve coping skills as much as possible.

In comparison with acute post-traumatic pain, far fewer chronic pain patients benefit from neural blockade. The basis for use of therapeutic neural blockade in chronic post-traumatic pain involves the following:

1. Interruption of ongoing nociceptive input
2. Interruption of abnormal neurogenic reflex mechanisms
3. Interruption of sympathetic overactivity
4. Relief of muscle spasm and abolition of trigger point activity.

The medications administered by regional block technique for these purposes primarily include local anesthetics, antisympathetic agents, and depot forms of corticosteroid. It cannot be overemphasized that, unlike acute pain, neural blockade is rarely sufficient treatment in and of itself in the chronic pain patient. Even when the aforementioned conditions are present, other methods of treatment should be used concomitantly.

The complexity of chronic pain mechanisms is such that, when compared to the acute pain syndromes previously described, one generally is forced to accept lesser degrees of therapeutic success. Reasonable goals should be discussed frankly with the patient at the onset of treatment and frequently reiterated. Chronic pain management should be directed toward pain control rather than cure, with specific goals that include the following:

1. Reduction in pain and elevation in pain threshold
2. Emphasis on improved function, rehabilitation, and education to prevent overuse injury
3. Finally, and perhaps most importantly, the acute pain model where the passive patient is healed by the active physician must be abandoned in the chronic pain situation. The patient must become the active component and accept the challenge of becoming well. The physician should provide guidance and work to preserve the patient's independent functioning.

DRUGS USED IN ACUTE AND CHRONIC TRAUMA PATIENTS

Narcotics

Narcotics are the mainstay of pain management of severely traumatized patients. The potency, speed of onset, and relative potencies are listed in Table 4.2. Apparent potencies, however, can change over time and can be a function of the route of administration. For example, morphine administered over a long period of time may seem to become more potent; this may be a result of gradual accumulation of active metabolites from the previously administered doses. The potencies listed are based on acute administration only. The potency of a drug used IV will differ from its potency when used by extravascular routes (e.g. oral, rectal), and this is a function of the drug's bioavailability. To convert from a parenteral dosage of a drug to its oral form, divide the parenteral dose by the bioavailability. So a 10 mg IV dose of morphine is approximately equivalent to a 30 mg oral dose based on a bioavailability of 0.3.

Probably of greatest importance in determining the speed of onset of analgesia of systemically administered analgesics is the gradient between blood and brain tissue. Although other factors such as percentage of free, unionized drug in blood and lipid solubility would appear to play a

Table 4.2 Relative potencies of opioid analgesics

Drug	Relative potency (IM)	Relative potency (oral)
Morphine	10	30
Hydromorphone	1.5	7.5
Meperidine	75	300
Methadone	10	12.5
Codeine	120	200
Levorphanol	2	4
Nalbuphine	10	
Oxycodone		30
Pentazocine	60	180

significant role in the rate of drug entry into the CNS, empirically these factors do not correlate to drug onset. For example, alfentanil is known to have a shorter time to onset of drug effect than either fentanyl or morphine. However, fentanyl is over 7 times more lipid soluble than alfentanil, and morphine has 16 times more unionized free drug available to enter the CNS for any given dose. Alfentanil's rapid onset is likely due to its small volume of distribution, which allows a greater blood to brain gradient to persist than either morphine or fentanyl.[78]

All of the opioid agonists have similar clinical effects that vary in degree from one drug to another. In addition to analgesia, sedation, respiratory depression, nausea, constipation, cough suppression, euphoria, dysphoria, and miosis are also known dose-dependent effects of the opioid agonists. The respiratory depression is likely to be the result of μ_2 receptors located in the brainstem.[79]

The gastrointestinal (GI) effects include constipation, nausea, and vomiting. Constipation is likely to be the result of decreased GI transit and an effect on μ_2 receptors within the brain and in the peripheral nerve plexus.[80] The nausea and vomiting are likely to be the result of stimulation of the chemoreceptor trigger zone in the medulla, but it is unclear whether it involves opioid receptors specifically.[81]

Increased tone of smooth muscle sphincters can also occur with opioid use. This has been reported in the sphincter of Oddi but study results conflict. One study demonstrated that morphine produces greater biliary sphincter spasm than meperidine, whereas another demonstrated no significant differences between morphine and meperidine; but fentanyl produced even larger increases in intrabiliary pressure.[82,83]

Typically, opioid agonists have few cardiovas-cular effects at the therapeutic doses in supine patients. At high doses, however, most opioids produce significant bradycardia, probably via medullary vagal stimulation.[84] An exception is meperidine, which can often cause tachycardia, either as a result of its similarity in structure to atropine or via a reflex response to hypotension.[85,86] Morphine may cause tachycardia as a reflex to hypotension resulting from histamine release.[87,88] Histamine release is less with meperidine, sufentanil, and fentanyl.[89]

NONSTEROIDAL ANTI-INFLAMMATORY ANALGESICS

The nonopioid analgesics most often used are the nonsteroidal anti-inflammatory drugs (NSAIDs). In 1984, it was estimated that one in seven Americans was treated with a NSAID.[89] The class of NSAIDs contains compounds that are often chemically unrelated, and they are grouped together based only on their therapeutic actions.[90] Unlike the opioids, NSAIDs do not demonstrate tolerance and are often more effective at controlling certain pain conditions with fewer side effects than the opioids.[91]

Mechanism of action

All NSAIDs have analgesic properties. Traditional teaching indicates that NSAIDs provide analgesia primarily through actions outside the CNS by inhibiting the formation of prostaglandins. When cell membranes are damaged, a class of substances called the *eicosanoids* (which includes arachidonic acid) is released. Arachidonic acid is then broken down by the lipooxygenase system or the cyclooxygenase (also called the prostaglandin synthetase) enzyme system. Although all NSAIDs inhibit cyclooxygenase, several also inhibit lipooxygenase.

The metabolites of the lipooxygenase system are the leukotrienes. Some of the leukotrienes are involved in affecting pain transmission: leukotriene B4 produces thermal hyperalgesia in humans. The cyclooxygenase system produces prostaglandins, which can sensitize nociceptors to respond to what are normally non-noxious stimuli, possibly by altering sodium channel permeability. Prostacyclin (PGI_2), prostaglandin (PGE_1), and PGE_2 are most likely involved in inflammatory pain via promotion of the response of nociceptors to other inflammatory mediators.

However, more research has been indicating that NSAIDs may produce analgesia at least partially through a mechanism in the CNS.[92–96] NSAIDs cross the blood–brain barrier to enter the CNS, sometimes in proportion to plasma concentrations.[97] The central mechanisms of NSAIDs to produce analgesia may involve facilitation of the descending pathways involved in pain inhibition or possible inhibition of peripheral inflammation through nonprostaglandin mechanisms in the CNS.[95,98] Furthermore, there is evidence that NSAIDs have cellular effects unrelated to the synthesis of prostaglandins, such as inhibiting the release of inflammatory mediators from neutrophils and macrophages.[99]

Evidence has indicated that the analgesic response to a particular NSAID will vary depending on the individual. The mean response of a population is the same for all NSAIDs, but the individual response can be highly variable. This is reflected in clinical situations where patients respond well to some NSAIDs and do not respond to others.[100,101] Some studies have stated that, because of the interpatient variability in side effects and efficacy, other drugs are necessary to provide a reasonable range of alternative therapy.[102]

Specific drugs
Salicylates

Aspirin. Aspirin is the most studied and commonly used NSAID. Aspirin has an elimination half-life that changes from 2.5 hours at low doses to 19 hours at high doses. It is well absorbed in the stomach and small intestine, with peak blood levels 1 hour after an oral dose. There is then rapid conversion of aspirin to salicylates from high first-pass effect, which occurs in both the wall of the small intestine and the liver.

Diflunisal. Diflunisal is possibly better tolerated in the GI system because it is not metabolized to salicylic acid in plasma. It has a short half-life relative to aspirin.

Choline magnesium trisalicylate and salsalate. Both are nonacetylated salicylates that have minimal effect on platelet function and less effect on GI mucosa than their acetylated counterparts. They produce similar analgesia and blood levels of salicylate to those of the acetylated class.

Acetaminophen. Acetaminophen is a para-aminophenol derivative with analgesic and antipyretic properties similar to those of aspirin. Antipyresis is likely from direct action on the hypothalamic heat-regulating centers via inhibiting action of endogenous pyrogen. Although equipotent to aspirin in inhibiting central prostaglandin synthesis, acetaminophen has no significant peripheral prostaglandin synthetase inhibition. Doses of 650 mg have been shown to be more effective than doses of 300 mg but little additional benefit is seen at doses above 650 mg, indicating a possible ceiling effect. It has few side effects in the usual dosage range; no significant GI toxicity or platelet functional changes occur with acetaminophen use. It is almost entirely metabolized in the liver, and the minor metabolites are responsible for the hepatotoxicity seen in overdose. Inducers of the P-450 enzyme system in the liver (such as alcohol) increase the formation of metabolites and therefore increase hepatotoxicity.

Acetic acid derivatives. This group of NSAIDs contains two subclasses: pyrroleacetic acids and phenylacetic acids (of which only diclofenac is approved for use in the USA so far).

Indomethacin. Indomethacin has good oral and rectal absorption although the extent of absorption varies widely between patients. There is also a large interpatient variability in elimination half-life, caused by extensive enterohepatic recirculation of the drug. Its clinical use is somewhat limited by a relatively high incidence of side effects.

Sulindac. Sulindac was the result of a search for a drug similar to indomethacin but with less toxicity. The lower GI toxicity with sulindac may be because sulindac is an inactive prodrug that is converted after absorption by liver microsomal enzymes to sulindac disulfide, which appears to be the active metabolite. However, one study demonstrated a relatively high rate of GI hemorrhage with sulindac.[103] As mentioned previously, sulindac was considered in previous studies to be the least nephrotoxic of the NSAIDs, but more recent studies have failed to support that contention.[104,105]

Tometin and etodolac. Both of these drugs claim fewer side effects than other NSAIDs.

Ketorolac. Ketorolac is currently the only parenteral NSAID for clinical analgesic use in the USA.

Although indomethacin has been available as an injectable form for years, it was pursued only in low dose as a treatment for patent ductus arteriosus. Ketorolac demonstrates analgesia well beyond anti-inflammatory properties that are between those of indomethacin and naproxen; but ketorolac can provide analgesia 50 times that of naproxen. It has antipyretic effects 20 times that of aspirin and thus can mask temperatures when given routinely to patients postoperatively. Several studies have demonstrated efficacy comparable to or exceeding that of morphine for moderate postoperative pain treatment but with fewer side effects.[106,107] Although ketorolac prolongs bleeding time, it does not do so excessively; however, case reports of postoperative bleeding associated with intraoperative ketorolac use have been reported.[108,109] Oral ketorolac was approved for use in the USA approximately 3 years after the parenteral form and has an efficacy similar to that of naproxen and ibuprofen.[110] However, the parenteral form is given in a loading dose of 60 mg followed by 30 mg IM every 6 hours, whereas the oral dose is limited to 10 to 20 mg because of GI toxicity.

Diclofenac. Diclofenac differs from the other NSAIDs by having a high first-pass effect and hence a lower oral bioavailability. As mentioned previously, it may also have a significantly higher incidence of hepatotoxicity than the other NSAIDs. A parenteral form has been used in Europe, and one study showed it is effective in reducing opioid requirements and pain after thoracotomies.[111]

Propionic acid derivatives. This class contains ibuprofen, fenoprofen, ketoprofen, flurbiprofen, and naproxen. A newer drug in this class is oxaprozin, which has received attention because it has a once-daily dosing; but it has no other distinct advantage over other NSAIDs.

Oxicam derivatives. The only NSAID in this class in clinical use is piroxicam. Unlike other NSAIDs, it has a slow time to peak serum concentration following oral dosing of 5.5 hours. It is also notable for its long elimination half-life of 48.5 hours, so it may take up to 1 week to achieve steady state blood concentrations, although it does also allow for once-daily dosing.

Pyrazolone derivatives. The only drug in clinical use in this class is phenylbutazone. Although phenylbutazone is a very effective anti-inflammatory and analgesic, it has been associated with aplastic anemias and agranulocytosis; therefore it

cannot be recommended for long-term use. It is thus not often clinically used.

Anthranilic acid derivatives. These NSAIDs are unique because they block prostaglandin synthesis and the tissue response to prostaglandins. Mefenamic acid has been associated with severe pancytopenia and many other side effects. Therefore therapy cannot be used for more than 1 week.[112] Meclofenamate also has a high incidence of GI toxicity, so it is not a first-line drug.

Naphthyl-alkanones. This new class of NSAID is most noted for being a nonacidic chemical structure unlike other clinically used NSAIDs. Some describe the structure as similar to naproxen. The only clinically available NSAID in this class is nabumetone. Studies have shown that its use results in fewer gastric lesions than aspirin, naproxen, or ibuprofen. Also, doses of 1 g/day for 7 days in volunteers resulted in no change in bleeding time. Only 35% of the drug is converted to its active form after oral administration. None of the parent drug can be measured in plasma after oral administration because of the rapid biotransformation that occurs during first-pass, which makes nabumetone a prodrug.[113]

COX 2 Inhibitors. NSAIDS work by inhibiting prostaglandin synthesis. As a result, an anti-inflammatory, analgesic, and antipyretic effect is seen after administration. While many patients benefit from the use of NSAIDS, at times their use is limited because of side effects such as platelet dysfunction, gastrointestinal distress, ulceration or bleeding, or renal dysfunction. The prevention of prostaglandin synthesis from NSAIDS is mediated through the inhibition of the cyclooxygenase pathway. There appear to be two cyclooxygenase pathways; cyclooxygenase 1 affecting platelet and GI function, and cyclooxygenase 2 that is associated with inflammation and pain. Specific cyclooxygenase 2 inhibitors (COX 2 inhibitors) have just been introduced. The hope is that the side effects of platelet dysfunction and gastrointestinal distress will be avoided when these drugs are utilized. Their ability to selectively block pain and inflammation without causing side effects remains to be seen as these drugs begin to be utilized by large numbers of patients. The effect on kidney function also remains to be determined.

ANTI-DEPRESSANTS

Most review articles conclude that either the use of anti-depressants for various pain states is widespread but not well supported[114–118] or that they have special utility in treating chronic pain.[117,118] All reviewers mention the relationship between the monoamine hypothesis of affective disorders and the role these compounds are thought to have in the descending pain inhibitory pathways.[114–120] In a review attempting to explain the mechanism of action of the anti-depressants in pain relief, Feinmann[119] postulated three possibilities:

1. alleviation of overlying depression, which intensified the suffering of the individual;
2. a common underlying biochemical substrate integral to the experience of pain and depression;
3. neuromodulatory effects of these drugs on the endogenous opioid systems. Despite much research, all three of these explanations have some merit, and the definitive answer awaits discovery.

Max et al[121] published an important article that employed an 'active' placebo, i.e. a formulation (anticholinergic, with sedative added in early part of study) that mimicked the side effects of amitriptyline. The two compounds were given to patients with diabetic neuropathy over a 6-week period. They found that amitriptyline was associated with significant improvement in pain of neuropathy, regardless of the affective state of the patient. The analgesia from amitriptyline was not associated with altered mood. A similar finding was obtained using low (30 mg) and high (150 mg) dose amitriptyline versus placebo in chronic facial pain.[122] This study found analgesia independent of mood effects. These studies would argue for a mechanism independent of depression alleviation.

Davis et al[123] published one of the first reports citing that amitriptyline or fluphenazine, alone or in combination, provided a significant reduction in pain. This series of eight cases showed that pain relief ensued within days (5 or less). The pain relief occurred much sooner than the usual lag time between instituting an antidepressant and the depression response, which is generally 1 to 2 weeks.

This brief overview of a few of the many studies that have been done would indicate that the antidepressants, alone or in combination with other drugs such as neuroleptics, can be beneficial to the patient suffering from a variety of painful conditions.

Guidelines for using anti-depressants

The monoamine oxidase inhibitors, although useful in some types of chronic pain, should not be recommended to patients by the nonpsychiatric physician because of their pharmacologic side effects and medicolegal ramifications. Concomitant use of these drugs with other anti-depressants has been associated with a syndrome of rigidity, hyperthermia, and seizures.

When selecting an anti-depressant for use in pain management, the problems experienced by the patient should be matched with the drug most likely to have an effect on that problem. Most pain patients will, for example, have poor sleep patterns. This would lead one to select a tertiary amine tricyclic or trazodone. As many chronic pain patients are very somatically focused, it is important to start the medications slowly and to inform the patient of what the future side effects are likely to be. It is also helpful to inform patients that, in general, anti-depressants are associated with 'nuisance' side effects as opposed to serious effects. Fortunately, most patients will develop rapid tolerance to the daytime sedation that is commonly experienced when starting a sedating antidepressant. Sleep effects are frequently noted on the first dose.

Antimuscarinic tolerance typically takes weeks and can be a reason for stopping the drugs. Tolerance to the analgesic effects has not been reported. Long-term use of these drugs is generally safe, but withdrawal must be gradual to avoid insomnia and abdominal discomfort. Gradually decreasing the dosage for 1 to 2 weeks is usually sufficient to obviate any significant withdrawal phenomena.

To institute anti-depressants for pain treatment, start with 25 mg of amitriptyline or an equivalent dosage of another compound, to be taken about 1 to 2 hours before sleep. If the individual is frail, elderly, or predisposed to untoward side effects, a starting dose of 10 mg would be appropriate. This should be monitored and increased every few days by 25 mg as needed. Any signs of toxicity should prompt a serum level determination. It must be stressed to pain patients that these drugs have some potential to reduce pain but are not typical analgesics, and must therefore be taken on a fixed schedule to have a predictable effect. For pain management the dose is 25–50 mg. However, if administered for depression higher doses are used.

To summarize, anti-depressants are used as one part of a comprehensive approach to the management of pain and its associated problems. They have analgesic activity, are nonaddicting hypnotics and anxiolytics, and may enhance ulcer healing. They have a myriad of pharmacologic actions, and this must be recognized by the prescribing physician. Serum levels are useful in determining compliance or toxicity but have not yet been correlated to efficacy in pain treatment. These drugs are highly protein bound. Therefore the potential for pharmacokinetic alterations by disease states and co-administration of other drugs must be considered.

NEUROLEPTICS

Few publications have speculated on the precise mechanism of action in regard to analgesia. Most studies that have shown some efficacy have been difficult to interpret as a result of small numbers, mixed diagnoses, or a variety of drugs and dosing schedules. There is a trend, however, to suggest that these drugs may have some usefulness in diabetic neuropathy[123,124] and postherpetic neuralgia.[116,125,126] Many studies employed a combination of an anti-depressant and a neuroleptic, making the therapeutic agent difficult to specify,[123,124,126,127] and it is possible that the neuroleptic exerted an effect by increasing serum levels of the anti-depressants.[128]

Clarke reviewed his experiences with the combination of amitriptyline and perphenazine in 120 patients with various diagnoses.[129] The daily dose was 25 mg of the anti-depressant and 2 mg of perphenazine each morning, and double doses of each at night. 10 patients were withdrawn because of unacceptable side effects (dry mouth, urinary retention, drowsiness, and dissociation). The remainder completed the 2-month study period. Of 13 patients, 7 had postherpetic neuralgia, and 10 of 19 patients with postsurgical scar pain were 'improved'. Results were not as good with failed laminectomies and other diagnoses. Overall, 33.6% of the patients improved to such a degree that no other treatment was deemed necessary.

Methotrimeprazine has been studied by numerous French investigators and has been felt to have analgesic properties. Montilla et al, in one of the earliest American studies, compared methotrimeprazine to morphine in 105 patients with a variety of diagnoses, from postherpetic neuralgia to cancer to coronary occlusion.[130] They used a double-blind design, and all assessments of pain in a given patient were done by the same investigator. Morphine 10 mg or methotrimeprazine 15 mg was

administered subcutaneously. In addition, 44 patients received the opiate and 61 patients received the neuroleptic during the study period. The methotrimeprazine group had a greater average pain score initially (3.18 versus 2.09 on a 0 to 4 scale) but had similar postdrug scores throughout the 4-hour observation period (approximately 1.5).

Guidelines for using neuroleptics

When choosing a neuroleptic for use in pain management, weigh the risk of side effects against possible benefit. Although this is sound policy for any medical decision, it is especially important here because tardive dyskinesia can be permanent. Prudence would dictate starting an anti-depressant first and adding a neuroleptic only if there was no change in pain after the patient's sleep pattern had normalized. At that point, there is no clear indication of which drug to add. Higher-potency drugs offer the advantage of little daytime sedation but have higher risks of side effects mediated through dopaminergic blockade. Low-potency drugs may enhance sleep but have high antimuscarinic and alpha-adrenergic blockade. Perphenazine can be co-administered with amitriptyline in one formulation, which may enhance compliance but decreases dosing flexibility. Methotrimeprazine can cause sedation and hypotension, but in a nonambulatory terminal cancer patient, this may not be an issue. All of the neuroleptics can raise prolactin levels over time.

Neuroleptics should be instituted gradually, starting at night and increasing the dose to include daytime doses only if nocturnal administration is inadequate for symptom control. Monitor frequently for the development of akathisia, cogwheel rigidity, and orthostatic hypotension. A family history of Parkinson's disease may indicate a greater propensity for these adverse reactions from these drugs.

To summarize, the neuroleptic drugs may have some benefit in pain management, especially in regard to neuropathic pain syndromes. Presently, there are no reasons to choose one particular drug; physician experience and side-effect profile appear to be the deciding factors.

ANTICONVULSANTS

Swerdlow has compiled the most extensive review of efficacy in pain management to date.[131] Hatangdi et al reported on the treatment of 34 patients with postherpetic neuralgia who had been symptomatic for months to years and half-experiencing symptoms for more than a decade.[132] Many of these patients had received neuroleptics without benefit. They used carbamazepine in therapeutic blood levels supplemented with nortriptyline 50–100 mg per day in divided doses. Of the 34 subjects, 18 (53%) had complete relief on this regimen, 9 had 'good' relief, 3 had 'partial' relief, and 4 discontinued the drugs because of side effects from either agent.

Young & Clarke used an algorithmic approach to the treatment of diabetic neuropathy, where clonazepam was the only anticonvulsant and the last drug employed and was used only after failure of simple analgesics, two different antidepressants, and one of two neuroleptics.[133] They studied 80 patients, and three progressed through the protocol to enter the clonazepam phase of the study. Two of the patients obtained relief and commented that clonazepam was useful in treating the syndrome of restless legs.

Bouckoms & Litman treated 21 patients who had symptoms suggestive of deafferentation pain, with clonazepam in a range of 1–4 mg per night.[134] Six of the study group responded with 'marked or complete' relief. Of the 12 who met several of their criteria for deafferentation pain, the 6 who responded to treatment had allodynia as a presenting finding, while 5 of the 6 who were nonresponders to clonazepam did not have allodynia. Based on these results, Bouckoms & Litman suggested that allodynia may be predictive of clonazepam responsiveness.

Summary

Even though anticonvulsants have significant potential side effects, they can be useful in the management of pain that has been refractory to other therapy. They appear to be particularly useful in the treatment of neuropathic pain states. Anticonvulsants are considered the treatment of choice in trigeminal neuralgia and are gaining status in the management of other neuralgias. Serum levels have generally not been correlated with pain response, but toxicity concerns mandate using established ranges as target levels.

SEDATIVE–HYPNOTICS AND ANXIOLYTICS

Few studies focus on the use of benzodiazepines in pain management. Diazepam is commonly used to treat the muscle spasm and pain presumed to arise from pain problems.[135,136]

Singh et al studied the effects of acute postoperative administration of diazepam in a group of 35 patients who underwent upper abdominal surgery.[137] After fully recovering from a standardized anesthetic technique, baseline pain ratings were obtained. They were randomized into groups receiving either morphine 10 mg, diazepam 10 mg, or a mixture of 5 mg of each IM. They found indistinguishable relief at 30 minutes postinjection, but thereafter diazepam alone was not as effective and caused more pain at the injection site than either of the other two treatment options.

Hollister et al studied 108 neurosurgical clinic patients who had been taking diazepam in doses of 5–40 mg per day for up to 16 years.[136] The drug was being taken for muscle spasms in 36% of the cases, as an analgesic in 30% and for nerves and to aid sleep in 34% of patients with pain and spasm.

Alprazolam appears to be unique among this class in that it seems to have particular efficacy in the treatment of panic disorder and has demonstrated an antidepressant efficacy in several placebo-controlled, double-blind, multicenter studies.[138–140] The mean doses for antidepressant action were 2.87 and 3.0 mg per day in two studies by Feighner and Rickels.[139,140] With the exception of drowsiness occurring in some patients, alprazolam was associated with fewer side effects than the tricyclic antidepressants used in the studies.

The anxiolytics are commonly used by patients suffering from chronic pain, despite little evidence to substantiate that use. The benzodiazepines are useful when given for a limited time for acute anxiety and insomnia. The risk of dependence and withdrawal may be greater in the chronic-pain population. Alprazolam appears to have some unique assets, but also has all of the drawbacks of this class, including the particular difficulty in discontinuing.[141] Buspirone lacks many of the disadvantages of the other drugs in this section but has not demonstrated any efficacy as an analgesic to date.

ANTIHISTAMINES AND MUSCLE RELAXANTS

Hydroxyzine has been studied as a potent analgesic that lacks respiratory depression. At the First

World Congress on Pain, Beaver & Feise reported their results of a study involving 96 postoperative patients who received placebo, 8 mg of morphine, 100 mg of hydroxyzine or the same doses of both active drugs simultaneously. All drugs were given IM on one occasion in the early postoperative period, and the patients were questioned hourly for pain ratings for 6 hours after placebo, but there was no significant difference between the response curves of morphine and hydroxyzine. Furthermore the combination had an additive rather than synergistic effect. This relationship also held when the patients were stratified by the severity of their baseline pain.[140]

Hydroxyzine 100 mg combined with morphine 10 mg provided superior analgesia over morphine alone in 82 postoperative patients who were enrolled in a double-blind, single-dose study.[142] The combination also provided better pain relief than morphine 5 mg by itself or combined with 100 mg of hydroxyzine. Larger doses of morphine and hydroxyzine in combination produced more drowsiness than any of the other treatments.

Studies of efficacy of the skeletal muscle relaxants generally showed some improvement in acute muscle problems versus placebo.[143] Evidence of effect in chronic cases is less convincing; only cyclobenzaprine showed possible benefit.[143] Elenbaas concluded that there was no evidence to suggest superiority of any particular drug, or to suggest superiority of these drugs over sedatives or analgesics.

Hydroxyzine has inherent analgesic properties that may be clinically relevant but has a ceiling effect that does not warrant the use of the drug in doses beyond 150 mg. The skeletal muscle relaxants have been inadequately studied, given their frequency of use. They are probably effective for acute muscle problems but do not appear to have utility in chronic pain syndromes. Care must be used in prescribing cyclobenzaprine because of its long half-life and its antimuscarinic effects.

LOCAL ANESTHETICS

The placement of local anesthetics at various sites along the neural axis to produce anesthesia or analgesia is classified as *regional anesthesia*. The application of these techniques is used for surgical

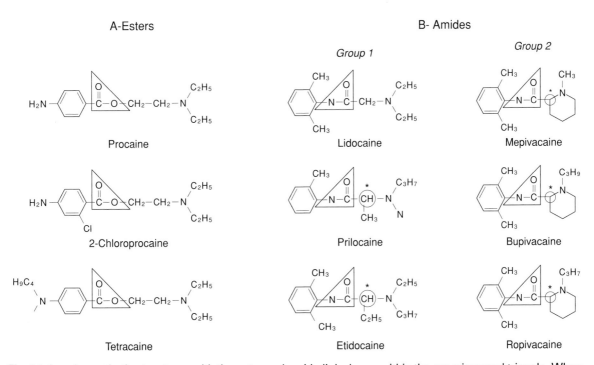

Fig. 4.1 Local anesthetic structures with the ester and amide link shown within the superimposed triangle. When present, the asymmetric carbon is circled, shaded, and marked with an asterisk (*). From DiFazio CA, Woods AM. Pharmacology of local anesthetics. In Raj PP (ed): Practical Management of Pain, 2nd ed. St. Louis, Mosby, 1992.

anesthesia and postoperative analgesia and as acute or chronic pain management modalities.

Local anesthetics can be used in combination or with other adjuvant medications in order to potentiate speed of onset and duration of action or to increase the intensity of anesthesia or analgesia. It is important to know the pharmacology of these medications in order to select the appropriate drug for a specific therapeutic task.

The chemical structure determines metabolism and elimination of these drugs from the body. Local anesthetics exist in two chemical forms, amino esters and amino amides (Fig. 4.1). Amino esters are ester derivatives of para-aminobenzoic acid and are metabolized by plasma cholinesterase. The metabolic byproduct is para-aminobenzoic acid, which is a known allergen; and allergic reactions are therefore not uncommon. On the other hand, amino amides are compounds with amide linkages and are metabolized for the most part by the liver. The potentials for allergic reactions are extremely rare.

Local anesthetics can also be classified on the basis of their clinical properties[144] into three basic categories:

1. Low potency/short duration, e.g. procaine, 2-chloroprocaine
2. Intermediate potency/intermediate duration, e.g. lidocaine, mepivacaine, prilocaine
3. High potency/long duration, e.g. bupivacaine, tetracaine, etidocaine.

The difference in clinical activities among the local anesthetics can be explained by both their inherent physicochemical properties.

Physical and chemical properties

Lipid solubility, protein binding, and pK_a of the local anesthetic agents are important factors that directly influence potency, onset of action, and duration of action (Table 4.3). In addition, some local anesthetics exist as chemical isomers (chiral forms) and may further create differences in their inherent activity and toxicity.

Lipid solubility

The potency of a local anesthetic is influenced in a nonlinear manner by its lipid solubility.[145] The more lipid soluble a local anesthetic is, then the more potent the local anesthetic effect. The major determinant of the lipid solubility is the aromatic group (benzene ring) found on the local anesthetic molecule. The measurement of solubility is performed by studying the base form's solubility in organic solvents. However, experimental evaluations of solubility differ from clinical effect in that local anesthetics' clinical potency increases to a point and then levels off. This leveling off occurs at a lipid partition coefficient of about four. The plateauing of clinical potency has been surmised to be related to the surrounding fat and blood vessel adjacent to the nerve. These may act as a depot and pull local anesthetic away thereby decreasing the total amount of drug available to the nerve.

Protein binding

Local anesthetics bind to both plasma proteins as well as tissue proteins. Local anesthetic with a high protein-binding capacity will stay on the protein receptor for a longer time, producing an increased duration of effect. Also, when these molecules are bound to the plasma proteins, they are not pharmacologically active; and this has implications on their activity, toxicity, and metabolism. The two main binding plasma proteins are albumin and α_1-acid glycoprotein. α_1-acid glycoprotein is described as having a high affinity, low

Table 4.3 Physical properties and equipotent concentrations of local anesthetics

	Procaine	Lidocaine	Mepivacaine	Bupivacaine	Etidocaine	Ropivacaine
Molecular weight	236	234	246	288	276	274
pK_a	8.9	7.7	7.6	8.1	7.7	8.0
Lipid solubility	1	4	1	30	140	2.8
Partition coefficient	0.02	2.9	0.8	28	141	9
Protein binding	5	65	75	95	95	90–95
Equipotent conc ck		2.0	1.5	0.5	1.0	0.75

From DiFazio CA, Woods AM. Pharmacology of local anesthetics. In: Raj PP, ed. Practical management of pain. 2nd ed. St Louis: Mosby; 1992.

capacity for binding with the local anesthetics; whereas albumin has a lower affinity and higher capacity. In other words, albumin, which has less affinity, will bind larger amounts of the local anesthetics long after the α_1-acid glycoprotein capacity to bind has been maximized. This capacity for binding the local anesthetics is concentration-dependent and decreases in a curvilinear manner as concentration increases. The clinical importance of this is that the potential for toxicity increases disproportionately with increased plasma concentrations.

Protein binding is also influenced by the pH of the plasma. The percentage of the bound drug decreases as the pH decreases. Therefore, in acidotic states, for a given total concentration there is an increase fraction of free active drug found in the circulation; and this potentiates the toxicity. This occurs at the receptor proteins in the sodium channels as well and may decrease duration of the local anesthetic effect.

Ionization

It is the amino acid group on the local anesthetic molecule that determines the ionization of the molecule and, thus, the hydrophilic activity. This amino group is capable of accepting a hydrogen ion (H^+), and in so doing converts the unionized base form of the drug into the cationic form of the drug. The proportions of these forms present in solution are determined by the pK_a of the drug and the pH of the solution. The pK_a is defined as the pH where 50% of the local anesthetic will remain in the uncharged (basic) form and 50% will exist in the charged (cationic) form. This relationship between the pH and the pK_a and the concentrations of the cation and the base forms is described by the Henderson–Hasselbach equation:

$$pK_a = pH + \log(\text{cation/base})$$

The pK_a is important in determining the speed of onset of the local anesthetic. It is believed that the unionized form is responsible for diffusion across the nerve membrane and the ionized form produces blockade of the sodium ion movement through the sodium channel by binding to the receptor proteins. Hence, both uncharged and charged forms are important for local anesthetic neural blockade. For local anesthetics the pK_a falls within a narrow range, 7.6 to 8.9; thus, these drugs at equilibrium exist predominantly in the cationic form at normal pH. Even still, agents with a pK_a closest to the body's pH will have the fastest onset of action since a major portion will exist in the uncharged forms.

Chiral forms

The identification of stereoisomers for some of the local anesthetics like bupivacaine, mepivacaine, etidocaine, prilocaine, and ropivacaine has led to further evaluations into potential differences in potency, toxicity, and duration between them. For stereoisomers to exist, an asymmetric carbon atom must be present in the molecule. The nomenclature used to describe these isomers has changed in recent years and now terms like 'D' and 'L' have been replaced by 'R' and 'S' respectively. Details for these differences are noted in Table 4.4, but as a rule the 'S' form is less toxic and has a longer duration of anesthesia.

Mechanisms of local anesthetic function

Local anesthetics act on the membrane by interfering with its ability to undergo the specific changes that result in the altered permeability to Na^+. Thus, local anesthetics increase the threshold for electrical excitation in the nerve, slow the propagation of the impulse, reduce the rate of rise of the action potential, and eventually block the conduction. Several theories have been postulated over the years as to the exact mechanism of local anesthetics.

Presently, the most popular theories are the combination of the receptor[146] and the membrane expansion theories[147] (Fig. 4.2) The membrane expansion theory states that local anesthetic in its uncharged base form dissolves in the nerve membrane, causing an expansion of the membrane. This produces conformational changes between the proteins and

Table 4.4 Anesthetic duration and toxicity of local anesthetic isomers

Drug	Duration Toxicity
Etidocaine	S = RS = R
Mepivacaine	S > RS = R
Bupivacaine	S > RS < R
Ropivacaine	S > RS < R

From DiFazio CA, Woods AM. Pharmacology of local anesthetics. In: Raj PP, ed. Practical management of pain. 2nd ed. St Louis: Mosby; 1992.

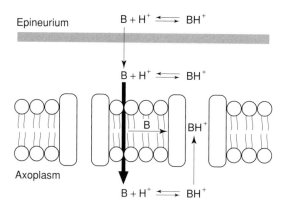

Fig. 4.2 Local anesthetic access to the sodium channel. The unchanged molecule diffuses most easily across lipid barriers and interacts with the channel through the axolemma interior. The charged species formed in the axoplasm gains access to a specific receptor via the sodium channel pore. From Carpenter RL, Mackey DC. Local anesthetics. In Barash PG, Cullen BF, Stoelting RK (eds): Clinical Anesthesia. Phildelphia, JB Lippincott, 1989, p. 510.

Table 4.5 Effects of dose and epinephrine on local anesthetic properties

	Increased dose (concentration or volume)	Addition of epinephrine
Onset time	↓	(Minimal effect for etidocaine)
Degree of motor blockade	↑	
Degree of sensory blockade	↑	
Duration of blockade	↑	
Area of blockade	↑	
Peak plasma concentration	↑	

↓, decrease; ↑, increase.
From Covino BG. Clinical pharmacology of local anesthetic agents. In: Cousins MJ, Bridenbaugh PO, eds. Clinical anesthesia and management of pain. Philadelphia: JB Lippincott; 1988.

their association with the membrane lipids; and results in the partial collapse of these ionic channels, thus impeding the passage of Na+ ions.

The receptor theories basically state that the local anesthetics bind to receptors at the cell membrane and prevent the opening of channels or pores for the passage of ions.

The local anesthetics are believed to diffuse through the lipid bilayer structure of the cell membrane in their lipid-soluble, uncharged base form. They then equilibrate in the axoplasm of the nerve into the charged cationic and uncharged form in accordance with the drug's pK_a and the pH of the axoplasm. It is the cationic form that then enters the Na+ channel from the intracellular side, binds to the anionic site within the Na+ channel, and physically or ionically blocks the movement of the Na+ ions. Therefore, the local anesthetic prevents the action potential from developing in the nerve by inhibition of the movement of Na+ into the cell. The resulting effect is a nondepolarization block, similar to the action of curare at the neuromuscular junction.

Factors that effect blockade
Volume and concentration

The total amount of agent will dictate the onset, quality, and duration of the block; such that with

increasing doses of local anesthetic one can make the onset faster and the duration longer (Table 4.5). Using the same volume, rapid onset, better quality, and duration of the block are observed with increasing concentration or volume of local anesthetics.[148,149] On the other hand, it has been shown with epidural blockade that, when the concentration is varied and the volume is adjusted in order to maintain the same milligram dosage, there is no difference noted in the onset, duration, and quality of the block; however, the spread of the block may be higher when using the larger volume. It must also be noted that the potential for increased serum levels and toxicity is also seen with increased dosage.

Addition of vasoconstrictor agents

The addition of epinephrine, norepinephrine and phenylephrine is frequently used with different local anesthetics to hasten onset and improve the quality and duration of the analgesia[150] (see Table 4.6). These drugs reverse the known intrinsic vasodilatation effects found among most of the local anesthetics. Vasoconstriction caused by these chemicals will reduce the absorption of the local anesthetics hence more agent is available for neural blockade.

Site of the injection

The proximity to the nervous tissues and the anatomical structures can influence onset, duration,

Table 4.6 Comparative onset times and analgesic durations of various local anesthetic agents and effects of epinephrine (5 microg/mL) on duration and peak plasma levels (C_{max})

Anesthetic technique	Anesthetic agent	Usual conc.(%)	Average onset time (min ± SE)	Average analgesic duration (min ± SE)	Addition of EPI* % Change	
					duration	C_{max}
Brachial plexus block	Lidocaine	1.0	14 ± 4	195 ± 26	+ 50	−20–30
(40–50 mL)	Mepivacaine	1.0	15 ± 6	245 ± 27	−	−20–30
	Bupivacaine	0.25–0.5	10–25	575	−	−10–20
	Etidocaine	0.5	9	572	−	−10–20
Epidural anesthesia	Lidocaine	2.0	15	100 ± 20	+ 50	−20–30
(20–30 mL)	Mepivacaine	2.0	15	115 ± 15	+ 50	−20–30
	Bupivacaine	0.5	17	195 ± 30	+ 0–30	−10–20
	Etidocaine	1.0	11	170 ± 57	+ 0–30	−10–20
Local infiltration	Lidocaine	0.5		75 (35–340)	+ 200	−50
	Mepivacaine	0.5		108 (15–240)	+ 120	−
	Bupivacaine	0.25		200 ± 33	+ 115	−

*5 microg/mL; C_{max}, peak plasma levels; SE, standard error.
From Carpenter RL, Mackey DC. Local anesthetics. In: Barash PG, Cullen BF, Stoelting RK, eds. Clinical anesthesia. Philadelphia: JB Lippincott; 1989, p. 522.

and peak serum levels. For example, the subarachnoid route of administration has a faster onset than an epidural placement.

Decreased duration of effect and increased serum levels of local anesthetics are related to the amount of blood flow at the site of injection. The potential for these effects is listed in decreasing order: intercostal, caudal, epidural, brachial plexus and then sciatic or femoral nerves.[151]

Bicarbonation and carbonation of local anesthetics

The addition of bicarbonate to local anesthetics is associated with faster onset and spread of the block. Local anesthetics are often supplied at low pH to prolong the shelf life. The addition of bicarbonate will increase the pH of these solutions and ultimately the percentage of the uncharged form that is important for diffusion through the nerve membrane.

The mixing of CO_2 (700 mmHg) with local anesthetic will also shorten the onset time, but by a different mechanism. The CO_2 diffuses rapidly across the axonal membrane and thus decreases the intracellular pH.[152] This will increase the concentration of the charged form of the local anesthetic, which is important for receptor binding and neural blockade.

Temperature

Warming local anesthetic has been observed to reduce the onset of epidural blockade because the elevation of the temperature decreases the pK_a of the drug.[153]

Pregnancy

The requirements for local anesthetic in parturients have been observed to be decreased compared to their nonpregnant counterparts.[154] Onset has been shown to be faster with the use of epidural and spinal anesthesia, or peripheral nerve blocks. Progesterone is suspected to possibly be a factor in this reported effect.[155]

Combination of local anesthetics

The combining of local anesthetics is utilized to hasten the onset of action, as well as to improve the quality of block. However, this may not always be the case. For example, the addition of 2-chloroprocaine with bupivacaine improves the onset and quality of the sensory block; however, the combination has been shown to shorten the duration of bupivacaine. This may occur from interference by 2-chloroprocaine or its metabolites with the binding of bupivacaine to the receptors.[156]

Specific local anesthetics

Esters

Cocaine is a rather complex alkaloid originally obtained from the Peruvian coca plant. Cocaine is used solely for topical anesthesia. Because of its unique vasoconstrictive action, which is related to its abilities to inhibit the reuptake of norepinephrine, it is especially useful during procedures on the oral and nasal cavities. Addiction and high toxicity are the main drawbacks to its use. Metabolism occur by two pathways of hydrolysis, but 20% is still excreted in the urine unchanged.

Amino amides

Lidocaine (Xylocaine, Lignocaine) remains the most versatile and commonly-used local anesthetic because of its inherent potency, rapid onset, and moderate duration of action. It is used in infiltration, peripheral nerve block, and epidural, spinal and topical anesthesia. Administered IV it acts as a systemic analgesic for blunting the response to intubation in the operating room and in the treatment of certain chronic pain syndromes secondary to its direct effects on the CNS. Generally, the duration of lidocaine is 1 to 3 hours for various regional anesthetic procedures; however, the addition of epinephrine to the dosage will increase its onset, extend the duration and at the same time decrease its toxicity by limiting peak levels in the serum. Lidocaine is metabolized in the liver and, although the metabolites are excreted by the biliary tree, they are reabsorbed by the circulation only to be excreted in the urine. Only a small portion of lidocaine is excreted in the urine unchanged.

Bupivacaine (Marcaine, Sensorcaine) is a butyl derivative of a ringed piperidine carboxylic acid amide. It is used in infiltration, peripheral nerve block and epidural and spinal anesthesia; but not for topical anesthesia. Bupivacaine has a duration that is two to three times longer then lidocaine but so is its toxicity. It is this severe toxic profile that prevents its use for IV regional anesthesia or as a systemic anesthetic. Because it offers excellent differential blockade between different nerve fibers, it has gained popularity for use in obstetric, acute postoperative, and chronic pain anesthetic techniques. Its longest duration of action occurs when it is used for peripheral nerve blockade and then it has been reported to last up to hours or even

longer. The addition of epinephrine does influence its vascular absorption and its effect on target sites. Other facts of interest are that, as an intrathecal agent, it has a better satisfactory anesthetic effect than tetracaine, and reportedly less potential for hypotensive side effects. Also, the degree of motor blockade is greater when isobaric solutions of bupivacaine are used as opposed to hyperbaric formulations.

Mepivacaine (Carbocaine) is a methyl derivative of a ringed piperidine rather than an alkyl-amino compound. Its duration is slightly longer than lidocaine. It is known to have some vasoconstrictive activity, but the addition of epinephrine affects the duration, onset, and potential for toxicity just as it does for lidocaine. It is used in infiltration, peripheral nerve, and epidural anesthesia in the USA; but it is not effective as a topical agent. Also, the metabolism is markedly decreased in the fetus and the newborn, so it is infrequently used in obstetric anesthesia.[157] Although it is eliminated by the same mechanism as lidocaine, the metabolites are also excreted by the salivary glands and gastric mucosa.

Prilocaine (Citanest, Propitocaine) is a secondary amine analogue of lidocaine. It is as potent as lidocaine, but it is the least toxic of all the amino amide local anesthetics. This is due to the fact that levels in the blood are cleared quickly secondary to rapid uptake by the tissues. It has a rapid onset, a moderate duration, and profound depth of conduction blockade. Prilocaine is used in infiltration, peripheral nerve blocks, and epidural anesthesia. No specific formulas for topical or spinal use are available because of its short duration of action. During metabolism it is biotransformed to an amino phenol end product. This compound can oxidize hemoglobin to methemoglobin that can result in cyanosis; thus, the total dose needs to be limited to 600 mg. Also, its use in obstetric anesthesia and IV analgesic techniques has been abandoned. The metabolism of prilocaine is via the lung, liver, and kidney.

Ropivacaine is a propyl derivative of an n-alkyl piperidine amide. Ropivacaine is a chiral drug, but in its production the racemic mixture exists almost as a pure solution of one isomer. It is believed that this isomer possesses the most therapeutic qualities and the safest cardiac profile.[158] In fact, one of the main advantages of ropivacaine over bupivacaine is its reduced cardiotoxic potential. The physicochemical properties of ropivacaine are similar to those of bupivacaine, except for the fact that it is less lipid soluble (Table 4.6). This may explain why, although ropivacaine and bupivacaine have equipotent effects on C-fiber action potentials, ropivacaine is less potent in blocking A-fiber activity. In other words, when compared with bupivacaine, the sensory anesthetic profiles of the two drugs were similar in onset, depth, and duration; but the depth and duration of the motor block were less with ropivacaine.[159] It is felt that ropivacaine may possess an even greater potential for a differential sensory motor blockade as compared to bupivacaine.

However, this differential blocking effect has been shown to be overcome by increasing the concentration of the ropivacaine. This would make ropivacaine superior to bupivacaine and an extremely useful agent for obstetrical anesthesia and postoperative epidural analgesia. Ropivacaine has been found to be an effective local anesthetic agent for infiltration, epidural, spinal, and brachial plexus anesthesia. Also, the addition of epinephrine has not been shown to alter the onset or duration of its action significantly because of its own inherent vasoconstrictive activity.[160] A clinical profile of local anesthetics is presented in Table 4.7.

Table 4.7   Clinical profile of local anesthetic agents

Agent	Concentration (%)	Clinical use	Onset	Usual duration (h)	Recommended maximum single dose (mg)	Comments	pH of pain solutions
Amides							
Lidocaine	0.5–1.0	Infiltration	Fast	1.0–2.0	300	Most versatile agents	6.5
	0.25–0.5	IV regional				3 mg/kg maximum 40 ml	
	1.0–1.5	Peripheral nerve blocks	Fast	1.0–3.0	500 + epinephrine		
	1.5–2.0	Epidural	Fast	1.0–2.0	500 + epinephrine		
	4	Topical	Moderate	0.5–1.0	500 + epinephrine		
	5	Spinal	Fast	0.5–1.5	100		
Prilocaine	0.5–1.0	Infiltration	Fast	1.0–2.0	600	Least toxic agents	4.5
	0.25–0.5	IV regional			600	Methemoglobinemia occurs	
	1.5–2.0	Peripheral nerve blocks	Fast	1.5–3.0	600	usually above 600 mg	
	2.0–3.0	Epidural	Fast	1.0–3.0			
Mepivacaine	0.5–1.0	Infiltration	Fast	1.5–3.0	400 / 500 + epinephrine	Longer duration of plain solutions than lidocaine without epinephrine	4.5
	1.0–1.5	Peripheral nerve blocks	Fast	2.0–3.0			
	1.5–2.0	Epidural	Fast	1.5–3.0		Useful when epinephrine is contraindicated	
	4.0	Spinal	Fast	1.0–1.5	100		
Bupivacaine	0.25	Infiltration	Fast	2.0–4.0	175 / 225 + epinephrine	Lower concentrations provide differential sensory/motor block.	4.5–6
	0.25–0.5	Peripheral nerve blocks	Slow	4.0–12.0	225 + epinephrine		
	0.25–0.5	Obstetric epidural	Moderate	2.0–4.0	225 + epinephrine	Ventricular arrhythmias and	
	0.5–0.75	Surgical epidural	Moderate	2.0–5.0	225 + epinephrine	sudden cardiovascular collapse reported	
	0.5–0.75	Spinal	Fast	2.0–4.0	20	following rapid IV injection	
Cocaine	4.0–10.0	Topical	Slow	30–60	150	Topical use only. Addictive, causes vasoconstriction. CNS toxicity marked excitation ('fight and flight' response). May cause cardiac arrhythmias owing to sympathetic stimulation.	

From Covino BG. Clinical pharmacology of local anesthetic agents. In: Cousins MJ, Bridenbaugh PO, eds. Clinical anesthesia and management of pain. Philadelphia: JB Lippincott; 1988.

Toxicity of local anesthetics

Allergic reactions to local anesthetics are known to occur mainly with the amino ester-linkage local anesthetics. This has been especially documented for procaine; but crossover hypersensitivity has also been seen with the other ester amide-linkage drugs. This is thought to happen because of a cross-sensitivity with para-aminobenzoic acid.[161] True allergic reactions to amino amide local anesthetics are extremely rare and are usually related, not to the drug, but to the preservative methylparaben.[162] Paraben esters have excellent bacteriostatic and fungistatic properties, and are widely used in multidose vials. In the past, skin testing of those suspected of possible allergic reactions to local anesthetics was felt to be the best way to identify these patients. However, this may not be scientifically reliable because only a small amount of drug is used; and there may need to be a conjugation of the drug with a carrier molecule before allergic reactions can occur. Also, the possibility of a severe anaphylactic reaction could put the patient's life at risk.

Local tissue toxicity

Tissue toxicity is rare when proper technique and concentrations of local anesthetics are used. However, serious neurotoxicity may result from intraneural injections, needle trauma, injections of large concentrations or volumes, chemical contamination, and neural ischemia produced by local neural compression or systemic hypotension.[163]

The neurologic deficits reported with the use of 2-chloroprocaine in epidural anesthesia are an example. Although the 2-chloroprocaine itself did not appear to have neurotoxic effects at clinical level, the preservative sodium bisulfite[164] and the low pH[165] of the solution were felt to be the culprit. This resulted in the reformulation of this local anesthetic.

There are recent reports of neurotoxicity with the administration of local anesthetics through small-gauged subarachnoid catheters.[166] At present, the proposed theory is that the use of these catheters results in a maldistribution of local anesthetic. This, in turn, leads to localized areas of the cauda equina being continuously exposed to high concentrations of local anesthetics, which results in direct local anesthetic neurotoxicity. Therefore, a ban on the use of these smaller catheters is in place until further investigation.

Systemic toxicity

The systemic effects of local anesthetic, ranging from therapeutic to toxic, can best be described as a continuum that is dependent on blood level concentrations. Systemic toxicity most frequently arises from one of two causes: (1) accidental vascular injections, or (2) administration of an excessive dose (Table 4.8). The main toxic effects occur in the CNS and cardiovascular systems, but the cardiovascular system is four to seven times more resistant to these effects, i.e. seizures will occur with lower concentrations than are required to produce cardiovascular collapse.

Table 4.8 Comparable safe doses of local anesthetics (mg/kg)*

Drugs	Peripheral blocks‡	Central blocks ± Plain	Central blocks ± With Epi 1:200 000	Intercostal blocks with Epi 1:200 000
2-Chloroprocaine	–	20	25	–
Procaine	–	14	18	–
Lidocaine	20	7	9	6
Mepivacaine	20	7	9	6
Bupivacaine	5	2	2	2
Tetracaine	–	2	2	–

*Estimated to produce peak plasma levels that are less than half the plasma levels at which seizures could occur.
‡Areas of low vascularity, i.e. axillary blocks using local anesthetic solutions containing 1:200 000 epinephrine.
§Areas of high vascularity i.e. intercostal blocks using local anesthetic solutions containing 1:200 000 epinephrine.
From Covino BG. Clinical pharmacology of local anesthetic agents. In: Cousins MJ, Bridenbaugh PO, eds. Clinical anesthesia and management of pain. Philadelphia: JB Lippincott; 1988.

CNS toxicity

The continuum of symptoms related to CNS toxicity appears to be not only related to concentration but also to the rate at which it presents itself to the nervous system.

For example, small amounts of local anesthetic can induce side effects, even seizures, if their application to the CNS is instantaneous, as with inadvertent intra-arterial injections. On the other hand, high blood concentrations can be tolerated without signs of systemic toxicity if they are applied over long periods of time with continuous perineural and epidural infusions. The progression of CNS toxic symptoms results from selective depression of inhibitory fibers or centers in the CNS that results in excessive excitatory input. Early signs of toxicity differ between the ester and amide-linkage local anesthetics. The former generally produces stimulant and euphoric symptoms, whereas the latter tends to produce sedation and amnesia. Beyond this, all the local anesthetics produce similar toxic symptoms. Commonly reported symptoms in association with rising blood levels are headache; lightheadedness; numbness and tingling of the perioral area or distal extremities; tinnitus; drowsiness; a flushed or chilled sensation; and blurred vision, or difficulty in focusing the eyes. Objectively, signs of obtundation, confusion, slurred speech, nystagmus, and muscle tremors or twitches can be observed. It is important to recognize these signs, as they can foreshadow an impending seizure. The seizures appear to arise from subcortical levels in the brain, mainly the amygdala and the hippocampus; and then subsequently spread, producing a generalized grand mal seizure.[167]

There are other factors that affect the CNS toxicity of local anesthetics. Increases in P_{CO_2} may possibly have an effect by increasing cerebral blood flow and therefore increasing delivery to the CNS, as well as enhancing excitatory effects on the brain tissue.[168] Similarly, a decrease in pH may increase the concentration of the active cationic form in the brain cells. Also it has been shown that cimetidine can increase the toxicity of local anesthetics by its slowing of their elimination.[169]

Likewise, the toxic effects of local anesthetics can be decreased by the effects of barbiturates, benzodiazepines, and inhalation anesthetics by raising the seizure threshold of the CNS.

Cardiovascular system toxicity

Although the cardiovascular system is more resistant to the toxic effects of local anesthetics, cardiovascular toxicity can be severe and difficult, if not impossible, to treat. Decreases in myocardial contractility, rates of cardiac electrical impulse conduction, and effects on smooth muscle contractual functions are dose-dependent. Cardiac arrhythmias and hypertension develop as dosages increase. At one time the potency of the local anesthetics was thought to be directly related to their cardiac toxicity. However, now it is known that bupivacaine and etidocaine have a more profound effect on the electrophysiology of the heart. Bupivacaine is approximately 70 times more potent than lidocaine in blocking cardiac conduction, yet it is only four times more potent in blocking the conduction of nerves.[170] This is due to the slower dissociation of bupivacaine from the cardiac Na^+ channels than that of lidocaine. This lack of complete dissociation leads to a progressive number of blocked Na^+ channels during diastole, which leads to subsequent cardiac depression and failure. Also, there is an indirect contribution to the cardiac toxicity by the local anesthetic's suppressive effects on the CNS. In addition, local anesthetics have both a direct and an indirect (via the autonomic system) effect on the vascular smooth muscle tone, resulting in either vasoconstriction and/or vasodilatation in different vascular beds, which is related to different levels of dosages. Cardiovascular toxicity is increased by hypoxia, acidosis, pregnancy, and hyperkalemia.[171]

SUMMARY

Post-traumatic pain encompasses acute post-traumatic and subsequent chronic pain states. The pathophysiology of pain varies with chronicity. Consequently, appropriate therapeutic intervention requires consideration of both prevailing perturbations in hemodynamic and respiratory physiology, as well as resultant alterations in pain mechanisms. Furthermore, post-traumatic complications and the late development of chronic pain states can be altered by the choice of analgesic technique.

Acute pain management should promote early mobilization and, therefore, a reduction in post-traumatic and postoperative complications. The complexity of chronic pain, however, requires a multidisciplinary approach to management, with an emphasis on improved function and rehabilitation.

REFERENCES

1. Bonica JJ. Pain research and therapy: Past and current status and future needs. In: Ng LKY, Bonica JJ, eds. Pain, discomfort and humanitarian care. New York: Elsevier; 1980.
2. American Pain Society, APS Bulletin 1997; 7.
3. Acute pain management: Operative or medical procedures and trauma. Rockville, Maryland: Agency for Health Care Policy and Research; 1989.
4. The necessity for early evaluation and treatment of the chronic pain patient: A consensus statement from the American Academy of Pain Medicine. Clin J Pain 1997; 13.
5. Management of acute pain: A practical guide. International Association for the Study of Pain. Seattle: IASP Publications; 1992.
6. Zoltie N, Cust MP. Analgesia in the acute abdomen. Ann R Coll Surg Engl 1986; 68: 209–210.
7. Carpenter RL, Abram SE, Bromage PR, Rauck RL. Consensus statement on acute pain management. Reg Anesth 1996; 21(6S): 152–156.
8. Cousins MJ, Wright CJ. Graft, muscle, skin blood flow after epidural block in vascular surgical procedures. Surg Gynecol Obstet 1971; 133: 59–69.
9. Bridenbaugh PO. Anesthesia and influence on hospitalization time. Reg Anesth 1982; 7: S151–155.
10. Noller DW, Gillenwater JY, Howards SS. Intercostal nerve block with flank incision. J Urol 1977; 117: 759.
11. Pflug AK, Murphy TM, Butler SH, et al. The effects of postoperative peridural analgesic on pulmonary therapy and pulmonary complications. Anesthesiology 1974; 41: 8–17.
12. Nimmo WS, Littlewood DG, Scott DB, et al. Gastric emptying following hysterectomy with extradural analgesia. Br J Anaesth 1978; 50: 559–561.
13. Shulman M, Sandler AN, Bradley JW, et al. Postthoracotomy pain and pulmonary function following epidural and systemic morphine. Anesthesiology 1984; 61: 569–575.
14. Yeager MP, Glass DD, Neff RK, et al. Epidural anesthesia and analgesia in high risk surgical patients. Anesthesiology 1987; 66: 729–736.
15. Halpern LM. Anxiety and pain in postoperative patients. In: Proceedings: Consideration in management of acute pain. New York: HP Publishing; 1977.
16. Taenzer P, Melzack R, Jeans ME. Influence of psychological factors on postoperative pain, mood and analgesic requirements. Pain 1986; 24: 331–342.
17. Benedikt RA, Kolb LC. Preliminary findings on chronic pain and posttraumatic stress disorder. Am J Psychiatry 1986; 143: 908–910.
18. Hartrick CT. Managing the difficult pain patient. In: Raj P, Erdine S, Niv D, Raja S, eds. Management of pain, a world perspective. Bologna: Monduzzi Editore; 1995.
19. Boisaubin EV. The assessment and treatment of pain in the emergency room. Clin J Pain 1989; S2: 19–24.
20. Kovi SH, Miller RP, Todd DD. Kinisophobia: A new view of chronic pain behavior. Pain Management 1990; 3: 35–43.
21. Schott GD. The relationship of peripheral trauma and pain to dystonia. J Neurol Neurosurg Psychiatry 1985; 48: 698–701.
22. Pecina MM, Bojanic I. Overuse injuries of the musculoskeletal system. Boca Raton: CRC Press; 1993.
23. Maron BR. Orthopedic aspects of sports medicine. In: Appenseller O, ed. Sports medicine. 3rd ed. Baltimore: Urban and Schwarzenberg; 1988.
24. Raj PP, Montgomery SJ, Bradley VH. Agents and techniques in anesthesia for surgery of trauma. Clin Anesth 1976; 11: 41.
25. Raj PP, Knarr D, Vigdorth E, et al. Difference in analgesia following epidural blockade in patients with postoperative or chronic low back pain. Pain 1988; 34: 21–27.
26. Mogensen T, Scott NB, Lund C, et al. The roles of acute and chronic pain in regression of sensory analgesia during continuous epidural bupivacaine infusion. Anesth Analg 1988; 67: 737–740.
27. Inbal R, Devor M, Tuchendler O, et al. Autotomy following nerve injury: Genetic factors in the development of chronic pain. Pain 1980; 9: 327–337.
28. Devor M, Raber P. Heritability of symptoms in an experimental model of neuropathic pain. Pain 1990; 42: 51–67.
29. Wiesenfeld-Hallin Z, Hao JX, Xu XJ, et al. Genetic factors influence the development of mechanical hypersensitivity, motor deficits and morphological damage after transient spinal cord ischemia in the rat. Pain 1993; 55: 235–241.
30. Mailis A, Wade J. Profile of caucasian women with possible genetic predisposition to reflex sympathetic dystrophy: A pilot study. Clin J Pain 1996; 10: 210–217.

31. Hagedorn SD, Maruta T, Swanson DW, et al. Premorbid MMPI profiles of low back pain patients: Surgical successes versus surgical failures. Clin J Pain 1985; 1: 177–179.

32. France RD, Krishnan KRR, Trainor M. Chronic pain and depression III: Family history study of depression and alcoholism in chronic low back pain patients. Pain 1986; 24: 185–190.

33. Bruehl S, Carlson CR. Predisposing psychological factors in the development of reflex sympathetic dystrophy: A review of the empirical evidence. Clin J Pain 1992; 8: 287–299.

34. Philips HC, Berkowitz J. The prevention of chronic pain and disability: A preliminary investigation. Behav Res Ther 1991; 29: 443–450.

35. Gatchel RJ, Polatin PB, Kinney RK. Predicting outcome of chronic back pain using clinical predictors of psychopathology: a prospective analysis. Health Psychol 1995; 14: 415–420.

36. Gatchel RJ, Polatin PB, Mayer TG. The dominant role of psychosocial risk factors in the development of chronic low back pain disability. Spine 1995; 20: 2702–2709.

37. Klenerman L, Slade PD, Stanley IM, et al. The prediction of chronicity in patients with an acute attack of low back pain in a general practice setting. Spine 1995; 20: 478–484.

38. Cats-Baril WL, Frymoyer JW. Identifying patients at risk of becoming disabled because of low back pain. Spine 1991; 16: 605–607.

39. Dworkin RH. Which individuals with acute pain are most likely to develop a chronic pain syndrome? Pain Forum 1997; 6: 127–136.

40. Jensen TS, Krebs B, Nielsen J, et al. Immediate and long-term phantom limb pain in amputees: Incidence, clinical characteristics and relationship to preamputation limb pain. Pain 1985; 21: 267–278.

41. Weiss SA, Lindell B. Phantom limb pain and etiology of amputation in unilateral lower extremity amputees. J Pain Sympt Manage 1996; 11: 3–17.

42. Bach S, Noreng MF, Tjellden NU. Phantom limb pain in amputees during the first 12 months following limb amputation, after preoperative lumbar epidural blockade. Pain 1988; 33: 297–301.

43. Kroner K, Krebs B, Skov J, et al. Immediate and long-term phantom breast syndrome after mastectomy: Incidence, clinical characteristics and relationship to premastectomy breast pain. Pain 1989; 36: 327–334.

44. Coderre TJ, Katz J, Vaccarino AL, et al. Contribution of central neuroplasticity to pathological pain: Review of clinical and experimental evidence. Pain 1993; 52: 259–285.

45. Dannenberg AL, Needle S, Mullady D, et al. Predictors of injury among 1638 riders in a recreational long-distance bicycle tour. Am J Sports Med 1996; 24: 747–753.

46. Heir T, Glomsaker P. Epidemiology of musculoskeletal injuries among Norwegian conscripts undergoing basic military training. Scand J Med Sci Sports 1996; 6: 186–191.

47. Heir T, Eide G. Age, body composition, aerobic fitness and health condition as risk factors for musculoskeletal injuries in conscripts. Scand J Med Sci Sports 1996; 6: 222–227.

48. Cowan DN, Jones BH, Frykman PN, et al. Lower limb morphology and risk of overuse injury among male infantry trainees. Med Sci Sports Exerc 1996; 28: 945–952.

49. Bennell KL, Crossley K. Musculoskeletal injuries in track and field: Incidence, distribution and risk factors. Aust J Sci Med Sport 1996; 28: 69–75.

50. Bennell KL, Malcolm SA, Thomas SA, et al. Risk factors for stress fractures in track and field athletes: A twelve-month prospective study. Am J Sports Med 1996; 24: 810–818.

51. Inklaar H, Bol E, Schmikli SL, et al. Injuries in male soccer players: Team risk analysis. Int J Sports Med 1996; 17: 229–234.

52. Lysens RJ, Ostyn MS, Vanden Auweele Y, et al. The accident-prone and overuse-prone profiles of the young athlete. Am J Sports Med 1989; 17: 612–619.

53. Sola A. Upper extremity pain. In: Wall PD, Melzack R, eds. Textbook of pain. New York: Churchill Livingstone; 1984.

54. Cooper DE, DeLee JC, Ramamurthy S. Reflex sympathetic dystrophy of the knee: Treatment using continuous epidural anesthesia. J Bone Joint Surg 1989; 71: 365–369.

55. Cousins MJ. Acute pain and the injury response: Immediate and prolonged effects. Reg Anesth 1989; 14: 162–179.

56. Stulz P, Pfieffer KM. Peripheral nerve injuries resulting from common surgical procedures in the lower portion of the abdomen. Arch Surg 1982; 117: 324–327.

57. Hartrick CT. Thermographic evaluation of post-surgical groin pain. Mich Osteo J 1987; 52: 20–24.

58. Hitchcock E, Alvarez RM. Incisional pain. Clin J Pain 1988; 4: 205–208.

59. Kelley JT. Chronic pain and trauma. Adv Psychosom Med 1986; 16: 141–142.

60. Fields HL. Sources of variability in the sensation of pain. Pain 1988; 33: 195–200.

61. Rosenfeld JP, Silvia R, Weitkunat R, et al. Operant control of human somatosensory evoked potentials alters experimental pain perception. In: Fields HL, et al, eds. Advances in pain research and therapy, vol 9. New York: Raven Press; 1985.

62. Duncan GH, Bushnell MC, Bates R, et al. Task related responses of monkey medullary dorsal horn neurons. J Neurophysiol 1987; S7: 289–310.

63. Noyes RJ, Andreasen NJ, Hartford CE. The psychological reaction to severe burns. Psychosomatics 1971; 12: 416–422.

64. Andreasen NC. Neuropsychiatric complications in burn patients. Int J Psychiatry Med 1974; 5: 161–165.

65. Mancusi-Ungaro HR, Tarbox AR, Wainwright DJ. Posttraumatic stress disorder in electrical burn patients. J Burn Care Rehabil 1986; 7: 521–525.

66. Geisser ME, Roth RS, Bachman JE, et al. The relationship between symptoms of post-traumatic stress disorder and pain, affective disturbance and disability among patients with accident and non-accident related pain. Pain 1996; 66: 207–214.

67. Kuch K, Cox BJ, Evans RJ. Posttraumatic stress disorder and motor vehicle accidents: A multidisciplinary overview. Can J Psychiatry 1996; 41: 429–434.

68. Muse M, Frigola G. Development of a quick screening instrument for detecting posttraumatic stress disorder in the chronic pain patients: Construction of the Posttraumatic Chronic Pain Test (PCPT). Clin J Pain 1987; 2: 151–153.

69. Chaney HS, Williams SG, Cohn CK, et al. MMPI results: A comparison of trauma victims, psychogenic pain, and patients with organic disease. J Clin Psychiatry 1984; 40: 1450–1454.

70. Wilson JF, Bennett RL. Coping styles, medication use, and pain score in patients using patient controlled analgesia for postoperative pain. Anesthesiology 1984; 61: A193.

71. Gourlay GK, Kowalski SR, Plummer JL, et al. Fentanyl blood concentration: Analgesic response relationship in the treatment of postoperative pain. Anesth Analg 1988; 67: 329–337.

72. Tamsen A, Sakurada T, Wahlstrom A, et al. Postoperative demand for analgesics in relation to individual levels of endorphins and substance P in cerebrospinal fluid. Pain 1982; 13: 171–183.

73. Grant IS, Nimmo WC, Clements JH. Pharmacokinetics and analgesic effects of IM and oral ketamine. Br J Anaesth 1981; 53: 805.

74. Gurnani A, Sharma PK, Rautela RS, et al. Analgesia for acute musculoskeletal trauma: Low-dose subcutaneous infusion of ketamine. Anaesth Intensive Care 1996; 24: 32–36.

75. Arendt-Nielsen L, Petersen-Felix S, Fischer M, et al. The effect of N-methyl-D-aspartate antagonist (ketamine) on single and repeated nociceptive stimuli: A placebo controlled experimental human study. Anesth Analg 1995; 81: 63–68.

76. Ready LB, Brown CR, Stahlgren LH, et al. Evaluation of intravenous ketorolac administered by bolus or infusion for treatment of postoperative pain: A double-blind, placebo-controlled, multicenter study. Anesthesiology 1994; 80: 1277–1286.

77. Brena SF, Chapman SL. Chronic pain states and compensable disability: An algorithmic approach. In: Benedetti C, ed. Advances in pain research and therapy, vol 7. New York: Raven Press; 1984.

78. Hill M, Mather L. Patient-controlled analgesia, pharmacokinetic and therapeutic considerations. Clin Pharmacokinet 1993; 24: 124–140.

79. Ling G, et al. Dissociation of morphine's analgesic and respiratory depressant actions. Eur J Pharmacol 1983; 86: 487–488.

80. Gintzler A, Pastemak G. Multiple mu receptors: Evidence for mu, sites in the guinea pig ilium. Neurosci Lett 1983; 39: 51–56.

81. Pastemak G. Multiple morphine and enkephalin receptors and the relief of pain. JAMA 1988; 259: 1362–1367.

82. Economou G, Ward-McQuaid W. A cross-over comparison of the effect of morphine, pethidine, pentazocine, and phenazocine in biliary pressure. Gut 1971; 12: 21X–221.

83. Radnay P, et al. The effect of equi-analgesic doses of fentanyl, morphine, meperidine and pentazocine on common bile duct pressure. Anaesthetist 1980; 29: 26–29.

84. Reitan J, et al. Central vagal control of fentanyl induced bradycardia during halothane anesthesia. Anesth Analg 1978; 57: 31–36.

85. Stanley T, et al. Cardiovascular effects of nitrous oxide during meperidine infusion in the dog. Anesth Analg 1977; 56: 836–841.

86. Freye E. Cardiovascular effects of high dosages of fentanyl, meperidine, and naloxone in dogs. Anesth Analg 1974; 53: 40–47.

87. Rosow C, et al. Histamine release during morphine and fentanyl anesthesia. Anesthesiology 1982; 56: 93–96.

88. Bovill J, Sebel P, Stanley T. Opioid analgesics in anesthesia: With special reference to their use in cardiovascular anesthesia. Anesthesiology 1984; 61: 731–755.

89. Clive D, Stoff J. Renal syndromes associated with nonsteroidal anti-inflammatory drugs. N Engl J Med 1984; 310: 563–572.

90. Flower R, Moncada S, Vane J. Analgesic-antipyretics and antiinflammatory agents; drugs employed in the treatment of gout. In: Gilman A, et al, eds. The pharmacological basis of therapeutics. 7th ed. New York: Macmillan; 1985.

91. Parr G, et al. Joint pain and quality of life: Results of a randomised trial. Br J Clin Pharmacol 1989; 27: 235–242.

92. Ferreira S. Prostaglandins: Peripheral and central analgesia. In: Bonica JJ, Lindblom U, Iggo A, eds. Advances in pain research and therapy, vol 5. New York: Raven Press; 1983.

93. Willer J, De Broucker T, Bussel B. Central analgesic effects of ketoprofen in humans: Electrophysiological evidence for a supraspinal mechanism in a double-blind and cross-over study. Pain 1989; 38: 1–7.

94. Carlsson K, Monzel W, Juma I. Depression by morphine and the nonopioid analgesic agents metamizol, lysine acetylate and paracetamol, of activity in rat thalamus neurons evoked by electrical stimulation of nociceptive afferents. Pain 1988; 32: 313–326.

95. Taiwo Y, Levine J. Prostaglandins inhibit endogenous pain control mechanisms by blocking transmission at spinal noradrenergic synapses. J Neurosci 1988; 8: 1346–1349.

96. Fabbri A, et al. Piroxicam-induced analgesia: Evidence for a central component which is not opioid mediated. Experientia 1992; 48: 1139–1142.

97. Bannwarth B, et al. Clinical pharmacokinetics of nonsteroidal antiinflammatory drugs in the cerebrospinal fluid. Biomed Pharmacother 1989; 43: 121–126.

98. Catania A, et al. Inhibition of acute inflammation in the periphery by central action of salicylates. Proc Natl Acad Sci USA 1991; 88: 8544–8547.

99. Abramson S. Therapy with and mechanisms of nonsteroidal antiinflammatory drugs. Curr Opin Rheumatol 1991; 3: 336–340.

100. Day R, et al. Variability in response to NSAIDs–fact or fiction? Drugs 1988; 36: 643–651.

101. Day R, et al. Clinical pharmacology of nonsteroidal antiinflammatory drugs. Pharmacol Ther 1987; 33: 384–433.

102. Dukes M, Lunde I. The regulatory control of nonsteroidal antiinflammatory drug preparations within individual rheumatology private practices. J Rheumatol 1989; 16: 1253–1258.

103. Carson J, et al. The relative gastrointestinal toxicity of the nonsteroidal antiinflammatory drugs. Arch Intern Med 1987; 147: 1054–1059.

104. Roberts D, et al. Sulindac is not renal sparing in man. Clin Pharmacol Ther 1985; 38: 258–265.

105. Quintero E, et al. Sulindac reduces the urinary excretion of prostaglandins and impairs renal function in cirrhosis with ascites. Nephron 1986; 42: 298–303.

106. Stouten E, et al. Comparison of ketorolac and morphine for postoperative pain after major surgery. Acta Anaesthesiol Scand 1992; 36: 716–721.

107. Brown C, et al. Comparison of repeat doses of intramuscular ketorolac tromethamine and morphine sulfate for analgesia after major surgery. Pharmacotherapy 1990; 10: 45S–50S.

108. Greer I. Effects of ketorolac tromethamine on hemostasis. Pharmacotherapy 1990; 10: 71S–76S.

109. Garcha I, Bostwick J. Postoperative hematomas associated with Toradol [letter]. Plast Reconstr Surg 1991; 88: 919–920.

110. Forbes JA, et al. Evaluation of ketorolac, ibuprofen, acetaminophen, and an acetaminophen-codeine combination in postoperative oral surgery pain. Pharmacotherapy 1990; 10: 94S–105S.

111. Rhodes M. Nonsteroidal antiinflammatory drugs for postthoracotomy pain. J Thorac Cardiovasc Surg 1992; 103: 17–20.

112. Medical Letter 1972; 14: 31.

113. Dahl S. Nabumetone: A 'nonacidic,' nonsteroidal antiinflammatory drug. Ann Pharmacother 1993; 27: 456–463.

114. Walsh TD. Antidepressants in chronic pain. Neuropharmacol 1983; 6: 271–295.

115. France RD, Houpt JL, Ellinwood EH. Therapeutic effects of antidepressants in chronic pain. Gen Hosp Psychiatry 1984; 6: 55–63.

116. Atkinson JH, Kremer EF, Garfin SR. Psychopharmacological agents in the treatment of pain. J Bone Joint Surg Am 1985; 67-A: 337–342.

117. Rosenblatt RM, Reich J, Dehring D. Tricyclic antidepressants in the treatment of depression and chronic pain: Analysis of the supporting evidence. Anesth Analg 1984; 63: 1025–1032.

118. Aronoff GM, Wagner JM, Spangler AS. Chemical interventions for pain. J Consult Clin Psychol 1986; 54: 769–775.

119. Feinmann C. Pain relief by antidepressants: Possible modes of action. Pain 1985; 23: 1–8.

120. Melzack R, Wall PD. Pain mechanisms: A new theory. Science 1965; 150: 971–979.

121. Max MB, et al. Amitriptyline relieves diabetic neuropathy pain in patients with normal or depressed mood. Neurology 1987; 37: 589–596.

122. Sharav Y, et al. The analgesic effect of amitriptyline on chronic facial pain. Pain 1987; 31: 199–209.

123. Davis JL, et al. Peripheral diabetic neuropathy treated with amitriptyline and fluphenazine. JAMA 1977; 238: 2291–2292.

124. Richards GA, et al. Unusual drug interactions between monoamine oxidase inhibitors and tricyclic antidepressants (letter). J Neurol Neurosurg Psychiatry 1987; 50: 1240–1241.

125. Kocher R. Use of psychotropic drugs for the treatment of chronic severe pain. In: Bonica JJ, Albe-Fessard D, eds. Advances in pain research

and therapy, vol 1. New York: Raven Press; 1976.

126. Taub A, Collins WF. Observations on the treatment of denervation dysesthesia with psychotropic drugs: Postherpetic neuralgia, anesthesia dolorosa, peripheral neuropathy. In: Bonica JJ, ed. Advances in neurology, vol 4. New York: Raven Press; 1974.

127. Mendel CM, et al. A trial of amitriptyline and fluphenazine in the treatment of painful diabetic neuropathy. JAMA 1986; 255: 637–639.

128. Linnoila M, George L, Guthrie S. Interaction between antidepressants and perphenazine in psychiatric inpatients. Am J Psychiatry 1982; 139: 1329–1331.

129. Clarke IMC. Amitriptyline and perphenazine (Triptafen DA) in chronic pain. Anaesthesia 1981; 36: 210–211.

130. Montilla E, Frederick WS, Cass LJ. Analgesic effect of methotrimeprazine and morphine. Arch Intern Med; 1963; 111: 91–94.

131. Swerdlow M. Anticonvulsant drugs and chronic pain. Clin Neuropharmacol 1984; 7: 51–82.

132. Hatangdi VS, Boas RA, Richards KG. Postherpetic neuralgia management with antiepileptic and tricyclic drugs. In: Bonica JJ, Albe-Fessard E, eds. Advances in pain research and therapy. New York: Raven Press; 1976.

133. Young RJ, Clarke BF. Pain relief in diabetic neuropathy: The effectiveness of imipramine and related drugs. Diabet Med 1985; 2: 363–366.

134. Bouckoms AJ, Litman RE. Clonazepam in the treatment of neuralgic pain syndrome. Psychosomatics 1985; 26: 933–936.

135. Greenblatt DJ, Shader RI, Abernethy DR. Current status of the benzodiazepines.(1). N Engl J Med 1983; 309: 410–416.

136. Hollister LH, et al. Long-term use of diazepam. JAMA 1981; 246: 1568–1570.

137. Singh PN, et al. Clinical evaluation of diazepam for relief of postoperative pain. Br J Anaesth 1981; 53: 831–835.

138. Drugs and insomnia: The use of medications to promote sleep. JAMA 1984; 251: 2410–2414.

139. Feighner JP, et al. Comparison of alprozalom, imipramine and placebo in the treatment of depression. JAMA 1983; 249: 3057–3064.

140. Rickels K, Feighner JP, Smith WT. Alprazolam amitriptyline, doxepin and placebo in the treatment of depression. Arch Gen Psychiatry 1985; 45: 134–141.

141. Choice of benzodiazepines. Med Lett Drugs Ther 1988; 30: 26–28.

142. Hupert C, Yacoub M, Turgeon LR. Effect of hydroxyzine on morphine for the treatment of postoperative pain. Anesth Analg 1980; 59: 690–696.

143. Elenbaas JK. Centrally acting oral skeletal muscle relaxants. Am J Hosp Pharm 1980; 37: 1313–1323.

144. Covino BG, Vassello HG. Local anesthetics, mechanism of action and clinical use. New York: Grune and Stratton; 1976.

145. Covino BG. Pharmacology of local anesthetic agents. Br J Anaesth 1986; 5: 701–706.

146. Hille B. Local anesthetics: Hydrophilic and hydrophobic pathways for the drug-receptor reaction. J Gen Physiol 1977; 69: 497–575.

147. Seeman P. The membrane expansion theory of anaesthesia. In: Fink BR, ed. Molecular mechanisms of anesthesia. Progress in Anesthesiology, vol 1. New York: Raven Press; 1975.

148. Littlewood DG, Buckley P, Covino BG, et al. Comparative study of various local anesthetic solutions in extradural block in labour. Br J Anaesth 1979; 51: 47.

149. Scott BD, McClure JH, Giasi RM, et al. Effects of concentration of local anaesthetic drugs in extradural block. Br J Anaesth 1980; 52: 1033.

150. Covino BG. Clinical pharmacology of local anesthetic agents. Neural blockade. In: Cousins MJ, Bridenbaugh PO, eds. Clinical anesthesia and management of pain. Philadelphia: JB Lippincott; 1988.

151. Tucker GT, Mather LE. Clinical pharmacokinetics of local anaesthetic. Clin Pharmacokin 1979; 4: 241.

152. Catchlove RFH. The influence of CO_2 and pH on local anesthetic action. J Pharmacol Exp Ther 1972; 181: 291.

153. Metha PM, Theriot E, Mehrotra D. A simple technique to make bupivacaine a rapid-acting epidural anesthetic. Reg Anesth 1987; 123: 135.

154. Fagraeus L, Urban BJ, Bromage PR. Spread of epidural analgesia in early pregnancy. Anesthesiology 1983; 58: 184.

155. Datta S, Lambert DH, Gregus J, et al. Differential sensitivities of mammalian nerve fibers during pregnancy. Anesth Analg 1983; 62: 1070.

156. Corke BC, Carlson CG, Dettbarn WD. The influence of 2-chloroprocaine on the subsequent analgesic potency of bupivacaine. Anesthesiology 1984; 60: 25.

157. DiFazio CA, Woods AM. Pharmacology of local anesthetics. In: Raj PP, ed. Practical management of pain. 2nd ed. St Louis: Mosby; 1992.

158. Arthur GR, Feldman HS, Covino BG. Acute IV toxicity of LEA-103, a new local anesthetic, compared to lidocaine and bupivacaine in the awake dog. Anesthesiology 1986; 65: 724.

159. Bader AM, Datta S, Flanagan H. Comparison of bupivacaine and ropivacaine induced conduction blockade in the isolated rabbit vagus nerve. Anesth Analg 1989; 68: 724.

160. Kopacz DJ, Carpenter RL, Mackey DC. Effects of ropivacaine on uterine blood flow in pregnant sheep. Anesthesiology 1989; 71: 69.

161. Fisher MM, Pennington JC. Allergy to local anesthesia. Br J Anaesth 1982; 54: 893–894.

162. Aldrete AJ, Johnson DA. Allergy to local anesthetic. JAMA 1969; 207: 356.

163. Kane RE. Neurologic deficits following epidural or spinal anesthesia. Anesth Analg 1981; 60: 150.

164. Wang BC, Hillman DE, Spielholz NI, et al. Chronic neurological deficits and nesacaine-CE–An effect of the anesthetic, 2-chloroprocaine, or the antioxidant, sodium bisulfite? Anesth Analg 1984; 63: 445.

165. Ravindran RS, Turner MS, Muller J. Neurologic effects of subarachnoid administration of 2-chloroprocaine-CE, bupivacaine, and low pH normal saline in dogs. Anesth Analg 1982; 61: 279.

166. Rigler M, Drasner K, Krejcie T, et al. Cauda equina syndrome after continuous spinal anesthesia. Anesth Analg 1991; 72: 275–281.

167. Wagman IH, DeJong RH, Prince DA. Effects of lidocaine on the central nervous system. Anesthesiology 1967; 28: 155.

168. Englesson S. The influence of acid-base changes on central nervous system toxicity of local anesthetic agents. Acta Anaesthesiol Scand 1974; 18: 79.

169. Kim KC, Tasch MD. Effects of cimetidine and ranitidine on local anesthetic central nervous system toxicity in mice. Anesth Analg 1986; 65: 840.

170. Clarkson CW, Hondeghem LM. Mechanism for bupivacaine depression of cardiac conduction: Fast block of sodium channels during action potential with slow recovery from block during diastole. Anesthesiology 1985; 62: 396.

171. Carpenter RL, Mackey DC. Local anesthetics. In: Barash PG, Cullen BF, Stoelting RK, eds. Clinical Anesthesia. Philadelphia: JB Lippincott; 1989.

5

Regional anesthesia and analgesia in trauma: advantages and disadvantages in specific medical and clinical situations

Mitchell H Marshall

Introduction

The patient with cardiovascular disease
Atherosclerotic cardiovascular disease
Valvular heart disease
Regional versus general anesthesia

The patient with pulmonary disease

The patient with hepatic disease
Gilbert's disease
Viral hepatitis
Alcoholic liver disease
Fatty liver
Cirrhosis
Cholestasis

The patient with endocrine disease
Diabetes mellitus
Thyroid disease
Adrenal suppression

The patient with renal and electrolyte disorders
Acute renal failure
Chronic renal insufficiency

The patient with coagulopathy and the anticoagulated patient
Coagulation tests
Use of regional anesthesia
Thromboprohylaxis

Regional anesthesia in the infected patient

Benefits of regional anesthesia/analgesia in trauma

Risks of regional anesthesia/analgesia in trauma
Spinal anesthesia
Peripheral nerve block

Summary

INTRODUCTION

The decision to use a regional technique in the perioperative care of the trauma patient requires a proper evaluation of the patient's underlying medical status and the extent of the underlying trauma. After an evaluation that takes into account the urgency of intervention, a coherent preoperative assessment will determine the need for relevant risk stratification. Frequently, trauma patients require urgent or semi-urgent operative care, limiting the scope of one's optimal assessment. It is in this setting that the decision to use a regional anesthetic or analgesic must be made. Intraoperative regional anesthesia is often continued postoperatively to maintain analgesia. Alternatively, one can utilize combinations of techniques to treat the patient intra- and postoperatively.

This review will look at specific advantages and disadvantages of regional anesthetic techniques in various common medical and clinical situations. This discussion will be of limited value in the management of the patient with severe polytrauma who is clinically unstable and requires emergent intervention. The luxury of time is usually not available in such a situation to allow anything other than an extremely limited evaluation, directed towards stabilizing the patient and bringing him safely through the perioperative period. Those situations where the traumatic injury is of a more limited nature, allowing for more specific analysis, are those where regional anesthesia and analgesia have a larger role.

Many decisions made by the anesthesiologist will be based on limited study data in a particular situation. Decisions may be based more on one's clinical judgement than on clear-cut evidence for the superiority of a given anesthetic. Specific outcome studies may look at factors not applicable to a given patient. Furthermore, not all benefits lead to long-term changes in morbidity and mortality. Trauma patients able to participate in the decision-making process may bring their own preconceptions about what is 'best' into the operating room (OR). These feelings have to be included in the final determination of the anesthetic plan. Clearly, many trauma patients will not be candidates for a regional technique. This discussion will refer to those patients where the possibility of a regional anesthetic is not immediately contraindicated by the surgical situation. These include patients with orthopedic, vascular, and abdominal injuries. Regional techniques for postoperative analgesia expand the list of possible situations that are applicable, e.g. thoracic trauma.

Studies of regional anesthetic outcome usually refer to major conduction anesthesia, i.e. spinal and epidural. Far less data are available on the use of other techniques, such as plexus anesthesia for upper and lower extremities, intravenous regional anesthesia, specific nerve blocks or limb blocks (e.g. wrist or ankle blocks), and monitored anesthesia care. Common sense and clinical judgement are major determinants of their use.

The following discussion will summarize the important preoperative considerations in patients with various medical conditions, their impact on regional anesthesia and analgesia, clinical situations where regional techniques may be utilized, and a summary of benefits and risks of these methods.

THE PATIENT WITH CARDIOVASCULAR DISEASE

As the prevalence of cardiac disease in the general population is high, patients will frequently present with concurrent cardiovascular conditions that must be considered in the preoperative evaluation. These can be divided into two general categories: atherosclerotic cardiovascular disease (ASHD) and valvular cardiac disease. The magnitude of the population at risk for perioperative cardiovascular morbidity is about 5% of the 25 to 30 million patients undergoing non-cardiac operative procedures annually. Some 50 000 will experience perioperative myocardial infarction (MI) and about half of these patients die from their ischemic insult.[1] This statistic would seem to justify the time, effort, and cost of trying to lower the incidence of cardiac complications.[2]

Atherosclerotic cardiovascular disease

The evaluation of patients with coronary artery disease has led to extensive study to determine which methods of risk stratification and preoperative intervention are optimal. Today's emphasis on cost containment, as well as the need for timely work-up, makes the proper utilization of potentially expensive and invasive testing essential. It may not be necessary to order a test on a given patient if the information gained will not have the potential to change the perioperative plan. Obtaining information for its own sake may or may not lead to improved patient outcome. In the trauma setting, the degree of urgency in proceeding to surgery must be included in the work-up algorithm.

There are many known risk factors for coronary artery disease, and many important conditions which affect the prediction of perioperative cardiac events. These include congestive heart failure (CHF), recent MI (within the preceding 3 to 6 months), unstable angina, left ventricular hypertrophy (LVH), male gender, age >65, smoking history, diabetes mellitus, hypertension, arrhythmias, significant aortic stenosis, elevated serum cholesterol, and peripheral vascular disease.[3]

To utilize these clinical data in a unifying manner, multifactorial indices have been developed to enable one to quantify risk more coherently. The first, and arguably the best known, multifactorial risk index was developed by Goldman et al in

1977.[4] In the original study of about 1000 patients undergoing non-cardiac surgery under general anesthesia, a cardiac risk index was developed which looked at nine factors, the presence of each contributing a number of points to a weight factor. The sum of the points determined the risk index class, stratified into four groups (I–IV). Increasing class number was associated with an increased risk of perioperative cardiac complications (myocardial infarction, pulmonary edema, ventricular arrhythmia, and cardiac death). Subsequent studies validated the reliability of the risk index concept. Detsky et al modified the risk index to take into account additional factors, especially the added risk of major vascular surgery.[5] His index stratified cardiac risk among three groups. The broad classification of the American Society of Anesthesiologists has some correlation with the risk of death and major complications in large groups of patients though not specific for cardiac complications.[6]

An implication of the cardiac risk indices is that intervention that brings a patient into a lower risk class will, in fact, lower the cardiac risk. However, none of these systems suggests the proper methods for evaluating a patient to modify cardiac risk.

Guidelines have recently been published by several internal medicine groups regarding preoperative cardiac evaluation. A joint task force of The American College of Cardiology and American Heart Association (ACC/AHA) recently published 'Guidelines for Perioperative Cardiovascular Evaluation for Noncardiac Surgery.'[7] The American College of Physicians (ACP) has also published a set of guidelines for assessing cardiac risk in the patient undergoing noncardiac surgery.[8]

The purpose of the ACP clinical guidelines[9] is to summarize available evidence on preoperative cardiac risk stratification so that the internist may:

1. Use clinical and electrocardiographic findings to stratify a patient's perioperative risk for myocardial infarction and death
2. Decide which tests provide useful additional risk-related information
3. Understand the benefits, risks, and evidence surrounding the decision to undertake coronary revascularization before elective noncardiac surgery.

The ACP modified cardiac risk index is shown in Table 5.1, and the management algorithm is illustrated in Figures 5.1 and 5.2.

Table 5.1 American College of Physicians' modified risk index

Variable	Points
Myocardial infarction within past 6 months	10
Myocardial infarction over 6 months ago	5
Class III angina	10
Class IV angina	20
Pulmonary edema within past week	10
Pulmonary edema at any time	5
Critical aortic stenosis	20
Rhythm other than sinus with or without APCs	5
More than 5 PVCs on baseline ECG	5
Poor general medical status ($PO_2 < 60$ mmHg, $PCO_2 > 50$ mmHg; $K^+ < 3.0$ mmol/L; BUN > 50 mmol/L; creatinine > 260 µmol/L; bedridden	5
Age > 70 years	5
Emergency surgery	10

Class 1 = 0–15 points; Class II = 20–30 points; Class III > 30 points; Class III angina = angina with walking 1–2 blocks or climbing one flight of stairs at normal pace. Class IV angina = angina with any physical activity; APC, Atrial premature contraction; PVC, premature ventricular contraction; ECG, electrocardiogram; BUN, blood urea nitrogen. From Palda VA, Detsky AS,[8] with permission.

As opposed to this evidence-based approach, the ACC/AHA guidelines are based on clinical risk variables and stratification according to perceived complexity and risk of the surgery. The algorithm is based on the available evidence and expert opinion. Four basic issues are addressed:

1. To what extent is the surgery elective or relatively urgent?
2. Which patients are most likely to experience cardiac ischemic events or death, and to what extent can risk be accurately stratified by simple clinical descriptors?
3. For patients who have not had recent prior coronary testing, what operations require additional evaluation, and which studies are most appropriate for a particular patient?
4. How will the results of these assessments alter the medical and surgical management? Finally, what is the optimal strategy for this patient, considering both the short-term and long-term perspectives?

The algorithm of the ACC/AHA is summarized in Figure 5.3. In the stepwise approach to evaluating the cardiac patient, the first consideration, clearly, is the degree of urgency of the surgery. If time is available, patients with unstable coronary

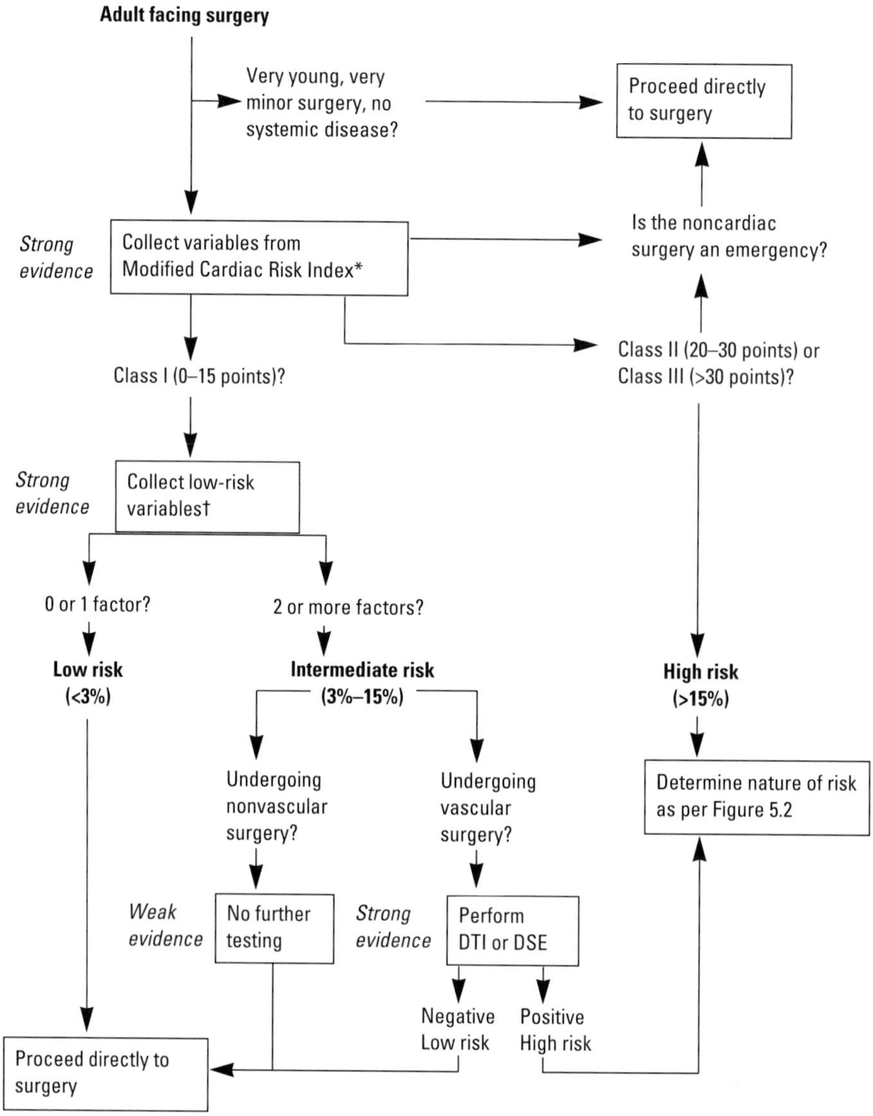

Adult facing surgery

Fig. 5.1 Algorithm for risk assessment and management of patients undergoing noncardiac surgery, at low and intermediate risk of perioperative cardiac events from the American College of Physicians' clinical guidelines. DTI, dipyridamole thallium imaging; DSE, dobutamine stress echocardiography. (From Palda VA, Detsky AS,[8] with permission.)

syndromes should be treated. A history of previous coronary evaluation or revascularization should be elicited.

Clinical predictors are then used to categorize the patient into one of three groups, representing low, intermediate, or high clinical risk. Depending on this risk, and the nature of the surgical procedure (Tables 5.2 and 5.3), the patient will either require no further evaluation and can proceed to the OR, or further testing will be indicated.

Testing may take the form of dipyridamole thallium imaging[10] and dobutamine stress echocardiography,[11] leading to the possibility of cardiac catheterization and angiography and consideration for coronary revascularization. There are no good studies, which specifically look at the effect of bypass surgery or angioplasty on changing cardiac morbidity and mortality for non-cardiac surgery. However, in patients who have had revascularization, the subsequent risk of surgery seems

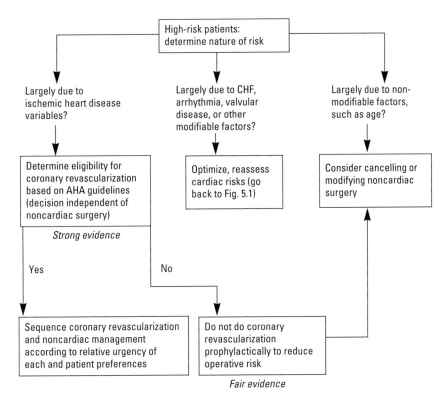

Fig. 5.2. Algorithm for management of patients at high risk for perioperative cardiac events, from American College of Physicians' clinical guidelines. CHF, congestive heart failure; AHA, American Heart Association. (From Palda VA, Detsky AS,[8] with permission.)

Table 5.2 Clinical predictors of coronary artery disease

Minor predictors	Intermediate predictors	Major predictors
Advanced age	Mild angina	Unstable coronary syndrome
Abnormal ECG	Prior MI	Decompensated CHF
Rhythm other than sinus	Compensated CHF	Significant arrhythmias
Low functional capacity	Diabetes mellitus	Severe vascular disease
History of stroke		
Systemic hypertension		

ECG, electrocardiogram; MI, myocardial infarction; CHF, congestive heart failure. Modified from Eagle KA, et al.[8]

Table 5.3 Degree of cardiac risk by surgical procedure

Low risk	Intermediate risk	High risk
Ophthalmologic	Intra-abdominal	Aortic surgery
Minor head and neck	Intrathoracic	Major vascular (intra-abdominal, infra-inguinal)
Minor prostate	Major orthopedic	Major emergency procedures
Most ambulatory surgery	Carotid endarterectomy	
Endoscopy	Major head and neck	
Superficial procedures	Radical prostatectomy	

Modified from Coley CM, Eagle KA. Perioperative assessment and perioperative management of cardiac ischemic risk in noncardiac surgery. Curr Probl Cardiol 1996; 21(5): 295–382.

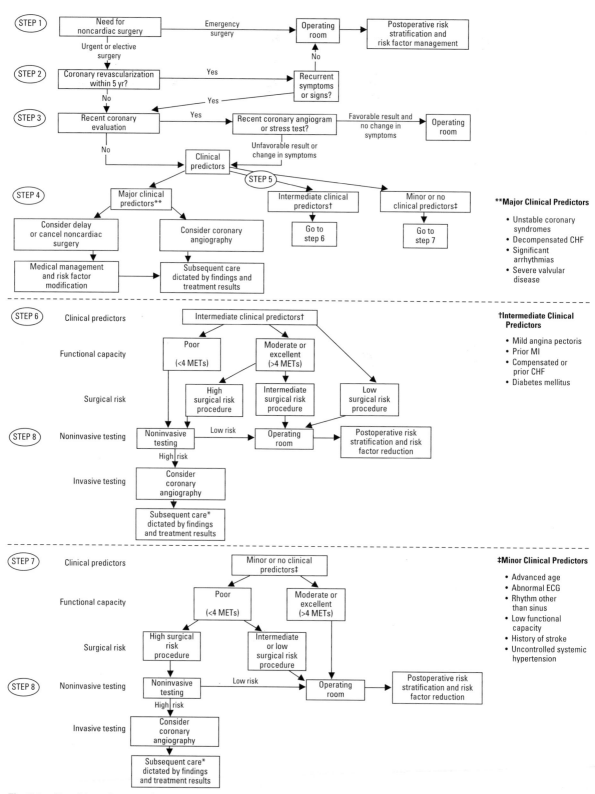

Fig. 5.3 Algorithm of a stepwise approach to preoperative cardiac assessment developed by the American Heart Association and American College of Cardiology joint task force on practice guidelines. Decisions are based on clinical predictors, urgency of surgical procedure and degree of exercise tolerance. CHF, congestive heart failure; MI, myocardial infarction; ECG, electrocardiogram; MET, metabolic equivalent. (From Eagle KA, et al[7] with permission.)

to be relatively low.[12,13] When considering a patient for revascularization, the overall risk must take into account the risk of the revascularization itself.

In the absence of clear-cut studies demonstrating the value of revascularization, Fleisher et al have constructed a decision-analysis tree.[14] This looks at the overall risk of the intervention itself (about 2.3% overall for patients in the Coronary Artery Surgery Study)[15] along with potential long-term benefit of the procedure.

For patients who are not candidates for revascularization, other therapies may be useful in the management of cardiac risk modification. Anti-ischemic medical therapy with β-blockers administered perioperatively has recently been shown to have a demonstrably positive effect.[16] Patients at risk in this study were judged to meet two of the following criteria: age > 65, hypertension, smoker, serum cholesterol > 240 mg/dL, and diabetes. Atenolol was given throughout the hospitalization. Mortality rates and rates of cardiovascular events were significantly reduced. This finding has been confirmed by a study showing a reduction in perioperative ischemia and risk of death for 2 years following short-term treatment with atenolol perioperatively.[17] In the absence of specific contraindication, β-blockade in the perioperative period may become increasingly important in the near future in the management of high-risk patients.[18] The effect of nitrates, digoxin, and calcium-channel blockers is less clear-cut.

Valvular heart disease

There are very few studies looking at non-coronary cardiac disease and cardiac risk, other than valvular aortic stenosis (AS). As is predictive of an increased risk of death and is included in the various cardiac risk indices. The presence of a suggestive murmur, even in the absence of symptoms, should lead to consideration of further evaluation with echocardiography, if possible. There are no pathognomonic findings which suggest critical AS, though left ventricular hypertrophy on ECG, cardiomegaly on chest X-ray, and the symptoms of angina, syncope and congestive failure may be present. Aortic valve replacement may be required in some cases before elective or semi-elective surgery. The hemodynamic goals while managing these patients include maintaining a relatively slow heart rate, avoiding drops in systemic vascular resistance (SVR) and preload, and preserving contractility and sinus rhythm. It would seem that this could best be accomplished by general anesthesia. Conduction anesthesia with central neuroaxial blockade and resultant sympathectomy, in the face of a fixed cardiac output, may lead to precipitous drops in SVR, preload, with hypotension and decreased coronary perfusion. This may induce ischemia and LV dysfunction, and lead to a cycle of rapid deterioration. However, epidural and continuous spinal anesthesia have been successfully utilized in such cases.[19] Plexus anesthesia, where appropriate, utilizing large volumes of local anesthetic with epinephrine may lead to tachycardia from systemic absorption or inadvertent intravascular injection. Though there is not a sympathetic blockade equivalent to that seen with neuraxial blockade, undesirable consequences may occur. Even local anesthesia in the setting of monitored anesthesia care may lead to morbidity, especially when used in a high-risk population.[20] Patients with undiagnosed critical AS may go into pulmonary edema when blood pressure control is attempted with β-blockade.

Aortic insufficiency is important to identify as long-term treatment with angiotensin-converting enzyme (ACE) inhibitors is of benefit. Patients with mitral stenosis (MS) and mitral regurgitation (MR) are at uncertain risk, although severe disease may require preoperative intervention. Severe MR may require afterload reducing agents, diuretics and pulmonary artery (PA) catheter monitoring. Patients with MS are at risk for pulmonary edema and right-heart failure and need to be monitored accordingly.

Regional versus general anesthesia

There are few randomized, controlled studies, which look at choice of anesthetic technique (general, spinal/epidural, regional or local) to be an independent risk factor for perioperative ischemic events. Various studies have given conflicting data. Most studies look at high-risk patients in the setting of vascular surgery.

Tuman et al[21] studied high-risk patients undergoing vascular surgery with either general anesthesia or general anesthesia supplemented with an epidural technique. Postoperative analgesia was obtained with parenteral narcotics or via an epidural catheter, respectively. They found marked reductions in cardiac morbidity (28% vs

10%), infectious complications (20% vs 5%), and thrombotic complications (28% vs 2.5%) in the epidural group compared with those only receiving general anesthesia. This confirmed earlier findings by Yeager et al[22] in a mixed surgical population. Conversely, later studies by Baron et al[23], Christopherson et al[24] and Bodie et al[25] in vascular surgery populations have shown no significant differences in cardiac morbidity between general and epidural or spinal anesthesia. Methodological limitations may account for the conflicting results seen in these studies. In patient populations different from the ones studied, theoretical benefits of regional anesthesia may ultimately be shown to significantly lower cardiac morbidity. Until then, there is no substitute for proper clinical evaluation and judgement in the utilization of anesthetic techniques. Practical considerations, such as the utility of an epidural for both intraoperative and postoperative management, are important parts of the clinical decision.

THE PATIENT WITH PULMONARY DISEASE

As in any acute trauma situation, the pulmonary evaluation must reflect the degree of urgency of the proposed intervention. In the case of immediate surgery, a limited assessment may consist of the history and physical exam (as always!), chest X-ray, arterial blood gases and limited spirometry, such as a peak expiratory flow measurement. With more time available to assess pulmonary function, formal pulmonary function testing (PFTs) may be utilized. PFTs with values 50% or more from normal may suggest a patient at increased risk.[26] Implied in pulmonary evaluation is the idea that this will lead to optimization of the patient's pulmonary status with the goal of minimizing the potential for perioperative pulmonary complications. This certainly applies for surgery involving the lung, but is true for non-pulmonary surgery as well. The choice of anesthetic, when options are available, may depend on data elicited by the work-up.

Typical pulmonary pathophysiology falls into the categories of obstructive and restrictive disease. Obstructive processes include asthma, chronic obstructive pulmonary disease (COPD – chronic bronchitis and emphysema) and sleep apnea. Restrictive lung diseases are seen less often, but include a large differential of fibrotic disorders, granulomatous diseases (e.g. scleroderma), obesity, skeletal and neuromuscular diseases (e.g. scoliosis and multiple sclerosis). The presence of infectious processes, such as upper and lower respiratory conditions, viral and bacterial, will also affect management decisions. Secondary vascular abnormalities, such as cor pulmonale and pulmonary hypertension, may also contribute to morbidity. Obviously, the traumatic injury may affect the lung directly by injuries to the chest wall, resulting in flail chest, pneumothorax and hemothorax, pulmonary contusion, diaphragmatic injury, and trauma-induced adult respiratory distress syndrome (ARDS).[27]

The discussion of pulmonary risk includes the possibility of postoperative hypoxia, atelectasis, bronchitis and pneumonia, bronchospasm, pulmonary aspiration, pulmonary edema (both cardiac and negative-pressure, non-cardiac), ARDS, and respiratory failure. Many patients will transiently develop some of these pulmonary 'complications' without developing long-term or serious morbidity. Studies looking at pulmonary issues related to general and regional anesthesia must consider the preoperative status of the patient, the type of surgery, and clearly define the end-points, which constitute pulmonary morbidity (e.g. postoperative mechanical ventilation or presence of pneumonia). Such considerations may make it difficult to apply study results to a given situation. Again, clinical judgement is essential to the proper management of such patients.

Factors causing patients to be considered at risk for perioperative pulmonary problems include age (over 70 years old), smoking, obesity, presence of COPD, lengthy surgical procedures (> 3 hours), abdominal, thoracic, and emergency surgery.[28] With the standard of operative pulse oximetry, all patients should have a baseline, room-air oxygen saturation determination, unless specific pulmonary evaluation has previously been carried out. An unexplained hypoxic reading should give cause for consideration of the differential diagnosis. The patient with mild decrease in saturation owing to preoperative sedation is not at increased pulmonary risk. However, failure to correct an abnormal value with simple maneuvers such as forced inspiration may suggest more ominous pathophysiology. In the setting of trauma and other high-risk situations, the presence of a pulmonary embolus (PE) or fat embolus cannot be ignored. Failure to rule this out may lead to significant perioperative morbidity.

It is tempting to assume an inherent superiority of regional anesthesia over general in the pulmonary patient, but this has not been borne out in clinical studies. In the absence of significant sedation, the patient maintains his own ventilation. This can be compromised, however, by a 'high spinal', where the level of spinal blockade affects the intercostal muscles and phrenic nerve. Interscalene blocks must be assumed to block the ipsilateral phrenic nerve, resulting in decreased ventilatory performance. The ability to cough in these instances will be diminished.

THE PATIENT WITH HEPATIC DISEASE

Most patients with significant liver disease will be identified by a thorough history and physical exam. In the days of 'shotgun' preoperative laboratory testing, many asymptomatic patients were noted to have isolated elevations of various liver-related enzymes, causing confusion among practitioners in how to proceed. In the absence of clinical evidence of liver disease by history or physical exam, there is little justification for such testing. Conversely, failure to adequately assess patients with suggestive clinical markers, by underutilization of specific testing, may result in significant missed pathology. In the setting of acute trauma, it may be reasonable to obtain various tests needed for assessment of hepatocellular injury, biliary tract integrity, and hepatic synthetic function. Balancing the need for urgent surgical intervention with the degree of hepatic risk requires understanding the implications of various patterns of abnormal hepatic data.

Various serum assays are used to delineate the type of hepatic disease present. None, by themselves, are definitive, but are useful when combined, and measured serially, in the diagnosis of liver disease. While often referred to as 'liver function tests', commonly available tests may or may not reflect derangements in hepatic function. Among the most widely utilized indices are the aminotransferases (aspartate aminotransferase – AST, SGOT, and alanine aminotransferase – ALT, SGPT), alkaline phosphatase, γ-glutamyltranspeptidase (GGTP), 5′-nucleotidase, bilirubin, serum proteins, and clotting factors (Table 5.4). Some commonly available tests,

Table 5.4 Serum hepatic testing abnormalities

Diagnostic category	Serum test	Findings
Hepatocellular injury (Acute and chronic hepatitis, cirrhosis, hepatic failure)	AST, ALT	↑ – ↑↑↑
	GGTP	± – ↑↑↑
	Bilirubin	± – ↑↑↑
	Albumin	± – ↓↓
	Prothrombin time	± – ↑↑↑
Biliary tract obstruction (Cholestasis, bile duct injury, choledocholithiasis)	AST, ALT	± – ↑
	GGTP	↑↑↑
	Alkaline phosphatase	↑↑↑
	5′-Nucleotidase	↑↑↑
	Bilirubin	± – ↑↑↑
	Albumin	±
	Prothrombin time	±

↑, increased; ↓, decreased; ±, normal or minimal change; AST, aspartate aminotransferase; ALT, alanine aminotransferase; GGTP, γ-glutamyl transpeptidase.

such as lactic dehydrogenase (LDH), are so non-specific that they are of little value. The GGTP alone lacks specificity, and may be elevated in pancreatic and renal disease. Elevations of AST may be due to non-hepatic sources, including neuromuscular disease and injury, myocardial infarction, neoplasms, and drug effect (e.g. antibiotics). The ALT is more specific for liver disease. In some patients, precise diagnosis may be required utilizing serologic testing, ultrasound, computed topography (CT), or percutaneous liver biopsy.

Serum bilirubin consists of two fractions:

1. direct reacting (with diazo reagent), water-soluble, conjugated (as mono- and diglucuronide) fraction,
2. indirect reacting, lipid soluble, unconjugated fraction.

Total bilirubin consists of the total of direct and indirect fractions. The conjugated form is the only one that appears in the urine.

The entities most often seen in patients with liver pathology include Gilbert's disease, viral hepatitis, alcoholic liver disease, fatty liver, cirrhosis, and cholestasis.

Gilbert's disease

This is a common disorder, seen in about 5% of the general population. A defect in bilirubin conjugation, it results in elevated levels of indirect bilirubin in the blood (unconjugated hyperbilirubinemia), but normal transaminases. The bilirubin tends to go up at times of stress and may cause mild jaundice, with total bilirubin generally under 3 mg/dL. It is a benign disorder and has no implications for anesthetic risk.

Viral hepatitis

Hepatitis may be either acute or chronic. Acute viral hepatitis may be due to Hepatitis A, B, C, D, E, F and G viruses, cytomegalovirus and Epstein–Barr virus. Hepatitis B, C and D viruses may lead to chronic hepatitis. Clinically, hepatitis A, B and C (formerly called non-A, non-B hepatitis) are most commonly encountered. Only serologic testing can reliably diagnose specific viral types; clinical features and routine labs can only *suggest* that hepatitis is present. In acute hepatitis transaminase levels are typically > 300 IU/L and may reach into the thousands, especially with hepatitis A and B. Intermittent laboratory testing may miss the peak enzyme elevations, however. The AST and ALT levels generally parallel each other. The bilirubin may rise to 15 to 20 mg/dL and the alkaline phosphatase and GGTP may show varying degrees of elevation. Hepatitis C, a growing public health problem, may have a more insidious nature. Most patients with hepatitis C do not present with an acute icteric illness. Diagnosis is most commonly made after routine testing reveals mild transaminase elevations. The prevalence of hepatitis C is approaching 2% of the general population and is most likely to be diagnosed in those with transfusion history prior to the mid-1990s. The majority of these patients will progress to a chronic hepatitis with subsequent cirrhosis and, possibly, hepatoma. Chronic hepatitis, aside from viral etiologies, may be due to autoimmune causes, cryptogenic, drug-induced, associated with Wilson's disease, α_1-antitrypsin deficiency, and cholestatic diseases. Transaminases may be minimally elevated, or reach into the mid-hundreds. The bilirubin tends to be normal in chronic viral hepatitis. Chronic hepatitis, defined as disease lasting for 6 months or more, may be classified as chronic persistent or chronic active (or aggressive), based on liver biopsy pathology.

Studies available on the risk of anesthesia in patients with acute hepatitis are very limited, but suggest very high mortality rates (ranging from 9–100%).[29,30] No satisfactory data are available on the relative merits of general or regional anesthesia in these patients. Surgery should only be contemplated in life-threatening situations. Patients with chronic hepatitis, however, appear to be at much lower risk for surgery. Again, no satisfactory outcome studies are available, but in the patient with stable transaminases and good hepatic synthetic function, the risk appears to be acceptable for necessary interventions. Arguments made about the superiority of regional anesthesia in these situations sound appealing, but are not based on firm data. In the absence of specific contraindications, regional techniques are reasonable modalities. In the consideration of maintenance of hepatic blood flow as a possibly desirable end-point, there seems to be no advantage of neuroaxial block over general anesthesia,[31] but peripheral nerve blocks may be less likely to cause reduction.

Alcoholic liver disease

Patients with alcoholic liver disease run the gamut from mild fatty infiltration of the liver, to severe alcoholic hepatitis, to cirrhosis. The GGTP may be elevated out of proportion to the transaminases. The AST/ALT ratio may be 2 or more (also increased in fatty liver of pregnancy). The scant evidence available suggests a high mortality is associated with surgery in patients with alcoholic hepatitis.[32]

Fatty liver

Patients with minimally elevated transaminases and variable elevations of GGTP may have diffuse fatty liver disease. This may present with minimal or no symptoms. It is often associated with alcohol intake, pregnancy, diabetes mellitus, obesity, glucocorticoid therapy, and drugs (e.g. methotrexate). An enlarged, non- or minimally tender liver may be present, and the diagnosis is usually made by abdominal ultrasound, CT or MRI scan. The anesthetic implications, in the presence of normal hepatic synthetic function, are minimal, unless associated with alcoholic hepatitis.

Cirrhosis

Patients with cirrhosis may be classified by the methods of Child or Pugh.[33] Mild cirrhosis, with low bilirubin, normal albumin, minimally prolonged PT and no ascites or encephalopathy (Class A) has a 5–10% mortality rate. Class C (bilirubin > 2, albumin < 2.8, PT > 6 seconds prolonged, ascites and encephalopathy present) has a very high potential mortality (> 50%). Class B falls in-between. As before, no good data are available regarding choice of anesthetic in the absence of specific contraindications, such as coagulopathy, for spinal or epidural anesthesia.

Cholestasis

Patients with cholestasis, or obstructive jaundice, frequently undergo surgery to correct the biliary obstruction. As an incidental finding in the trauma patient, the presence of cholestasis increases the probability of perioperative sepsis and acute renal failure. In the presence of a high bilirubin level (> 10 mg/dL) mortality levels are significantly increased regardless of anesthetic choice.[34] Cholestatic liver disease may also be a result of specific drug injury, such as anabolic steroids, oral contraceptives, calcium-channel antagonists (e.g. verapamil), and the immuno-suppressive cyclosporine.

THE PATIENT WITH ENDOCRINE DISEASE

The most common endocrine abnormalities encountered are diabetes mellitus, thyroid diseases, and adrenally-suppressed patients. While no good studies exist which specifically look at regional anesthesia in these settings, optimization regardless of the anesthetic choice should be a clinical goal.

Diabetes mellitus

In the acute setting, the goal of management is to reasonably control the glucose level by administration of insulin and fluids, and control any apparent acid–base and electrolyte abnormalities. Preoperative evaluation should also be directed towards the assessment of associated end-organ disease, including cardiac, renal, peripheral vascular, and peripheral and autonomic neuropathies. The potential for diabetic gastric paresis, particularly in the trauma patient, may significantly increase the possibility of aspiration. In the insulin-dependent diabetic patient, the stress of a traumatic injury may lead to the development of diabetic ketoacidosis (DKA) with its associated metabolic abnormalities. Hyperglycemia, acido-sis, hyperkalemia, hyponatremia and volume depletion are hallmarks of DKA. Induction of general anesthesia in such a patient, even with agents considered to provide hemodynamic stability, such as etomidate, may lead to marked hypotension. The total body water deficit may approach 10 L or more. Correction of these abnormalities should be done before surgical intervention, if possible. Fluid replacement should be with normal or half-normal saline (Ringer's lactate may transiently increase the potassium and glucose levels). Invasive monitoring may be useful, particularly in the management of vascular volume status. The use of continuous infusions of regular insulin (5–10 units per hour) until the acidosis and hyperglycemia are resolved may help simplify management. While hyperkalemic when acidemic, these patients tend to be potassium-depleted, and may require repletion with potassium chloride or potassium phosphate appropriately administered (never as a bolus injection). Insulin may need to be administered with glucose until the acidosis resolves. Patients may be at increased risk of cardiovascular morbidity, as a result of both the associated increased risk of cardiac disease and the associated acute stress response to DKA. The vast majority of diabetic patients have non-insulin-dependent, or Type-II, diabetes, with an incidence in the general population of around 6%. Many of these patients will be on oral- hypoglycemic agents either alone or in combination with insulin. No standard therapy for control of perioperative glucose is mandated, but coverage of elevated glucose levels with regular human insulin is the goal. The frequency of glucose determination should be guided by the patient's clinical parameters.

Thyroid disease

Most patients with significant thyroid disease will present with varying degrees of hypothyroidism. Thyroid storm, while a metabolic crisis, is rare and usually seen in hyperthyroid patients with Grave's disease in the setting of thyroid surgery or secondary to some particular precipitant, such as infection or trauma. It constitutes a medical emergency with a high mortality and must be aggressively treated via a multi-stage approach:

• correct the hyperthyroidism
• normalize the homeostatic decompensation
• treat the precipitating event.

Patients with hypothyroidism who are being treated with thyroid hormone replacement rarely present a problem. Mild hypothyroidism is not generally considered a contraindication to surgery,[35] although limited data have suggested otherwise.[36,37] Only instances of severe hypothyroidism leading to myxedema is there clear reason to delay surgery, if possible.[38] Myxedema may lead to CHF, coma, and circulatory collapse perioperatively. Acute treatment with thyroid replacement may precipitate angina and MI. Preoperative assessment with thyroid stimulating hormone (TSH) levels and triiodothyronine (T_3) and thyroxine (T_4 or free T_4) measurements may be needed.

In patients with evidence of hypothyroidism who require urgent surgery, there are theoretical advantages to regional anesthesia, though none proven in clinical studies. Thyroid goiter may lead to airway compromise, which may lead one to use a regional anesthetic in mild cases. Myxedema may cause swelling of the upper airway with macroglossia and vocal cord edema. Where severe airway abnormalities exist, however, a secured airway is of paramount importance. The question of postoperative respiratory depression following general anesthesia with hypothyroidism may suggest using a regional technique. Coagulation abnormalities may be present and should be assessed with appropriate testing.

Adrenal suppression

While there are many entities leading to adrenal insufficiency (Addison's disease, infectious processes), most cases will be secondary to adrenal suppression as a result of steroid treatment. This is especially likely in those with rheumatic diseases, asthma and COPD. 'Stress' doses of cortisone or its equivalents (Table 5.5) are essential parts of the

Table 5.5 Glucocorticoid equivalencies

Drug	Equivalent dose (mg)	Duration of action (half-life)
Cortisone	25	Short (< 8 h half-life)
Hydrocortisone	20	Short (< 8 h)
Cortisol	20	Short (< 8 h)
Prednisone	5	Intermediate (12–24 h)
Prednisolone	5	Intermediate (12–24 h)
Methylprednisolone	4	Intermediate (24–36 h)
Dexamethasone	0.7	Long (48–72 h)

All have similar mineralocorticoid potency (about 0.5% of fludrocortisone) except dexamethasone, which has no mineralocorticoid effect.

Table 5.6 Perioperative steroid coverage for patients on exogenous glucocorticoid therapy

Degree of surgical stress	Suggested regimen (daily hydrocortisone equivalent)
Minor surgery	25–50 mg, or baseline dose
Intermediate stress	50–75 mg
Major surgery	100–300 mg (typical regimen: 100 mg IV q 8 h)

IV, intravenous.

perioperative medical regimen (Table 5.6). The use of steroids (including topical preparations) for a week or longer within the year preceding surgery suggest perioperative steroid supplementation.[39] Some patients on long-term steroid therapy may remain suppressed for up to 2 years after termination of therapy.

THE PATIENT WITH RENAL AND ELECTROLYTE DISORDERS

As renal function is intimately involved with regulation of electrolyte and acid–base balance, significant disorders tend to be noted during evaluation of laboratory testing routinely obtained in most trauma patients. The 'SMA-6', or standard test for electrolytes (sodium, potassium, chloride and bicarbonate) with blood, urea, nitrogen (BUN) and serum creatinine, can reveal the presence of acute or chronic renal failure. While acute renal failure may be seen in trauma and critically ill patients, the role of regional anesthesia tends to be limited to those presenting with various degrees of chronic renal insufficiency, including patients on dialysis. However, anesthetic interventions should be utilized with consideration towards preventing the development of acute renal failure in high-risk patients.

Acute renal failure

Patients at risk for acute renal failure perioperatively include elderly patients with preexisting renal insufficiency, congestive failure, trauma patients with shock or sepsis, massive blood transfusion, cholestasis, rhabdomyolysis, those undergoing vascular surgery, and those receiving radiographic contrast media or nephrotoxic drugs (e.g. amphotericin B).[40] Intensive care unit patients are at

Table 5.7 Causes of acute renal failure

Class	Etiologies
Prerenal failure	Hypovolemia (hemorrhage, dehydration, GI loss, diuresis, burns)
	↓Cardiac output (cardiomyopathy, valvular disease, pulmonary hypertension)
	↑Renal vascular resistance (sepsis, cirrhosis, antihypertensives, anesthetics)
	Drug effects (cyclooxygenase inhibitors, angiotensin converting enzyme inhibitors)
Intrinsic failure	Acute tubular necrosis (ischemia, trauma, free hemoglobin, myoglobin, direct toxic effects of drugs, e.g. radiocontrast, aminoglycosides, cyclosporin A)
	Interstitial nephritis (infectious, allergic)
	Glomerulonephritis
	Renovascular disease (vasculitis, direct injury, thrombosis)
	Systemic disease (lupus, scleroderma, sickle cell disease)
Postrenal failure	Ureteral obstruction (calculi, tumor)
	Bladder neck obstruction (cancer, prostate disease, neurogenic bladder)
	Urethral obstruction (phimosis, strictures)

↓, decreased; ↑, increased.

Table 5.8 Clinical findings in chronic renal failure and uremia

System	Findings
Fluid and electrolytes	Hypervolemia, metabolic acidosis, hyperkalemia, hyperphosphatemia, hypocalcemia
Cardiovascular	Hypertension, pericarditis, cardiomyopathy, pulmonary edema
Hematologic	Anemia (normocytic, normochromic), platelet dysfunction, hypersplenism
Metabolic	Renal osteodystrophy, secondary hyperparathyroidism, hyperuricemia
Gastrointestinal	Anorexia, peptic ulcer disease, nausea
Neuromuscular	Lethargy, asterixis, neuropathy, seizures

particular high risk for development of acute renal disease. Proper management requires identification of the major causes, divided into prerenal failure, intrinsic acute renal failure, and postrenal obstructive failure (Table 5.7). Modalities for prevention of acute renal failure include maintenance of cardiac output, prevention of reflex vasoconstriction (by maintaining intravascular volume, use of calcium channel blockers and ACE inhibitors), renal vasodilatation (e.g. via dopamine) and preservation of tubular flow.[41] The presence of specific electrolyte disorders in the absence of clear-cut renal disease must also be addressed to optimize the patient's status perioperatively. Patients at particularly high risk for renal disease are those where systemic disease leads to end-organ damage, as in hypertension, diabetes, and various collagen vascular diseases (such as rheumatoid arthritis and systemic lupus erythematosus).

Chronic renal insufficiency

Chronic renal insufficiency and failure represent a spectrum of diseases, from multiple etiologies, characterized by a steady decrease in the number of functioning nephrons. This results in decreased glomerular filtration rate (GFR), ultimately leading to end-stage renal disease and the need for dialysis in severely affected patients. Advanced stages of renal disease may lead to metabolic acidosis, hyperkalemia, hypocalcemia, hyperphosphatemia, hypervolemia, hypertension, and disorders of platelet and immune function (Table 5.8). Drugs dependent on renal excretion will require modification of dosing based on the GFR (e.g. digoxin). Anemia and associated increased cardiac index may result in decreased duration of local anesthetic activity.[42] Erythropoietin therapy is generally utilized to minimize the severe anemia usually seen. Patients on dialysis should be dialyzed within the 24 hours preceding surgery, if possible, especially in the presence of marked electrolyte imbalance and fluid overload. Assessment of coagulation status should be considered for patients who are candidates for regional anesthesia, especially major conduction blocks.

THE PATIENT WITH COAGULOPATHY AND THE ANTICOAGULATED PATIENT

When discussing the presence of a coagulopathy, we usually refer to the presence of abnormal coagulation test results obtained during preoperative testing. These may be due to an actual disorder of the coagulation pathway (generally abnormal factor concentration or biologically inactive factors), leading to clinical bleeding abnormalities. There may be circulating anticoagulants, or inhibitors, which cause abnormal test results but do not increase the clinical risk of bleeding and may lead to a hypercoagulable state (lupus anticoagulant). Other inhibitors are associated with hemorrhage, such as an anti-factor VIII antibody seen with autoimmune disorders. Patients may be receiving anticoagulant medication designed to achieve full or partial anticoagulation or prevent thromboembolic complications related to high-risk situations such as surgery and trauma. Platelet number and function may be abnormal resulting in abnormal coagulation. The role of regional anesthesia and analgesia depends on the specifics of a given clinical picture.

Evaluating a patient starts with a history directed towards uncovering episodes of bleeding or thrombosis. Specifically, questions regarding a history of easy bruisability, epistaxis, patterns of bleeding (e.g. petechial or mucosal bleeding), bleeding associated with dental work or other surgical interventions, menstrual pattern and specific drug use should be asked. Drugs with anti-platelet activity as well as warfarin-type drugs are associated with increased bleeding tendencies. Conversely, patients with hypercoagulability may give a history of thrombosis and thromboembolic phenomena. This may be seen in patients with deficiencies of Antithrombin-III, protein-C and protein-S. In patients with suggestive histories, coagulation tests (Table 5.9) typically include the prothrombin time (PT) and activated partial thromboplastin time (PTT or aPTT). A complete blood count with platelet count should be done. Other tests available are the thrombin time (TT),

reptilase time (RT), bleeding time, specific tests of platelet function, and specific factor analyses. Details on the normal coagulation pathway can be found elsewhere[43] (Fig. 5.4).

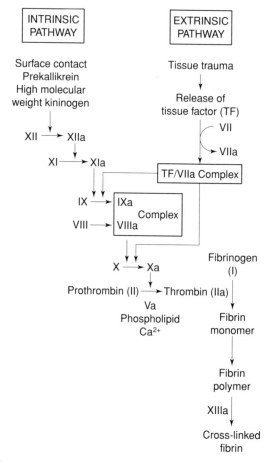

Fig. 5.4 Schematic of the coagulation cascade, delineating the intrinsic and extrinsic pathways. Refer to text for correlation with coagulation testing.

Table 5.9 Coagulation testing

Test	Factors measured	Normal range	Elevated in
Protime (PT)	Extrinsic pathway– I, II, V, VII, X	9–12 s	Coumadin therapy
Partial thrombo-plastin time (PTT)	Intrinsic pathway–I, II, V, VIII, IX, X, XI	25–35 s	Heparin therapy
Thrombin time (TT)	I, II	15–16 s	Heparin, DIC
Reptilase time	I	15 s	DIC, dysfibrinogenemia (normal with heparin)
Bleeding time	Platelet aggregation	<9–10 m	Disorders of platelet function, thrombocytopenia, cyclooxygenase inhibitors

DIC, disseminated intravascular coagulation.

Coagulation tests

PTT

The PTT is a test of the intrinsic coagulation pathway. Kaolin is added to whole plasma 6 minutes prior to the test, to provide a foreign surface and maximally activate factors XII and XI. Cephalin, a platelet lipid surrogate, is then added and the time to produce fibrin is noted. The test is sensitive to deficiencies of procoagulant activation preceding factor X activation. It is very sensitive to the action of heparin (which inhibits activation of factors II, IX, X and XI via the Heparin–Antithrombin III complex).

PT

This test of the extrinsic pathway of coagulation is done by adding thromboplastin (tissue factor) to plasma measuring the time to fibrin formation (usually 10 to 11 seconds). It measures deficiencies of factors I, II, V, VII and X. Factors II, VII, IX and X are vitamin-K dependent procoagulants, which require vitamin-K for γ-carboxylation of glutamic acid residues to achieve activation. As factor VII has the shortest biologic half-life, the PT is sensitive for clinically utilized vitamin-K antagonists, such as coumadin. Different commercially available thromboplastins have varying sensitivity to the effects of these agents on procoagulant activity. This makes it difficult to translate specific study results to clinical practice. The World Health Organization (WHO) has established the International Normalized Ratio (INR) for interlaboratory comparisons. A standard reference thromboplastin has been developed for calibration of individual thromboplastins, enabling the reporting of prothrombin time ratios to assess clinical effects on the PT. The clinically useful range of INR to manage coumadin therapy is 2.0 to 3.0 for treatment and prophylaxis of deep venous thrombosis and pulmonary embolism. Patients receiving stroke prophylaxis in the presence of atrial fibrillation are maintained between 2.0 and 3.5,[44] while those with mechanical valves should have INR values of 3.0 to 4.0. Values below 2.0 lead to increased risk, while increased risk of hemorrhage is associated with values above 4.0 to 4.5.[45]

TT

The thrombin time tests for abnormalities in the conversion of fibrinogen to fibrin. Dilute preparations of thrombin are added to plasma to obtain a normal TT of about 15 seconds (pure thrombin, being very active, would give a TT of about 5 seconds and overwhelm inhibitor activity). Prolongations of the TT, representing inhibition of fibrinogen to fibrin conversion, are due to Heparin–Antithrombin III complex and fibrin degradation products (FDPs). It is therefore a sensitive indicator of heparin activity and disseminated intravascular coagulation (DIC). It may also be prolonged by dysfibronogenemias and paraproteinemias.

Other tests

The bleeding time tests platelet count and function. It increases as the platelet count decreases below 100 000 in the presence of normal platelets. It is increased in the presence of abnormal platelet function when the platelet count is above 100 000. Drugs affecting platelet function, such as aspirin and nonsteroidal anti-inflammatory agents, will prolong the bleeding time, but an abnormal test does not reliably predict the risk of hemorrhage.[46] It is particularly useful in screening for, and in following the treatment of, von Willebrand's disease (the most common inherited disorder of hemostasis). Specific tests of platelet function measure platelet aggregation to various reagents, and are generally the province of the hematology consultant. The RT uses reptilase, a thrombin-like enzyme that converts fibrinogen to fibrin. Unlike the TT, it is not affected by Heparin–Antithrombin-III complex. It is more sensitive to dysfibrinogenemias than the TT. In the presence of heparin, one would expect a prolonged TT and a normal RT.

Use of regional anesthesia

The question of how safe it is to utilize a regional technique in the patient with a coagulation disorder can be broken down into several categories:

- Are we dealing with a minor local anesthetic, a major plexus block, or a spinal or epidural block?
- Is there a difference in a patient who is partially or fully anticoagulated?
- Is there any problem in a patient with a treated coagulopathy, or one with a circulating anticoagulant?

Clearly, any uncontrolled bleeding is a potential problem at any regional anesthesia site. The spinal canal is particularly vulnerable to bleeding because of complications associated with an epidural or subarachnoid bleed. However, the risk of such a bleed is relatively low owing to several factors.[47] Quantifying the risk and carrying out adequate studies to compare groups is difficult because of the need for large patient groups. Meta-analysis and case reports have been used to evaluate these complications. A review by Vandermeulen et al has looked at the many clinical studies published.[48] One issue frequently presenting in the acute setting is the use of conduction anesthesia in patients on aspirin. Use of the bleeding time in this situation needs to be critically evaluated, as there is no good correlation between bleeding time and hemorrhage.[49] Platelet aggregation may be abnormal in the face of a normal bleeding time. However, the risk of significant bleeding in patients receiving epidural or spinal anesthesia while on aspirin appears to be quite low.[50] The entire clinical picture for a given patient must be considered when making this choice.

Thromboprophylaxis

Patients who may present for surgery in the trauma setting, especially with long-bone trauma, may be receiving prophylaxis against venous thromboembolism (to prevent deep venous thrombosis and pulmonary embolism) (Table 5.10). This may consist of mechanical modalities as well as pharmacologic agents. Elastic compression stockings and intermittent or sequential pneumatic compression devices are commonly utilized with or without specific drug therapy. In the past, pharmacologic measures included the use of volume expanders such as dextran, warfarin, intravenous heparin and low fixed dose

Table 5.10 Modalities of venous thromboembolism prophylaxis

Mechanical methods: compression stockings, intermittent pneumatic compression boots
Low-dose (mini) heparin
Low molecular weight heparins
Dextran
Warfarin (coumadin)

(minidose) heparin, usually given subcutaneously. More recently, low molecular weight heparin (LMWH) preparations have replaced unfractionated heparin for prophylaxis, first in specific clinical settings, such as following total hip and knee replacements, and then more generally. Minidose heparin and aspirin have tended to be used in patients undergoing thoracoabdominal surgery or in elderly and debilitated patients. There is a growing trend to administer prophylaxis to patients in the intensive care unit setting. Many patients being so treated will present for surgery having received minidose heparin or LMWH within the preceding 12 hours. A question of major importance is how safe is it to administer a central neural block in these patients, and, further, what are the implications of indwelling catheters in terms of the risk of bleeding complications?

LMWH, unlike standard heparin, has long-acting anti-X activity (2 to 4 times its anti-II activity), which is about 50% of peak activity 12 hours after dosing. There is no simple test readily available to indicate the degree of residual anticoagulant activity present. This has led to increased complication rates.

Recent reports to the Food and Drug Administration (FDA) have described cases of spinal hematomas in patients receiving spinal and epidural anesthetics in patients on LMWH. The FDA issued a health advisory on the use of LMWH, marketed as Lovenox (enoxaparin sodium, Rhone-Poulenc-Rorer Pharmaceuticals, Inc.) and others, stating, in part:

The FDA is advising doctors to carefully monitor patients receiving low molecular weight heparins or heparinoids for possible spinal or epidural bleeding.

The risk for bleeding or hematomas is increased by use of catheters placed in the spinal canal to administer pain medication or by the use of other drugs that can affect blood clotting such as non-steroidal anti-inflammatory drugs, platelet inhibitors, or other anticoagulants. The risk of adverse effects also appears to be increased by traumatic or repeated spinal or epidural punctures.[51]

A review by Horlocker & Heit on standard heparin (SH) and LMWH provides some guidelines in this area.[52] A more recent editorial review[53] adds to the recommendations:

1. IV heparin should not be started for at least 60 minutes after needle placement and anticoagulation status is acceptable (PTT 1.5 to 2.0 times control).

2. The smallest effective dose of LMWH should be used (e.g. 40 mg once a day of enoxaparin). Therapy should be delayed as long as possible postoperatively (12 to 24 hours).
3. Antiplatelet or oral anticoagulants given with LMWH may increase the risk of spinal hematoma.
4. Indwelling catheters may increase the risk of spinal hematoma while on LMWH. Removal should occur before LMWH therapy, if possible. Catheters should be removed only when heparin activity is low or completely reversed. If on subcutaneous heparin (SH), needle placement and catheter removal should wait for at least 4 hours following previous dose. If on LMWH, 10 to 12 hours should elapse prior to removal.
5. In patients on LMWH, a single shot spinal technique is probably the safest neuroaxial block. The procedure should not be done until 10 to 12 hours after the last administered dose has elapsed. Subsequent doses should not be given for at least 2 hours after needle insertion.
6. Increased vigilance in patients with indwelling catheters receiving LMWH is recommended to detect neurological changes, which may suggest hematoma formation. This can be achieved more easily by the use of opioids or dilute local anesthetic concentrations. Monitoring for neurological dysfunction should include observing for increasing degree of block, changes in bowel and bladder function, and presence of back pain. If suspected, hematoma may be diagnosed by MRI, and should be treated within 8 hours by decompressive laminectomy to prevent irreversible damage.

It is essential, therefore, to have precise knowledge of a patient's medical regimen, including all drugs and a record of administration, when planning a regional anesthetic. The same, certainly, can be said of any anesthetic, but is of particular concern in the above situations. The use of neuroaxial techniques in patients with coagulopathy, or on anticoagulants, should be carefully weighed with the potential for serious side effects before final selection. Little data exists on the safety of other forms of regional anesthesia, but it seems that reasonable caution in these settings should guide the practitioner in their safe use.

REGIONAL ANESTHESIA IN THE INFECTED PATIENT

The question of whether regional anesthesia and analgesia is safe in the patient with infection is not one that can be definitively answered by randomized, prospective studies. The question has many sub-categories, and the ultimate solution rests with proper clinical judgement based on the particulars of a given patient. Is the patient considered septic, infected but with stable hemodynamics, or at risk for bacteremia? Is there a difference between major conduction anesthetics and plexus anesthesia, and is a single shot technique safer than one involving an indwelling catheter? We need to establish how infection, in particular, leads to increased risk by nature of the regional technique, as opposed to general anesthesia. Clinical studies that look into these questions are generally concerned with spinal or epidural anesthetics. The issue addressed is usually related to risk of epidural abscess and meningitis. Exceedingly rare is the risk of vertebral osteomyelitis. Presumably, these risks are of substantially greater significance than potential infection at the site of a peripheral block.

In vitro studies of local anesthetics have demonstrated deleterious effects on various areas of immune function. These include decreased chemotaxis,[54] phagocytosis,[55] and macrophage function.[56] However, at the plasma levels of local anesthetics found with typical doses used in spinal and epidural anesthesia, these effects appear of little significance.[57] Additionally, the routine use of antibiotics in the hospitalized patient undergoing surgery, especially in the face of a known infection or bacteremia, may limit the risk.[58] Yeager et al have demonstrated a lower incidence of infection when using epidural analgesia postoperatively when compared to parenteral opioids.[59]

Diagnostic lumbar punctures in pediatric populations have shown no increased risk for subsequent meningitis in the presence of bacteremia.[60] Retrospective studies of epidural anesthesia in obstetric patients show only rare episodes of epidural infection, but with no obvious relationship to bacteremia.[61] In obstetric patients with chorioamnionitis, one study of 319 women showed an 8% incidence of bacteremia but no infectious complications in those receiving epidurals.[62] A more recent study showed similar findings in a group of 517 women.[63]

Limited data from animal models have suggested that dural puncture in the presence of bacteremia without antibiotics is associated with a high risk of meningitis.[64] A small group of patients with systemic infections who had indwelling epidural catheters and died from other causes showed a high incidence (7/9) of signs of epidural infection, but no abscesses.[65]

From this and similar data, it seems reasonable to include regional anesthetic techniques in the trauma patient with signs of infection. For those with infections that are more serious or sepsis, and those with multiple risk factors, such as diabetes, HIV, steroid suppression and other immunosuppressed states, careful consideration to the type of regional procedure should be given. The probable increased risk associated with indwelling catheters, especially epidural ones, should be factored into the final decision. Obvious infection at the site of injection should be taken as a potential contraindication. Cellulitis at the site of epidural injection has been associated with an increased risk of meningitis.[66] The ultimate anesthetic choice should balance the potential advantages of a regional anesthetic in a given clinical situation with the possibility of infectious complications.

BENEFITS OF REGIONAL ANESTHESIA/ANALGESIA IN TRAUMA

Discussions of the specific benefits of regional anesthesia (Table 5.11) are usually given in terms of a 'general versus regional' context. The question of which technique is 'safer' may have little relevance in most clinical situations. Certain preferences for particular techniques may result from the biases of a given team, including the anesthesiologist, surgeon and patient. A few limited circumstances may proscribe the utilization of a given method, as we have noted. However, most situations must be analyzed without the benefit of study results conclusively demonstrating superiority of a given method. This may be due to study limitations, absence of adequate prospective research, or to a true absence of superiority of technique. Practitioners of anesthesia must utilize their skills to assess the needs of a patient with a particular set of clinical and surgical parameters and synthesize an anesthetic plan which will be as safe as possible. Benefits of regional anesthesia are just that, and should not always be thought of in context of 'versus general'.

By simple avoidance of general anesthesia associated with tracheal intubation, regional anesthesia avoids risks associated with laryngoscopy and the endotracheal tube. In the trauma patient with 'full stomach' considerations, regional anesthesia, when appropriate, preserves protective airway reflexes. In the absence of concurrent sedation, the likelihood of drug-induced nausea and vomiting is decreased, as is the presence of early lethargy. Other benefits to the gastrointestinal system include decreased likelihood of postoperative ileus and delayed gastric emptying as a result of sympathetic blockade with conduction anesthesia.[67] Regional blocks, which persist into the recovery period, give pain relief without immediate need for separate modes of analgesia. Certainly, for the patient unwilling to undergo general anesthesia, or for the one who desires to be awake, regional anesthesia should be offered if clinically appropriate.

RISKS OF REGIONAL ANESTHESIA/ANALGESIA IN TRAUMA

Risks of regional anesthesia may be specific to the trauma situation, e.g. in a patient acutely hypovolemic, or to the risks related to specific regional techniques which may apply to any patient. There may also be relative and absolute contraindications to regional techniques in any given clinical situation (Table 5.12).

Technique-specific risk can be broken down into risk from peripheral nerve block and from spinal/epidural block.

Table 5.11   Benefits of regional anesthesia in trauma

Suppression of surgical stress response (↓sympathetic tone)
↓ Blood loss
↓ Incidence of venous thromboembolism
Improved peripheral vascular circulation
Improved gastrointestinal function
Reduced pulmonary complications
Supplement to general anesthesia
Postoperative analgesia
Improved mental status

↓, decreased.

Table 5.12 Contraindications to regional anesthesia in trauma

Hemodynamic instability (shock, multisystem trauma)
Coagulopathy
Patient/surgeon refusal
Uncooperative patient (alcohol withdrawal, psychiatric illness)
Infection at site of injection
Specific medical conditions (e.g. severe aortic or mitral stenosis and spinal)
Anesthesiologist inexperience and inability to perform block
Inability to secure airway if necessary (failure of block, prolonged procedure)

Spinal anesthesia

The risks of spinal anesthesia are secondary to the needle puncture itself, and the effects of local anesthetic in the spinal canal. The use of various size needles with different bevels and orifice locations has had varying effects on the incidence of postdural puncture headache (PDPH). While PDPH is the most common significant side effect of lumbar puncture, the potential for significant complications in susceptible patients exists (Table 5.13).

Neurologic complications may be due to spinal anesthesia or non-anesthetic factors related to surgical technique, positioning, or tourniquet use.

Despite the use of lidocaine for spinal anesthesia for many decades, recently concern has developed over association of intrathecal lidocaine with transient radicular irritation[68] and cauda equina syndrome.[69] Initial concern was over the use of hyperbaric lidocaine solutions, but reports of problems with isobaric solutions have been published.[70] Tetracaine and bupivicaine may be

Table 5.13 Complications of lumbar puncture

Headache
Back pain
Nerve root irritation
Vasovagal syncope
Cauda equina syndrome (adhesive arachnoiditis)
Cranial neuropathies
Infection (epidural abscess, meningitis)
Anterior spinal artery syndrome
Implantation of epidural tumors
Herniation (tonsillar or uncal)
Seizures

less problematic. Isobaric solutions of 0.5% bupivicaine, with or without vasoconstrictors, especially in orthopedic trauma, have the advantages of reliability, less prominent sympathetic blockade and less likelihood of radicular symptoms postoperatively.

Epidural anesthesia may lead to intrathecal or intravascular injections of local anesthetics leading to total spinal or seizures. The consequences may be minimal or severe if rapid securing of the airway and control of hemodynamic alterations are delayed. The potential for epidural hematoma, especially in those receiving thromboembolic prophylaxis, has been noted. Hemodynamic effects, including hypotension and bradycardia, are well known. Volume loading to offset decreases in blood pressure may lead to central volume overload in patients with cardiac compromise when sympathetic blockade resolves.

Peripheral nerve block

In any clinical setting, and especially in trauma, the skillful administration of a nerve block is required to achieve the goals of adequate anesthesia with a low incidence of side effects. Practitioners who are not adept at a particular technique are likely to require significantly more time to administer the anesthetic compared with general anesthesia. This may be compounded by an unacceptably high failure rate to achieve an effect. The need to be familiar with regional anesthetic techniques and maintain clinical proficiency will minimize the need for block supplementation by general anesthesia.

Direct nerve injury from the needle may lead to mild, transient paresthesias, or, when severe, pain and paralysis which may persist for months or longer. Controversy exists over the superiority of the paresthesia versus nerve stimulator technique as far as safety is concerned. Whichever method is utilized, careful attention to performance of the block is necessary for maximal safety.

Because of the near-toxic levels of local anesthetic agents utilized in major nerve blocks, inadvertent vascular injection or larger then toxic amounts of local anesthetic may lead to seizures (see Chap. 4). Inability to strictly control the duration of a block, in the absence of continuous catheter techniques, may be problematic in patients where the duration of surgery is highly variable. This is less of a factor with continuous epidural methods.

SUMMARY

The role of regional techniques for anesthesia and analgesia in the trauma patient requires a thorough evaluation of the many clinical parameters present in a given patient. The nature of the trauma determines the urgency of intervention. Whether regional anesthesia is appropriate is based on the type of the procedure to be performed, the hemodynamic, neurological, and medical status of the patient, the balancing of the potential benefits and disadvantages of the technique, the attitudes of the patient and surgeon, and the skill of the anesthesiologist.[71] The role of a proper medical evaluation, given the constraints of the time available preoperatively, has been discussed. The significant advantage of regional techniques being utilized for perioperative analgesia may be of major benefit in the appropriate patient.

REFERENCES

1. Mangano DT. Perioperative cardiac morbidity. Anesthesiology 1990; 72: 153–184.
2. Eagle KA, Coley CM. Preoperative assessment and perioperative management of cardiac ischemic risk in noncardiac surgery. Curr Probl Cardiol 1996; 21(5): 298.
3. Goldman L. Cardiac risk in non-cardiac surgery: An update. Anesth Analg 1995; 80: 810–820.
4. Goldman L, Caldera DL, Nussbaum SR, et al. Multifactorial index of cardiac risk in non-cardiac surgical procedures. N Engl J Med 1977; 297: 845–850.
5. Detsky A, Abrams H, McLaughlin J, et al. Predicting cardiac complications in patients undergoing non-cardiac surgery. J Gen Intern Med 1986; 1: 211–219.
6. Cohen MM, Duncan PG. Physical status score and trends in anesthetic complications. J Clin Epidemiol 1988; 41: 83–90.
7. Eagle K, Brundage B, Chaitman B, et al. Guidelines for perioperative cardiovascular evaluation for noncardiac surgery. Circulation 1996; 93: 1278–1317.
8. Palda VA, Detsky AS. American College of Physicians. Guidelines for assessing and managing the perioperative risk from coronary artery disease associated with major noncardiac surgery. Ann Intern Med 1997; 127: 309–328.
9. Eagle KA, Rihal CS, Mickel MC, et al. Cardiac risk of noncardiac surgery: influence of coronary disease and type of surgery in 3368 operations. Circulation 1997; 96: 1882–1887.
10. Fleisher LA, Rosenbaum SH, Nelson AH, et al. Preoperative dipyridamole thallium imaging and Holter monitoring as a predictor of perioperative cardiac events and long-term outcome. Anesthesiology 1995; 83: 906–917.
11. Lane RT, Sawada S, Seger DS, et al. Dobutamine stress echocardiography for assessment of cardiac risk before noncardiac surgery. Am J Cardiol 1991; 68: 976–977.
12. Nielsen J, Page CP, Mann C, et al. Risk of major elective operation after myocardial revascularization. Am J Surg 1992; 164: 423–426.
13. Huber KC, Evans MA, Bresnahan JF, et al. Outcome of noncardiac operations in patients with severe coronary artery disease successfully treated preoperatively with coronary angioplasty. Mayo Clin Proc 1992; 67: 15–21.
14. Fleisher LA, Skoloick ED, Holroyd KJ, Lehmann HP. Coronary artery revascularization before abdominal aortic aneurysm surgery: a decision analytic approach. Anesth Analg 1994; 79: 661–669.
15. Foster ED, Davis KB, Carpenter JA, et al. Risk of noncardiac operation in patients with defined coronary disease: The Coronary Artery Surgery Study (CASS) registry experience. Ann Thorac Surg 1986; 41: 42–50.
16. Mangano DT, Layug EL, Wallace A, Tarco I. Effects of atenolol on mortality and cardiovascular morbidity after noncardiac surgery. The Multicenter Study of Perioperative Ischemia Research Group. N Engl J Med 1996; 335: 1713–1720.
17. Wallace A, Layug B, Tateo I, et al. Prophylactic atenolol reduces postoperative myocardial ischemia. Anesthesiology 1998; 88: 1–7.
18. Warltier D. Beta-adrenergic blocking drugs – incredibly useful, incredibly under-utilized. (Editorial) Anesthesiology 1988; 88: 2–4.
19. Collard CD, Eappen S, Lynch E, Conception M. Continuous spinal anesthesia with invasive hemodynamic for surgical repair of the hip in two patients with severe aortic stenosis. Anesth Analg 1995; 81: 195–198.
20. Cohen M, Duncan PG, Tate RB. Does anesthesia contribute to operative mortality? JAMA 1988; 260: 2859–2863.
21. Tuman KJ, McCarthy RJ, March RJ, et al. Effects of epidural anesthesia and analgesia on coagulation and outcome after major vascular surgery. Anesth Analg 1991; 73: 696–704.
22. Yeager MP, Glass D, Neff RK, et al. Epidural anesthesia and analgesia in high-risk surgical patients. Anesthesiology 1987; 66: 729–736.
23. Baron JF, Bertrand M, Barre E, et al. Combined epidural and general anesthesia versus general anesthesia for abdominal aortic surgery. Anesthesiology 1991; 75: 611–618.

24. Christopherson R, Beattie C, Frank SM, et al. Perioperative morbidity in patients randomized to epidural or general anesthesia for lower extremity vascular surgery: Perioperative Ischemia Randomized Anesthesia Trial Study Group. Anesthesiology 1993; 79: 422–443.

25. Bodie RH, Lewis KP, Zarich SW, et al. Cardiac outcome after peripheral vascular surgery: Comparison of general and regional anesthesia. Anesthesiology 1996; 84: 3–8.

26. Milledge JS, Nunn JF. Criteria of fitness for anaesthesia in patients with chronic obstructive lung disease. BMJ 1975; 3: 670–673.

27. Domino KB. Pulmonary function and dysfunction in the traumatized patient. Anesth Clin N/A 1996; 14(1): 59–84.

28. Pederson T, Viby-Mogensen J, Ringsted C. Anaesthetic practice and postoperative pulmonary complications. Acta Anaesthesiol Scand 1992; 36: 812–818.

29. Harville DD, Summerskll WHJ. Surgery in acute hepatitis: Causes and effects. JAMA 1963; 184: 257–261.

30. Powell-Jackson P, Greenway B, Williams R. Adverse effects of exploratory laparotomy in patients with unsuspected liver disease. Br J Surg 1982; 69: 449–451.

31. Effects of anesthetics on hepatic blood flow. In: Brown BR, ed. Anesthesia in hepatic and biliary tract disease. Philadelphia: FA Davis; 1988.

32. Greenwood SM, Leffler CT, Minkowitz S. The increased mortality rate of open liver biopsy in alcoholic hepatitis. Surg Gynecol Obstet 1972; 134: 600–604.

33. Pugh RNH, Murray-Lyon IM, Dawson JL, et al. Transection of the oesophagus for bleeding oesophageal varices. Br J Surg 1973; 60: 646–649.

34. Pitt HA, Cameron JL, Postier RG, et al. Factors affecting mortality in biliary tract surgery. Am J Surg 1981; 141: 66–72.

35. Weinberg AD, Brennan MD, Gorman CA, et al. Outcome of anesthesia and surgery in hypothyroid patients. Arch Intern Med 1983; 143: 893–897.

36. Litt L, Roizen MF. Anesthetic and surgical risk in hypothyroidism. Arch Intern Med 1984; 144: 657–660.

37. Ladenson PW, Levin AA, Ridgeway EC, Daniels GH. Complications of surgery in hypothyroid patients. Am J Med 1984; 77: 261–266.

38. Weinberg AD, Ehrenwerth J. Anesthetic considerations and perioperative management of patients with hypothyroidism. Adv Anesthesiol 1987; 4: 185–212.

39. Wall RT. Unusual endocrine problems. Anesth Clin of N/A 1996; 14(3): 471–493.

40. Novis BK, Roizen MF, Aronson F, Thisted RA. Association of preoperative risk factors with postoperative acute renal failure. Anesth Analg 1994; 78: 143–149.

41. Sladen RN, Prough DS. Perioperative renal protection. Problems in Anesthesia 1997; 9(3): 314–331.

42. Bromage PR, Gertel MD. Brachial plexus anesthesia in chronic renal failure. Anesthesiology 1972; 36: 488–493.

43. Lake CL. Normal hemostasis. In: Lake CL, Moore RA, eds. Blood: hemostasis, transfusion, and alternatives in the perioperative period. New York: Raven Press; 1995: 3–16.

44. Rosendaal FR. The scylla and charybdis of oral anticoagulant treatment. (Editorial) N Engl J Med 1996; 335: 587–589.

45. Hylek EMM, Skates SJ, Sheehan MA, Singer DE. An analysis of the lowest effective intensity of prophylactic anticoagulation for patients with non-rheumatic atrial fibrillation. N Engl J Med 1996; 335: 540–546.

46. The bleeding time. (Editorial) Lancet 1991; 337: 1447–1448.

47. Rauck RL. The anticoagulated patient. Reg Anesth 1996; 21(6S): 51–56.

48. Vandermeulen EP, Van Aken H, Vermylen J. Anticoagulants and spinal-epidural anesthesia. Anesth Analg 1994; 79: 1165–1177.

49. Rodgers RPC, Levin J. A critical reappraisal of the bleeding time. Semin Thromb Hemost 1990; 16: 1–20.

50. Horlocker TT, Wedel DJ, Offord KP, et al. Preoperative antiplatelet drugs do not increase the risk of spinal hematoma associated with regional anesthesia. (Abstract) Reg Anesth 1994; 19(Suppl): 8–13.

51. FDA Talk Paper. Health advisory for certain anticoagulant drugs. December 1997.

52. Horlocker T, Heit J. Low molecular weight heparin: Biochemistry, pharmacology perioperative prophylaxis regimens, and guidelines for regional anesthetic management. Anesth Analg 1997; 85: 874–885.

53. Horlocker TT, Wedel DJ. Spinal and epidural blockade and perioperative low molecular weight heparin: Smooth sailing on the Titanic. (Editorial) Anesth Analg 1998; 86: 1153–1156.

54. Moudgil GC, Allan RB, Russell RJ, et al. Inhibition, by anesthetic agents, of human leukocyte locomotion towards chemical attractants. Br J Anaesth 1977; 49: 97–105.

55. Hoidal JR, White JG, Repine JE. Influence of cationic local anesthetics on the metabolism and ultrastructure of human alveolar macrophages. J Lab Clin Med 1979; 93: 857–866.

56. Kijlstra A, Van Dorp W, Daha MR, et al. The effect of lidocaine on the processing of soluble immune aggregates and immune complexes by

peritoneal macrophages. Immunology 1980; 41: 237–244.

57. Stanley TH, Hill GE, Hill HR. The influence of spinal and epidural anesthesia on neutrophil chemotaxis in man. Anesth Analg 1978; 57: 567–571.

58. Cafferkey MT, Falkiner FR, Gillespie WA, Murphy DM. Antibiotics for the prevention of septicaemia in urology. J Antimicrob Chemother 1982; 9: 471–477.

59. Yeager MP, Glass DD, Neff RK, Brinck-Johnsen T. Epidural anesthesia and analgesia in high-risk surgical patients. Anesthesiology 1987; 66: 29–36.

60. Shapiro ED, Aaron NH, Wald ER, Chiponis D. Risk factors for development of bacterial meningitis among children with occult bacteremia. J Pediatrics 1986; 109: 15–19.

61. Scott DB, Hibbard BM. Serious non-fatal complications associated with extradural block in obstetric practice. Br J Anaesth 1990; 64: 537–541.

62. Bader AM, Gilbertson L, Kirz L, Datta S. Regional anesthesia in women with chorioamnionitis. Reg Anesth 1992; 21: 84–86.

63. Goodman EJ, DeHora E, Taguiam JM. Safety of spinal and epidural anesthesia in parturients with chorioamnionitis. Reg Anesth 1996; 21: 436–441.

64. Carp H, Bailey S. The association between menin-

gitis and dural puncture in bacteremic rats. Anesthesiology 1992; 76: 739–742.

65. Wulf H, Strieling E. Postmortem findings after parturients with chorioamnionitis. Reg Anesth 1996; 21: 436–441.

66. Ready LB, Helfer D. Bacterial meningitis in parturients after epidural anesthesia. Anesthesiology 1989; 71: 988–990.

67. Nimmo WS, Littlewood DG, Scott DB, Prescott LF. Gastric emptying following hysterectomy with extradural analgesia. Br J Anaesth 1978; 50: 559–561.

68. Pollock JE, Neal JM, Stephenson CA, et al. Prospective study of the incidence of transient radicular irritation in patients undergoing spinal anesthesia. Anesthesiology 1996; 84: 1361–1367.

69. Rigler M, Drasner K, Krejcie T, et al. Cauda equina syndrome after continuous spinal anesthesia. Anesth Analg 1991; 72: 275–281.

70. Hampl KF, Schneider MC, Bont A, Pargger H. Transient radicular irritation after single subarachnoid injection of isobaric 2% lidocaine for spinal anesthesia. Anaesthesia 1996; 51: 178–181.

71. Desai SM, Bernhard WB, McAlary B. Regional anesthesia: management considerations in the trauma patient. Crit Care Clin 1990; 6: 85–101.

LOCATION-BASED PAIN MANAGEMENT: CONCEPTS AND CONSIDERATIONS

6

Pain management in the pre-hospital/emergency medical service environment: on-site and transport

Torben Wisborg and Hans Flaatten

Introduction	Ketamine
Pre-hospital working conditions	**Pre-hospital induction of anesthesia** Monitoring for pre-hospital anesthesia
Monitoring	**Inhalational analgesics** The role of nitrous oxide/oxygen
Assessment of pain	
Parenteral and enteral analgesics Opioids Non-narcotic analgesics	**Regional anesthesia in the field** Blocks in the lower extremity Blocks in the upper extremity

INTRODUCTION

Pain is an inevitable companion of trauma, and is the immediate concern of patients and relatives, even before long-term consequences of an injury are considered. The public expects trauma patients to be in pain, and emergency medical service (EMS) providers to be able to offer relief from the pain. Yet many patients arrive at the hospital still in pain, and not all EMS systems effectively provide analgesia in the pre-hospital setting.[1] It seems that even in Emergency Rooms and Accident and Emergency Departments knowledge of rational pain management is lacking.[2]

In this chapter we shall suggest several techniques for pre-hospital pain relief. Our aim is to offer safe, simple and reliable techniques, based on our own experience as air ambulance anesthe-siologists.[3,4] Others may have favorable experiences with different techniques, and this chapter does not claim to be a complete review of all possible means of providing pre-hospital pain relief.

Advances in pre-hospital pain management are based on experience mainly achieved in operating rooms and intensive care units (ICU). This is a reasonable way of extending new techniques, from an environment with good monitoring capabilities, to a less controlled setting. Nevertheless, research in pre-hospital pain management has to be performed in the pre-hospital setting.[5]

PRE-HOSPITAL WORKING CONDITIONS

Depending upon the local organization, pre-hospital trauma care will be provided by a combination of anesthesiologists, other physicians, and non-physician emergency medical technicians, paramedics, ambulance personnel and nurses/nurse anesthetists. As a rule the number of these professionals present at the trauma scene will be limited, with a reduced amount of equipment as well. Assuming the pre-hospital emergency service is delivered by an anesthesiologist, there will seldom be any on-line medical direction, so the physician present has to make decisions alone. In addition, helpers such as ambulance personnel, paramedics and nurses will be few and may well be occupied with other casualties. Therefore one has to become more or less self-sufficient, not only concerning equipment, but in decision-making as well (Table 6.1).

One of our French colleagues from the Service D'Aide Medicale Urgente concluded a review of

the pre-hospital use of propofol by stating: 'Any contraindication and precaution recommended from the hospital use should be strictly adhered to and amplified because of the difficult circumstances...'[6] We agree with this statement, and extend these words of caution to the entire pre-hospital range of analgesic techniques (Fig. 6.1).

MONITORING

Most advanced pre-hospital EMS units will carry equipment comparable to that of a sophisticated ICU including monitors, infusion pumps, drugs, and airway/circulation support equipment. In EMS systems employing anesthesiologists, anesthetic drugs and a ventilator will also be part of the armamentarium. Nevertheless, the use of monitors in the pre-hospital setting is intended only as a supplement to what is visible and audible without any equipment.

Desirable qualities in a monitor constructed for pre-hospital use are listed in Table 6.2.

The software should allow for configuration by the user to give only significant information. Alarms should be configurable to react only to variables considered significant for the situation. Alarms should be both audible and visual. In the helicopter or ambulance little or nothing will be heard from audible alarms, so it is vitally important that visible alarms are sufficient to attract attention.

For practical reasons it is desirable to assemble as many functions as possible in one monitor, although the EMS is then much more vulnerable in case of equipment failure. A back-up unit should always be available.

Table 6.1   Differences between in-hospital and pre-hospital working conditions

	In-hospital	Pre-hospital
Physical access to patient	Unlimited	Restricted
Noise	Little	Extensive
Light	Plenty	Little
Extra supplies	Extensive	Restricted
Manpower	Unlimited	Restricted
Supervision	As needed	Absent
Consultation and advice	As needed	Absent

Table 6.2   Desirable qualities for pre-hospital monitors

Lightweight	Battery-operated, long durability
Good visibility of display	Rechargeable with 12/24/220 V
Adjustable alarms, audible and visual	Selective display, only monitored variables*
Trend recording	Multi-parameter in one monitor
ECG	Blood pressure (automatic oscillometric and invasive)
Pulse oximetry	End-tidal CO_2
Temperature	

*i.e. the monitor should only display information from connected equipment; if no ECG-leads are attached, it should not show a flat line ECG.

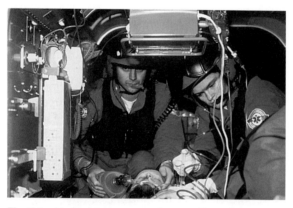

Fig. 6.1   Limited space, even in a medium-sized ambulance helicopter, makes working conditions different from in-hospital. A Norwegian Air Ambulance anesthesiologist together with a paramedic is treating a trauma victim in a Eurocopter BK-117 helicopter. (Photo: T. Hillestad.)

ECG has been an established, natural component of all patient-monitoring schemes. This has mainly been for the need to detect arrhythmia and cardiac ischemia. ECG-monitoring is highly susceptible to electrical noise and motion, and may thus be misinterpreted and cause confusion. However, the ECG is included in most monitors, but should not be the first variable monitored.

Blood pressure monitoring is very important in trauma patients, and it is desirable to have a reliable, automatic oscillometric blood pressure cuff as part of the monitor. This equipment will give systolic, mean and diastolic blood pressure through direct measurement of oscillations in the cuff. It is the most power-consuming part of most monitors, and the measurement interval has to be easily adjustable. *Invasive blood pressure* is relevant for secondary transports (i.e. 'critical care transports', interfacility transports etc.), but seldom is used in the primary pre-hospital setting.

Pulse oximetry provides an instant picture of the oxygenation of arterial blood, and if combined with a graphic display of the plethysmographic wave may give qualitative information comparable to that of an arterial wave. The pulse oximeter reports *only* the difference between oxy- and deoxyhemoglobin. It is necessary to emphasize that *a high oxygen saturation shown by pulse oximetry does not indicate adequacy of ventilation*, which is indicated only by the carbon dioxide level in the arterial blood.

End-tidal CO_2 (ETCO$_2$) gives an indication of the arterial level of carbon dioxide. It confirms endotracheal tube position, and gives early warnings about greater changes in circulation.

ASSESSMENT OF PAIN

Pain is a subjective feeling, with no accurate objective way to measure it. Therefore pain is often underestimated and undertreated. In this respect, the pre-hospital setting is probably not very different from in-hospital experience.

However, intensity of pain can be assessed in different ways using different scaling methods. The most widely used is the Visual Analog Scale (VAS) in which pain intensity is marked by the patient using a 10 cm scale: zero indicates no pain at all, and 10 the worst pain imaginable. The patient places a mark somewhere between these two limits. With modification, such an approach to pain assessment can be used in the pre-hospital setting. Since using pen and paper may be impractical outside hospital, the conscious patient may simply be asked to verbally rate the pain on the 0 to 10 scale – 'If 10 is the worst pain you can imagine and 0 is no pain at all, how intense is your pain?' This number may then be noted by the EMS doctor or nurse. Applying this method before starting treatment of pain, and reassessing every 10 to 15 minutes during transport can provide an easy and useful method to evaluate efficacy of pain management.

When patients are unconscious this method cannot be employed. Nonetheless, since patients may experience severe pain while unconscious, the Glasgow Coma Scale (GCS) may be used to decide whether the patient is experiencing pain. In the component of the GCS assessing motor response (scoring from 6 to 1), a score of ≥ 3 indicates preserved reaction to pain stimuli. The GCS should always be documented in unconscious patients, and using this information in pain assessment should be part of the standard responsibility for EMS personnel. If the patient suffers an injury likely to give moderate to severe pain, is unconscious but with GCS motor response ≥ 3, administering pain relief should be considered.

PARENTERAL AND ENTERAL ANALGESICS

Opioids

Opioid analgesics are the cornerstone of pre-hospital pain management. These drugs may be categorized according to their origin as follows:

- naturally-occurring opium derivatives: morphine and codeine
- semi-synthetic derivatives of morphine: heroin and oxymorphone
- synthetic compounds: fentanyl, alfentanil, sufentanil, meperidine, methadone, propoxyphene
- agonist–antagonists: pentazocine, buprenorphine, butorphanol and naloxone.

Several opioid receptors have been identified, and differences in affinity for each of the opioids explains differences in effects and side effects.

The action of opioids depends on the concentration of the drug at receptor sites in the central nervous system. Thus despite the routes of administration, effect ultimately depends on absorption into the systemic circulation. Enteral administration, whether oral or rectal, depends on the splanchnic circulation, and may expose the absorbed drug to degradation by first-pass liver metabolism. Intramuscular and subcutaneous injections are subjected to variations in peripheral circulation, such as caused by hypotension, hypothermia and regional vasoconstriction. Absorption will therefore be unpredictable and slow, and may result in unsatisfactory levels initially, and subsequent overdosage when peripheral circulation is improved. Sublingual administration depends on sufficient moisture to dissolve tablets and is thus unsuitable for patients in respiratory distress. It is however independent of splanchnic blood flow, and owing to the lack of need for IV access this route may be attractive. A summary of possible routes of drug administration is given in Table 6.3.

Morphine is the 'gold standard' opioid, to which all comparisons are made. The IV loading dose is 0.08–0.12 mg/kg, which has a duration of action of approximately 2 to 3 hours. The onset is very rapid, but not as fast as fentanyl. Supplemental doses should be withheld for a few minutes. As a result of morphine's profile of affinity for opioid-receptors, it can cause histamine release, biliary colic, pruritus, nausea and vomiting. Most of these side effects are preventable by slow injections of small incremental doses, in addition to the simultaneous administration of a combined central and peripheral anti-emetic as metoclopramide. Respiratory depression is moderate as compared to other opioids.

Fentanyl has a shorter half-life (duration of action approximately 30 minutes) and greater analgesic and respiratory depressant properties than morphine. Initial dose is 0.5–1 microg/kg which has almost immediate action. It will seldom be chosen as a first analgesic, but is very useful for obtunding the hypertensive response to intubation. It should be used only when continuous monitoring of respiration can be achieved. Under these circumstances it has proven safe in the pre-hospital setting.[7,8] However, fentanyl has a tendency to increase muscular tone in the chest wall, which may lead to significant difficulties in ventilation. This is mainly seen after large doses, and may be relieved by administration of small doses of a neuromuscular blocking drug – not something considered very desirable in the pre-hospital setting.

Nalbuphine is an agonist–antagonist opioid with proven pre-hospital experience.[9,10] It may be administered intravenously and normal dosages of 10–20 mg produce analgesia comparable to 10 mg of morphine. In contrast to the latter, nalbuphine has a ceiling effect on respiratory depression. Initially a dose-dependent respiratory depression will be seen, equivalent to the respiratory depression seen after morphine, but with increasing doses of nalbuphine this depression will reach a ceiling beyond doses of 30 mg.

Buprenorphine is an agonist–antagonist opioid, 25 to 50 times more potent than morphine. 0.4 mg buprenorphine is equivalent to 10 mg of morphine. Duration of analgesia is somewhat longer than morphine. It is available in a sublingual preparation.

Respiratory depression is the major side effect of all opioids. Although seen to a lesser degree in the agonist–antagonists, it is encountered in a dose-dependent manner after the agonists with some variation between drugs. The depression is mainly in the respiratory rate, and to a lesser extent in the tidal volume. It is thus easily measurable, and in the spontaneous breathing patient the respiratory rate ought to be documented. This respiratory depression will of course increase the end-tidal CO_2, and thus $PaCO_2$. In closed head injury this will increase the intracranial pressure and is best avoided, unless the breathing is controlled.

All the opioids reduce sympathetic tone. The reason is probably less perceived pain, and thus less sympathetic 'drive', combined with no intrinsic sympathetic activity in the opioids. This may lead to hypotension in the patient with hypovolemia compensated for by increased sympathetic activity. Small incremental doses guided by the clinical response will reduce the danger of circulatory collapse.

Table 6.3 Routes of administration of opioid analgesics

Intravenous	'Gold standard' with almost instantaneous effect
Intramuscular	Slower, unpredictable absorption
Subcutaneous	Very slow, and highly unpredictable absorption in hypovolemia/hypothermia
Oral, rectal	Dependent on splanchnic blood flow, first-pass effect in liver
Sublingual	Fast absorption, unsuitable for respiratory distress
Topical, transdermal	Very slow, highly dependent on peripheral blood flow
Intraosseous	Comparable to intravenous

All of the effects and side effects of opioid ago-nists may be reversed by a competitive, reversible, receptor-site antagonism with naloxone. The dose depends on the intensity of the respiratory depres-sion, with 1–2 microg/kg as a suitable initial dose. The half-life of naloxone is approximately 1 hour, which indicates a need for supplemental doses in patients with overdosage of morphine, heroin, meperidine and compounds with similar duration of effect. Care should be taken with the opioids in the agonist–antagonist class, where naloxone may be only partially effective.

Suggested strategy

> Morphine 0.05 mg/kg IV, supplemented with 50–100% of initial dose after 2–3 minutes. Consider prophylactic metoclopramide.
>
> If under close, continued supervision, fentanyl is the most effective drug. Initial dose 0.5–1 microg/kg, supplemented with 50–100% of initial dose after 2–3 minutes.

Our strategy for the patient in which we do not intend to induce anesthesia is to use *morphine*, in incremental intravenous bolus injections com-mencing with 0.05 mg/kg, supplemented with 50 to 100% of the initial dose according to patient response after 2 to 3 minutes (allow a little longer circulation time for low cardiac output/shock). The unpredictability of the required dose is illus-trated by one of our personal experiences.

Case study

A man (aged 24, weight 80 kg) was riding a motorbike with his sister (aged 18, weight 55 kg) and lost control of the bike. When the air ambulance helicopter arrived they were both conscious. The brother sustained a deep lac-eration to his right thigh. He was given 5 mg morphine IV and taken to hospital by an ordi-nary ambulance. His sister had a right pelvic fracture with proximal dislocation of the femur. She was taken by the ambulance heli-copter, and received a total of 20 mg mor-phine IV en route. On arrival at the trauma center the brother was drowsy, but responded to commands. The sister was still screaming, and obviously undertreated with analgesics.

Non-narcotic analgesics

A number of non-narcotic, non steroidal anti-inflammatory drugs (NSAIDs) have been synthe-sized during the last decade. Many of these are claimed to have analgesic properties comparable to morphine, and some may be administered intravenously. They all lack the respiratory depressant effects of opioids, and might thus be attractive for pre-hospital use. Unfortunately, they all share a number of unwanted side effects: mainly gastrointestinal hemorrhage, reduction of the hemostatic effects of blood platelets, and reduced renal blood flow in hypovolemia. The administration of these drugs in hypovolemia may induce acute renal failure, and in patients with congestive heart failure it may precipitate pul-monary edema due to sodium retention.[11] Patients hypersensitive to acetylsalicylic acid may have an allergic reaction to NSAIDs.

In our opinion these drugs are presently not indicated in the pre-hospital phase of pain man-agement for trauma patients, because these patients are all prone to deterioration in their hemostatic mechanisms. In addition gastrointesti-nal hemorrhage owing to stress ulceration is not uncommon, and the bleeding trauma patient is almost invariably also hypovolemic. NSAIDs may prove very efficient and valuable for these patients after surgery when hypovolemia, bleeding, and other contraindications have been ruled out.

Ketamine

Ketamine is an anesthetic in the sense that it has ability to induce amnesia, analgesia, and sleep (or, at least, a non-perceiving state of mind), but it does not reduce reflexes or muscular tonus. This is why ketamine has been considered the most suitable in-field and wartime, single-drug anes-thetic.

Ketamine has intrinsic sympathetic activity, and will increase heart rate and blood pressure. It does also increase the intracranial and intraocular pres-sure. Ketamine does not reduce the minute venti-lation, although the respiratory pattern after anesthetic doses may change, and become some-what irregular. A short period of respiratory arrest may occur after rapid intravenous boluses.

Pharyngeal reflexes are thought to be intact after ketamine administration, and the insertion of pharyngeal airways or other devices should be avoided. The reflexes are however not considered sufficiently protective against pulmonary aspiration of gastric contents, and in cases of general anesthesia the risk of pulmonary aspiration should be weighed against the advantages of maintaining spontaneous ventilation without endotracheal intubation.

For induction of anesthesia, initial doses are 2 mg/kg IV or 10 mg/kg IM. After IV injection the onset is within 1 minute; after IM induction the onset time is 3 to 5 minutes. Duration of a single dose should be expected to be 10 to 15 minutes after IV administration and 15 to 25 minutes after IM administration.

The excellent analgesic properties of ketamine in sub-anesthetic doses are less well-known. Used as an analgesic, the IV dose is 0.3 mg/kg or 25 mg IV for an adult. This dose will produce intense analgesia for 15 to 30 minutes without significant reduction of consciousness, although the patient may experience vivid dreams. Patients should be warned about this before the ketamine is administered. Concomitant administration of a small dose of benzodiazepine will reduce these psychomimetic effects.

Side effects of ketamine are intracranial and intraocular hypertension, and ketamine should thus be used with caution in closed head injury and open bulbar injury. The hallucinations experienced after ketamine anesthesia may be avoided by benzodiazepine administration, and by reducing visual, audible, and tactile stimulation of the patient during emergence. Ketamine induces an intense salivation, which is seen to a lesser extent in analgesic doses. It is wise to administer an anticholinergic at the anesthetic induction to reduce salivation.

PRE-HOSPITAL INDUCTION OF ANESTHESIA

At a certain level the provision of pre-hospital 'analgesia' actually turns into 'anesthesia'. Although it may be difficult to define this point exactly, it is important to bear it in mind. When respiration or protective reflexes of the throat are sufficiently depressed, the patient is no longer able to maintain the necessary alveolar ventilation and/or protect his airway against vomit. At this point anesthesia (in the sense of lost airway control) has de facto been induced. This transition from analgesia to anesthesia ought to be a planned process, and not a surprising side effect of the analgesic administration. The indications for pre-hospital induction of anesthesia are listed in Table 6.4.

For simplicity and safety the pre-hospital approach to induction of anesthesia must be uniform with respect to drugs, equipment, and technique. All intravenous agents are theoretically possible to use. We suggest using a barbiturate (we use thiopental), a benzodiazepine (we use midazolam), an analgesic (we use morphine and fentanyl) and two neuromuscular blocking agents (we use succinylcholine and vecuronium).[12] Equipment includes a laryngoscope with two blades, Magill's forceps, various endotracheal tubes and tape/gauze for fixation, a field intubation kit with cricothyrotomy equipment, self-inflating ventilation bag, oxygen, a hand/foot-operated suctioning device with large capacity, and in the helicopter a pressure-driven ventilator.

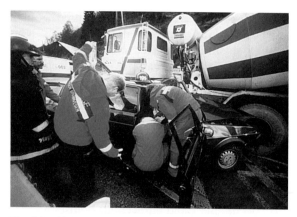

Fig. 6.2 Ketamine was used in this situation as an analgesic for the entrapped patient before extrication. (Photo: T. Hillestad.)

Table 6.4 Indications for pre-hospital induction of anesthesia

Depressed consciousness (GCS < 8)	Insufficient ventilation
Lack of protective airway reflexes	Injury to the face or upper airways
Insufficient pain relief by analgesics	Combative, uncontrollable patient
Before prolonged painful extrication	Possible carbon monoxide poisoning

When indicated, patients are primarily induced where they are found, although it is preferable to have them on stretchers. The equipment listed above must be present. Adverse environmental conditions may dictate the transfer of patients to an ambulance/helicopter prior to induction, although space in vehicles often hampers optimal cervical spine stabilization.

All trauma patients should be considered as having an unstable cervical spine and a full stomach placing them at risk for gastric aspiration until definitively ruled out. They should also be considered to be hypovolemic, and if unconscious or confused should be assumed to have a closed head injury. The anesthetic technique should therefore reduce the risk of cervical movement during intubation, prevent gastric aspiration, prevent increases in intracranial pressure, and maintain cardiovascular stability.

Monitoring for pre-hospital anesthesia

Monitoring during induction in the pre-hospital phase reflects the concerns discussed above. Monitoring should *at least* include ECG, non-invasive, automatic blood pressure measuring and pulse oximetry. Capnography is highly desirable. A complete discussion of pre-hospital monitoring appears previously in this chapter.

As in the hospital, an anesthetic plan is made prior to induction. Our 'ideal' anesthetic technique includes the participation of at least two well-trained and experienced persons. It is important that all personnel involved are well aware of the plan. After the primary survey and resuscitation are complete, the patient is ventilated with 100% O_2 via bag and mask. Infusions are in place and going, and monitoring is as previously described, with the monitors visible to the anesthesiologist. Drugs are prepared in syringes. A trained assistant correctly applies cricoid pressure. The anesthesiologist ventilates and administers the drugs intravenously. Intubation is done in a rapid-sequence procedure with administration of hypnotic and muscular relaxant almost simultaneously. We prefer direct orotracheal intubation. Confirmation of tube position is done by auscultation with a stethoscope and, if present, capnography. The endotracheal tube is *secured well* (we recommend adhesive tape in a circular fashion around the neck, allowing the tape to adhere to itself, but avoiding compression of the jugular veins).

After intubation vital signs are re-checked, bearing in mind that a simple asymptomatic pneumothorax may develop into a tension pneumothorax after positive pressure ventilation (especially with some altitude changes experienced in the air ambulance), and that circulation may be disturbed by the altered intrathoracic pressures as well as the anesthetic drug effects.

INHALATIONAL ANALGESICS

The role of nitrous oxide/oxygen

Nitrous oxide (N_2O) is a medical gas widely used as a part of general anesthesia. The gas is a strong anxiolytic with some sedative properties as well. The effects of N_2O are probably related to the central nervous system (CNS) blunting of painful stimuli. N_2O has, however, weak analgesic properties, and the MAC-50 (mean alveolar concentration when 50% of the individual does not react to a surgical incision) is 105%. This can never be achieved in isobaric conditions when 79% is the maximal concentration of N_2O if a normal oxygen fraction (21%) is to be given. Obviously, hypobaric conditions (altitude) weaken the analgesic properties of N_2O. If the patient requires increased amounts of oxygen, this additionally reduces the amount of N_2O that can be administered.

Outside the hospital a special mixture of 50% N_2O and 50% O_2 (Entonox) is the way nitrous oxide is usually given. This way of providing pain relief has been widely used for women in labor, and is utilized in several EMS systems. The advantage is a patient-administered system with few side effects. The disadvantages are several. As previously described, N_2O is a very weak analgesic, and its effects have been questioned. It may lead to inadequate pain relief, through the withholding of more efficient therapies. If there is need for > 50% oxygen, the method cannot be used, and in high altitudes (> 5000 feet) at least 70% N_2O must be given. In addition there has been a growing concern about the global polluting properties of N_2O, specifically the effects on the atmosphere. N_2O is not degraded in nature.

If the EMS service uses medical doctors, nurses or trained paramedics, other methods of pain relief are more flexible and efficient and should be considered before utilizing N_2O. Finally, there are no controlled studies concerning the effects of

N_2O in the pre-hospital settings, and the few available controlled studies conducted in hospital have not demonstrated significant pain relief.[13]

REGIONAL ANESTHESIA IN THE FIELD

Regional anesthetic techniques can be very useful in the EMS setting. Regional anesthesia blocks pain stimuli entering the CNS, and provides excellent pain relief if the injured region is completely blocked. It does not have any effect on consciousness, rendering a completely cooperative and non-sedated patient. Effects on respiratory functions are minimal, more often leading to improved function. However, several of the techniques require experience and training which is difficult to obtain outside the operating room.

The central blocks (spinal and epidural anesthesia) are not suitable as they are too complicated to perform, and there is a risk of hypotension from simultaneous sympathetic blockade. There is also a risk of toxic reactions if large doses of local anesthetics are accidentally administered intravenously. In spite of this, some of the peripheral blocks may be extremely useful to the EMS practitioner. In particular, the femoral nerve block which is easy to perform without extensive training is a valuable block to provide pain relief.

Blocks in the lower extremity

Femoral nerve block

The femoral nerve enters the thigh under the inguinal ligament. Usually its several components gather just before entering the thigh, but occasionally it consists of two or more parts. It lies just lateral to the femoral artery which is an important landmark when performing the block (Fig. 6.3). The femoral nerve brings motor nerves to the sartorius and the quadriceps muscles and sensory nerves from anterior thigh, and inside of the calf down to the medial malleolus (saphenous nerve). The most important bony structure receiving sensory fibers from the femoral nerve is the femoral bone. This is why this block is of great interest in the EMS setting. The distal two-thirds of the femur is totally supplied by the femoral nerve, and the upper third partially so (together with the obturator nerve). In addition parts of the fibula are also supplied by the femoral nerve.

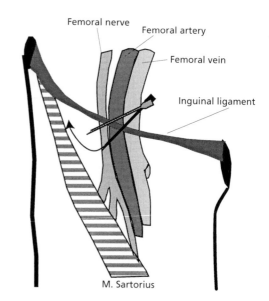

Fig. 6.3 The anatomical landmarks for the femoral nerve block in the right inguinal region. The needle is moved in a fan-wise direction as described in the text. (Graphics: H Flaatten.)

Indications The main indication for performing a femoral nerve block in the EMS setting is fracture of the femur (shaft fractures). Everyone who has encountered a patient with such a fracture knows how painful this injury can be, making even smooth transport excruciating. Even high doses of opioids are frequently insufficient to relieve pain, and certainly insufficient to attempt reduction of the fracture if necessary.

Technique Free access to the inguinal area on the injured side is necessary. In addition it is necessary to locate the femoral artery. The block can be performed using any local anesthetic, but bupivacaine 5 mg/mL is preferred because of its long duration (4 to 6 hours). The normal dose in adults is 15–20 mL (75–100 mg). Table 6.5 gives dose recommendations for bupivacaine and lidocaine in children and adults.

Local anesthesia is drawn into a 20 mL syringe. A 21G needle (0.8 mm), 4–5 cm long is necessary. After locating the femoral artery, the needle is inserted just lateral to the artery, immediately distal to the inguinal ligament. The needle is introduced about 2–2.5 cm. If the patient feels a paresthesia to the knee, it confirms correct

Table 6.5 Recommended safe maximal doses of bupivacaine and lidocaine given as mg/kg body weight

Clinical setting	Bupivacaine	Lidocaine
Nerve block and infiltration	3	8
Infiltration in highly vascular areas	2 (with epinephrine)	6 (with epinephrine)
Small children		5

position (but this is not necessary in order to perform the block). After careful aspiration, the local anesthetic is injected while the needle is slowly withdrawn 1–1.5 cm, and then redirected a bit more laterally. A fan-wise injection must be made reaching 3–4 cm lateral to the femoral artery (Fig. 6.3). In this way all parts of the femoral nerve will be blocked. Frequent aspiration is mandatory. Using bupivacaine, the effects usually begin within 5 minutes, with full effect achieved within 15 to 20 minutes. No manipulation of the patient should occur until the block is satisfactory. Frequently the patient will spontaneously state that the pain has diminished. When the block is satisfactory, full manipulations of the femoral shaft are usually possible, such as correction of malposition, application of traction, and lifting and transporting. When using bupivacaine, often the block will last until definitive surgery can be performed, thus making other forms of preoperative analgesia unnecessary.

Ankle block

Providing pain relief from injuries to the foot with regional anesthetic techniques is also relatively simple. The foot is innervated by nerve fibers from the tibial nerve (posteriorly), superficial and deep peroneal and saphenous nerve (anteriorly). These nerves travel very superficially near the malleolus, where they can be effectively blocked. Using the medial malleolus as a reference, 4–5 mL local anesthetic solution (e.g. bupivacaine 5 mg/mL) is injected near the posterior tibial artery (dorsal to the malleolus) in order to block the tibial nerve, and the same amount is injected behind the lateral malleolus to block the sural nerve. From the frontal side, the saphenous nerve is blocked anterior to the medial malleolus, and the superficial peroneal nerve is blocked immediately above the talocrural joint. As all nerves lie near to vascular structures, frequent aspiration must be performed in order to avoid intravascular injection. It is

important to be aware of the total dose of local anesthetic when all four nerves are blocked.

Blocks in the upper extremity

Blocks in the upper extremity may also be performed in the pre-hospital setting, but training is essential because these blocks are frequently more difficult to perform. Blockade of the brachial plexus can be of value in several injuries to the upper extremity. However, supraclavicular blocks, are not recommended outside the hospital because of the possibility of creating an iatrogenic pneumothorax.

Block of the axillary nerve where it travels in the vascular sheath with the axillary artery and vein is a more appealing approach outside the hospital, and the reader is referred for detailed discussion of this technique.

REFERENCES

1. Chambers JA, Guly HR. The need for better pre-hospital analgesia. Arch Emerg Med 1993; 10: 187–192.
2. Reichl M, Bodiwala GG. Use of analgesia in severe pain in the accident and emergency department. Arch Emerg Med 1987; 4: 25–31.
3. Wisborg T, Guttormsen AB, Sørensen MB, Flaatten HK. The potential of an anaesthesiologist-manned ambulance service in a rural/urban district. Acta Anaesthesiol Scand 1994; 38: 657–661.
4. Wisborg T, Strand T. Trauma anesthesia practices throughout the world: Norway. In: Grande CM, ed. Textbook of trauma anesthesia and critical care. Philadelphia: Mosby–Yearbook; 1992: 245–250.
5. Proceedings from the First International Symposium on Pain Research in Emergency Medicine in Montreal, October 1994. Ann Emerg Med 1996; 27: 399–474.

6. Petit P. Utilisation du Diprivan pour les urgences préhospitalières. Ann Fr Anesth Reanim 1998; 13: 643–646.
7. Thomas SH, et al. Safety of fentanyl for analgesia in adults undergoing air medical transport from trauma scenes. Air Medical Journal 1996; 15: 57–59.
8. Poulton TJ. Use of fentanyl confirms experiences. Air Medical Journal 1996; 15: 154.
9. Stene JK, Stofberg L, MacDonald G, Myers RA, Ramzy A, Burns B. Nalbuphine analgesia in the prehospital setting. Am J Emerg Med 1998; 6: 634–639.
10. Chambers JA, Guly HR. Prehospital intravenous nalbuphine administered by paramedics. Resuscitation 1994; 27: 153–158.
11. Smith CM, Reynard AM, eds. Textbook of pharmacology. Philadelphia: WB Saunders; 1992: 424–429.
12. Smith CE, Grande CM. The use of neuromuscular blocking agents in the trauma patient. Baltimore: International Trauma Anesthesia and Critical Care Society; 1995.
13. Sprehn M, Trautner S, Wiingaard S, Sørensen MB. Prehospital pain relief with nitrous oxide (Entonox). Ugeskr Laeger 1994; 156: 5830–5835.

7

Pain management in the emergency room: initial evaluation and interventions

Andreas R Thierbach, Markus D W Lipp and Monika Daubländer

Introduction
  Missed or delayed diagnosis
  Pain assessment

**Use of local and regional anesthesia techniques in
  the emergency room**
  Infiltration
  Minor nerve blocks
  Major nerve blocks
  Central nerve blocks

Systemic drug application
  Analgesics
  Sedatives and hypnotics

Adjuvant medication
Analgesia and sedation techniques

Choice of techniques

Safety and monitoring

Pain management for special patient groups
  Thermal injuries
  Patients in shock
  Head injuries
  Fractures of the lower extremity

Summary

INTRODUCTION

The provision of adequate analgesia is an often neglected aspect of primary and secondary care in many emergency rooms (ER). Analgesia issues outside the trauma room also apply to acute traumatized patients who must tolerate diagnostic and therapeutic measures before surgery. Some risk factors for ER underutilization of analgesics have been published. Selbst & Clark showed that children in general are less likely to receive analgesics under acute, painful conditions, and that children less than 2 years old receive analgesics less often than older children.[1] Todd et al reported that in Los Angeles, ethnic Hispanics are less likely than non-Hispanics to receive analgesics in the ER for isolated long-bone fractures.[2]

Reichl & Bodiwala concluded in their 1978 study of pain management procedures in British ERs that a significant number of patients with acute painful conditions are undertreated with analgesics.[3] They stated that a large percentage of patients in the ER receive an inappropriate drug, a drug via an inappropriate route of administration (i.e. intramuscular), or suffer from long intervals between analgesic administration. Similar statements have been published from various authors in the USA.[4]

Only when immediate treatment of cardiorespiratory instability is required, or if a competent patient declines treatment, should analgesia be withheld for a painful procedure.[5] The presence of an injury that could eventually result in cardiovascular, hemodynamic, neurologic, or pulmonary instability (e.g. femur fracture, pneumothorax, skull fracture) is not an absolute contraindication to systemic analgesia, although careful titration and monitoring must be provided. Though pain control may not be needed for certain procedures (e.g. diagnostic computerized imaging or ultrasound examination), providing analgesia is likely to enhance the accuracy of these examinations by reducing patient writhing or restlessness because of pain.

In the ER setting, some procedures can be safely performed under local or regional anesthesia, but systemic analgesia or even general anesthesia may be required to provide optimal pain control.

Well-judged and appropriately administered pain therapy includes a variety of measures and techniques, which only can be performed by experienced and well-trained physicians. Anesthesiologists, as advocates of pain therapy, have much to offer in this respect. But anesthesiologists and surgeons (and even other emergency physicians) have to interact to accomplish optimal pain treatment in the ER, the operating room (OR) as well as the intensive care unit or trauma ward.

Missed or delayed diagnosis

Inappropriate doses and routes of narcotics may result in respiratory depression or interfere with the patient's assessment, but this concern should not be overemphasized. Proper monitoring can detect overdosage (see Safety and monitoring). Despite the variety of diagnostic methods available to identify all significant injuries in the trauma patient at the time of admission (computerized tomography, ultrasound or radiological examinations), in many instances the initial performance of these studies will depend on the findings of a careful, initial, physical examination in the field as well as in the ER. In addition to the initial examination, careful follow-up examinations are vitally important for the early diagnosis of certain types of injuries. Both systemic and particularly regional anesthesia techniques may potentially mask the physical signs of serious underlying injury. If analgesic methods are to be employed that put the patient at risk for a diminished response of developing signs of injury, serious consideration should be given to first reliably excluding injuries using all available diagnostic methods.[6] For example, repeated ultrasound examinations should be considered in all patients with multiple rib fractures who are candidates for epidural catheters in order to exclude the presence

of a significant intra-abdominal injury. Protocols that rely on serial physical examination as a means of diagnosing injury may not be compatible with the institution of certain analgesic methods.

Pain assessment

Optimal application of pain control methods depends on cooperation among different members of the health care team throughout the patient's course of treatment. To ensure that this process occurs effectively, formal protocols must be developed and used within each institution to assess pain management practices and to obtain patient feedback to calibrate the adequacy of pain control.

Assessment of pain in the ER should be frequent and simple. Factors that influence analgesic requirement and consumption include:

- Age of the patient: elderly patients usually require smaller doses
- Sex
- Co-existing medical condition (such as substance abuse or withdrawal, hyperthyroidism, anxiety disorder, affective disorder, hepatic or renal impairments)
- Cultural factors and personality (Personal, cultural, and language factors can affect patient's attitude towards pain. Identifying these factors is an essential part of the patient's history.)
- The evidence that pain is influenced by cultural factors leads naturally to an examination of the role of early experience in adult behavior related to pain. It is commonly accepted that children are deeply influenced by the attitudes of their parents toward pain.
- Site of injury (i.e. bone injuries are associated with the most oppressive pain)
- Individual variation in response and pain threshold.

Very little has been written about the assessment of pain in the ER. Obviously, pain assessment in critically injured patients is often hindered by the fact that many patients are unable to communicate effectively because of the extent of trauma (e.g. head injury, facial trauma, shock, intubation, lack of physical reserves or mental capability).

Usually, physicians treat pain based on the patient's non-verbal behavior, general verbal complaints, and physiologic changes. This practice compounds the problem of undermanagement of pain, since studies show that a patient's reports of pain in relationship to the physician's or nurse's perception of the degree of pain the patient is experiencing do not correlate.[7]

Several pain assessment tools are available that are designed to allow a patient to assess the intensity of her or his pain.[8] Additional testing of these tools, such as the Visual Analog Scale, in this special trauma population is necessary to establish reliability; however, their use in clinical practice can and has benefited other surgical patients.[9]

USE OF LOCAL AND REGIONAL ANESTHESIA TECHNIQUES IN THE EMERGENCY ROOM

The techniques that can be used will be divided into infiltration, minor, major, and central nerve blocks.

Infiltration

Using regional anesthetic techniques for acute traumatic pain relief does not, by any means, always involve the major forms of nerve blockade. Many minor traumas, for example, amputation of fingers, can be very painful, although the acute pain is of relatively short duration. In these, excellent analgesia can be achieved by using a local anesthetic method for diagnostic procedures and as well as for the operation itself, relying on the duration of the block to outlast the most painful period.

Infiltration of local anesthetic into a wound can produce analgesia at the site lasting several hours, particularly if epinephrine is added. Adequate time, at least 10 minutes, is necessary for the local anesthetic agent to have full effect. Intracutaneous and subcutaneous infiltration with a suitable dilute concentration (0.5% or 1%) of an intermediate-acting anesthetic drug is sufficient for removal of superficial scars or lesions.

In more major trauma, irrigation of wounds with local anesthetic solutions has been administered successfully.[10] For this procedure, a multihole catheter is left in place under the skin and the muscle layers of the incision, and injections of local anesthetic, for example, bupivacaine 0.125%, are made intermittently. Good analgesia of the wound is claimed, and the method may be augmented by parenteral opioids.

An expansion of this technique is the 'field block', achieved by subcutaneous infiltration blocking of nerves that supply a particular area. This procedure is usually performed by a surgeon and provides good pre- and postoperative analgesia as well as good intraoperative anesthesia. The addition of epinephrine as a vasoconstrictor can be helpful in obtaining hemostasis, although it is contraindicated in injuries close to the terminal capillary system (e.g. nose tip, digits, penis).

Intravenous regional anesthesia (Bier's block)

This technique, which is a form of infiltration, is always unsuitable when a tourniquet is contraindicated, as in amputations or vascular trauma. Local anesthetics such as lidocaine or prilocaine provide only a rather short period of analgesia, which is limited by the pressure-induced pain of the tourniquet to approximately 60 minutes. It has been suggested that bupivacaine be used for intravenous regional anesthesia could give a useful period of analgesia. However, the dose required for this was prohibitively high and cannot be recommended.[11,12]

Minor nerve blocks

Although many medical centers, particularly in the USA, will perform 30% to 40% of surgical procedures on an outpatient basis, either in special ambulatory care centers, ERs, or physicians' offices, it is important to keep a proper perspective when selecting regional anesthesia as the pain treatment technique in acute traumatized patients.

Compared to a fully equipped OR, the ER may be rather primitive in smaller hospitals. Specific peripheral nerve blocks would be, therefore, appropriate and have a definite advantage if the physician is capable of performing them. Many small nerves not only are anatomically easy to block, but will also remain blocked for many hours with standard doses of local anesthetic.

Digital nerve blocks of fingers and toes are easily performed by ring blocks at the proximal end of the digit.[13] If a ring block is performed well, the amount of general anesthetic would be greatly reduced, and several hours of analgesia would be provided (see Ch. 14).

Wrist blocks, although simple to do, are also

infrequently used in ERs. Nevertheless, in many patients, the blockade of the terminal parts of the median, radial, and ulnar nerves at the wrist will give significant analgesia for traumatized hands and fingers. There is little to be gained by blocking the nerves at the elbow as opposed to the wrist. The wrist block is usually simpler to perform. Only hand anesthesia results from blocking the three major nerve trunks at the elbow because the forearm cutaneous nerves arise in the upper arm and are quite separate at this level.

Ankle blocks are in a similar category. The saphenous, deep and superficial peroneal, sural, and plantar nerves are all readily available for blockade, which will decrease the requirement for systemic analgesics and provide several hours of increased patient comfort (see Ch. 14).

Major nerve blocks

Brachial plexus block

If more profound, deep anesthesia of the upper extremity is required, regional block of the brachial plexus should be favored. The plexus can be approached in the interscalene groove, as it crosses the first rib, or in the axilla.

Each technique has its advantages and proponents. The *supraclavicular* and *interscalene* approaches pose a small but disabling incidence of pneumothorax. They are particularly suited for analgesia for shoulder and upper arm injuries. The axillary approach provides good anesthesia to the forearm, as long as care is taken to block the musculocutaneous nerve by infiltration. The main problem of the axillary block for painful lesions is that it may take 15 to 20 minutes to achieve adequate levels of analgesia. Alternatively, an infraclavicular nerve block can be utilized (see Ch. 13).

Brachial plexus blockade can be indefinitely extended for pain therapy by the simple method of leaving a plastic cannula within the neurovascular sheath of the plexus (see Ch. 13).

Blocks of the lower extremity

The '*3 in 1*' *block* (the perivascular approach to the lumbar plexus) is of particular benefit in fractured lower limbs. This technique includes a femoral nerve block, a lateral femoral cutaneous nerve block, and an obturator nerve block for analgesia after lower limb trauma.

A *femoral nerve block* yields almost total analgesia to the patient with a fractured shaft of the femur, so that it may be of value for pain relief while the patient is awaiting more definitive therapy in the ER.

Femoral nerve block is a relatively simple procedure and produces analgesia of the shaft of the femur. Patients who require traction or who have to undergo surgery for a shaft fracture will benefit from such a block. Again, if it is necessary, a cannula can be left in place for repeated injection (see Ch. 13).

Central nerve blocks

Epidural analgesia is a simple and useful technique for the relief of pain in acutely traumatized patients because a catheter can be used to maintain analgesia in the postoperative period.

As described earlier, the use of regional anesthetic approaches may be beneficial for particular operative sites, when not contraindicated by sepsis, coagulopathy, or cardiorespiratory instability. For example, discomfort and splinting caused by flail chest injury may improve with thoracic epidural analgesia, and borderline perfusion of an injured lower limb can increase with a sympathetic blockade by a lumbar epidural local anesthetic (see Ch. 12).[14]

For major lower limb trauma, central nerve blocks offer the easiest method of producing widespread analgesia; however, they are also associated with a greater degree of autonomic block, which can have a profound physiologic effect on the patient. Thus a balance must be found between effective pain relief and possible danger. Autonomic dysfunction will affect cardiovascular control, gastrointestinal function, and micturition.

Patients having epidural blocks must be monitored carefully: there is the risk of hypotension (sympathetic blockade) and the risk of respiratory arrest (spread of local analgesic solution).

SYSTEMIC DRUG APPLICATION

Analgesics

Systemic treatment modalities available for pain control include intramuscular, subcutaneous, intravenous, oral, rectal, transdermal, transmuscular, epidural, or intrathecal application of analgesics.

The intravenous (IV) route is the preferred delivery mode because of its rapid onset and easy reliable dosing. Using an IV route sidesteps the pain and the unpredictable absorption, onset, and duration of action associated with most of the other systemic treatment modalities.

Nonsteroidal anti-inflammatory drugs

The use of nonsteroidal anti-inflammatory drugs (NSAIDs) in the trauma patient remains controversial. They are undoubtedly of value in the patient with minor trauma, but the risk of excessive bleeding and gastric stress ulcers may prohibit their use following closed head injury, burn injury, or other multisystem injuries.

NSAIDs have several advantages over opioids. They do not have hemodynamic effects, cause respiratory depression, or slow gastric emptying or small-bowel transit time.

NSAIDs currently have a limited role in the management of acute, traumatic pain. These agents may control mild to moderate pain after relatively minor trauma (e.g. minor injuries of limbs). Even when insufficient alone to control pain, NSAIDs have significant opioid dose-sparing effects on postoperative pain, and hence can be useful in reducing opioid side effects.

Ketamine

Intravenous ketamine has a rapid onset of action and produces a state of conscious sedation in which patients respond to verbal commands and maintain airway reflexes but experience analgesia. It is a unique drug evoking intense analgesia at subanesthetic doses for moderate to severe pain following trauma.

Possible side effects include dysphoria, tachycardia, increased salivary and tracheal secretions. It may increase both intracranial and systemic vascular pressures, and cause myocardial ischemia in patients with pre-existing cardiac disease and thus should not be applied in these situations.

A variety of drugs used in preoperative medication or as adjuvants during maintenance of anesthesia have been evaluated in attempts to prevent emergence delirium following administration of ketamine. Benzodiazepines have proven the most effective in the prevention of this phenomenon, with midazolam being more effective than diazepam.[15,16] Nevertheless, ketamine is a very

useful analgesic for patients in shock because it causes only little reduction in blood pressure.

Opioids

Opioid analgesics are the cornerstone of pharmacological pain management, especially for trauma causing moderate to severe pain.

Opioids may be administered by a variety of routes. As described earlier, the IV route is the preferred delivery mode. When IV access is problematic, sublingual and rectal routes should be considered as alternatives to traditional intramuscular or subcutaneous injections.

Proper use of opioids involves selecting a particular drug and route of administration and judging:

- Suitable initial dose
- Frequency of administration
- Optimal doses of non-opioid analgesics (if these are also to be given)
- Incidence and severity of side effects
- Whether the analgesic will be given in an inpatient or ambulatory setting.

Titration of opioids in the ER should be based on the patient's analgesic response and side effects. Remember that patients vary greatly in their analgesic dose requirements and responses to opioid analgesics. Opioids are often significantly underdosed because of the diffuse, dominant fear for patient safety. Most often, IV titration of an opioid like *morphine*, with observation for 5 to 10 minutes between doses, will provide safe and adequate analgesia.[17]

Several studies have demonstrated the analgesic efficacy of *tramadol* after IV application, both in adults and children. Moreover, negligible respiratory depressant activity and only minor side effects have consistently been shown.[18] IV and intramuscular tramadol offers sufficient analgesia in treating moderate pain, e.g. for fractures and burns.

Fentanyl may be preferable when cardiovascular stability is an issue and patients are closely monitored and/or intubated. This drug may be used in small doses (25 microg increments) but carries a higher risk than morphine of inducing chest wall rigidity that must be immediately managed by administering a quick-onset muscle relaxant and supporting ventilation.

New strong-acting opioids such as *alfentanil* in sub-anesthetic doses have to be taken into consideration for future pain management as well.[19]

Respiratory depression secondary to opioids.
Since respiratory depression is strongly correlated with the degree of sedation, stimulation of the patient as well as the administration of small doses of naloxone (e.g. 0.04 mg) may be adequate to reverse mild degrees of hypoventilation. Of course, assisted ventilation by bag and mask, or (ultimately) endotracheal intubation and repetitive naloxone dosing, may be required to reverse more severe degrees of respiratory depression. If such respiratory depression does occur, the patient should be observed until well after the naloxone effect has worn off (usually after 1 hour). Nausea, bradycardia, and hypotension are other side effects to watch for in the ER. Contraindications to opioid analgesia include altered sensorium, lung disease, near-term pregnancy, or an inability to monitor and manage the previously mentioned side effects.

Opioid tolerance physiologic dependence.
Opioid tolerance or physiological dependence is unusual in short-term use in opioid naive patients. Likewise, psychologic dependence and addiction are extremely unlikely to develop in patients without prior drug abuse histories who receive opioids for acute pain.

Sedatives and hypnotics

Benzodiazepines

As fear and anxiety are an almost universal response to burn injury and trauma of any kind, sedatives such as benzodiazepines are useful to supplement opioid analgesics. Although they lack analgesic properties for treatment of pain caused by acute tissue injury, benzodiazepines diminish skeletal muscle spasm (e.g. during orthopedic reduction), reduce anxiety, and in higher doses, provide amnesia.

These agents can be given either orally or intravenously. Like opioids, IV benzodiazepines are given in increments and titrated to sedative effect. Benzodiazepines provide sedation, not analgesia, and hence they are often used with opioids for painful procedures.

Typically, in a 70 kg adult, midazolam is used in incremental doses of 1 mg intravenously. Midazolam, 0.1–0.15 mg/kg infused over 3 to 5 minutes, produces sedation and amnesia without significant cardiorespiratory depression. Co-administration of an opioid and a benzodiazepine carries a substantially higher risk of inducing respiratory depression than administration of either drug individually, so particular vigilance and monitoring are necessary.

Propofol

This relatively new agent is an emulsion in soybean oil, glycerol, and purified egg phosphatide offering a strictly dose-dependent depression of the central nervous system. Its pharmacological characteristics make it appropriate for sedation with combined use of analgesics in trauma patients in a variety of clinical situations.

Propofol sedation offers advantages over the other sedative-hypnotics (including midazolam) because of its rapid recovery and favorable side-effect profile. This drug has no analgesic effect and is used with analgesics for painful procedures. In addition, the degree of sedation is readily changeable from 'light' to 'deep' levels by varying the infusion rate.

As with benzodiazepines, close observation for respiratory depression is essential, particularly if an opioid is co-administered.

Adjuvant medication

Nitrous oxide

Nitrous oxide/oxygen mixtures are safe and effective sedative/analgesic agents for use in the ER. Inhalation of a nitrous oxide/oxygen mixture can provide prompt anxiolysis and moderate analgesia. As a precaution, the patient should breathe through a face mask that he or she is holding, so that the mask will drop away if the patient becomes somnolent.[20]

Risks and side effects of its use are listed in Table 7.1.

Table 7.1 Nitrous oxide – contraindications and side effects

Contraindications
Inhalation of pure nitrous oxide (without a minimum of 30% oxygen)
Entrapped air (pneumothorax or pulmonary blebs, bowel obstruction, air embolism, chronic pulmonary disease, or suspected decompression sickness)
Side effects
Environmental contamination (scavenging system necessary)
Patients with altered sensorium (aggravation likely)

Analgesia and sedation techniques

Conscious sedation

During 'conscious sedation', a minimally depressed level of consciousness that retains the patient's ability to maintain the airway and to respond appropriately to physical stimulation and verbal command, medication is administered to provide amnesia and sedation, to reduce anxiety, and to control pain.

Agents commonly used in adults for sedation include benzodiazepines for anxiety reduction and amnesia, opioids to control pain, and low doses of IV or inhalation anesthetics to provide sedation. Benzodiazepines, such as midazolam, or the IV anesthetic propofol may be used alone because both reduce anxiety and cause amnesia. For more painful trauma, or where a regional block does not seem to be working well, opioids (e.g. fentanyl, 25–50 microg/70 kg) are usually added.

Deep sedation

Deep sedation is defined as 'a controlled state of depressed consciousness, accompanied by partial loss of protective reflexes, including inability to respond purposefully to verbal commands; produced by pharmacologic or nonpharmacologic methods, alone or in combination.' The state of deep sedation may be reached easily by frequent titration of opioid agents and sedatives.

In deeply sedated traumatized patients the risks of hypoventilation and aspiration of gastric contents rise unquestionably. Therefore, general anesthesia with endotracheal intubation should be commenced if the analgesic and sedative requirements are expected to or do exceed conscious sedation.

CHOICE OF TECHNIQUES

Especially in emergencies, the traumatologist has to reflect on different aspects before selecting an appropriate pain treatment technique:

- Does the airway have to be secured? In case of a compromised airway or insufficient oxygenation, then induction of general anesthesia with endotracheal intubation is the method of choice.
- What are the cardiopulmonary effects of the technique selected?
- Is the patient in a hemodynamically stable condition? Massive blood loss, shock and/or coagulopathy may contraindicate the use of epidural catheters or other regional anesthetic techniques in which the risks of hemodynamic instability are increased.
- What is the patient's level of consciousness?
- Is there any need to avoid central acting drugs? If there is any doubt about the patient's level of consciousness, this has to be evaluated first before the application of sedatives or analgesics. Furthermore, adequate monitoring and surveillance have to be provided.
- Is there any need for checking the patient's neurologic status frequently? Local and regional anesthesia techniques offer the unique advantage of acting only at the traumatized limb or body area, and not compromising central functions and thus facilitating continued neurologic evaluation. In drug addicts, local or regional anesthesia techniques usually are superior to central-acting drugs because of the more predictable peripheral effect.
- What is the individual incidence of nausea, vomiting, and aspiration? Many patients who come to the ER are at risk for aspiration pneumonitis. The classic example is the multiple traumatized patient with acute pain and a 'full stomach' who must have anesthesia induction for securing the airway and treating the pain. In these patients, endotracheal intubation is often required to minimize the risk of aspiration following adverse-effects of central-acting drugs.
- What is the individual likelihood of myalgia, backache, headache, or sore throat?
- Will there be enough time to perform a regional anesthesia technique? The necessary time for proper administration of local anesthetic is usually several times as long as the administration of IV analgesia or general anesthesia.
- What is the individual physician's success rate for the selected technique? In general, but especially in emergencies, no anesthetic or analgesic agent should be used unless the clinician understands the proper technique of administration, dosage, contraindications, side effects, and treatment of overdose.
- Are the required safety standards (personnel and monitors) for the selected technique available?

SAFETY AND MONITORING

In general, no anesthetic or analgesic agent should be used unless the clinician understands the proper technique of administration, dosage, contraindications, side effects, and treatment of overdose. Close monitoring of heart and respiratory rates, respiratory effort, blood pressure, and responsiveness to stimuli is mandatory in all trauma patients.

Skilled supervision is necessary whenever systemic pharmacologic agents are used for conscious sedation (i.e. the patient maintains a response to verbal, and physical stimuli). A separate health care provider, not involved in performing the procedure, should monitor for conscious sedation including frequent assessment of heart rate, respiratory rate and effort, blood pressure, level of consciousness, and oxygen saturation.

The monitoring capabilities and anesthesia equipment in the non-operating room environment (e.g. the ER) should be similar to the standard OR. The American Society of Anesthesiologists (ASA) has established guidelines for non-operating room anesthetizing locations.[21] Uniformity of anesthesia equipment enhances safety and constant maintenance of this equipment is essential because the location often makes immediate help from OR personnel unlikely. The physician unfamiliar with the monitors and layout in the ER location should spend additional time ensuring proper functioning of this equipment.

In addition, equipment should be available to promptly treat any untoward complication in trauma patients. Apart from the mentioned monitoring devices, such emergency equipment includes supplemental oxygen, devices to maintain airway patency (e.g. oral and nasal airways, face masks, endotracheal tubes, laryngoscopes, and a bag–valve–mask device), suction, drugs for resuscitation (e.g. atropine, naloxone), and an electrical defibrillator. Most important, there must be a physician or other provider on site who is skilled in resuscitation, particularly airway management.

Further, whenever monitored anesthesia care, regional or general anesthesia techniques are being performed, the ASA standards for basic anesthetic monitoring should be adjusted to the ER. These standards apply to all anesthesia care, although, in emergency circumstances, appropri-

Table 7.2 ASA guidelines for non-operating room anesthetizing locations (in excerpts)

Qualified anesthesia personnel shall be present in the room throughout the conduct of all general anesthetics, regional anesthetics, and monitored anesthesia care.
During all anesthetics, the patient's oxygenation, ventilation, circulation, and temperature shall be continually evaluated.

ate life support measures take precedence. These standards may be exceeded at any time based on the judgement of the responsible anesthesiologist.

This set of standards addresses only the issue of basic monitoring, which is only one component of anesthesia care. In certain rare or unusual circumstances, (1) some of these methods of monitoring may be clinically impractical, and (2) appropriate use of the described monitoring methods may fail to detect untoward clinical developments (especially in emergencies).

After completion of any procedure, monitoring should continue until the patient is fully awake and has resumed the former level of function. In any case, machines cannot substitute for skilled and frequent assessment and observation by the experienced health care provider.

Regular assessment of vital signs and level of consciousness is necessary when parenteral opioids are used for managing acute traumatic pain. Because of wide inter- and intraindividual variations in response to opioids, an occasional patient will have an adverse reaction despite even the most careful titration of doses and intervals. Serum levels of opioids may increase many hours after a one-time intramuscular or subcutaneous dose, presumably as a result of late release from tissue stores. The practitioner should be aware of this.

PAIN MANAGEMENT FOR SPECIAL PATIENT GROUPS

The choice of techniques for analgesia and sedation of the individual patient is influenced by many factors such as the following:

- Patient-dependent factors (e.g. age, weight, ability to understand and to cooperate with treatment, co-existing medical and psychological problems)

- Patient's cardiovascular or respiratory instability that mandates immediate life-saving procedures (e.g. endotracheal intubation, defibrillation, cut-down, and chest tube insertion), without analgesia or anesthesia
- Physician's preferences and skills
- Available equipment and monitoring devices.

Once the patient is resuscitated, and requires diagnostic and/or definitive surgical procedures, analgesia should be provided as outlined in the following guidelines for the various injured sites.

Thermal injuries (see also Ch. 20)

Pain associated with thermal injuries, especially second degree burns or scalds, is at least as severe as other trauma pain. The serious burn injury will require very special pain control after the initial resuscitation. The myth that 'third degree burns never hurt' unfortunately still serves as a basis for widespread institutional denial of pain assessment and treatment for burned patients. Furthermore, thermal injuries often represent psychologically very agonizing events for patients.

Ketamine in analgesic doses (0.5–1.0 mg/kg IV) in combination with the amnestic properties of midazolam (0.05–0.1 mg/kg IV) or propofol (1.0–4.0 mg/kg per hour as continuous infusion) provides analgesia superior to that achieved with opioids and ensures near-total amnesia.

The almost universal presence of hypotension and vasodilatation (with or without sepsis) generally precludes the use of epidural analgesia for pain control until the burn wound is closed.

Patients in shock

Patients with hypovolemia are particularly susceptible to the cardiovascular and respiratory depression associated with analgesia and sedation. Therefore, in hypovolemic patients the decreased volume of distribution for the parenteral application of drugs has to be considered. Incremental doses of midazolam together with ketamine or fentanyl offer the advantage of minimal cardiovascular instability.

Head injuries (see also Ch. 22)

Injuries of the head pose the problem of interpretation. Not only does the analgesic reduce the level of consciousness, but also, by constricting the pupils, it may reduce or confuse the value of eye signs.

In several studies, patients with an associated minor head injury are less likely to receive analgesics than those with isolated fracture. In a study of 99 children who did not undergo endotracheal intubation in the ER, only 31% of those with a combined limb and head injury received analgesics.[22] Several authors even advocate this policy.[23,24] Concern exists that respiratory depression will lead to increased $PaCO_2$ and central blood flow (see Chs 6 and 22).

The practice of not applying adequate pain therapy to patients with appreciable head injuries and pain should not be acceptable any longer. The securing of the airway, adequate oxygenation, and pain therapy may be achieved for patients with depressed level of consciousness, at least in all patients with a GCS < 8, by general anesthesia with endotracheal intubation and appropriate ventilation. Usually, decisions regarding further therapeutic measures (including operations) are made using computerized tomography scans, but not clinical neurologic examinations.

Fractures of the lower extremity

The blocking of the lumbar plexus via the inguinal perivascular approach deserves special mention. This technique provides excellent analgesia within 10 to 15 minutes for patients with femoral or tibial fractures, including the hip and thigh. This block allows comfortable transportation and movement for diagnostic measures before operation. A catheter should be left in place to permit intermittent or continuous infusion of local anesthetics during the perioperative period (see Ch. 13).

SUMMARY

The adequate management of pain in ERs depends on knowledge of the pharmacology of analgesic drugs and regional anesthesia techniques. Physiologic responses of the traumatized patient to pain have to be considered when assessing pain and when prescribing a particular analgesic and/or anesthetic agent or technique to relieve pain. Especially in the ER, ongoing systematic assessment and monitoring are critical so that all patients receive the maximal effects to keep them above their particular pain thresholds bearing in mind the risk of cardiorespiratory depression.

Table 7.3　Suggestions of a differentiated pain management in the ER

Condition	Regional or local anesthesia technique	IV agents	Comments
Head injury		Opioids	General anesthesia with et intubation if GCS < 8
Burn injury		Ketamine or opioids + benzodiazepine	General anesthesia with et intubation if severe inhalational trauma is suspected
Fractured ribs (more than 4 in number)	Thoracic epidural	Opioids + benzodiazepine	General anesthesia with et intubation if pulmonary contusion is suspected
Fractured ribs (up to 4 in number)	Intercostal nerve block just posterior to fracture	Opioids + benzodiazepine	
Axial spine injury		Opioids or ketamine + benzodiazepine	
Fractured upper extremity (proximal of elbow)	Interscalene or supracavicular brachial plexus block	Opioids or ketamine	
Fractured upper extremity (distal of elbow)	Axillary brachial or infraclavicular plexus block	Opioids or ketamine	
Isolated hand injury	Wrist or digital nerve block	NSAID; opioids	
Fractured lower extremity (proximal of ankle)	'3 in 1' block	Opioids or ketamine	
Isolated foot injury	Ankle block or digital nerve block		

et, endotracheal; GCS, Glasgow Coma Scale.

Table 7.3 lists suggestions of a differentiated pain management plan in the ER. Therapeutic intervention for the control of pain in complex, multisystem injuries must be carefully incorporated within the overall management plan. A 'cookbook' approach to the individual patient is impossible because of the diversity of patient and clinical scenarios.

REFERENCES

1. Selbst SM, Clark M. Analgesic use in the emergency department. Ann Emerg Med 1990; 19: 1010–1013.
2. Todd KH, Samaroo N, Hoffmann JR. Ethnicity as a risk factor for inadequate emergency department analgesia. JAMA 1993; 269: 1537–1539.
3. Reichl M, Bodiwala GG. Use of analgesia in severe pain in the accident and emergency department. Arch Emerg Med 1987; 4: 25–31.
4. Dempster E. Pain relief in accident and emergency? Accid Emerg Nurs 1995; 3: 3–6.
5. Acute pain management: operative or medical procedures and trauma, Part 2. Agency for Health Care Policy and Research. Clin Pharm 1992; 11: 391–414.
6. Mackersie RC, Karagianes TG. Pain management following trauma and burns. Crit Care Clin 1990; 6: 433–449.
7. Teske K, Daut R, Cleeland C. Relationships between nurses' observations and patient's self reports of pain. Pain 1983; 16: 289–296.
8. Acute pain management: operative or medical procedures and trauma, Part 1. Agency for Health Care Policy and Research. Clin Pharm 1992; 11: 309–331.

9. Kaiser KS. Assessment and management of pain in the critically ill trauma patient. Crit Care Nurs Q 1992; 15: 14–34.

10. Thomas DFM, Lambert WG, Lloyd-Williams K. The direct perfusion of surgical wounds with local anaesthetic solutions: An approach to postoperative pain. Ann R Coll Surg Engl 1983; 65: 226.

11. Committee on Safety of Medicines: Bupivacaine (Marcain Plain) in intravenous regional anaesthesia (Bier's Block). Current Problems 1983; 12.

12. Hollingworth A, Wallace WA, Dabir R. Comparison of bupivacaine and prilocaine used in Bier's Block: A double-blind trial. Injury 1982; 13: 331.

13. Hahn MB, McQuillan PM, Sheplock GJ, eds. Regional anesthesia: An atlas of anatomy and techniques. St Louis: Mosby–Yearbook; 1996.

14. Cousins MJ, Bridenbaugh PO, eds. Neural blockade in clinical anesthesia and management of pain. 2nd ed. Philadelphia: Lippincott-Raven; 1997.

15. Cartwright PD, Pingel SM. Midazolam and diazepam in ketamine anaesthesia. Anaesthesia 1984; 59: 439–442.

16. Toft P, Romer U. Comparison of midazolam and diazepam to supplement total intravenous anaesthesia with ketamine for endoscopy. Can J Anaesth 1987; 34: 466–469.

17. Whipple JK, Lewis KS, Quebbeman EJ, et al. Current patterns of prescribing and administering morphine in trauma patients. Pharmacotherapy 1995; 15: 210–215.

18. Lehmann KA. Tramadol for the management of acute pain. Drugs 1994; 47 Suppl 1: 19–32.

19. Tarantino DP, Baker CR, Bower TC. Patient-administered alfentanil for wound dressing changes in a non-intensive care unit setting. Anesth Analg 1995; 80: 191–193.

20. Stewart RD. Nitrous oxide sedation/analgesia in emergency medicine. Ann Emerg Med 1985; 14: 139–148.

21. Guidelines of the American Society of Anesthesiologists: Directory of Members, American Society of Anesthesiologists. Park Ridge, Illinois: American Society of Anesthesiologists; 1995: 393.

22. Friedland LR, Kulick RM. Emergency department analgesic use in pediatric trauma victims with fractures. Ann Emerg Med 1994; 23: 203–207.

23. Lloyd Thomas AR, Anderson I. ABC of major trauma. Paediatric trauma: secondary survey. BMJ 1990; 301: 433–437.

24. Genge M. Musculoskeletal emergencies. In: Kitt S, Kaiser J, eds. Emergency nursing, 2nd ed. Philadelphia: WB Saunders; 1990.

8

Pain management in the operating room: regional anesthesia for operative intervention and to augment general anesthesia

Noor M Gajraj and Adolph H Giesecke

Introduction	**General considerations**
Benefits of regional anesthesia	**Potential problems**
Airway and respiratory function	
Cardiovascular function	**Summary**
Cerebral function	
Gastrointestinal/nutritional effects	
Neuroendocrine function	
Musculoskeletal function	

INTRODUCTION

Trauma patients may require surgery for many types of injury including limb fractures, vascular injuries, skin grafts, limb reimplantations, and limb amputations. During these procedures, regional anesthesia may be used as a supplement or replacement for general anesthesia. The provision of good quality analgesia in the perioperative period is important not only for humanitarian reasons but also to reduce cardiovascular and respiratory complications. In addition to reducing the adverse effects of general anesthetic techniques, regional anesthesia may also reduce the stress response associated with trauma and surgery. Reduction of the stress response may provide additional benefits to the patient with extremity trauma by possibly modulating blood flow dynamics in a positive way. Regional techniques may therefore have an important role in minimizing morbidity and mortality and improving patient outcome.[1,2]

BENEFITS OF REGIONAL ANESTHESIA

Regional anesthesia can provide several benefits to the trauma patient (Table 8.1).

Table 8.1 Advantages of regional anesthesia

Good quality analgesia
Avoids airway difficulties
Decreased respiratory complications
Decreased risk of pulmonary aspiration
Decreased cardiovascular complications
Decreased incidence of thromboembolism
Increased limb blood flow
Decreased blood loss
Less impairment of cognitive function
Decreased gastrointestinal complications
Decreased stress response
Provision of postoperative analgesia
Earlier mobilization
Decreased hospital stay

Airway and respiratory function

Regional techniques may avoid the need for tracheal intubation. The risk to patients with cervical spine injuries may therefore be minimized. Between 1.5 and 3% of major trauma patients have a cervical spine injury, and 25 to 75% of these are unstable. Trauma patients often have full stomachs. The risk of pulmonary aspiration may also be reduced by the use of regional techniques.

Avoiding positive pressure ventilation may decrease the possibility of pneumothorax in patients with chest injuries. However, tracheal intubation and mechanical ventilation may be required for the management of airway obstruction, pulmonary aspiration, thoracic injury, or raised intracranial pressure.

Postoperatively, the most important alteration of respiratory function is a decrease in functional residual capacity. The role of regional anesthesia in preserving pulmonary function has been studied extensively. The incidence of pulmonary complications (infection, atelectasis, hypoxemia) following upper abdominal and thoracic surgery is reduced when effective regional anesthetic blocks are used for postoperative analgesia.

Cardiovascular function

Major surgery and trauma are associated with a hypercoagulable state that persists well into the postoperative period.[3,4] Vaso-occlusive and thromboembolic events may result in postoperative morbidity and mortality. Although the etiology of the hypercoagulable state is not fully understood, the stress response appears to be an important factor. Postoperative changes occur in all arms of the coagulation cascade and include increased concentrations of coagulation factors, decreased concentration of coagulation inhibitors, enhanced platelet activity, and impaired fibrinolysis. Epidural anesthesia is associated with a reduced incidence of thromboembolism probably as a result of a reduction in postoperative coagulability and increased lower limb blood flow.[5,6] Blood loss following orthopedic surgery is also reduced as a result of dilatation of venous capacitance beds, which results in lower venous pressures.[7,8]

During anesthesia and surgery, activation of the sympathetic nervous system can result in a tachycardia and increased myocardial oxygen demand. It may also result in a reduction in myocardial oxygen supply because of coronary vasoconstriction or thrombosis. Use of regional anesthesia may obtund these sympathetically-mediated effects and thereby preserve myocardial oxygen balance.

Cerebral function

In the short-term, regional anesthesia has been shown to have advantages over general anesthesia in terms of cerebral function. Chung et al showed that patients undergoing transurethral resection of the prostate or pelvic floor repair with spinal anesthesia had better mental function scores than those undergoing the procedure with general anesthesia at 6 hours, 1 day, 3 days, and 5 days postoperatively.[9] The transient postoperative mental disturbance affected mainly recent memory recall, attention, and calculation. These differences may have implications in terms of recovery and rehabilitation.

In head-injured patients, use of regional techniques as an alternative to general anesthesia allows the level of consciousness to be assessed as an indication of raised intracranial pressure. However, sympathetic blockade may result in a Horner's syndrome and pupillary constriction, which can confuse the neurologic evaluation.

Gastrointestinal/nutritional effects

Epidural anesthesia for patients undergoing abdominal surgery can reduce the duration of postoperative ileus. Evidence suggests that this may result from improved quality of analgesia, systemic absorption of the local anesthetic, blockade of sympathetic innervation of the bowel, and a reduced requirement for systemic opioids. In addition, protein catabolism and nitrogen loss are also reduced.

Neuroendocrine function

The metabolic response to trauma and surgery involves the release of neuroendocrine hormones and cytokines that may result in detrimental physiologic responses (see Chs 3 and 4). Regional anesthesia may attenuate these effects as demonstrated by reduced levels of catecholamines and cortisol and a reduction of insulin-resistant hyperglycemia. Prevention of hyperglycemia may benefit the head-injured patient with possible brain ischemia. Under ischemic conditions, oxidative metabolism of glucose is impaired and glycolysis occurs which results in lactate production and cerebral acidosis.

Either intraoperative or postoperative administration of epidural local anesthetics and opiates can decrease the stress response. However, only pre-incisional establishment of epidural anesthesia with local anesthetics can prevent the stress response and maintain mediator concentrations at preoperative values. Once the stress response is initiated, postincisional administration of epidural anesthesia can only attenuate the response. Extension of epidural anesthesia into the postoperative period may be critical, as maximal increases in the stress response continue for as long as 5 days.

Musculoskeletal function

The systemic effects of local anesthetics on the peripheral vasculature are biphasic.[10] In low concentrations they produce vasoconstriction, whereas in the higher concentrations that are used clinically they are vasodilators. Mechanisms causing vasodilatation include a direct action on vascular smooth muscle (cocaine is an exception) and sympathetic blockade. Sympathetic blockade associated with the use of regional anesthesia, particularly for limb surgery, may contribute significantly to preservation of blood flow. Thus, if the blood supply to a limb has been compromised by surgery or trauma, the improvement in regional flow may prevent ischemia provided that an adequate perfusion pressure, hematocrit, and hemoglobin saturation is maintained.

By blocking sensory input and decreasing sympathetic overactivity, regional anesthesia may decrease the incidence of phantom limb pain and reflex sympathetic dystrophy observed in the extremities after injury and surgery (see Ch. 24).[11]

GENERAL CONSIDERATIONS

Trauma patients must be carefully assessed by history, physical examination, and appropriate investigations.

Pre-existing disease states and the presence of multiple injuries are of particular importance. The procedure must be explained to the patient and consent obtained. Any preoperative neurological deficits must be carefully documented. Although regional anesthetic techniques are not necessarily contraindicated in patients with peripheral nerve injuries, there may be an increased medicolegal risk if neurologic function has not been thoroughly documented.

Contraindications to regional techniques include local anesthetic allergy, local or systemic infection, hypovolemia, or coagulation defects (Table 8.2). Coagulation defects may, for example, be present in patients who have received large quantities of blood. Coagulation studies may be necessary and hypovolemia must be corrected. The use of 'single-shot' spinal or epidural anesthesia should be avoided in hypovolemic patients because absolute hypovolemia is exacerbated by vasodilatation which may result in severe reductions in venous return, cardiac output, and arterial blood pressure. Additionally, patients with fixed cardiac output states as a result of valvular heart disease (e.g. aortic or mitral stenosis) may be unable to compensate for the reduction in afterload produced by spinal or epidural anesthesia.

All equipment and drug dosages must be checked before the anesthetic procedure. Equipment for emergency airway management must also be available (Table 8.3). The patient

Table 8.2 Contraindications to regional anesthesia in the trauma patient

Patient refusal
Coagulopathy
Hypovolemia
Fixed cardiac output states
Sepsis

Table 8.3 Equipment for emergency airway management in the trauma patient

Assortment of oral and nasal airways
Variety of laryngoscope blades
Variety of endotracheal tubes
Stylets
Gum elastic bougie
Light wand
Laryngeal mask airway
Combitube
Fiberoptic bronchoscope
Wire for retrograde techniques
Cricothyroidotomy needle

who is undergoing a regional technique must be monitored as carefully as one undergoing a general anesthetic, including the use of invasive monitoring when indicated. Adequate venous access is essential. If sedation is used, the patient should receive supplemental oxygen via nasal cannulae or a face mask. During peripheral or plexus blocks, a nerve stimulator is especially useful for patients who are drowsy, have altered levels of consciousness or who cannot communicate with the anesthesiologist because of a language barrier.

Treatment of hypotension during spinal or epidural anesthesia may require use of intravenous fluids, a change in posture, and administration of oxygen. Vasopressors are more effective than administration of intravenous fluids and should be readily available.

The majority of lower abdominal and limb surgeries can be performed under regional anesthesia either as the sole technique or in combination with general anesthesia. Continuous catheter techniques allow analgesia to be extended into the postoperative period. The adequacy of the block must be tested prior to surgical incision. During the surgery, the anesthesiologist should remain in close contact with the awake patient and ensure his or her comfort. Operating personnel need to bear in mind that the patient is conscious and provide a reassuring atmosphere.

POTENTIAL PROBLEMS

The use of regional techniques in the trauma patient is not without potential problems (Table 8.4). It may be difficult to position the patient because of pain. Small doses of opiates, e.g. fentanyl 25–50 micrograms or ketamine 10–20 mg, may be administered to the patient to make positioning and performance of the regional technique more comfortable.

The trauma patient may have injuries at multiple sites. It may not be possible to use local anesthetic techniques without exceeding the maximum recommended dose. Use of major regional blocks at more than one site may increase the risk of cardiovascular collapse.[12] Needle trauma can result from the regional technique. For example, brachial plexus block via the supraclavicular route carries a risk of pneumothorax which may cause serious morbidity and even mortality in the already traumatized patient.

Table 8.4 Potential problems during regional techniques in the trauma patient

Patient positioning
Local anesthetic toxicity
Needle trauma (e.g. pneumothorax)
Alcohol intoxication
Uncooperative patient
Horner's syndrome may confuse neurologic exam
Prolonged surgical time
Occult blood loss
Hypotension

Alcohol intoxication may be present in up to 60% of trauma patients. Sedatives, which are used to help an intoxicated patient cooperate and tolerate surgery, may act synergistically with the alcohol, increasing the risk of airway obstruction and pulmonary aspiration.

If the surgical procedure is noisy or the patient reports slight discomfort, then small doses of intravenous opiates, benzodiazepines or propofol may be administered. Amputation of limbs and insertion or removal of hardware requiring force on the part of the surgeons are examples of such procedures. However, sedation should not be used to compensate for an inadequate regional technique. Sedation in this situation may only increase the patient's agitation and depression of respiration and airway reflexes can easily occur. If necessary, the patient should receive a general anesthetic.

Use of drapes to screen out unpleasant sights and playing background music may be helpful. Patients may become uncomfortable when lying on an operating table for prolonged periods of time as occurs during reimplantation procedures and reconstructive surgery. In these situations, it may be advisable to administer a light general anesthetic.

Regional anesthesia may be harmful to patients if provided incorrectly.

In an awake patient, hypotension may result in nausea and vomiting. For this reason, regional techniques are avoided if large blood loss is anticipated. Hypotension may occur after an intrathecal or epidural block for several reasons. In addition to vasodilatation, sympathetic blockade may result in bradycardia if the block is high enough to affect the cardiac accelerator nerves (T1–T4).

Systemic absorption of local anesthetic may result in myocardial depression. Additional considerations in the trauma patient include:

- Unrecognized or untreated hypovolemia caused by the main or associated injury – potential sites for occult loss of intravascular volume include the chest, pelvis, and femur
- Chest or abdominal injuries may produce hypoxia and hypercarbia, and the resulting myocardial depression may contribute to the development of hypotension
- Cardiac injuries such as myocardial contusion and hemopericardium may initially produce minimal hemodynamic disturbance until the onset of sympathetic blockade and decreased venous return
- Vasodilatation caused by alcohol.

Caplan et al have reported 14 cases of unexpected cardiac arrest during spinal anesthesia.[13] On the basis of their study, three recommendations for the management of routine spinal anesthesia were made. First, a pulse oximeter should be employed whenever sedative agents are administered or when the ability to communicate with the patient is impaired. Second, epinephrine should be considered early in the treatment of sudden bradycardia, especially if conventional doses of atropine or ephedrine are not effective. Third, a full dose of epinephrine should be given immediately upon the recognition of cardiac arrest. The chronotropic effect of epinephrine may be more effective than ephedrine in preventing bradycardia from progressing to cardiac arrest. Epinephrine is also a much more potent α-agonist than ephedrine. By promoting peripheral vasoconstriction, α-agonists may increase venous return to the heart and thereby improve cardiac output during external cardiac compression. Additionally, peripheral vasoconstriction may increase diastolic blood pressure and coronary perfusion, resulting in faster recovery of cardiac function.

CASE STUDY

A 68-year-old, 76 kg man presented for internal fixation of left humeral fractures following a motor vehicle accident. He also had fractures of the left 5th and 6th ribs. Past history included chronic obstructive pulmonary disease and hypertension. In the operating room, standard monitors were applied consisting of a pulse oximetry, electrocardiogram, and an automatic blood pressure device. After sedation with intravenous midazolam 2 mg, a left interscalene block was performed with the aid of a peripheral nerve stimulator. 40 mL of mepivacaine 1.5% with adrenaline 1:200 000 was injected resulting in a good sensory and motor block of the left arm. During the surgery, additional doses of midazolam were given (total 7 mg) and the patient received 2 L of oxygen via nasal cannulae continuously. The surgery was completed satisfactorily and the patient made an uneventful recovery without respiratory complications.

SUMMARY

The trauma patient may be a challenge to the anesthesiologist for many reasons including multiple injuries, drug intoxication, prolonged operative procedures, and severe postoperative pain. Regional anesthesia may be used with sedation as an alternative to general anesthesia. Regional anesthesia can also be used in combination with general anesthesia, allowing a reduction in total general anesthetic requirement. However, safe use of regional techniques requires a high degree of vigilance if morbidity and even mortality are to be avoided.

REFERENCES

1. Liu S, Carpenter RL, Neal JM. Epidural anesthesia and analgesia. Their role in postoperative outcome. Anesthesiology 1995; 82: 1474–1506.
2. Scott NB, Kehlet H. Regional anesthesia and surgical morbidity. Br J Surg 1988; 75: 299–304.
3. Collins GJ, Barber JA, Zajtchuk R, Vanek D, Malogne LA. The effects of operative stress on the coagulation profile. Am J Surg 1977; 133: 612–616.
4. Donadoni R, Baele G, Devulder J, Rolly G. Coagulation and fibrinolytic parameters in patients undergoing total hip replacement: Influence of anesthetic technique. Acta Anaesthesiol Scand 1989; 33: 588–592.
5. McKenzie PJ, Wishart HY, Gray I, Smith G. Effects of anesthetic technique on deep vein thrombosis: a comparison of subarachnoid and

general anesthesia. Br J Anaesth 1985; 57: 853–857.

6. Modig J, Malmberg P, Karlstrom G. Effect of epidural versus general anesthesia on calf blood flow. Acta Anaesthesiol Scand 1980; 24: 305–309.

7. Keith I. Anaesthesia and blood loss in total hip replacement. Anaesthesia 1977; 32: 444.

8. Rosberg B, Fredin H, Gustaform C. Anaesthetic techniques and surgical blood loss in total hip arthroplasty. Acta Anaesthesiol Scand 1982; 26: 189.

9. Chung F, Meier R, Lautenschlager E, Carmichael FJ, Chung A. General or spinal anaesthesia: which is better in the elderly? Anesthesiology 1987; 67: 422–427.

10. Johns RA, DiFazio CA, Longnecker DE. Lidocaine constricts or dilates rat arterioles in a dose dependent manner. Anesthesiology 1986; 65: 186.

11. Bach S, Noreng MF, Tjellden NU. Phantom limb pain in amputees during the first 12 months following limb amputation, after preoperative lumbar epidural blockade. Pain 1988; 33: 297–301.

12. Ngan-Kee WD, Lee BB. Cardiovascular collapse after combined spinal anesthesia and interscalene brachial plexus block. Anaesthesia and Intensive Care 1995; 23: 212–214.

13. Caplan RA, Ward RJ, Posner K, Cheney FW. Unexpected cardiac arrest during spinal anesthesia. A closed claims analysis of predisposing factors. Anesthesiology 1988; 68: 5–11.

9

Pain management and sedation in the intensive care unit

Laureen L Hill and Ronald G Pearl

Introduction

Goals of sedation and analgesia

Assessment of sedation
  Scoring scales
  Electroencephalogram

Non-pharmacologic interventions

Analgesics
  Nonsteroidal anti-inflammatory drugs
  Opioid drugs
  Remifentanil

Benzodiazepines

Barbiturates

Ketamine

Etomidate

Propofol

Inhalational anesthetics

Delirium and neuroleptics

Pharmacologic approach

Conclusion

INTRODUCTION

Pain and agitation frequently occur in critically-ill and -injured patients. The intensive care unit (ICU) can be a frightening environment, and critical illness is an extremely stressful event. Postoperative pain, invasive procedures, and the presence of endotracheal tubes and indwelling lines and catheters are common in the ICU. Patients who are mechanically ventilated cannot communicate their discomfort and pain to their caregivers. Patients experience stress and agitation resulting from loss of control, inability to communicate, concern for personal survival, disorientation, and physiologic responses to their critical illness. Awareness of the potential for pain and agitation, and an understanding of the pharmacologic properties of the analgesic, sedative–hypnotic, and neuroleptic agents available are essential in caring for critically-ill and -injured patients. This chapter will review the current strategies for assessing, monitoring, and treating pain and agitation in the ICU.

GOALS OF SEDATION AND ANALGESIA

The purpose of pain and sedation management in the ICU is to improve patient comfort, reduce anxiety, facilitate sleep, and minimize undesired physiologic responses to illness and its therapy. Before designing a treatment regimen, one must first determine the specific needs of the patient. Agitation may result from pathologic conditions which must be ruled out before providing drugs which may mask the symptoms. Hypoxia, hypercarbia, electrolyte disturbances, metabolic perturbations, withdrawal from alcohol, sedative or opiate drugs, and acute drug reactions can produce agitation.

While pain is acknowledged as a source of significant distress to patients, it continues to be underrecognized and inadequately treated. In a survey conducted by Loper et al many healthcare providers had significant misunderstandings about the sedative and analgesic properties of various drugs used for treatment of anxiety.[1] For example, 80% of physicians and 43% of nurses surveyed thought that diazepam had analgesic properties, and 5% of physicians and 10% of nurses believed that pancuronium relieved anxiety. Many physicians have misguided fears of opiate addiction in critically-ill patients.

Most critically-ill and -injured patients are unable to communicate their discomfort owing to endotracheal intubation, pharmacologic paralysis, or altered levels of consciousness as a result of their underlying illness/injury (e.g. head trauma) and may be inadequately treated. Pain stimulates the stress response and increases levels of catecholamines and other stress hormones. The effects of the stress response may be deleterious in critically-ill and -injured patients with organ system dysfunction and poor reserve (see Ch. 4.) In their study of epidural analgesia and the stress response in high risk patients, Yeager et al demonstrated that patients with well-controlled pain have decreased stress responses and improved outcomes.[2]

The next important consideration in designing a treatment regimen for analgesia and sedation is airway assessment and the need for mechanical ventilation. Intubated patients generally require both analgesic and sedative interventions to improve tolerance of endotracheal intubation and mechanical ventilation. Despite the provision of adequate minute ventilation, some intubated patients experience dyspnea and have difficulty breathing in synchrony with the ventilator. The use of opiate analgesics to depress respiratory efforts can facilitate ventilatory management and improve patient comfort. The selection of a particular agent(s) depends on the intended duration of intubation and plans for weaning from mechanical ventilatory support.

The use of neuromuscular blocking agents (NMBAs) in an awake patient is an absolute indication for the use of sedating drugs. One of the most frightening experiences a patient can suffer is to be paralyzed and awake. Following his experimental 'curarization' in 1947, Smith reported the physical discomfort and mental distress of being unable to move, swallow, or take a deep breath despite adequate artificial ventilation.[3] Even when his own ventilation returned to normal, he experienced ongoing concern over the discomfort of residual paralysis. Because paralyzed patients appear relaxed and are unable to move in response to stimuli, signs of awareness and inadequate sedation may be absent or difficult to assess. Unrecognized awareness can have significant consequences, including hypertension, myocardial ischemia, and post-traumatic stress disorder.[4] In a retrospective evaluation of the incidence and patient perception of recall in trauma victims undergoing surgery, Bogetz et al found the incidence of recall of surgery in victims of major trauma considerable. Those patients with intraoperative recall considered such awareness their worst hospital experience. Repeated verbal reassurance and a regular schedule of sedative agents, particularly sedative drugs with amnestic properties, e.g. benzodiazepines, should be provided to this high risk group of patients. It is also recommended, whenever possible, that patients be allowed to recover from paralysis on a daily basis to assess for adequacy of analgesic and sedative therapies.

The desire to minimize metabolic demands and oxygen consumption in critically-ill patients has led to increased use of sedation, particularly during stimulating interventions such as dressing changes, physiotherapy, and chest percussive therapy (CPT). For example, CPT can increase oxygen consumption by up to 40 to 50% with related increases in heart rate and minute ventilation.[5] A number of studies have shown that adequate sedative therapy can attenuate this response and lower O_2 consumption to levels 10 to 15% below those of unstimulated awake patients.[6,7] This decrease in oxygen consumption can also be observed in patients receiving NMBAs; however, for the reasons discussed above, careful attention to adequate sedation therapy must be provided concurrently.

The degree of desired sedation must also be determined to tailor therapy. The ideal level of sedation is generally one in which the patient is calm, but easily aroused with minimal stimulation. This may not always be appropriate, however, depending on the underlying pathology. For example, patients with severe lung injury, hypoxia, and decreased tissue oxygen delivery may require deep levels of sedation with or without paralysis to decrease oxygen demand. On the other hand, patients with neurologic injury may require a sedation regimen which allows for frequent neurologic assessment. The anticipated duration of sedation therapy may also affect the choice of drugs used.

The potential side effects of medications must be considered in selecting a sedation regimen. Agents with myocardial depressant effects would obviously be undesirable in patients with poor cardiac function. Likewise, drugs with respiratory depressant effects must be used cautiously in non-intubated patients. Other effects such as histamine release, adrenal suppression, altered cerebral perfusion and sympathetic stimulation must be considered.

Lastly, the underlying pathophysiologic processes may affect the choice of medication. Altered renal function and hepatic dysfunction will alter the dosing and/or selection of agents used for pain management and sedation. One must also consider that critical illness alone may change the way a given individual will respond to a certain drug, requiring careful titration of dosage to achieve the desired effect.

ASSESSMENT OF SEDATION

Our ability to titrate drugs to achieve the desired level of sedation requires frequent assessment of a patient's level of consciousness and response to stimuli. Certain clinical parameters such as resting heart rate and blood pressure variations, spontaneous respiratory rate, general muscle tone, and facial tension can provide some useful information regarding the level of sedation. Several sedation scoring systems have been developed in order to provide a more consistent and objective means of assessing a patient's level of sedation.

Scoring scales

The Ramsay sedation scale was developed in the 1970s for the purpose of assessing level of sedation in experimental studies. A patient's degree of wakefulness or response to stimulation is graded on a numeric scale from 1 to 6.[8] The Observer's Assessment of Alertness/Sedation Scale is another scale developed for research purposes that involves assessing responsiveness to verbal and physical stimulation, speech, facial expression, and eye appearance.[9] The Faces Pain Scale is a simple self-reporting method for children in which children's drawings of facial expressions of pain are used as an index of pain.[10] An observer-reported faces scale has been compared with the self-reported visual analog scale in adult patients in the ICU following thoracoabdominal procedures for esophageal cancer, and was found to be potentially useful for pain evaluation in the ICU.[11] These and other clinical scales are relatively easy to use, but have limited utility in patients who are receiving NMBAs. Methods of assessing cortical brain activity are desirable because they can provide continuous, objective data regarding the brain's function, and are not affected by the presence of NMBAs.

Electroencephalogram

The electroencephalogram (EEG) is a measurement of the spontaneous electrical activity of the brain and is recorded using pairs of scalp electrodes placed over specific areas of the cerebral cortex. The waveforms displayed represent the electrical activity of each electrode pair, plotted as voltage versus time. The pattern of waveform frequency and amplitude allows interpretation of the raw EEG data. Low amplitude, high frequency beta waves (>13 Hz) are seen during wakeful states with mental alertness, while alpha waves (8–13 Hz) are typically seen in awake, restful states and during light sedation. During general anesthesia, theta (4–8 Hz) waves predominate. The high voltage, slow delta waves (0–4 Hz) are seen with deep sleep, deep anesthesia, and in the presence of ischemia or severe metabolic disturbances. In contrast to the spontaneous electrical activity recorded in the EEG, evoked potentials (EP) are recorded following external sensory stimulation. The type of stimulus may be somatosensory, visual, or auditory. Anesthetic drugs will predictably change the amplitude and latency of the EP responses.

The collection and interpretation of massive amounts of raw EEG data are prohibitive in the ICU environment where physicians must monitor many other physiologic variables.

The EEG data can be compressed and reduced by a number of signal processing techniques to provide a simplified interpretation of cortical brain activity for clinical application. The EEG is a complex signal comprised of sine waves or sinusoids which are defined by amplitude, frequency, and phase angle. Most processed EEG parameters have been based on power spectral analysis (PSA) which describes amplitude or power distribution as a function of frequency, ignoring phase information. One such example is the compressed spectral edge, a derived parameter representing the frequency below which 95% of the power in the EEG signal is located. Because PSA does not take into account the phase angle of constituent sinusoids, two complex waveforms with different phase information (i.e. different EEG signals) may have the same power spectra.

Bispectral analysis is a method of signal processing which considers the phase information of complex waveforms and the relationships between signal components. By quantifying more of the information available from the EEG signal, bispectral analysis may more accurately describe brain function.[12,13] Bispectral analysis is a signal processing technique which quantifies the degree of phase coupling between components of the EEG signal. The bispectral index (BIS) is a numeric index ranging from 0 to 100 which is derived from bispectral and other EEG features. Several investigators have demonstrated the ability of BIS to provide useful information regarding anesthetic effects on the central nervous system, depth of sedation, and loss of consciousness.

A number of processed signals have been found to have good correlation with blood concentrations of centrally-acting drugs and have been used extensively in pharmacologic research.[14–17] The processed EEG is used widely in the operating room (OR) as a monitor of central nervous system (CNS) activity during anesthesia;[18] however, it has not been proven to provide clinically meaningful information regarding the level of sedation in patients in the ICU.[19] Likewise, evoked potentials are used perioperatively to monitor spinal cord, brainstem, and visual cortex function, but their use for monitoring level of sedation in the ICU is not established.

NON-PHARMACOLOGIC INTERVENTIONS

A great source of distress for patients in the ICU is the loss of control they experience. Often they are intubated and unable to speak. Patients are usually supine and visually isolated. They undergo a variety of procedures and interventions without always understanding what is being done or why it is necessary. Physical restraints are often used to prevent accidental extubation, and visiting policies are generally restrictive. By establishing eye-

to-eye contact when applicable, and developing effective communication strategies, caregivers can make patients feel less isolated and vulnerable. Physical restraints should be used judiciously, and visiting policies should be as flexible as possible. Relaxation methods such as imagery and deep breathing exercises may be effective in patients who are able to cooperate. Lastly, music therapy can be useful in relieving stress in ICU patients. While these measures will not completely alleviate symptoms of pain and agitation, they are simple, effective strategies which should be employed in the delivery of critical care.

ANALGESICS

Pain is an unpleasant emotional experience, which arises in the periphery from tissue injury and the secondary release of biochemical mediators. The pain impulses are carried to the spinal cord via afferent C and A-δ fibers, and ultimately to the cerebral cortex by ascending sensory tracts. Analgesia may be achieved by attenuating the effect of biochemical mediators in the periphery, by interfering with nerve transmission, or by altering pain perception in the brain.

Regional anesthetic techniques can be useful in managing pain in critically-ill patients; this topic is well-covered elsewhere in this text.

Nonsteroidal anti-inflammatory drugs

Nonsteroidal anti-inflammatory drugs (NSAIDs) decrease prostaglandin synthesis by inhibiting cyclooxygenase. Ketorolac is the first parenteral NSAID available for treatment of acute pain. It exhibits analgesic, anti-inflammatory and antipyretic properties with no ventilatory, cardiovascular, or central nervous system depression. Like all NSAIDs, ketorolac reversibly inhibits platelet aggregation, decreases protective barriers to gastric acidity, and can cause renal insufficiency by decreasing synthesis of vasodilator renal prostaglandins. The duration of ketorolac use should not exceed 5 days. Therefore its use in the ICU is generally limited to treatment of acute postoperative pain.

Opioid drugs

The most commonly used analgesics in the ICU are the opioid drugs. Opiates are powerful analgesics which act at opioid receptors in the CNS and other tissues to produce pain relief without inhibiting conduction of nerve impulses or altering responsiveness of afferent nerve endings. The drugs are classified as agonist, agonist–antagonist, or antagonist based on their activity at a given receptor. There are several types of opioid receptors, each with different pharmacologic effects. μ_1-receptors primarily provide supraspinal analgesia, while μ_2-receptors are responsible for the undesirable side effects of hypoventilation, ileus, nausea, pruritus, euphoria, and physical dependence.

Unfortunately, purely μ_1-agonists are not available for clinical use at this time. Delta receptors modulate μ receptor activity. κ receptor activation results primarily in spinal analgesia with few side effects, and σ receptor activation leads to dysphoria, hypertonia, tachycardia, and tachypnea. Pure agonists primarily activate the μ receptor, while mixed agonist–antagonists act as agonists at the κ and σ receptors and antagonists at the μ receptor. Pure opioid antagonists competitively inhibit opioid agonists, resulting in reversal of their effects. Opioid antagonists should be used with caution as they may precipitate significant side effects including hypertension, excitement, pulmonary edema, myocardial ischemia, and acute withdrawal.

The duration and effect of opiates are determined by a number of factors including lipid solubility, protein binding, pK_a, duration and route of administration, and underlying hepatic or renal disease. Lipid solubility determines the rapidity with which the drug can cross the blood–brain barrier and thus the onset and offset of drug effect, while protein binding and pK_a influence the amount of drug available for activity. Drugs administered via intramuscular, transdermal, or transmucosal routes have variable and unpredictable absorption in critically-ill patients, so IV administration is preferred. Continuous infusion of drug leads to accumulation, particularly in fat stores, and alters drug elimination. Most opiates are hepatically metabolized and renally excreted, so disease states affecting the kidneys or liver will alter the clearance of drug.

Morphine and fentanyl are the two opiate drugs used most commonly in the ICU. A new, short-acting synthetic opioid, remifentanil, differs significantly from the other opiates to be discussed and will be reviewed separately.

Morphine is poorly lipid soluble, and enters the brain slowly with peak effect achieved 10 to 30 minutes after IV administration. It undergoes conjugation in the liver to form water-soluble glucuronides which are eliminated by the kidneys. One of the metabolites, morphine-6-glucuronide is more potent than the parent compound, and has a duration of action twice that of morphine. In contrast, fentanyl is a synthetic opioid which is highly lipid soluble and has a rapid onset of CNS effects. It is metabolized to inactive compounds which are renally excreted. Meperidine is another synthetically-derived opiate which is not used commonly in critically-ill patients because its metabolite, normeperidine, is potentially toxic. Normeperidine is a cerebral stimulant which can cause tremor, myoclonus, or grand mal seizures, and may accumulate with prolonged meperidine administration, particularly in renal failure.

Side effects of opioid analgesics

The major side effects of opioid analgesics include respiratory, cardiovascular, and gastrointestinal depression. Respiratory depression results from activation of μ_2-receptors which blunts the ventilatory response to increasing levels of carbon dioxide in the CNS, shifting the CO_2 response curve down and to the right. This is of greatest concern in patients who are not intubated or those being weaned from mechanical ventilation. Morphine and meperidine may produce histamine release and thus hypotension and bronchospasm. Fentanyl and dilaudid do not cause histamine release and are preferred in patients at significant risk. Severe chest wall rigidity has been associated with the use of fentanyl and its derivatives, particularly with rapid administration. Neuromuscular blockade may be necessary to reverse the rigidity and allow adequate ventilation of the patient.

While generally mild, the cardiovascular effects of opiates include a slight decrease in blood pressure owing to sympatholysis caused by all opiates, and some degree of myocardial depression and vasodilatation related to histamine release by morphine and meperidine. These effects are potentiated in patients receiving concurrent sedative–hypnotics and in hypovolemic patients and may lead to significant hypotension. Meperidine has vagolytic properties which can produce tachycardia that may be undesirable in patients with cardiac disease, while fentanyl can cause profound bradycardia, especially at higher doses.

Opioids are known to cause a decrease in gastrointestinal motility leading to constipation. The delay in gastric emptying, as well as stimulation of the chemotrigger zone of the brain can lead to the nausea and vomiting seen in patients treated with opioid drugs. In addition, opiates can cause spasm of the sphincter of Oddi leading to symptoms of biliary colic and pancreatitis. This effect can be reversed with naloxone, although the use of glucagon can reverse the biliary spasm without reversing the analgesic opiate effect.

Tolerance and dependence occur with prolonged or continued use of opiates, necessitating increasing amounts of drug to achieve the same desired effect. Withdrawal reactions may occur when the drug is discontinued, so gradual weaning from continuous infusion is recommended.

Remifentanil

Remifentanil is a novel, synthetic, mu-receptor agonist which is metabolized by non-specific blood esterases. This property allows for rapid systemic elimination independent of hepatic and renal function, and predictable termination of effect, even with continuous administration. The contact sensitive half-time (i.e. the time to reach a 50% decrease in effective site concentration) was estimated to be 4 minutes independent of infusion duration.[20] Because of its unique pharmacokinetics, remifentanil offers the ability to provide potent analgesia with rapid recovery; however, rapid offset of analgesia may not be desirable as it may precipitate acute pain and elevated catecholamine levels with untoward cardiovascular effects including hypertension, left ventricular failure, myocardial ischemia, and pulmonary edema. One potential use in the ICU would be to provide analgesia for brief, painful procedures. Constant vigilance must be used to ensure the infusion is not unintentionally interrupted.

The side effect profile for remifentanil is similar to other opiates, i.e. respiratory depression and apnea, decreased GI motility, nausea, vomiting, and pruritus. Like fentanyl, it can cause bradycardia and a secondary decrease in blood pressure. Chest wall rigidity may be profound, especially with bolus administration. In a multicenter evaluation of remifentanil for postoperative analgesia, Bowdle et al reported that adverse respiratory events including respiratory depression (SpO_2 < 90% or respiratory rate < 12 breaths/minute)

and apnea occurred in 29% of patients receiving remifentanil according to an extremely detailed protocol, with apnea occurring in 7% of patients.[21] The administration of such a potent, rapidly acting opioid should be done with extreme caution and under the supervision of individuals trained in the use of anesthetic drugs and skilled in airway management techniques.

BENZODIAZEPINES

Benzodiazepines are commonly used for their sedative and anxiolytic properties, and have desirable amnestic and anticonvulsant effects as well. They have no analgesic activity. A relatively new indication is for the management of acute cocaine intoxication,[22] and they have been a mainstay in the treatment of alcohol withdrawal.[23]

Benzodiazepine agonists bind to specific benzodiazepine receptors in the CNS which form part of the γ-aminobutyric acid-(GABA) receptor complex, and enhance the action of GABA, the predominant inhibitory transmitter in the brain. Antagonists bind to the benzodiazepine receptor and competitively inhibit the effects of the agonists by displacing them from the receptor site. The benzodiazepines are lipophilic compounds which penetrate the CNS rapidly. Continuous infusion leads to drug accumulation, particularly in fat stores, which results in prolonged effects. Benzodiazepines undergo hepatic metabolism with renal excretion of the metabolites. Midazolam and diazepam undergo microsomal oxidation which is affected by increasing age, liver disease, and drugs such as cimetidine and isoniazid which inhibit microsomal enzyme activity. Both produce active metabolites which may accumulate in the presence of renal dysfunction. Lorazepam undergoes glucuronide conjugation to produce inactive metabolites.

Side effects

The major side effects of benzodiazepines are respiratory and cardiovascular depression. Benzodiazepines depress and shift the CO_2 response to the right, and blunt hypoxic drive, although the degree of respiratory depression varies with the particular agent, and is enhanced in the presence of opioids and other CNS depressants. Mild to moderate decreases in blood pressure may occur as a result of sympatholysis, direct cardiac depression, and systemic vasodilatation. Hypotension is greater in the presence of hypovolemia and with concomitant use of opioids and other CNS depressants.

As with opiates, tolerance and dependence are seen with prolonged benzodiazepine administration. Gradual decreases in drug dosage are recommended to avoid precipitating acute withdrawal.

BARBITURATES

Barbiturates work through barbiturate receptors which form part of the GABA-receptor complex, and enhance the activity of GABA. Unlike benzodiazepines, barbiturates can directly activate chloride channels, an action which is responsible for their ability to produce anesthesia with increasing levels. While barbiturates are popular induction agents in the OR, their use in the ICU is limited to treating elevated intracranial pressure and status epilepticus. They have the desirable properties of reducing cerebral blood flow and oxygen consumption, but they have profound cardiorespiratory depressant effects, limiting their use in critically-ill patients. In addition, they induce a hyperalgesic response to pain.

KETAMINE

Ketamine is a derivative of phencyclidine which produces a state of dissociative anesthesia in which the patient appears awake but is noncommunicative and amnestic. Ketamine produces intense analgesia even at subanesthetic doses. It is highly lipid soluble, and therefore has a rapid onset of action. Ketamine is metabolized by hepatic microsomal enzymes to produce an active metabolite which undergoes conjugation to form inactive water-soluble glucuronide metabolites. Prolonged administration may lead to drug accumulation, but also causes enzyme induction which may accelerate metabolism of ketamine and lead to the increased dose requirements observed in patients receiving repeated administration.

Side effects

The side effect profile of ketamine differs from the other sedative hypnotic agents previously discussed. Ketamine produces sympathetic stimulation with elevations in blood pressure, heart rate, cardiac output, and myocardial oxygen demand.[24,25] Ketamine does not produce significant respiratory depression, and upper airway muscle tone and reflexes remain relatively intact; however, patients are still at risk for aspiration and appropriate precautions must be taken. Ketamine stimulates oral and upper respiratory secretions so use of antisialagogues such as glycopyrrolate is recommended. Ketamine is a potent bronchodilator and may be useful in patients with reactive airway disease.

Ketamine increases cerebral blood flow by causing cerebral vasodilatation, placing patients with intracranial pathology at risk for elevations in intracranial pressure (ICP). Emergence from ketamine anesthesia has been associated with hallucinations, bad dreams, and delirium with a reported incidence ranging from 5 to 30%.[26] Benzodiazepines are very effective in reducing the incidence of emergence delirium, and should be used when possible.

ETOMIDATE

Etomidate is a hypnotic agent with no analgesic properties. It is moderately lipid soluble and has rapid onset of effect. The drug is metabolized to inactive compounds by both hepatic microsomal enzymes and plasma esterases. Etomidate depresses ventilation to a lesser degree than the barbiturates, although apnea may occur following bolus administration. Therapeutic doses have minimal effects on heart rate and stroke volume, although blood pressure is reduced secondary to decreases in systemic vascular resistance. Changes in mean arterial pressure are more pronounced in patients with hypovolemia. Myoclonic movements may occur with induction doses and are not related to epileptiform activity in the EEG. They are thought to be due to disinhibition of normal subcortical suppression of extrapyramidal activity. Etomidate decreases cerebral blood flow and metabolism, and therefore decreases intracranial pressure. The one side effect of etomidate limiting its usefulness for ICU sedation is adrenocortical suppression. Following even a single IV dose, etomidate inhibits the enzyme 11-β-hydroylase for up to 8 hours; therefore repeated administration or continuous infusion is not recommended.

PROPOFOL

Propofol is a phenolic derivative hypnotic agent which is formulated in a lipid emulsion because of its hydrophobic properties. Propofol has no analgesic activity. Because of its high lipid solubility, it penetrates the blood–brain barrier rapidly for fast onset of effect. Recovery from propofol is equally fast as a result of redistribution to peripheral tissues and rapid metabolism. The clearance of propofol exceeds hepatic blood flow, indicating extrahepatic elimination. The presence of renal or hepatic dysfunction does not alter the pharmacokinetics of propofol. Continuous infusion leads to some cumulative effect, although recovery is still significantly faster with propofol than with other sedative–hypnotic agents. Once an infusion is discontinued, patients generally recover within 30 minutes.[27] This property allows for frequent evaluations of CNS function and shorter times to extubation.

Side effects

Propofol is a profound depressant of ventilation, producing apnea following bolus injection. Reductions in blood pressure occur because of both direct myocardial depression and a decrease in systemic vascular resistance. As with most of the drugs previously discussed, these depressant effects are greater in the elderly and in patients with hypovolemia or poor cardiac function. Decreased cerebral blood flow, metabolic rate and ICP occur with propofol. Both proconvulsant and anticonvulsant activity has been described. Although the reason for this discrepancy is not clear, it has been suggested that the convulsions do not represent true epileptiform activity on the EEG.[28] Aseptic technique during preparation and administration of the drug is essential to prevent bacterial contamination and sepsis. The lipid vehicle for propofol contains no antimicrobial preservatives. Cases of Gram-positive, Gram-negative, and fungal infections have been reported in patients receiving contaminated propofol.[29,30] Long-term infusions of propofol may be associated with a progressive increase in serum triglyceride levels, predisposing patients to complications of elevated triglycerides including pancreatitis. The caloric content of propofol should be considered when determining the lipid requirements in patients receiving parenteral nutrition.

Case reports of cardiac arrest and unexplained metabolic acidosis occurring in children with respiratory infections receiving propofol for ICU sedation have appeared in the literature.[31] While the United States Food and Drug Administration was unable to establish a link between the use of propofol and the fatal outcomes, the unrestricted use of propofol in the pediatric ICU is not advised.

INHALATIONAL ANESTHETICS

An alternative to intravenous agents for sedation and analgesia is the use of inhalational anesthetics in mechanically-ventilated patients. They are delivered in the inspired gases provided by the ventilator and eliminated from the expiratory limb of the breathing circuit by active piped scavenging systems or adsorptive charcoal canisters. Both the inspired and expired concentrations can be easily monitored by mass spectroscopy or infrared absorption. Inhalational anesthetics have well-defined relationships between inspired concentrations, alveolar concentrations, and anesthetic effects. In subanesthetic concentrations, inhalational agents may be titrated to rapidly achieve the desired level of sedation, and recovery is significantly faster when compared to intravenous agents. Inhaled anesthetic agents produce analgesia, amnesia, and muscle relaxation at anesthetic levels, but analgesia will likely need to be supplemented at levels used for sedation in the ICU.

Isoflurane is the inhalational agent of choice for use in the ICU. Nitrous oxide inhibits methionine synthase activity leading to bone marrow depression and polyneuropathy. Prolonged use of nitrous oxide in critically-ill patients is not advised. Halothane produces myocardial depression and sensitizes the myocardium to the dysrhythmic effects of catecholamines. Additionally, halothane has been implicated in the development of hepatic dysfunction which may progress to fulminant hepatic failure. The etiology of halothane-mediated hepatotoxicity is multifactorial, but it is believed that inadequate hepatocyte oxygenation owing to decreases in both portal vein and hepatic artery blood flow and enzyme induction increasing oxygen demand is the principal mechanism. Critically-ill patients with underlying liver disease or compromise are at greater risk for the depressant effects of halothane on liver blood flow and oxygenation. Enflurane lowers the seizure threshold and increases both the rate of production and resistance to reabsorption of cerebrospinal fluid leading to an increase in ICP, making it unsuitable for patients with intracranial pathology.

Isoflurane produces less myocardial depression than halothane. Decreases in systemic blood pressure are due to decreases in systemic vascular resistance while cardiac output is maintained. It has no dysrhythmogenic properties. Isoflurane has minimal effects on cerebral blood flow, and seizure activity is not induced with its use. While portal blood flow is decreased with all volatile anesthetic agents, isoflurane use is associated with an increase in hepatic artery flow, thus maintaining overall hepatic blood flow. Like all volatile agents, isoflurane relaxes bronchial smooth muscle making it useful in patients with reactive airway disease and bronchospasm.

DELIRIUM AND NEUROLEPTICS

Delirium is a clinical state characterized by disorganized thinking, short-term memory deficits, and altered perceptions including delusional thinking and hallucinations. Delirium is usually precipitated by derangements in cerebral blood flow and oxygen delivery, systemic metabolic factors, neurohumoral responses to acute stress, and sleep/wake cycle disruption, all of which are common in critically-ill patients. Dopaminergic activity is increased in acute stress, and leads to the sensory and cognitive impairments seen in patients suffering from delirium.[32]

Treatment of delirium must be tailored carefully because inappropriate drug selection can interfere with therapy and may further confuse the clinical picture. Of course, careful management of hemodynamics, tissue perfusion and oxygenation, metabolic abnormalities, and an attempt to restore or maintain day/night sleep cycles is the first appropriate step in treating delirium. Opiates are not indicated unless the patient requires analgesics for pain management. The use of CNS depressants such as benzodiazepines can lead to increasing obtundation without any effect on the underlying brain disturbance.

Neuroleptic drugs such as haloperidol are useful at improving symptoms by decreasing the dopaminergic hyperactivity that is present in ICU delirium. Haloperidol reduces dopaminergic neurotransmission and prevents reuptake of dopamine in the CNS. It has variable sedative effects and produces little change in blood pressure, heart rate, and ventilation. Patients may develop extrapyramidal reactions necessitating discontinuation of the drug or treatment with an anticholinergic agent, although this occurs less frequently with intravenous administration. Neuroleptic malignant syndrome is a rare but potentially fatal side effect which presents with hyperpyrexia, muscle rigidity, and autonomic instability which requires prompt recognition, discontinuation of haloperidol, supportive therapy, and dantrolene.

PHARMACOLOGIC APPROACH

The optimal dosing strategy for sedatives and analgesics in the ICU depends on several factors. Choice of drugs should be guided by the patient's specific needs. Agents such as fentanyl and morphine are appropriate selections for pain management, while the sedative–hypnotic drugs are useful in treating agitation and anxiety. As noted above, delirium is a common phenomenon in the ICU and can be successfully managed with neuroleptic drugs such as haloperidol. Combinations of agents can be used as needed to provide the desired effects.

Intermittent bolus administration may be adequate for patients whose needs are likely to be short-term i.e. less than 48 hours. Examples include patients requiring ICU admission for close observation in the immediate postoperative period such as those undergoing carotid endarterectomy, uvulopalatopharyngoplasty, and reconstructive microvascular surgery. Typically these patients only require small doses of analgesics for perioperative pain control because excessive sedation is undesirable. Nursing personnel can administer appropriate medications in this setting based on patient reporting. Another alternative for pain control in the awake, postoperative patient is patient-controlled analgesia (PCA) in which analgesics are self-administered via a programmed pump delivery system. The physician determines the rate and amount of drug to be delivered upon patient request. This modality is covered in greater detail in Chapter 11.

Continuous intravenous infusion of both analgesics and sedatives may be most appropriate in patients who are intubated, pharmacologically paralyzed, and those whose needs are likely to be longer than 48 hours. Careful attention to the pharmaco-kinetic properties of the agents selected is important to avoid overdose or prolonged drug effect. Most pharmacokinetic models for analgesic and sedative drugs have been derived from studies in young, healthy volunteers receiving single bolus injections. These models may poorly predict the pharmocoki-netic profile of the same drugs administered by con-tinuous infusion to critically-ill patients.

Continuous infusion of sedative and analgesic agents may lead to peripheral tissue saturation with drug, and a slow decline in plasma drug con-centration following its discontinuation. For example, following a single IV bolus injection of midazolam, the duration of sedative effects ranges from 30 to 120 minutes. When midazolam is administered by continuous IV infusion for 3 days, the sedative effects may last for 24 hours or longer following discontinuation of the infusion.[33] Propofol has a long elimination half-life in ICU patients receiving continuous infusions for up to several days, but plasma propofol concentrations fall quickly to subtherapeutic concentrations because of the high metabolic clearance of propo-fol and continued redistribution into peripheral tissues. Sedative effects generally resolve within 30 minutes following discontinuation of the infu-sion. A useful strategy when planning to wean patients from deeper levels of sedation and/or mechanical ventilation is to discontinue longer-acting agents approximately 24 hours prior to the desired weaning time and substitute with propofol to allow for faster recovery from drug effect.

Continuous exposure to opiate analgesics can lead to drug tolerance, and increasing doses may be necessary to achieve the desired effect. For patients with extended ICU courses and pro-longed need for sedation/analgesia, one alternative to increasing IV infusions is to convert to enter-ally-administered, long-acting agents such as diazepam or methadone.

Discontinuation of opiates and benzodiazepines can lead to withdrawal. Slow weaning from these agents may be necessary, particularly following extended periods of exposure. Clonidine may be a useful adjunct in treating the sympathomimetic responses to opiate or benzodiazepine withdrawal.

CONCLUSION

Physicians caring for critically-ill and -injured patients must be aware of the potential for pain,

discomfort, and anxiety in their patients. Besides the obvious humanitarian reasons for providing analgesia and anxiolysis, adequate therapy can lead to decreased neurohumoral stress responses and improved outcomes. Understanding the phar-macologic properties of drugs commonly used for sedation in the ICU is necessary to provide appro-priate treatment and manage the inherent side effects, particularly in critically-ill or -injured patients with organ system compromise. The use of neuromuscular blocking agents only heightens the importance of continual assessment of a patient's state of awareness and level of pain, and adjustment of therapy accordingly.

REFERENCES

1. Loper KA, et al. Paralyzed with pain: the need for education. Pain 1989; 37(3): 315–316.
2. Yeager MP, et al. Epidural anesthesia and analge-sia in high-risk surgical patients. Anesthesiology 1987; 66(6): 729–736.
3. Smith SM, b.h., Toman Jep, et al. The lack of cerebral effects of d-tubocurarine. Anesthesiology 1947; 8: 1–14.
4. Bogetz MS, Katz JA. Recall of surgery for major trauma. Anesthesiology 1984; 61(1): 6–9.
5. Weissman C, Kemper M. Stressing the critically ill patient: the cardiopulmonary and metabolic responses to an acute increase in oxygen consump-tion. J Crit Care 1993; 8(2): 100–108.
6. Klein P, et al. Attenuation of the hemodynamic responses to chest physical therapy. Chest 1988; 93(1): 38–42.
7. Boyd O, Grounds M, Bennett D. The dependency of oxygen consumption on oxygen delivery in criti-cally ill postoperative patients is mimicked by vari-ations in sedation. Chest 1992; 101(6): 1619–1624.
8. Ramsay MA, et al. Controlled sedation with alphaxalone-alphadolone. BMJ 1974; 2(920): 656–659.
9. Chernik DA, et al. Validity and reliability of the Observer's Assessment of Alertness/Sedation Scale: study with intravenous midazolam. J Clin Psychopharmacol 1990; 10(4): 244–251.
10. Bieri D, et al. The Faces Pain Scale for the self-assessment of the severity of pain experienced by children: development, initial validation, and pre-liminary investigation for ratio scale properties. Pain 1990; 41(2): 139–150.
11. Terai T, Yukioka H, Asada A. Pain evaluation in the intensive care unit: observer-reported faces scale compared with self-reported visual analog scale. Reg Anesth Pain Med 1998; 23(2): 147–151.

12. Sigl JC, Chamoun NG. An introduction to bispectral analysis for the electroencephalogram. J Clin Monit 1994; 10(6): 392–404.

13. Avramov MN, White PF. Methods for monitoring the level of sedation. Crit Care Clin 1995; 11(4): 803–826.

14. Buhrer M, et al. Electroencephalographic effects of benzodiazepines. I. Choosing an electroencephalographic parameter to measure the effect of midazolam on the central nervous system. Clin Pharmacol Ther 1990; 48(5): 544–554.

15. Mandema JW, Danhof M. Electroencephalogram effect measures and relationships between pharmacokinetics and pharmacodynamics of centrally acting drugs. Clin Pharmacokinet 1992; 23(3): 191–215.

16. Scott JC, Ponganis KV, Stanski DR. EEG quantitation of narcotic effect: the comparative pharmacodynamics of fentanyl and alfentanil. Anesthesiology 1985; 62(3): 234–241.

17. Stanski DR, et al. Pharmacodynamic modeling of thiopental anesthesia. J Pharmacokinet Biopharm 1984; 12(2): 223–240.

18. Levy WJ, et al. Automated EEG processing for intraoperative monitoring: a comparison of techniques. Anesthesiology 1980; 53(3): 223–236.

19. Spencer EM, Green JL, Willatts SM. Continuous monitoring of depth of sedation by EEG spectral analysis in patients requiring mechanical ventilation. Br J Anaesth 1994; 73(5): 649–654.

20. Westmoreland CL, et al. Pharmacokinetics of remifentanil (GI87084B) and its major metabolite (GI90291) in patients undergoing elective inpatient surgery [see comments]. Anesthesiology 1993; 79(5): 893–903.

21. Bowdle TA, et al. A multicenter evaluation of remifentanil for early postoperative analgesia. Anesth Analg 1996; 83(6): 1292–1297.

22. Williams RG, Kavanagh KM, Teo KK. Pathophysiology and treatment of cocaine toxicity: implications for the heart and cardiovascular system. Can J Cardiol 1996; 12(12): 1295–1301.

23. Turner RC, et al. Alcohol withdrawal syndromes: a review of pathophysiology, clinical presentation, and treatment [see comments]. J Gen Intern Med 1989; 4(5): 432–444.

24. Stanley TH. Blood-pressure and pulse-rate responses to ketamine during general anesthesia. Anesthesiology 1973; 39(6): 648–649.

25. Traber DL, Wilson RD, Priano LL. Blockade of the hypertensive response to ketamine. Anesth Analg 1970; 49(3):420–426.

26. White PF, Way WL, Trevor AJ. Ketamine – its pharmacology and therapeutic uses. Anesthesiology 1982; 56(2): 119–136.

27. Beller JP, et al. Prolonged sedation with propofol in ICU patients: recovery and blood concentration changes during periodic interruptions in infusion. Br J Anaesth 1988; 61(5): 583–588.

28. Bevan JC. Propofol-related convulsions [editorial; comment] [see comments]. Can J Anaesth 1993; 40(9): 805–809.

29. Bennett SN, et al. Postoperative infections traced to contamination of an intravenous anesthetic, propofol [see comments]. N Engl J Med 1995; 333(3): 147–154.

30. Postsurgical infections associated with an extrinsically contaminated intravenous anesthetic agent–California, Illinois, Maine, Michigan. MMWR 1990; 39: 426–427, 433.

31. Strickland RA, Murray MJ. Fatal metabolic acidosis in a pediatric patient receiving an infusion of propofol in the intensive care unit: is there a relationship? [see comments]. Crit Care Med 1995; 23(2): 405–409.

32. Simon P, Panissaud C, Costentin J. Anxiogenic-like effects induced by stimulation of dopamine receptors. Pharmacol Biochem Behav 1993; 45(3): 685–690.

33. Barr J, Donner A. Optimal intravenous dosing strategies for sedatives and analgesics in the intensive care unit. Crit Care Clin 1995; 11(4): 827–847.

10

Pain management in the rehabilitation center

Frank J E Falco, P Prithvi Raj, Daniel Breitstein, Kenneth J Abrams and Christopher H Grande

Introduction	Vertebral fractures
Contractures	Compartment syndrome
Spasticity	Nerve entrapment syndromes
Pressure ulcers	Myofascial pain

INTRODUCTION

The trauma patient is at risk for developing a variety of conditions that can lead to pain. This chapter will focus on rehabilitative methods to treat and, more importantly, to prevent and to minimize painful conditions that can develop in the trauma patient. The following discussion will focus on treating the acutely-injured patient and not the trauma patient who develops chronic pain. Each condition will be reviewed and rehabilitation techniques will be discussed that are used to treat and prevent pain, impairment, and disability that can result from these disorders.

CONTRACTURES

The lack of full active or passive range of motion (ROM) owing to joint, muscle, or soft tissue restrictions is known as a contracture. Pain, paralysis, capsular or periarticular soft tissue fibrosis, and muscle damage are conditions that can lead to the development of a contracture. The absence of joint mobilization throughout the full physiologic range is the common denominator for the formation of a contracture despite the primary etiology. Understanding this point is important in the prevention of contractures in the trauma patient who

initially may be unconscious, disoriented, or purposely under sedation.

Contractures can be categorized into three basic groups: arthrogenic, myogenic, and soft tissue. These categories are based upon whether the primary pathology exists at the joint, muscle, or involves other soft tissues. Loss of ROM regardless of the pathological site can lead to significant functional deficits such as gait abnormalities and dependence in performing activities of daily living such as bathing, feeding, and dressing.

Every possible effort should be made by the medical team to prevent the formation of contractures. *Prevention* is *started immediately* with bedside therapy as soon as the patient has been stabilized. Proper positioning of the extremities with splints to maintain full ROM along with active or passive ROM exercises by a therapist is the main thrust of preventing contractures. ROM exercises are then combined with early mobilization which helps to maintain and restore ROM through functional activities.

The mainstay of rehabilitation of contractures once they have formed is through active and passive ROM exercises combined with stretching. In *active range of motion* (AROM) the patient is able to move the joint to some degree within its physiologic range. *Passive range of motion* (PROM) is when the therapist alone moves the joint without the assistance of the patient. This is done when the patient is unable to move the joint because of unconsciousness, disorientation, weakness, or pain. The therapist is required to stretch joint structures in order to maintain or to increase the range of motion which is often necessary in order to make progress with AROM and PROM exercises.

Stretching is accomplished by the therapist in several different ways. Most of the time the therapist manually stretches the joint. Therapeutic heat is often applied to the joint and muscles around the joint to relax soft tissues and maximize the degree of stretching.[1] Stretching can be combined with static splinting to maintain the large or small joints of the upper and lower extremities in a functional position. The therapist can then actively range the patient and use splints to maintain the position (Fig. 10.1). Serial casting is used in a similar fashion to maintain ROM at different degrees. This method is often used in conjunction with peripheral nerve blocks that allow for a further

increase in ROM by reducing muscle tone. The joint position is increased between castings until full ROM is accomplished. Dynamic splints use elastic or spring tension to maintain ROM with passive stretching but also allow for volitional movement by the patient to perform functional activities.

Continuous passive motion (CPM) machines are also useful in the prevention and treatment of contractures much in the same way as extremity braces. The distinction between the use of CPM versus bracing is that the former utilizes AROM while the latter is a passive modality. The CPM machine provides continuous AROM for long periods of time that would be impractical for the therapist to provide to the trauma patient. Typical patients who benefit from CPM are those with knee fractures, total knee replacements, contractures, and ligamentous repair of the knee or hand.[2]

Nerve blocks may assist contractures of myogenic etiology such as increased tone secondary to spasticity. The injections are directed to peripheral nerves providing innervation of muscles involved in moving the joint. An anesthetic is first used to determine the effect of the block on reducing the contracture. If there is a significant improvement with ROM from the anesthetic block, the injection can be repeated with alcohol to provide a longer lasting effect. Alternatively, the extremity can be placed in a position of maximum extension, as a result of the anesthetic effect, and casted or splinted in that position in order to reduce the contracture.

SPASTICITY

Spasticity is a condition that results from an upper motor neuron (UMN) insult or injury. Clinical syndromes commonly associated with spasticity are cerebral vascular accidents (stroke), spinal cord, and traumatic brain injuries. These are conditions that involve disorders of the UMN either as part of a disease process or from trauma.

The mechanism for spasticity is a complex combination of hyperactive spinal and supraspinal pathways that are not completely understood. Spasticity is defined as resistance to passive movement resulting from the hyperactive spinal and supraspinal reflexes. The patient with spasticity often presents clinically with hyperactive reflexes,

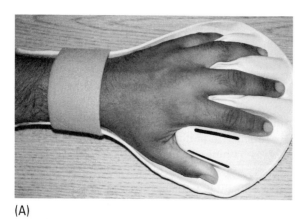

(A)

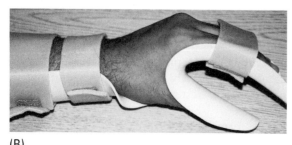

(B)

Fig. 10.1 Upper extremity splints (wrist–hand orthoses). (A) Splint to maintain wrist, hand, and fingers in a neutral position. (B) Splint to maintain wrist, hand, and fingers in a functional grip position.

uncontrollable spasms, increased muscle tone, clonus (repetitive muscle contractions to rapid and maintained stretch), and UMN reflexes such as the Babinski sign (plantar reflex). The effects of spasticity increase either with noxious stimuli such as a urinary tract infection or from a decubitus ulcer. These findings of spasticity typically are not present initially but rather develop over a period of weeks to months.[3,4] The patient acutely will exhibit a loss of reflexes and loss of tone which increases over time as reflexes return and become hyperactive.

Decorticate and decerebrate rigidity are hypertonic states often seen immediately following trauma or lesions to the midbrain, pons, or bilateral forebrain. These conditions are not related to spasticity and should not be classified in that manner. These are states of hypertonus associated with distinct posturing. Decorticate rigidity occurs from bilateral cortical insults and presents as bilateral upper extremity flexion and lower extremity extension. Decerebrate rigidity results from injury to the midbrain, pons, or to the diencephalon bilaterally and is characterized as extension of all four extremities and often the neck. Rigidity, like spasticity, is also increased with nociceptive stimuli. The presence of decorticate and decerebrate rigidity carries a poor prognosis and a high mortality rate.[5]

Although spasticity does not occur immediately after an acute UMN lesion, steps can be taken initially that may help reduce the severity of spasticity development. Placing muscles in a stretched posture and reducing noxious stimuli may reduce the degree of hyperactivity. Early and aggressive use of motor point and nerve blocks with splinting or casting may reduce the severity of spasticity.

The treatment of spasticity can be difficult and frustrating. Spasticity will be present to some level with UMN disorders and will continue to varying degrees despite treatment. Spasticity will not develop acutely in the trauma patient but will be a problem to contend with weeks to months after the injury. The physician must remember that optimizing function is the goal when treating spasticity. Therefore, the benefits and disadvantages of treating spasticity must be considered before treatment. Other effects of UMN disorders or injuries include paralysis, weakness, and altered sensation. A patient with a stroke and lower extremity weakness may be able to ambulate independently with an assistive device (walker or cane)

because of knee stability provided by extensor spasticity. Reducing lower extremity spasticity in these circumstances could lead to unstable knee biomechanics and an inability to ambulate.

The treatment of spasticity like many other conditions is addressed by using a stepped approach with conservative care at first, progressing to more invasive treatment (Fig. 10.2). Rehabilitation efforts are followed in increasing order by medications, motor point and nerve blocks, orthopedic limb surgery consisting of tendon lengthening and joint arthodesis, and neurosurgical procedures such as rhizotomies, cordectomies, and cordotomies.

Rehabilitation begins with treating any reversible cause of increased spasticity such as noxious stimuli that can occur from local infection, constipation, bowel obstruction, decubitus ulcers, sepsis, or fracture. Prevention of contractures from spasticity is extremely important because of the functional implications. Treatment consists of stretching, splinting, and/or serial casting as described earlier in this chapter. Spastic equinovarus is a common manifestation of spasticity in those with UMN disorders or injuries. The use of a splint known as an ankle–foot orthosis can help to maintain proper ankle–foot alignment which is important during the stance phase of gait as well as to provide clearance of the lower

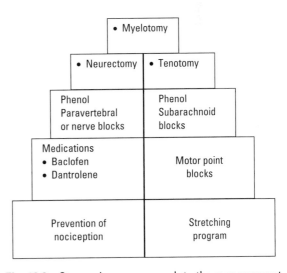

Fig. 10.2 Stepped care approach to the management of spasticity. (From Merritt JL. Management of spasticity in spinal cord injury. Mayo Clin Proc 1981; 56: 614–622, with permission.)

extremity during the swing phase of gait (Fig. 10.3). Peripheral electrical stimulation of muscle or nerve as well as biofeedback have been helpful in reducing spasticity.

As mentioned above, patients with spasticity often will have other neurological deficits such as weakness, sensory abnormalities, and bowel/bladder dysfunction that require treatment. The therapist works on exercising weak muscles, muscle re-education techniques, and functional stimulation to improve strength. The patient is also instructed on how to avoid triggering the spasticity. Treatment is then extended to gross functional activites such as transferring from a sitting to standing position and ambulation on level ground as well as managing inclines, declines, and stairs. The patient with insensate areas requires instruction on proper skin care to prevent breakdown and infection which in turn will reduce the aggravation of the spasticity. Patients need education and training on bowel and bladder care. This will also help to prevent exacerbations of spasticity from bowel impaction or bladder infection.

The use of assistive devices helps the spasticity patient to improve function despite the presence of the spasticity. Devices are used to assist with ambulation as well as activities of daily living. Ambulation aides such as foot–ankle orthoses, canes, crutches, walkers, and wheelchairs provide independence to these patients (Fig. 10.4).

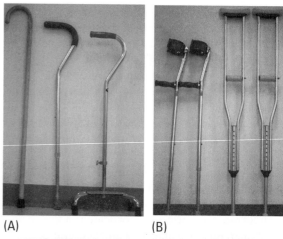

(A)   (B)

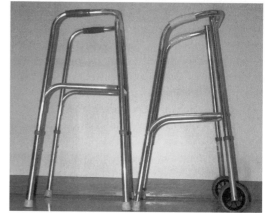

(C)

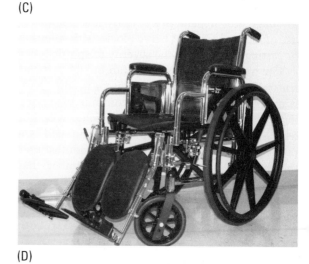

(D)

Fig. 10.4 Ambulation aids. (A) Canes. (B) Crutches. (C) Walkers. (D) Wheelchair.

Fig. 10.3 Ankle–foot orthoses. (A) Thermoplastic molded ankle–foot orthosis (MAFO) with foot and calf Velcro straps which is worn with a shoe. (B) Klenzak ankle–foot orthosis with metal medial and lateral upright supports, ankle joint, padded leather calf band, leather strap, and Velcro strap.

(A)   (B)

Devices to assist with activities of daily living include reachers, adaptive eating utensils, writing aides, wrist–hand orthoses, and dressing devices (Fig. 10.5). The patient confined to a wheelchair will require a pressure-relief seat cushion, and possibly a lapboard and forearm trough if there is upper extremity involvement.

There are interventional options available for treating spasticity other than major surgical procedures such as a rhizotomy or cordotomy when more conservative care is unsuccessful. As discussed earlier with contractures, peripheral nerve blocks and motor point blocks can be performed first with an anesthetic for diagnostic purposes and later with alcohol for a more permanent outcome. Radiofrequency lesioning of nerve roots and intrathecal baclofen for spasticity of cerebral origin are relatively new techniques for treating spasticity. Percutaneous rhizotomies at the dorsal root ganglion level utilizing radiofrequency allow for selective reduction of spasticity in affected limb(s). Intrathecal baclofen delivery via a subcutaneous pump, which has been used to treat spasticity of spinal cord origin, has also been approved to treat spasticity of cerebral etiology such as in stroke victims and traumatic brain injury patients. All of these modalities have the capability to reduce spasticity and improve function without the need for oral medications and their potential side effects.

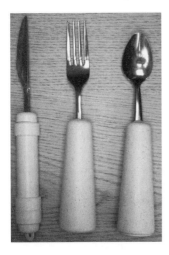

Fig. 10.5 Adaptive eating utensils. These utensils have 'built-up' handles which enable their use with a wider, weaker grip.

PRESSURE ULCERS

Pressure ulcers also known as decubitus ulcers or bed sores are areas of localized tissue necrosis that typically result from prolonged pressure over a small area such as a bony prominence. The exact mechanism for the development of pressure ulcers is not well understood. Many factors that predispose to the formation of decubitus ulcers are pressure, shear, moisture, age, reduced sensation, nutrition, surface area, weakness, and general condition of the skin and soft tissue structures.

Patients who have suffered trauma inherently are exposed to many of these factors and are thus predisposed to the formation of pressure ulcers. The normal individual will naturally shift their weight or position while awake or asleep when tissue pressures reach a subtle level of discomfort well before any deleterious effects leading to tissue breakdown. The unconscious or sedated trauma patient is in a state where he or she is unable to move or to reposition the body or extremities in response to pressure. In the awake trauma patient, factors such as reduced nutrition, poor bed positioning, generalized weakness, and any associated tissue injury from trauma contribute to ulcer formation. Keeping the skin dry in the trauma or any patient is an important preventive factor in the development of decubitus pressures. Urinary and/or fecal incontinence or poor bowel/bladder hygiene can lead to wet skin resulting in ulcer formation as well as infection. There are several areas on the body where there are bony prominences that require special attention including the occiput, scapula, sacrum, ischial tubercles, greater trochanters, heels, and lateral malleoli. These sites are especially predisposed to ulcer formation because of the lack of soft tissue covering the bony prominences which leads to a lower pressure tolerance.

There is a five grade classification system typically used to describe decubitus ulcers (Table 10.1).[6] A Grade I ulcer is defined as erythema and induration over a bony prominence. A Grade II ulcer is tissue necrosis extending into the dermis and a Grade III ulcer extends into the subcutaneous tissue. A Grade IV ulcer extends into the muscle down to the bone and a Grade V ulcer involves the joint and body cavities such as bowel or bladder.

Prevention is the best means of treatment for decubitus ulcers. Skin inspection on a regular

Table 10.1 Decubitus ulcers classification system (adapted from Daniel RK, Hall EJ, MacLeod M. Pressure sores: a reappraisal. Ann Plastic Surg; 1979; 1: 53–63)

Grade	Description
I	Superficial ulcer with skin erythema
II	Ulcer penetration into dermis
III	Ulcer penetration into subcutaneous fat
IV	Ulcer penetration into muscle and down to bone
V	Ulcer penetration into joint or body cavity

basis is imperative to identify the beginning of tissue breakdown. Trauma patients need proper positioning in bed. Particular attention is paid to bony prominences where additional cushioning or padding is helpful in preventing tissue breakdown. Changing posture in bed consisting of turning from side to side at scheduled intervals will assist in preventing ulcers until skin tolerance develops.[7] Therapeutic mattresses and beds such as the air-fluidized bed can also be used to reduce pressure and shear forces. Pressure-relieving cushions are used for the trauma patient who needs to spend significant time in a wheelchair. Other factors such as supplemental nutrition and bowel/bladder care are important in the prevention of ulcers. Patient education regarding ulcer formation and prevention begins as soon as possible by the physician, nurses, and therapy staff.

Treatment of pressure ulcers incorporates prevention measures as well as direct care. Correction or relief of mechanical forces alone can reverse Grade I or II ulcers. Grade II ulcers will also require superficial debridement and dressing changes. Topical agents for debridement of these ulcers include antibiotics, antiseptics, enzymes, and saline. Galvanic stimulation of the ulcer itself can enhance healing of Grade II and some Grade III ulcers.

Grade III to V ulcers typically require surgical treatment with ulcer excision and closure with a skin graft or a variety of soft tissue flaps. The patient will need intravenous antibiotics if there is bone involvement with Grade IV and V ulcers. Postoperative treatment includes many of the same preventive measures discussed earlier such as positioning, turning, skin inspection/care, and bowel/bladder management.

VERTEBRAL FRACTURES

Several different mechanisms of injury can lead to vertebral fractures. The type of injury leading to a vertebral fracture will have a profound effect on which part of the spinal column (anterior, middle, posterior) becomes disrupted leading to biomechanical failure and potential instability (Table 10.2). Hyperflexion is the most common mechanism of injury resulting in a vertebral body fracture. The point of force in hyperflexion injuries is focused at the middle of the intervertebral disc.[8] The discs in the upper thoracic spine are thinner and, as a result, hyperflexion forces are transferred to the vertebral bodies resulting in a true compression fracture. In the lower thoracic and lumbar spine the intervertebral discs are larger and better shock absorbers. Therefore, hyperflexion injuries are more likely to cause a herniation into the cartilaginous endplate rather than a fracture in these

Table 10.2 Vertebral fracture types and their effects on the spinal column (from Denis F, Armstrong EW, Searls K, et al. Acute thoracolumbar burst fractures in the absence of neurological deficit: A comparison between operative and non-operative treatment. Clin Orthop 1984; 189: 142–149, with permission)

Type	Column		
	Anterior	Middle	Posterior
Compression	Compression	None	None or distraction (severe)
Burst	Compression	Compression	None or splaying of pedicles
Flexion–distraction	None or distraction	Distraction	Distraction
Fracture/dislocation	Compression	Distraction	Distraction
	Rotation	Rotation	Rotation
	Shear	Shear	Shear

areas of the spine.[9] Compression fractures are graded by quarters as greater or lesser than 25, 50, or 75% of normal vertebral height. 50% or greater compression fractures are more likely to produce long-term problems such as delayed instability.[8]

Burst fractures involve the entire vertebral spine including the body, posterior arch, and spinal canal. These types of fractures are due to longitudinal compression without flexion although they may occur with severe hyperflexion injuries without longitudinal compression. Herniation into the endplate may occur, but disc or fracture fragments usually retropulse into the spinal canal. Retropulsed fragments can be associated with neurological injury.[10]

Flexion rotation injuries are relatively rare, but are some of the most unstable of spinal injuries. Most injuries by this mechanism occur at the thoracolumbar junction because of the rapid transition of facet joint orientation. This injury is associated with a high incidence of neurologic injury.[8] The extent of osseous injury will determine treatment. Hyperflexion injuries involve the anterior column (vertebral body) alone and typically are stable. Burst and flexion rotation fractures commonly involve all three spinal columns (vertebral body, posterior arch, spinal canal) and are therefore unstable.

Bracing is an important method for treating vertebral fractures. Anterior vertebral compression fractures are treated in a Jewett extension brace or similar brace (Fig. 10.6). This type of brace prevents further flexion posturing of the spine which aids healing. Immobilization in the brace is continued for 1 to 6 months depending on the degree of injury and pain. Neurologically-intact burst fractures can generally be immobilized with a brace in extension with careful neurologic follow-up. Burst fractures with neurologic compromise or fractures involving all three aspects of the spinal column require surgical stabilization.

Rehabilitation can be instituted while the patient is fitted with a brace as long as the fracture has been deemed stable. With open chain exercises (distal extremity is stationary and able to move through a range of motion) there in no aggravation of back pain. More aggressive therapy begins once the patient becomes pain free. Therapy emphasizes general upper and lower extremity flexibility and strength. Strengthening the abdominals and hip extensor muscles helps maintain trunk stability and posture. These exer-

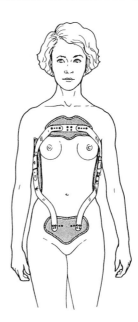

Fig. 10.6 Jewett hyperextension (thoracolumbosacral [TLSO]) orthosis. This type of brace is designed to prevent spinal flexion in a patient with a vertebral compression fracture. (From DeLisa JA, ed. Rehabilitation medicine: Principles and practice. Philadelphia: JB Lippincott; 1988, with permission.)

cises may be done in the brace. Light aerobic activities may be pursued that do not cause excessive axial loading. This prevents a prolonged reconditioning process after coming out of the brace. Non-loading aerobic activities might include cycling, stair climbing, or walking. After a period of brace immobilization the trauma patient may have lost a significant amount of neuromuscular control which will have to be remedied using a variety of muscle re-education techniques.

Nerve blocks to the gray rami communicans nerve, which provides innervation to the vertebral body, can reduce pain from a compression fracture. If a patient has a temporary but significant response to the nerve block(s), radiofrequency lesioning of the nerves can provide longer-term pain relief. This can aid in maximizing rehabilitation efforts over a shorter period of time during the recovery period. This is a procedure that requires further investigation to determine its efficacy for pain control in patients with vertebral compression fractures.

COMPARTMENT SYNDROME

A compartment syndrome is a condition in which increasing intracompartmental pressure surpasses a critical level resulting in decreased circulation, tissue ischemia, and compromised neuromuscular function. This syndrome can develop anywhere in the body where a fascial envelope is noncompliant and cannot accommodate a rise in intracompartmental pressure. This can lead to a complicated pathophysiologic cascade that can result in irreversible tissue necrosis and contracture (Fig. 10.7). Compartment syndromes are classified as either acute or chronic. Acute compartment syndrome (ACS) occurs from progressive and irreversible ischemia which must be treated promptly and aggressively to prevent permanent loss of function. Chronic compartment syndrome (CCS) is secondary to reversible ischemia related to exertional or exercise activities and resolves with rest.

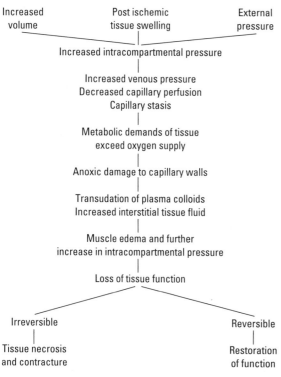

Fig. 10.7 Pathophysiologic events in acute and chronic compartment syndromes. (From Weinik MM, Falco FJE. Acute and chronic compartment syndromes of the lower leg. J Back Musculoskel Rehabil 1992; 2: 17–25, with permission.)

The primary factor in developing compartment syndrome is increased intracompartmental tissue pressure. The increase in pressure may be due to intrinsic or extrinsic causes.[11] Intrinsic causes such as hemorrhage from vascular injury, fracture, or coagulopathies lead to an increase in compartment volume. Postischemic tissue swelling may occur after tissue anoxia associated with surgical procedures that require prolonged tourniquet application after vascular reconstruction. Extrinsic causes lead to a reduction in compartment volume or compliance such as tight bandages, casts, or antishock garments.

The intensity and duration of rehabilitation depend on the severity of the compartment syndrome. When compartment syndrome is diagnosed early and muscle edema is minimal, therapy efforts can begin once hyperemia and swelling resolve. Passive ROM exercises may begin even though fasciotomy wounds are open. Active ROM activites are avoided since they may cause muscle hyperemia and progressive muscle swelling. If there is minimal muscle necrosis, rehabilitation still can be started at a minimal level. When there is excessive myonecrosis or an unstable fracture, however, therapy efforts are delayed which can subsequently lead to the formation of a contracture.

Delayed primary closure or split-thickness skin grafting usually is performed approximately 5 to 10 days postoperatively. The limb should be splinted and elevated if split-thickness skin grafting is performed and all ROM activities should be withheld until assurance of tissue viability. After delayed closure, low-level active exercises may begin as long as there is no stress at the surgical incision site. The exercise intensity can be increased in about 14 to 21 days. Weight-bearing activities are begun as soon as possible, approximately 1 month after surgery.

Contractures and permanent peripheral nerve injury will require a more prolonged duration of treatment. ROM and stretching exercises along with deep heating modalities may be necessary for several months after the injury for treatment of contractures. Ankle–foot orthotics and gait retraining are necessary in those patients who develop permanent neuromuscular injury.

Spinal cord stimulation (SCS) should be considered as a treatment option for patients who develop chronic leg pain from acute or chronic compartment syndrome if all other forms of treatment, including surgery, fail to relieve the pain. Pain coverage is easily accomplished with SCS in these patients since the pain is located in the distal lower extremity.[12]

NERVE ENTRAPMENT SYNDROMES

Entrapment of peripheral nerves by injured myofascial structures is an important source of persistent post-traumatic pain. Nerve entrapments occur at vulnerable points along the course of the nerve because of compromise within a fibrous or osseofibrous tunnel or constriction by a fibrous or muscular band. Other factors may contribute to the development of entrapment neuropathy such as repetitive motion, space-occupying lesions, systemic disorders, body habitus, external pressure, and trauma. Entrapment typically leads to focal nerve demyelination but may progress to axonal loss depending on the severity of the injury. There are many different nerve entrapment syndromes and a complete review is beyond the scope of this chapter. The following is a discussion of a few commonly encountered nerve entrapment syndromes.

Thoracic outlet syndrome (TSO) is a term used to describe pain, paresthesias, and vascular insufficiency from compression of the neurovascular bundle of the upper extremity as it leaves the neck. Compression may result from muscular or bony impingement at several levels along the course of the brachial plexus.

Entrapment in the *scalene triangle* (formed by the anterior scalene muscle, the middle scalene muscle, and the first rib) typically results in paresthesias along the postaxial border of the upper extremity owing to compression of the inferior trunk of the brachial plexus. The presence of a cervical rib with an associated elongated C7 transverse process and fibrous band predisposes to this condition. Adson's maneuver (neck hyperextension while turning the head toward the affected side during deep inspiration) often simultaneously demonstrates a diminution of the radial pulse with reproduction of the patient's pain when the anterior scalene is causative. When pain is reproduced while Adson's maneuver is performed with the head turned to the contralateral side, the middle scalene is implicated.

The *costoclavicular space* is a second site of potential neurovascular compression in the thoracic outlet syndrome. Deep inspiration while thrusting the shoulders inferiorly and posteriorly induces pain when the clavicle compresses the brachial plexus divisions in its descent towards the first rib. The third site of constriction occurs beneath the pectoralis minor muscle. The Allen test (raising the arm to the horizontal during external rotation with the head turned away), the Wright maneuver (elevation of the arm above the head with external rotation), or elevation with hyperabduction all may reproduce characteristic pain as the cords of the brachial plexus are compressed between the pectoralis minor insertion on the coracoid process and the chest wall. The pectoralis minor or hyperabduction syndrome is seen in swimmers as a result of repetitive hyperabduction and muscular hypertrophy.

Rehabilitation efforts at treating TSO involve stretching and ROM exercises of the scalene and pectoralis minor muscles. Patients are educated in proper body mechanics of the upper extremities and to avoid activities that exacerbate symptoms. The arms can be placed on rests when sitting or supported by placing hands on the waist when standing. The shoulders can be adjusted in an abducted and elevated posture with pillows while sleeping. Patients are instructed to avoid repetitive above-shoulder activities and not to carry heavy objects that will depress their shoulders. Neck posturing and positioning can also be helpful in alleviating symptoms. Strengthening of the shoulder girdle muscles can result in increasing the thoracic outlet. Blocking the C8 and T1 nerve roots or the medial cord of the brachial plexus can assist in reducing symptoms and maximizing rehabilitation efforts. Surgical decompression is considered if all conservative means of treatment fail to provide any significant relief of symptoms.

Carpal tunnel syndrome (CTS) is the most common peripheral entrapment neuropathy and results from compression of the median nerve beneath the transverse carpal ligament at the wrist (Fig. 10.8). Repetitive and forceful activities have been singled out as causing carpal tunnel syndrome in industry.[13] Several disorders have been known to lead to carpal tunnel syndrome such as pregnancy, gout, hypothyroidism, ganglion cysts, rheumatoid arthritis, myxedema, and amyloidosis. Several factors that increase the risk for developing carpal tunnel syndrome include gender (women > men), square-shaped wrist, increasing age, and hand dominance. Numbness in the

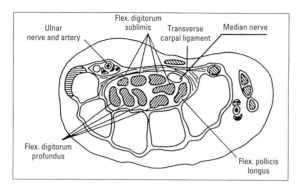

Fig. 10.8 Carpal tunnel. (From Primer on the rheumatic diseases, 9th ed. Atlanta: Arthritis Foundation; 1988, with permission.)

median nerve distribution to the radial three-and-a-half digits with or without thumb weakness are presenting symptoms. Thenar atrophy can occur in advanced cases.

Conservative treatment of CTS includes the use of nonsteroidal anti-inflammatory drugs (NSAIDs), splinting, carpal tunnel injections, light duty, and sometimes complete rest. Myofascial release and tendon stretching are other treatments. Any one of these measures alone or in combination can be effective in treating early CTS. Job modification or ergonomic redesign of the worksite can be helpful in reducing repetitive trauma. Surgery is indicated in cases of advanced CTS with objective sensory loss and/or weakness or atrophy of the abductor pollicis brevis.

The *axillary nerve* is most frequently damaged as a result of anterior shoulder dislocation. It also can be damaged from surgery. Weakness of shoulder abduction may be present on examination as well as decreased sensation over the lateral deltoid. Prognosis is good with partial versus total nerve involvement. Nerve conduction studies and needle electromyogram help to establish the diagnosis and to rule out other possible causes. Treatment consists of rest, NSAIDs, and modified activity. Symptoms and recovery time can be reduced by performing axillary nerve blocks in combination with conservative treatment. Surgical decompression may be required if there is no improvement after 6 to 12 months of conservative care.

Radial nerve entrapment occurs less frequently in comparison to the other upper extremity

nerves. The radial nerve is vulnerable to traumatic injury as it courses through the spinal groove in the arm and it is involved in 10 to 15% of humeral fractures.[14] Compression may occur in the axilla from prolonged pressure such as in the use of crutches. Patients present with wrist and finger extension weakness along with numbness in the first web space of the hand. Compression relief, rest, splinting, and NSAIDs typically result in a successful outcome. Surgical decompression may be considered if there is no improvement with conservative treatment over 2 to 3 months.

Ulnar nerve entrapment at the elbow, *cubital tunnel syndrome*, is the second most common peripheral nerve entrapment of the upper extremity. This condition is seen in individuals with fractures or soft tissue injuries to the elbow region. Heavy lifting, prolonged flexion, and repetitive lifting are predisposing factors to cubital tunnel syndrome. Hand weakness such as an inability to grip or pinch and numbness in the ulnar two-and-a-half digits are common presenting symptoms. Conservative care includes relative rest, NSAIDs, work activity modification, splinting, and elbow pads. Surgery is indicated in patients with significant pain and/or weakness.

Lumbar nerve root entrapment can occur from a disc herniation, vertebral compression fracture, or sacral fracture secondary to trauma. Initial treatment can be conservative if there is no spinal instability or profound neurological deficits. Treatment consists of NSAIDs, muscle relaxants, physical therapy with an emphasis on a muscular stabilization program, epidural injections, and nerve root blocks. Surgery is indicated in cases of spinal instability and considered in those who have failed conservative treatment. Some patients can develop lumbar nerve root entrapment from epidural scarring and fibrosis after surgery for spinal stabilization or disc resection. Conservative care is the first line of treatment. Spinal cord stimulation may be indicated for controlling intractable radicular leg pain in those who have failed conservative treatment.[12] Newer treatment modalities requiring further investigation such as epidural catheters and epiduroscopy may also provide relief of lower extremity radicular pain secondary to epidural fibrosis.

Pelvic trauma with associated fracture or hematoma can lead to *entrapment of the femoral and obturator nerves*. Patients with both types of nerve injuries have pain in the groin area. Femoral neuropathy results in hip flexion weakness, knee extension weakness, decreased patellar reflex, and decreased sensation of the anterior thigh and anterior medial leg. Obturator nerve insults lead to weakness of hip adduction and numbness along the medial thigh and knee. Treatment consists of rest, NSAIDs, restriction of hip extension (femoral nerve entrapments) or abduction/external rotation (obturator nerve entrapments), and nerve blocks. Surgical decompression is sometimes necessary to alleviate symptoms that do not respond to conservative care.

Peroneal nerve entrapments occur most commonly at the fibular head where the nerve travels near the lateral side of the knee. The most common mechanism of injury is acute compression, traction, or laceration at the fibular head. Other possible causes of neuropathy include bed positioning, squatting, casting, and tight boots. The nerve can also be injured during pelvic surgery or total hip arthroplasties. Foot numbness along the dorsum of the foot and dorsiflexion ankle weakness (foot drop) can be presenting symptoms. Foot drop can interfere with ambulation and climbing stairs. The mainstay of conservative treatment consists of NSAIDs, local nerve blocks, corrective shoes to maintain an eversion posture, and an ankle–foot orthosis for foot drop. Surgical release of the peroneal nerve may be indicated if there is no improvement with conservative care.

MYOFASCIAL PAIN

Perhaps the most common persistent pain following trauma is that emanating from myofascial structures (i.e. muscle, bone, tendon, ligament, and other soft tissues). Nonmuscular structures such as tendons, ligaments, and fasciae are common sources of musculoskeletal pain. Thoracic fasciitis following thoracotomy, bursitis, tenosynovitis, and ligamentous strains are a few examples of painful, soft tissue conditions. Other musculoskeletal conditions such as temporomandibular syndrome and whiplash injury result from injury to multiple tissue structures.

Myofascial pain dysfunction is characterized by specific changes within affected muscles. Following trauma, discrete regions within a muscle may develop lesions called *trigger points*. These trigger points clinically appear as palpable taut bands of muscle that elicit tenderness when stimulated by direct pressure, and depending on the severity of the stimulus, elicit referred pain.[15] These regions of muscle present a limitation to active and passive motion with apparent shortening and weakening of the involved musculature. Pain from deep somatic structures is typically dull and diffuse. The ability to localize precise trigger areas decreases with increasing tissue depth. Diffusion and radiation can be indicators of severity, with muscle spasm and tenderness in *zones of reference* (as distinguished from trigger points) often appearing at sites distant from the lesion.

Clinically, objective quantification of trigger points can be accomplished with thermography or measurement using pressure algometry or tissue compliance meters. Electromyography, however, frequently demonstrates electrical silence within the trigger points. Clearly, these regions are not the result of a simple muscle spasm but possibly an inflammatory process within the fascia resulting from mechanical damage to the muscle as the source of pain.

The musculotendinous unit can become injured from overuse, as it is under the greatest strain during muscular contraction. The tendon adapts more slowly than the muscle, and, therefore, is susceptible to aseptic inflammatory changes. Inflammation at the tendon–muscle junction is termed *myotendinitis*, whereas *paratendinitis* or *peritendinitis* refers to inflammation of the tendon sheath. *Enthesitis* refers to osteotendinitis, or reactive changes at the bony insertion. Chemotactic influences of the inflammatory mediators released produce an exudative infiltration that, if prolonged, may result in metaplastic changes leaving calcific deposit within the musculotendinous unit.

The response to connective tissue injury has been divided into stages. The first stage in the healing process is the inflammatory response. This phase typically extends through the first 2 days, during which time chemotactic mechanisms induce cell mobilization and infiltration. The second stage lasts from the third day through the fifth and is characterized by ground substance proliferation in preparation for collagen deposition. Collagen formation begins in the third proliferative phase, lasting through the second week following injury. The final stage is the formative stage, occurring from 14 days onward when the cross-linking of collagen organizes into functional fibrils in the healed tissue.

The timing of therapeutic intervention can affect the quality of the reparative process. The mainstay of conservative treatment includes the use of NSAIDs, stretching, soft tissue and joint mobilization, and manual posturing techniques. Stretching and mobilization in combination with a topical coolant spray to the affected area(s) are sometimes more beneficial than either therapy alone. Local injections with an anesthetic or dry needling of trigger points can reduce pain and enhance rehabilitation when combined with physical therapy. Botulinum toxin type A (BTXA) injections, which have been used successfully in treating blepharospasm and focal dystonias, are being used to treat myofascial pain with mixed results.[16,17] Radiofrequency is another promising modality for treating localized cervical and lumbar myofascial pain in patients who have had diagnostic and temporary relief from facet joint nerve blocks.[18,19] Additional investigation of BTXA and radiofrequency is necessary in order to further define their role in treating myofascial pain syndromes.

REFERENCES

1. Gersten JW. Effect of ultrasound on tendon extensibility. Am J Phys Med 1955; 34: 360–362.
2. Bentham JS, Brereton WDS, Eng P, et al. Continuous passive motion device for hand rehabilitation. Arch Phys Med Rehab 1987; 68: 248–250.
3. Michaelis LS. Spasticity in spinal cord injuries. In: Vinken PJ, Bruyn GW, eds. Handbook of clinical neurology, injuries of the spine and cord. New York: Elsevier; 1976: vol 26.
4. Twitchell T. The restoration of motor function following hemiplegia in man. Brain 1951; 74: 443–480.
5. Plum F, Posner JB. The diagnosis of stupor and coma. 3rd ed. Philadelphia: FA Davis; 1982.
6. Daniel RK, Hall EJ, MacLeod M. Pressure sores: a reappraisal. Ann Plastic Surg 1979; 1: 53–63.
7. Pinel C. Pressure sores. Nurs Times 1976; 2: 172–174.
8. Denis F. The three column spine and its significance on classification of acute thoracolumbar spine injuries. Spine 1983; 8: 817–831.
9. Berquist H, Gehweiler JA, Osborne RL, Becker RF. The radiology of vertebral trauma. Philadelphia: WB Saunders; 1980.
10. White AA III, Panjabi M. Clinical biomechanics of the spine. 2nd ed. Philadelphia: JB Lippincott; 1990.
11. Willis RB, Rorabeck CH. Treatment of compartment syndrome in children. Orthop Clin North Am 1990; 21: 401–412.
12. Ohnmeiss DD, Rashbaum RF, Bogdanffy GM. Prospective outcome evaluation of spinal cord stimulation in patients with intractable leg pain. Spine 1996; 21: 1344–1351.
13. Occupational disease surveillance: Carpal tunnel syndrome. Centers for Disease Control. JAMA 1989; 262: 88.
14. Parker JW, Foster RR, Garcia A, et al. The humeral fracture with radial nerve palsy: Is exploration warranted? Clinical Orthop 1972; 88: 34–38.
15. Travell JG, Simons DG. Myofascial pain and dysfunction–The trigger point manual. Baltimore: Williams & Wilkins; 1983.
16. Cheshire WP, Abashjan SW, Mann JD. Botulinum toxin in the treatment of myofascial pain syndrome. Pain 1994; 59: 65–69.
17. Wheeler AH, Goolkasian P, Gretz SS. A randomized, double-blind, prospective pilot study of botulinum toxin injection for refractory unilateral, cervicothoracic, paraspinal, myofascial pain syndrome. Spine 1998; 23: 1662–1667.
18. Lord SM, Barnsley L, Wallis BJ, et al. Percutaneous radio-frequency neurotomy for chronic cervical zygopophyseal-joint pain. NEJM 1996; 335: 1721–1739.
19. North RB, Han M, Zahurak M, et al. Radiofrequency lumbar facet denervation analysis of prognostic factors. Pain 1994; 57: 77–83.

PERIOPERATIVE PAIN MANAGEMENT IN TRAUMA: TECHNIQUES AND APPLICATIONS

11

Patient-controlled analgesia

Andrew D Rosenberg, Burdett R Porter and Joel F Lupatkin

Introduction

The patient-controlled analgesia paradigm
  Advantages and disadvantages

Terminology
  Bolus or loading dose
  Demand dose
  Lockout or dosage interval
  Basal infusion rate
  Total hourly dose

Patient selection criteria
  Age/autonomy
  Mental acuity
  Social history
  Allergy/contraindications

The technology

Starting patient-controlled analgesia

The ideal patient-controlled analgesia medication

Side effects of patient-controlled analgesia
  Respiratory depression and hypoxia
  Nausea and vomiting
  Confusion
  Urinary retention

Patient-controlled analgesia in the trauma setting

Conclusion

INTRODUCTION

Obtaining adequate postoperative pain relief has been a problem facing physicians, nurses and patients for many years. In general, lack of perioperative pain control is a complaint that occurs too frequently. A number of reasons exist to explain this phenomenon. These include inadequate dosing schedules, a lack of understanding of the best management modality for a given condition, a misunderstanding of the pharmacology of prescribed medications, delay from the onset of pain until the injected dose reaches adequate plasma levels, and concern that overmedication will result in significant complications.[1-4]

Patients are undermedicated in hospital settings. This is true at the physician, nurse, and patient level. Physicians tend to underprescribe pain medications utilizing standard intramuscular (IM) doses at fixed intervals often without considering variables such as age, type of surgery, concurrent medical problems, or prior history of drug use. Nurses also tend to undermedicate. When faced with medication options, nursing personnel frequently choose a lower dose leaving patients with inadequate pain relief. Finally, patients tend to underutilize the available pain medications sometimes fearing addiction or believing that pain is a necessary byproduct of their surgical experience.[1-3] Inadequate pain relief is a frequent experience in the postoperative period but it also occurs early during hospitalization. For example, in a study in Costa Rica only 11% of adults and 4% of children received pain medication in the emergency department (ER) and 25% of children and 50% of adults left the ER with no decrease in pain scores.[5]

Significant postoperative pain can prolong hospital stay, increase morbidity and mortality, and prevent adequate rehabilitation. Although traditional IM injections satisfy some clinical situations they fall short of providing adequate pain relief in far too many circumstances.

New modalities exist to provide pain relief. One such method is via patient-controlled analgesia (PCA). It is now recognized that allowing patients to receive pain medications 'on demand' or at their will provides more effective pain relief. By establishing acceptable parameters, physicians empower patients to obtain pain relief at their own discretion. In addition to obtaining pain medication as desired, the patient gains psychologically from being 'in control'. While conventional on-demand or patient-controlled analgesia is typically thought of as intravenously-(IV-) administered PCA, any potential entry point for pain medication in which the patient is empowered to control his own medication dose be it (IM) intravenous, subcutaneous, epidural, etc. can be termed as PCA.[1–4,6] In fact, Hocking & deMello recommend IM-PCA (self or buddy–buddy) injections as a basic approach to providing battlefield analgesia. Morphine 10 mg can be self-administered every 2 hours to obtain relief (Fig. 11.1).[7]

While the concepts and actual practice of IV-PCA are not difficult to understand or implement it is important to be aware of the potential pitfalls of administering pain medications at the discretion of the patient who is receiving them. This chapter will outline the general concepts of IV-PCA, how to initiate it for a patient, and methods for assessing treatment, adjusting doses, and treating problems that arise with its use. The emphasis in this chapter is IV-PCA. Epidural PCA is covered in Chapter 13.

THE PCA PARADIGM

The disadvantage of IM injections is that they are associated with varying opioid plasma levels.[1,2] As plasma levels vary from low to high concentrations and then decrease again, they result in a recurring cycle of pain, analgesia, and sedation and then the return of pain. The peaks and valleys of pain relief reflect the serum concentration of the administered analgesic and the prescribed dosing interval. Ferrante described this phenomenon pictorially (Fig. 11.2).[1,8] The sequence occurs as follows:

1. Pain occurs at serum concentrations below minimal analgesic concentrations. At this point the patient requests pain medication. As the serum drug concentration increases after IM pain medication is administered, the patient will reach the minimal analgesic concentration necessary to obtain pain relief.
2. The patient then enters an analgesic zone in which they are awake but relatively pain-free. However, since large doses of opioids are administered into the intramuscular depot at fixed intervals, the opioid plasma concentration continues to increase passing through the ideal analgesic range often sedating the

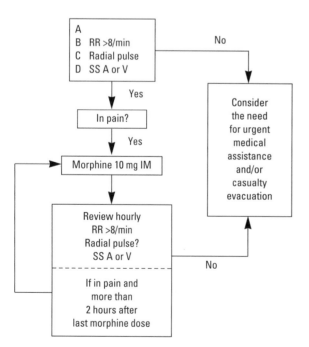

Fig. 11.1 Basic approach to battlefield analgesia. RR, respiratory rate; SS, secondary survey; A, alert; V, verbally responsive. (From Hocking & deMello,[7] with permission.)

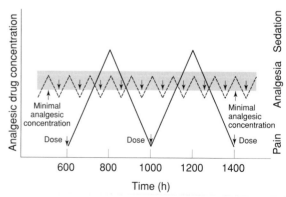

Fig. 11.2 PCA paradigm demonstrating the relationship of plasma opioid concentration to degree of analgesia. (From Ferrante et al,[8] with permission.)

patient, in addition to providing adequate pain relief. While the sedation stage is often viewed as salutary since the patient is 'finally resting comfortably', it is often accompanied by inadequate respiratory efforts and inability to continue proper rehabilitation and ambulation.

3. The pain medication then 'wears off' and the patient once again is in pain.

In contrast to the large doses administered with individual IM injections, with its associated peaks and valleys of sedation and pain relief, PCA allows the patient to receive small predetermined doses at fixed intervals in order to obtain the desired level of pain relief and remain in an analgesic zone without causing sedation.[1,8]

The approach of administering small IV doses in order to obtain pain relief and keep the patient in the analgesic zone was initiated by researchers such as Sechzer and others.[9,10] Medications were administered at the patient's request. If pain occurred as a result of the plasma concentration falling below the minimal analgesic concentration; or, if a situation that would result in pain, such as a dressing change, log rolling, or intense physical therapy were to occur, the patient could request pain relief. Nurses then provided smaller than the usual IM injections doses via the IV route. Sechzer was able to demonstrate improved pain relief in the patient population treated in this fashion. By utilizing small IV doses of opioids at shorter time intervals, patient satisfaction was increased and the chances of oversedation decreased.

The advent of technology that could replace the nurse and administer a prescribed dose intravenously at fixed desired intervals has provided a shortcut in obtaining adequate pain relief. This can be understood by comparing the multiple steps necessary for a given patient to obtain their IM doses of medication compared with obtaining a dose of IV-PCA medication (Fig. 11.3).

IV-PCA provides pain relief to the patient when the patient activates a button that signals that the patient is demanding a dose of medication. The administration system can be programmed so that the patient receives: (a) a dose only upon demand, (b) a background infusion rate without the patient's request, or (c) a combination of a demand dose and a background infusion can be ordered. The use of PCA is intended to give the patient personal control over pain relief, deliver a defined dose of pain medication at a fixed minimal lockout inter-

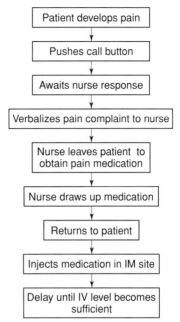

Fig. 11.3   Traditional method of IM injection.

val prescribed by the physician, and permit the patient to vary the amount received based upon the current level of pain.[1,2,8]

For a PCA program to be successful, it is important that physicians, nurses, and patients be adequately educated about the technique, that enough automated pump systems be available to provide pain relief to all who desire PCA, and sufficient staff be present to modify the dosing schedule should such modifications become necessary.

Advantages and disadvantages

There are numerous advantageous and potential disadvantages from the use of PCA and these are shown in Table 11.1.

Table 11.1   Potential advantages and disadvantages of PCA

Advantages	Potential disadvantages
Rapid pain relief	Machine cost
Patient in control	IV must be in place
Avoids excess drowsiness	Nausea and vomiting
No IM injections necessary	Respiratory depression
Physician still prescribes dose schedule	Drowsiness
Relieves nursing staff of excess work	Confusion
	Patient must understand technology
	Potential machine failure

TERMINOLOGY

It is important that those utilizing PCA be familiar with the terminology.

Bolus or loading dose

Definition

This is the dose that is administered at the start of PCA to provide rapid relief.[1–3]

Comment. It is intended to provide a dose sufficient enough to rapidly achieve analgesia. For example, in a 70 kg male in pain after major surgery 1–3 mg morphine may be considered an appropriate loading dose. If insufficient, another dose can be administered in 5 minutes until pain relief is obtained. Bolus-dosing rapidly increases the plasma opioid concentration into the analgesia zone. Remember that the patient who has just completed surgery may still have significant residual plasma concentration of narcotics and sedatives and thus be 'sensitive' to additionally administered opioids.

Demand dose

Definition

The dose the patient receives when the button is pressed for pain relief.[1–3]

Comment. This is programmed by the physician and is usually 0.5–1 mg morphine. If demand doses are inadequate they can be increased, but first make certain the patient is using the PCA activation button properly. The patient's history and narcotic 'sensitivities' should be considered prior to determining the demand dose. In general the demand dose is lower in geriatric patients than in patients in the 20 to 60 year age range.

Lockout or dosage interval

Definition

The lockout or dosage interval is the time during which a patient is unable to receive a demand dose even if the demand button is pushed.

Comment. The purpose of the lockout or dosage interval is to provide a time period during which

the patient can begin to feel the effects of the administered dose without allowing the patient to overdose himself. The time interval should not be too long so the patient avoids suffering while waiting for the next dose. Lockout intervals for morphine vary from 5 to 15 minutes depending on the patient. In general, when smaller demand doses are administered, a shorter lockout interval can be employed. If the patient complains of inadequate pain relief it is often worthwhile to determine the number of attempts for pain relief, not just the total dose of medication received and then adjust the lockout accordingly. (This data is available from the PCA apparatus or from the nursing flow sheet.) It is not uncommon to note that the patient complaining of inadequate pain relief made only three to four attempts for pain medication in an hour when they could have potentially received much more medication. The patient needs to be properly educated to push the button at specific intervals in order to actually receive medication. Conversely, someone who is constantly pushing the PCA button and is legitimately not obtaining adequate relief will need to have the demand dose increased or lockout decreased.

Basal infusion rate

Definition

This is the dosage of medication that is administered to the patient during the course of an hour, whether or not the patient pushes the demand button.[1–3]

Comment. By administering a basal infusion rate it is hoped that the concentration of the pain medication will remain in the analgesic range. The goal of a basal infusion rate is to maintain patient comfort, even allowing the patient to sleep and not awaken just to push the PCA button for more pain relief. Typically when basal infusion rates are used with morphine as the PCA medication, they are prescribed at 1 mg/h. Remember that with a basal rate of 1 mg/h morphine, the patient will receive 24 mg of morphine per day even if the demand button is not pushed. This total dose per day is increased to 48 mg if the basal rate is increased to 2 mg/h. (Be careful!) The literature does not provide evidence that basal rates improve pain control, but in fact they may be associated with episodes of respiratory depression (see side effects).[11,12] Parker et al found that basal infusions did not improve analgesia but did increase the risk of hypoxia.[11] McNeely & Trentadue evaluated the effectiveness of night-time PCA morphine in 36 school age children who underwent elective lower extremity surgery.[12] Compared to the PCA-only group the PCA-plus-basal-infusion group had equal visual analogue pain scores and sedation scores, but significantly more time was spent with the $SpO_2 \leq 90\%$ in patients who had basal infusions[12] (see Fig. 11.4). In a study of 6000 patients who received IV-PCA in New Zealand the use of a background PCA opioid infusion was also associated with a significantly higher complication rate.[13,14] However, there are physicians who believe that patients have improved analgesia with the use of a basal infusion.

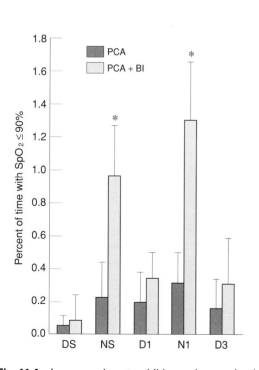

Fig. 11.4 In comparison to children who received just PCA, those who received PCA and a basal infusion (PCA + BI) spent more time with oxygen saturations <90%. DS, day of surgery; NS, night of surgery; D1, day of postoperative day (POD) 1; N1, night of POD1; D2, day of POD2. (From McNeely & Trentadue,[12] with permission.)

Total hourly dose
Definition

The total dose of medication the patient can possibly receive each hour – combination of total demand dose possible (consider lockout) and basal infusion rate.[13,14]

Comment. When administrating PCA it is important to know the total dose the patient can receive each hour. This is calculated by adding the basal infusion rate to the total number of demand doses possible.

Example. If the basal infusion rate of morphine is 1 mg/h and the patient is allowed 1 mg demand doses with a lockout of 6 minutes, then the total hourly dose is 11 mg of morphine.

PATIENT SELECTION CRITERIA

Age/autonomy

Patients must be old enough to understand how to operate a PCA pump. While some institutions use minimal age criteria of 10 to 12 years, others employ PCA in children as young as 5 years of age when there is a 'rooming-in' parent.[15] It is crucial that the patient presses the PCA button, and *not* a concerned 'guardian' trying to administer adequate sedation. This can result in overdose and respiratory arrest. In general, children who can play complicated video games can understand the concepts involved in PCA. On occasion with proper training nurse or parent PCA can be utilized.

Mental acuity

Patients must be mentally alert, not have suffered recent head trauma, and be able to comprehend and comply with the instructions for use of the pump.

Social history

While some consider narcotic abuse history a contraindication it is used by others in this situation. There is a level of complexity added in these patients since dosing is often inadequate and supplemental medications are often required.

Allergy/contraindications

Allergy to morphine is a contraindication to using it for PCA.

THE TECHNOLOGY

PCA devices may incorporate a syringe pump with a motor to drive the plunger of the syringe, or may have a modified peristaltic pump that draws solution from a supply cassette or infusion bag. The pumps deliver a bolus of analgesia when a push button is activated by the patient (Fig. 11.5). This button can be mounted on the pump, or on a cable for remote operations. Electronic units use a microprocessor to coordinate controls and alarms. The infusion pumps can operate using a PCA-only mode or a basal-infusion-only mode or basal-infusion-plus-PCA mode. PCA devices can be designed for mounting on IV poles or ambulatory use or both (see Useful addresses). Many PCA devices have a lock syringe or cassette compartment to secure controlled substances. The parameters for bolus, lockout, basal rate, and demand dose can be programmed. Anti-reflux valves are recommended for connection to a carrier IV solution. Most infusion pumps can display a history recording the number of attempts made, number of actual injections received, basal rate, and total volume of dose infused. Alarms can signal occlusion or tampering with the device.

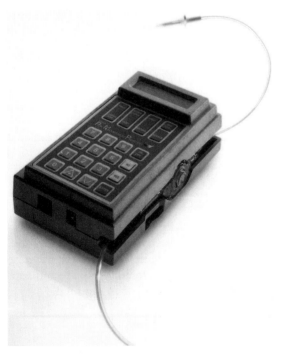

Fig. 11.5 PCA pump.

STARTING PATIENT-CONTROLLED ANALGESIA

PCA can be employed before or after surgery. When starting PCA first determine if a bolus is required. Bolus dose is based on the level of pain, age, weight, and physiologic factors. While initial doses are frequently 1–3 mg this should be modified based on foregoing matters. The basal infusion rate is either avoided or ordered at 1 mg/h. A demand dose of 0.5–1.0 mg is ordered with an appropriate lockout of 6 to 10 minutes. If pain relief is inadequate the lockout can be decreased slightly or the demand dose increased.

A PCA Order Sheet is completed when initiating PCA[3]: orders must be entered for bolus dose, basal infusion dose, PCA or demand dose, lockout interval, and 1-hour limit. Vital signs are ordered to ensure that the patient is observed carefully and medications are prescribed to treat potential side effects or complications (e.g. naloxone for respiratory depression, compazine for nausea and vomiting, and diphenhydramine for itching). Two examples of PCA order sheets from different institutions have been included to provide the reader with some notion of the necessary components of PCA administration (Figs 11.6A, B).

An excellent method of adequately assessing PCA effectiveness is accomplished by talking with the patient and reviewing a PCA Flow Sheet completed by the nursing staff[3] (Fig. 11.7). The flow sheet lists the basic ordered PCA parameters, e.g. dose, basal rate, 1-hour limit, the amount of medication received, the total number of injections received, and the total number of attempts made. Comparing the total number of attempts with the number of injections is important since a patient in severe pain who is using the activation button properly will demonstrate multiple attempts and approach maximal prescribed dosing, whereas someone who is complaining of pain but has made minimal attempts to receive pain medication may instead need proper education so they push the PCA button more often. Vital signs can also be recorded on the Flow Sheet as can level of pain, level of consciousness, and level of anxiety.

THE IDEAL PATIENT-CONTROLLED ANALGESIA

Since the goal of PCA is to obtain quick relief with small intermittent doses the ideal analgesic would

---

Patient-Controlled Analgesia (IV-PCA) Order

1. Give no other analgesic/sedative while patient on PCA
2. Meds: Morphine 1 mg/mL
3. Mode: PCA with basal rate
   a. Bolus dose: _____ mg (loading dose)
   b. PCA dose: _____ mg/injection
   c. Delay interval: _____ min (lock-out interval)
   d. Basal rate: _____ mg/hr (continuous rate)
   e. 1-hour limit: _____ mg
4. Tylenol: 2 325 mg tablets q4h PRN for the duration of treatment. If unable to take PO, give Tylenol 650 mg suppository per rectum
5. Narcan 0.4 mg available on unit for Rx side effects.
6. For nausea and vomiting, given Compazine 25 mg suppository per rectum or Compazine 10 mg IM
7. Call MD if patient is difficult to arouse, is confused, or if respiratory rate is <10 breaths/min.
8. Monitor vital signs (blood pressure, pulse, respiratory rate) and assess level of pain, level of consciousness, and level of anxiety q15min the 1st hr, q1h for 4hr, then q2h for 4 hr, and then q4h while patient is on PCA
9. Continuous IV LR 50 mL/hr infusion (unless otherwise specified) for the duration of treatment
10. PCA may run in an IV line containing blood, Kefzol, vancomycin, or dextran
11. Discontinue PCA at patient's or orthopedist's request, maximum 72 hr

Fig. 11.6A PCA order sheet from the Hospital for Joint Diseases Orthopedic Institute, New York City, NY. LR, lactated Ringer's solution.

---

1. DRUG: (   ) Morphine sulfate 1 mg/mL
            (   ) Hydromorphone 0.2 mg/mL
            (   ) Other

2. PCA Dose (circle):   OFF   0.2 mL   0.5 mL   0.7 mL
   1 mL   1.5 mL   2 mL   2.5 mL   3 mL   4 mL   5 mL   6 mL

3. Delay/Lockout Interval (circle)
   3 min   5 min   6 min   8 min   10 min   12 min
   15 min   20 min   25 min   30 min   45 min   60 min

4. Basal/Continuous Rate (circle):
   None(OFF)   0.5 mL/hr   1 mL/hr   1.5 mL/hr
   2 mL/hr   2.5 mL/hr   3 mL/hr   4 mL/hr
   5 mL/hr   7 mL/hr   8 mL/hr   9.9 mL/hr
   (   ) Use basal rate only during sleeping
         hours, i.e., only from 2200 to 0600

5. 1-Hour Limit Not to Exceed (circle):
   1 mL   3 mL   5 mL   8 mL   10 mL
   15 mL   20 mL   25 mL   30 mL

No IM, IV, or PO opioids, sedatives, CNS depressants to be given.

Monitoring and documentation: PCA settings, respiratory rate (RR), blood pressure, pulse, pain rating, sedation rating – Q 2 HRS for 8 HRS, then Q 4 HRS while patient is on PCA. Record hourly injections and attempts for duration of PCA. Documentation on Patient-Controlled Analgesia Flowsheet.

Naloxone (Narcan) 0.4 mg at bedside.

Notify Responsible Service for:

A. Ramsey Sedation Score > 2.
B. Respiratory rate of 10 or less.
C. Inadequate level of analgesia.

Management of side effects:

A. Naloxone – 0.1 mg IV for respiratory rate < 8.

B. Nausea/Vomiting

   Yes _____ No _____ Droperidol (Inapsine) 0.5 mg in 50cc 0.9 NaCl IVPB over 20 min Q6 HRS PRN X 2 doses.
   Yes _____ No _____ Metaclopramide (Regian) 10 mg in 50cc 0.9 NaCl over 20 min IVPB Q6 HRS PRN.
   Yes _____ No _____ Promethazine (Phenergan) 25 mg IM Q4-6 HRS PRN.
   Yes _____ No _____ Ondansetron 4 mg IV over 20 min Q6 HRS PRN, may repeat X 1

C. Pruritus: Diphenhydramine (Benadryl) 25 mg in 50 cc 0.9 NaCl over 20 min IVPB Q6 HRS PRN.

D. Urinary Retention: In and out bladder catheter PRN X 2. If second catheterization required notify Responsible Service.

E. Insomnia

   Yes _____ No _____ Triazolam (Halcion) 0.125 mg Q HS PRN. May repeat X 1.

Fig. 11.6B PCA order sheet from the University of Iowa.

PATIENT-CONTROLLED ANALGESIA FLOW SHEET

PCA Dose: _____

Basal Rate: _____

1-Hour Limit: _____

Level of Pain
1 = None
2 = Slight
3 = Tolerable
4 = Moderate
5 = Severe

Level of Consciousness (LOC)
1 = Awake/Alert
2 = Awakes w/ Stimulus
3 = Disoriented
4 = Sleeping
5 = Stupor

Level of Anxiety (LOA)
1 = Calm/Relaxed
2 = Mild Anxiety
3 = Moderate Anxiety
4 = Restless
5 = Agitated

| DATE | TIME | PCA DOSE INTERVAL | TOTAL MG DELIVERED | TOTAL # INJECTIONS | TOTAL # ATTEMPTS | VITAL SIGNS | | | ASSESSMENT | | | COMMENTS | INITIAL |
						RESP. RATE	PULSE	BP	PAIN RATING	LOC 1–5	LOA 1–5		

Fig. 11.7 PCA flow sheet from Hospital for Joint Diseases Orthopedic Institute.

have a rapid onset, be highly efficacious in providing pain relief, have an intermittent duration of action to improve control, not produce tolerance or dependence, and not have side effects or produce adverse drug interactions.[16] Table 11.2 provides a listing of agents which are currently being used for PCA, although morphine remains the mainstay. Table 11.3 lists the ordering range for PCA morphine and hydromorphone at the University of Iowa.

SIDE EFFECTS OF PATIENT-CONTROLLED ANALGESIA

Side effects such as hypoxia, respiratory depression, nausea, vomiting, sedation, and pruritus can occur with PCA.[1-4] As mentioned, basal infusion rates are associated with a higher incidence of complications. The incidence of complications decreases during the time period patients are on PCA[13] (Table 11.4).

Table 11.2   Guidelines for Opioid Administration via IV-PCA*

Drug (concentration)	Demand dose	Lockout interval (min)
Morphine (1 mg/mL)	0.5–3.0 mg	5–12
Meperidine (10 mg/mL)	5–30 mg	5–12
Fentanyl (10 microg/mL)	10–20 microg	5–10
Hydromorphone (0.2 mg/mL)	0.1–0.5 mg	5–10
Oxymorphone (0.25 mg/mL)	0.2–0.4 mg	8–10
Methadone (1 mg/mL)	0.5–2.5 mg	8–20
Nalbuphine (1 mg/mL)	1–5 mg	5–10

*Analgesic requirements vary widely among patients. Adjustment of dosage because of age, severe disease, or the idiosyncracies of individual drug handling is always necessary.
(Reproduced from Ferrante, with permission.[1])

Table 11.3   Dosage guidelines utilized at the University of Iowa

Dosing guidelines	Morphine sulfate 1 mg/mL	Hydromorphone HCl 0.2 mg/mL
Adults		
PCA dose	0.5–1.5 mg	0.1–0.3 mg
Lockout time	6–15 minutes	6–15 minutes
Basal (continuous) rate	None, or 1–2 mg/h	None, or 0.1–0.2 mg/h
1-hour limit	3 to 5 mg/h	0.6 to 1 mg/h
Pediatrics		
PCA dose	0.01–0.03 mg/kg	0.0015–0.0045 mg/kg
Lockout time	10–15 minutes	10–15 minutes
Basal (continuous) rate	None, or 0.01–0.03 mg/kg/h	None, or 0.0015–0.0045 mg/kg/h
1-hour limit	0.04–0.06 mg/kg/h	0.006–0.009 mg/kg/h

Table 11.4   Incidence of adverse side effects on the first 3 postoperative days

	Day 1 (N = 300)	Day 2 (N = 255)	Day 3 (N = 179)
Oximetry			
Hypoxemia (SpO_2 < 89%)	11 (3.6%)	6 (2.3%)	3 (1.6%)
Severe hypoxemia (SpO_2 <85%)	1 (0.3%)	3 (1.2%)	nil
Nausea	84 (28%)	43 (16.9%)*	14 (7.8%)*
Sedation	84 (28%)	28 (10.9%)*	10 (5.5%)*
Respiratory depression	6 (2%)	nil	nil
Other			
Pruritus	1 (0.3%)	nil	nil

*Indicates $P < 0.05$ compared with day 1 result.
From Sidebotham & Dijkhuizen.[13]

Respiratory depression and hypoxia

The major concern about the use of IV narcotics is their propensity to cause respiratory depression. While this can definitely occur, one of the 'built-in' safety mechanisms with IV-PCA is that the patient will become sedated and then not push the demand button prior to reaching the serum opioid level sufficient to cause respiratory depression or arrest. This 'safety feature' may be lost when a basal infusion rate is ordered.[14] (Fig. 11.8).

Although it might not be the best method to determine the onset of respiratory depression, the respiratory rate is frequently followed as an indication of sedation and effects of opioids on the respiratory system. In the New Zealand study referred to earlier, 6% of patients developed hypoxia and 2% developed respiratory depression while on PCA.[13] There were three risk factors present in these patients: (a) the demand dose was greater than 1 mg, (b) the patient's age was over 65 years, or (c) the patient underwent intra-abdominal surgery.[13] Other studies have provided additional reasons for respiratory depression, including relatives using PCA on the patient while the patient is asleep, unrecognized co-morbidity in the patient, flushing of the IV line with already present morphine in the IV line, basal infusion rates, machine failure, or programming errors.[1–4, 11–14] Naloxone should be readily available to treat respiratory depression, and standing orders to address this complication should be included in the PCA Order Sheet.

Nausea and vomiting

Stimulation of the chemoreceptor trigger zone is known to initiate nausea and vomiting in patients who have been administered opioids. This is exacerbated by motion. Nausea and vomiting are fairly patient-specific, and incidence increases in patients with a propensity toward motion sickness, women under 60 years of age, pediatric patients, obese patients, and after specific surgical procedures (e.g. head and neck, gynecological surgery).[4,17]

Anti-emetic medications should be prescribed as standing orders on the PCA Order Sheet so patients can receive rapid relief if necessary.

Confusion

Confusion, especially among the elderly, can occur with patients receiving PCA.[4] If confusion occurs it might be advisable to choose other methods for obtaining pain relief such as regional anesthesia or changing the medication used.

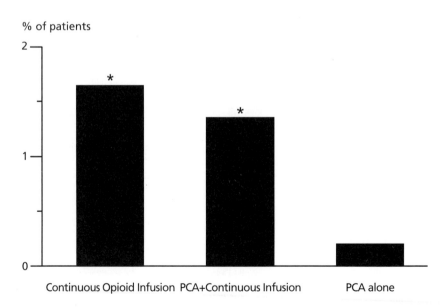

Fig. 11.8 Distribution of incidence of respiratory depression over techniques of opioid administration (*$P < 0.05$ versus PCA alone).

Urinary retention

As with any narcotic administration, and although seen more frequently with epidural and spinal narcotics, PCA morphine can produce urinary retention.

PATIENT-CONTROLLED ANALGESIA IN THE TRAUMA SETTING

Use of PCA in battlefield conditions has already been briefly mentioned. Other uses in trauma patients include routine postoperative care and for multiple dressing changes. One medication utilized for multiple dressing changes is alfentanil. Tarantino, Baker & Bower described use of PCA alfentanil at the R. Adams Cowley Shock Trauma Center.[18] 31 patients who required multiple dressing changes per day were placed on a PCA protocol (Table 11.5). After an initial dressing change with an anesthesia care provider, who titrated the alfentanil until the dressing change could be tolerated, alfentanil was subsequently administered on demand for dressing changes. The lockout interval was very long so the patient could not obtain multiple doses. In the 31 patients there were no incidents of respiratory depression, hypotension, bradycardia, or excess sedation.[18]

Table 11.5 PCA protocol for use of alfentanil during multiple dressing changes

---

Analgesia for initial dressing change by anesthesia care provider via stepwise titration to determine dose for infusion
Initial dressing changes in intensive care unit (ICU) or postanesthesia care unit–subsequent dressing changes *do not* require ICU setting
Alfentanil infusion prepared by pharmacy at 100 microg/cc concentration
Infusion delivered via Abbott 5500™ PCA: lockout set for interval between dressing changes
Baseline assessment documented by nursing and every 15 min for 1 h after dressing change
  Blood pressure, pulse, respiratory rate
  Cardiac rhythm
  Sao_2
  Level of alertness
Continuous monitoring of level of alertness and Sao_2 during dressing changes
O_2 delivered via face mask or nasal cannula
Resuscitative capabilities readily available

From Tarantino, Baker & Bower.[18]

IV-PCA has been utilized in the intensive care unit in both ventilated and non-intubated patients.[16]

Another medication utilized for PCA is tramadol.[19] Tramadol is used in Europe for IV-PCA pain relief. It is a centrally acting, weak, opioid analgesic which is equipotent to meperidine and has one-tenth the potency of morphine.[19] Tramadol is effective in both IM and IV formulations. Only rare episodes of respiratory depression occur when compared to morphine and meperidine.[19] It was very effective as a PCA medication in an evaluation by Lehmann.[19]

CONCLUSION

PCA is an effective method of obtaining pain relief both prior to and following surgery. The patient is empowered to help treat and control the pain being experienced. By following the basic orders, observing the patient, and evaluating the pain scores many patients have received excellent pain relief using this method.

Useful addresses-PCA pump manufacturers

Abbott Laboratories Hospital Products Division North Chicago, IL 60064 1-800-222-6883

Baxter Healthcare Corporation IV Systems Division Route 120 & Wilson Road Round Lake, IL 60073 1-800-933-0303

Deltec SIMS Deltec, Inc. St Paul, MN 55112 1-800-426-2448.

REFERENCES

1. Ferrante MF. Patient controlled analgesia: A conceptual framework for analgesic administration. In: Ferrante FM, VadeBoncouer TK, eds. Postoperative pain management. New York: Churchill Livingstone; 1993: ch 10.
2. Intravenous patient-controlled analgesia. Traditional postoperative pain management, In: Sevarino FB, Preble LM, eds. A manual for acute postoperative pain management. New York: Raven Press; 1922: 122–136; Tables 8.5, 8.8.
3. Bernstein RL, Rosenberg AD. Manual of orthopedic anesthesia and related pain syndromes. New York: Churchill Livingstone; 1993: ch 6.
4. Hauer M, Cram E, Titler M, Alpen M, Harp J. Intravenous patient-controlled analgesia in critically ill postoperative trauma patients: Research-

based practice recommendations. Dimensions in Critical Care Nursing 1995; 14(3) May–June: 144–153.

5. Jantos TJ, Paris PM, Menegazzi, JJ, Yealy DM. Analgesic practices for acute orthopedic trauma pain in Costa Rican Emergency Departments. Ann Emerg Med 1996; 28(2): 145–150.

6. Nolan JP, Dow MC, Parr MJA, Dauphinee K, Kalish M. Patient controlled epidural analgesia following post traumatic pelvic reconstruction. Anesthesia. 1992; 47: 1037–1041.

7. Hocking G, de Mello WF. Battlefield analgesia–A basic approach. JR Army Med Corps 1996; 142: 101–102.

8. Ferrante FM, Orau EJ, Rocco AG, Gallo J. A statistical model for pain in patient-controlled analgesia and conventional intramuscular opioid regimens. Anesth Analg 1988; 67: 457.

9. Sechzer PH. Objective measurement of pain. Anesthesiology 1968; 29: 205.

10. Sechzer PH. Studies in pain with analgesic-demand system. Anesth Analg 1971; 50: 1.

11. Parker RH, Holtmann B, White PF. Effects of a nighttime opioid infusion with PCA therapy on patient comfort and analgesic requirements after abdominal hysterectomy. Anesthesiology 1992; 76(3): 362–367.

12. McNeely JK, Trentadue NC. Comparison of patient controlled analgesia with and without nighttime morphine infusion following lower extremity surgery in children. J Pain Symptom Manage 1997; 13(5): 268–273.

13. Sidebotham D, Dijkhuizen MRJ, Schug SA. The safety and utilization of patient controlled analgesia. J Pain Symptom Manage 1997; 14(4): 202–209.

14. Schug SA, Torrie JJ. Safety assessment of postoperative pain management by an acute pain service. Pain 1993; 55: 387–391.

15. Broadman LM, Brown RE, Rice LJ, et al. Patient controlled analgesia in children and adolescents: A report of postoperative pain management in 150 patients. Anesthesiology 1989; 71: A1171.

16. Kroll W, List WF. Pain treatment in the ICU: Intravenous, regional or both? Eur J Anesthesiol 1900; 14(Suppl. 15): 49–52.

17. Watcha MF, White PF. Postoperative nausea and vomiting. Anesthesiology 1992; 77: 162–184.

18. Tarantino DP, Baker R, Bower TC. Patient-administered alfentanil for wound dressing changes in a non-intensive care setting. Anesth Analg 1995; 80: 191–193.

19. Lehmann KA. Le tramadol dans les douleurs aigues. Drugs 1997; 53(Suppl 2): 25–33.

12

Epidural and spinal techniques including patient-controlled epidural analgesia

Sassan Hassassian and Hagop Tabakian

Introduction

Indications
  Analgesia after thoracic trauma
  Analgesia after abdominal and pelvic trauma
  Analgesia after extremity trauma

Contraindications
  Central nervous system pathology
  Infections
  Major coagulation disorders/anticoagulation
    therapy
  Increased intracranial pressure
  Patient's lack of cooperation with positioning
  Uncorrected hypovolemia

Techniques
  Epidural
  Vertebral column
  Mechanism of epidural blockade
  Lumbar epidural techniques
  Thoracic epidural techniques
  Cervical epidural tecniques
  Caudal epidural techniques
  Spinal techniques

Pediatric epidurals

Pharmacologic agents
  Local anesthetics
  Opioids

Dosages

Other agents

Continuous epidural protocols

Advantages and disadvantages of epidural analgesia

Effects and complications of epidural analgesia
  Respiratory effects
  Circulatory effects
  Urinary retention
  Gastrointestinal effects
  Neurologic sequelae
  Local anesthetic toxicity
  Accidental subarachnoid injection
  Post-dural puncture headache

Complications of spinal anesthesia
  Hypotension
  Extensive spread of spinal anesthesia
  Nausea and vomiting
  Backache
  The 'failed' spinal
  Major neurologic sequelae

Special situations
  Patients with known or suspected history of
    substance abuse

Conclusion

INTRODUCTION

Successful management of pain in the trauma patient can be a challenging task. However, as in the majority of postoperative patients, neuroaxial pain management, specifically, epidural pain control remains as one of the most effective means by which trauma patients can be treated. Analysis of pain control of trauma patients by traditional methods (e.g. PO, IM injections) conducted in several major trauma centers reveals a major disparity in perception of pain between patients and caregivers. The discrepancy leads to undertreatment of the vast majority of patients.[1] Negative connotations associated with opioid analgesics, fear of addiction, federal and local regulations associated with prescribing opioids, and difficulty assessing pain are some of the factors underlying this trend.[2] Alternatively the neuroaxial method of providing analgesia has been employed in a number of different situations regardless of the site of the pain, be it from the upper extremity, torso, or the lower extremity, and has been shown to decrease the stress response to surgery.[3]

Our goal in this chapter is to provide a practical approach to understanding epidural pain control as well as techniques that might be useful to clinicians who deal with trauma patients. Spinal techniques and management will be explained briefly since these are not the mainstay of pain control. We will focus our attention initially on specific situations where epidural pain control can be of significant importance to overall patient management. Various indications and contraindications to using this technique will be discussed. We will then present practical hints on performing these procedures in both adult and pediatric patients. A discussion on common and new promising pharmacological agents will follow. Dosages, advantages, complications, and various epidural protocols will be provided.

INDICATIONS

Pain originating from any part of the body below the upper thoracic level is amenable to epidural analgesia. The intensity and the relatively discrete segmental analgesia produced by epidurally-administered drugs provide an advantage over systemically-administered drugs, with their higher side effect profile.

Analgesia after thoracic trauma

Patients with closed chest trauma with rib fracture, flail chest, and pulmonary contusion often present with respiratory distress and splinting because of pain, and may require immediate intubation and mechanical ventilation. However, if the pain is kept under adequate control, intubation in these patients may be avoided. Administration of systemic opioids often depresses respiration before adequate analgesia is achieved, especially in the elderly. This defeats the objectives of having the patient cough, and use the incentive spirometer effectively. Regional techniques in these patients can provide the necessary conditions to achieve these objectives.

The application of regional techniques has revolutionized the management of pain in thoracic trauma.[4–6] Epidural catheters for continuous administration of narcotics, local anesthetics, or a mixture thereof, are the most reliable and effective method to manage thoracic pain both within and outside intensive care settings. Studies comparing epidural with other modes of postoperative analgesia after thoracotomies have found: epidural analgesia with hydromorphone to be superior to intrapleural bupivacaine;[7] epidural morphine infusion after thoracotomy to be superior to extrapleural intercostal nerve block followed by an infusion of bupivacaine;[8] and post-thoracotomy epidural meperidine to be superior to intravenous patient-controlled meperidine with improved recovery of postoperative pulmonary function.[9]

Although improved outcome with epidural analgesia has not been directly documented, subjective patient comfort, early extubation, and mobilization with improved pulmonary parameters compared to other modalities of analgesia have been demonstrated.[10] The incidence of serious side effects has been quite low, provided that standard protocols for dosing guidelines are adhered to, and patients are evaluated and followed daily by the postoperative analgesia service.

Analgesia after abdominal and pelvic trauma

As in thoracic surgery, epidural analgesia after abdominal surgery offers more patient comfort, fewer side effects, and early ambulation when compared to intravenous opioids. Using various medications with an epidural infusion of bupivacaine and fentanyl provided better analgesia with a slightly lower side effect profile compared to intravenous patient-controlled analgesia (IV-PCA) after gynecological laparotomies.[11] Moreover, using epidural anesthesia intraoperatively and continuing it postoperatively for analgesia has resulted in decreased blood loss and shorter hospital stay than general anesthesia with systemic opioids for postoperative analgesia.[12]

Epidural analgesia with a mixture of local anesthetic and opioid has been shown to improve pulmonary function when compared with systemic opioids.[13] Improvements included a higher Pao_2, vital capacity, and peak expiratory flow.[14] In morbidly obese patients undergoing gastroplasty, epidural analgesia improved pulmonary function and provided early ambulation.[15] It has also been demonstrated that in patients with two or more risk factors for coronary artery disease the incidence of postoperative tachycardia, ischemia, and possibly infarction were decreased.[16] Similarly, in patients undergoing abdominal aortic aneurysm repair, the use of epidural analgesia in the postoperative period was associated with a shorter duration of intubation. Time in the intensive care unit, and the number of pulmonary and cardiac complications were also reduced leading to an overall decrease in hospital charges compared to the group which received parenteral opioids for postoperative analgesia.[17] In addition, following radical hysterectomies, bowel function recovery was faster and the hospitalization period was shorter in patients who were administered epidural bupivacaine/morphine for analgesia compared to patients who had IV-PCA with morphine.[18] Allowing patients to obtain pain relief through patient-controlled epidural analgesia (PCEA) is another important method of providing postoperative analgesia. In fact, PCEA seems to be a safer and more efficient way to control postoperative pain than with a continuous epidural infusion. In one study, patients used less morphine in the PCEA group than the continuous infusion group (6.87 +/– 0.27 mg vs 9.0 mg) over a 24-hour period, with similar pain and sedation scores, and a lower frequency of nausea and vomiting (33% vs 63%).[19] A comparison between PCEA and IV-PCA in patients undergoing upper abdominal surgery revealed the PCEA group had lower pain scores at rest and with coughing, as well as a higher patient satisfaction level than PCA patients. However, PCEA was also more time-consuming (407 vs 299 min) and expensive (cost: $71 vs $40 per day).[20]

Analgesia after extremity trauma

Early recovery after lower extremity procedures depends on adequate pain control, early physiotherapy, and exercise,[21] which can be effectively provided by epidural analgesia. Efficacy has been demonstrated in adult, geriatric, and pediatric populations with no serious side effects.[22]

One group that can particularly benefit from epidural analgesia are patients with traumatic amputation who need daily dressing changes or revisions of their stump. It is generally believed that epidural analgesia may prevent the development of phantom limb pain. This is based on studies that demonstrated a significant decrease in the incidence of phantom limb pain in patients who had pre-emptive epidural analgesia that was continued postoperatively for 3 days.[23] However, Nikolajsen et al did not find a difference in the incidence of stump and phantom limb pain between the two groups in 1-year follow-up.[24]

CONTRAINDICATIONS

As with any other procedure and treatment modality, there are some absolute and relative contraindications to the use of neuroaxial treatment of pain. Before instituting any form of therapy, it is the physician's obligation to thoroughly explain the intended procedure to the patient. If any patient or custodian candidly expresses refusal of an invasive procedure, it is our belief that the intervention should be avoided as much as possible to respect the patient's wish, and also to comply with medicolegal issues. Obviously, in trauma situations where the patient may not be able to give proper informed consent (e.g. alcohol intoxication) this would not present a significant issue as long as the interventional technique is clearly advantageous to the patient's overall level of care. If the practitioner believes that an invasive technique is superior and less risky than other modalities when the patient does not agree, he or she should try to seek legal approval from the respective institution's administration before proceeding with the procedure.

Central nervous system pathology

A significant number of neurologic sequelae which have been attributed to the injection of local anesthetics into the subarachnoid space are really just an exacerbation of pre-existing neurologic diseases (see Complications of spinal anesthesia). Therefore, unless there is a compelling indication, the administration of central neuroaxial anesthesia is best avoided in the presence of a pre-existing neurologic disorder.

Infections

Infection at the site of the proposed needle insertion, or a systemic infection with bacteremia are both considered absolute contraindications for placement of epidural catheters. Cutaneous infections at sites remote from the catheter entry site have been implicated as the source of spinal space infection,[25] but these complications are rare.

Major coagulation disorders/anticoagulation therapy

For detailed discussion of this topic, refer to the section on anticoagulant therapy.

Increased intracranial pressure

The issue of increased intracranial pressure (ICP) is one that could occur in trauma patients, particularly in those with head injury. Dural puncture during placement of an epidural catheter or performance of invasive procedures on the spinal cord can be quite detrimental to the patient. If an elevated ICP is present, the concern is that, by suddenly reducing pressure at the level of spine, the brainstem may herniate, thereby leading to cardiovascular, neurologic, and respiratory compromise. In addition, Grocott showed that epidural injection of a lidocaine solution in a porcine model with increased ICP resulted in a significant reduction in cerebral and spinal cord blood flow.[26] However, as long as ICP is not increased, the presence of head injury in itself is not considered a contraindication to epidural analgesia, and such patients have been successfully treated.[27]

Patient's lack of cooperation with positioning

Patients who are uncooperative or agitated secondary to head injury or unconsciousness, or who are simply uncooperative with the positioning, represent a relative contraindication for placement of neuroaxial block. They have a higher risk of sustaining injury during the block. Such patients are better served by alternate means of anesthesia and postoperative pain control.

Uncorrected hypovolemia

Hypovolemic patients rely on their sympathetic system to maintain their blood pressure and, hence, tissue perfusion. Neuroaxial block can also block their sympathetic outflow, and therefore neutralize the most important compensatory mechanism. This could expose them to cardiovascular collapse.

TECHNIQUES

Epidural

Intimate knowledge of the anatomy of the vertebral column is essential, not only for the safe and successful performance of spinal and epidural blocks, but also for the understanding of the spread of the local anesthetic or opioid in the subarachnoid and epidural space.

It is beyond the scope of this section to discuss the detailed anatomy of the vertebral column, thus only some of the practical aspects relevant to the epidural and subarachnoid spaces will be discussed.

Vertebral column

The vertebral column consists of 33 vertebrae: 7 cervical, 12 thoracic, 5 lumbar, 5 sacral (fused), and 4 coccygeal. It has four curves; the cervical and lumbar are convex anteriorly, and the thoracic and sacral are convex posteriorly. These curves are important to remember in relation to the spread of local anesthetic, especially in the subarachnoid space (Fig. 12.1). The vertebral column is held together by several ligaments:

Supraspinous ligament. This ligament connects the apices of the spinous processes together from the sacrum to C7, then continues upward as the ligamentum nuchae.

Interspinous ligament. Connects the spinous processes together.

Ligamentum flavum. Connects the adjacent laminas – the caudal edge of the vertebra above to the cephalad edge of the lamina below.

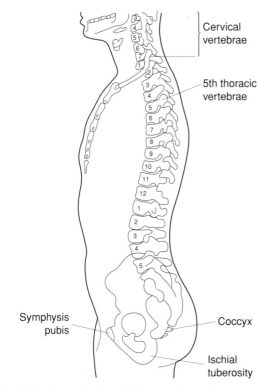

Fig. 12.1 Lateral view of the vertebral column.

Longitudinal ligaments. Anterior and posterior ligaments bind the vertebral bodies together.

Epidural space. This space surrounds the spinal meninges, and extends from the foramen magnum to the sacral hiatus, which is covered by the sacrococcygeal ligament. It is bound anteriorly by the posterior longitudinal ligament, laterally by the pedicles and the intervertebral foramina, and posteriorly by the ligamentum flavum. The space is widest posteriorly. In the cervical region it ranges from 1.0–1.5 mm, 2.5–3.0 mm at T6, and 5.0–6.0 mm at L2. In addition to the nerve roots, it contains fat, areolar tissue, and an extensive internal vertebral plexus of Batson, arteries, and lymphatics. Three layers of connective tissue, the meninges, protect the spinal cord.

Dura mater. It is a tough, fibroblastic tube, with fibers running longitudinally. Superiorly, it is attached to the circumference of the foramen magnum; caudally, it ends at the lower border of S2, where it is pierced by the filum terminale (the terminal thread of the pia mater). The dura pro-

vides a thin cover for the nerve roots as they emerge from the intervertebral foramina. It continues as epineurium and perineurium of the peripheral nerve.

Arachnoid mater. It is a delicate, nonvascular membrane closely attached to the dura. The subdural space is a potential space between the dura and the arachnoid that does not communicate with the subarachnoid space. It is wider laterally adjacent to the nerve roots and extends into the cranial cavity. Injection of local anesthetic into this space, the subdural space, after getting 'some' fluid, explains at least some of the failed spinals.

Pia mater. It is a delicate, highly vascular membrane, which is closely attached to the brain and the spinal cord. The space between the arachnoid and the pia is filled with cerebrospinal fluid (CSF) and is called the subarachnoid space. It contains the spinal nerves, blood vessels, and trabeculi that run between these two membranes. Lateral projections of the pia, the denticular ligaments, are attached to the dura and help hold the spinal cord in place.

Subarachnoid space. This space is bounded internally by the pia, externally by the arachnoid, and extends from the cranium to the spinal cord and further to the nerve roots. As the nerve roots leave the spinal cord, they are bathed in CSF.

Cerebrospinal fluid. The CSF is an ultrafiltrate of the plasma, formed by the choroid arterial plexuses of the lateral, third, and fourth ventricles. It circulates in the ventricles around the brain and the spinal cord, and is resorbed through the arachnoid villi. The rate of absorption and resorption are the same at equilibrium, at about 0.35 mL/min, or 500 mL/day. The total volume in an average adult ranges from 120–150 mL, of which 25–35 mL lies in the spinal subarachnoid space, mostly in the area of cauda equina. In supine position, CSF pressure ranges from 60–80 mmH$_2$O.

Mechanism of epidural blockade

Local anesthetics in the epidural space produce their effect by blocking the Na-channels in the neural membrane, consequently inhibiting Na-influx and initiation of neural action potential. The fate of the local anesthetic, or for that matter, any agent in the epidural space is absorption into the blood vessels, diffusion and retention into the fatty tissue of the epidural space, and diffusion into the target nerve fibers within the nerve roots.

The dura mater and the connective tissue around the nerve fibers offer a barrier to the local anesthetic reaching the nerve membranes, but this barrier is not an absolute one. Higher doses of the local anesthetic do eventually cross the dura; hence, the higher dose requirement for epidural blockade compared to subarachnoid blockade. In fact, there is evidence to suggest that epidurally-injected local anesthetic not only reaches the nerve roots, but also the spinal cord itself through diffusion into the subarachnoid space.[28] The contribution of this mode of action of the epidurally-injected local anesthetic to the overall effect is not yet known.

Neurophysiologic studies on the effect of opioids on the spinal cord demonstrate that morphine selectively suppresses dorsal horn neurons in laminas I and V, which mediate noxious input, but has no effect on lamina IV neurons, which process light touch and proprioceptive input.[29] Administration of opiates directly into the substantia gelatinosa results in selective inhibition of postsynaptic transmission of primary nociceptive afferent impulses.[30] Further evidence for the site of opiate action in the spinal cord was provided by the fact that enkephalin-containing neurons are exclusively localized in the substantia gelatinosa, and their activation attenuated the release of substance P and other nociceptive transmitters.[31]

Lumbar epidural techniques

Midline approach

Lumbar midline approach is the most common approach used to enter the epidural space. This level of block can provide adequate postoperative analgesia for genito-urinary and lower extremity surgeries, with minimal disruption of baseline hemodynamics.

Positioning. The importance of positioning of the patient cannot be overemphasized. In most instances, it makes the difference between a failed and successful attempt in entering the epidural space. Taking the time to carefully position the patient pays manifold in saving multiple attempts and avoiding a situation where patient, anesthesiologist, and the surgeon are frustrated.

There are two basic positions that may be chosen. The choice depends on the condition of the patient (some patients may not be able to sit up), and the comfort level of the anesthesiologist with one or the other position.

1. *Lateral decubitus position*, whereby the spine is maximally flexed with the knees drawn up towards the abdomen and the head is bent forward.
2. *Sitting position*, whereby the patient is on a firm surface, feet resting on a stool, elbows resting on the thighs, with the spine maximally flexed (i.e. 'the shrimp position').

In most circumstances, the sitting position is the most convenient for the anesthesiologist to identify the midline, and maintain sterility of the procedure field, especially in obese patients. This positioning may not always be possible, especially in trauma patients, in whom other injuries might interfere with proper positioning. Therefore, it is recommended to practice both positioning methods in elective patients to become comfortable in performing them under a variety of circumstances (Figs 12.2, 12.3).

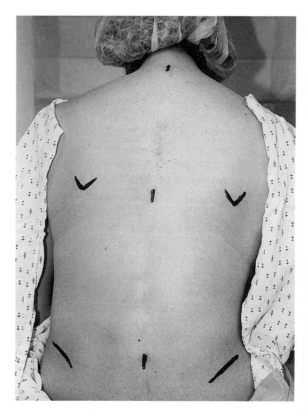

Fig. 12.2   Markings show the spinous process of T6, L4, posterior superior iliac spines, inferior tips of scapulae, and iliac crests.

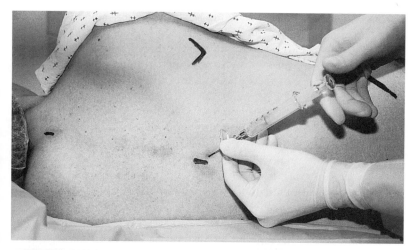

(A)

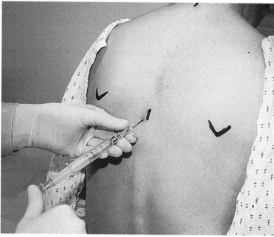

(B)

Fig. 12.3   Paramedian approach for thoracic epidural technique with patient in (A) lateral decubitus location at T6–T7 interspace; (B) sitting position at T6–T7 interspace.

Landmarks

Palpation of the iliac crests is relatively easy. A line connecting the iliac crests should pass through the L4 vertebra and the spinous process. Palpating the spinous processes moving upwards can identify the spinous processes of L3, L2, L1, etc. The appropriate intervertebral space is chosen and marked. If the area of surgery is known, the level corresponding to the dermatome covering the surgical site is chosen. This will be the most efficient way to provide intraoperative anesthesia and postoperative analgesia, since the target dermatomes will be covered with the least amount of drug mixture, thus avoiding significant side effects and unnecessary hemodynamic instability.

Needle insertion

It is a good practice to explain the procedure to the patient before starting, so he or she has an idea

of what to expect. Aseptic technique is used to prepare a wide area of the skin around the point where needle placement is planned with an appropriate antiseptic, usually Betadine. Time is allowed for the Betadine to dry. A skin wheal is raised at the center of the chosen interspace with local anesthetic. The epidural needle is then inserted and directed slightly cephalad but otherwise strictly in the midline through the interspinous ligament (Figs 12.3, 12.4, 12.5). The needle is then advanced onward in a controlled movement until the resistance of the ligamentum flavum is felt. At that point the stylet is removed, and a syringe is attached (usually filled with air, or saline with an air bubble). The non-dominant hand grasps the needle hub, with the back of the hand anchored against the skin. The syringe is attached to the hub, and the dominant hand attempts to depress the plunger to inject the contents of the syringe. This method is commonly

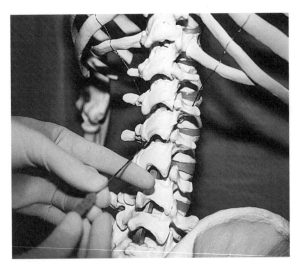

Fig. 12.4 Midline approach for lumbar epidural technique at L4–L5 interspace.

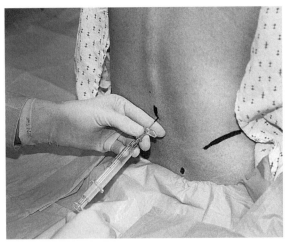

Fig. 12.5 Midline approach for lumbar epidural at L4–L5 interspace with needle tip in the epidural space.

known as the 'loss-of-resistance' method. The resistance at the tip of the needle will prevent the plunger from advancing until the epidural space is entered. The needle is advanced slowly and in a controlled movement a millimeter at a time, while keeping the pressure on the plunger. An alternate method is to tap on the plunger multiple times while advancing the needle in increments. As the needle enters the epidural space, the plunger will lose the resistance offered by the ligament, and will move forward easily in the syringe barrel.

It is important to test the syringe prior to attaching it to the hub to ensure that no resistance is encountered between the plunger and the syringe while attempting to move the plunger within the syringe. The movement back and forth should be fluid without any resistance. Some anesthesiologists prefer to irrigate the plunger and the syringe to ensure smooth movement, others prefer to keep the unit dry, so that any fluid in the syringe will alert them to the possibility of a wet tap, indicating a dural puncture. It is up to the individual anesthesiologist to develop his or her own method and know the possible implications of each.

In cases where difficulty is anticipated (obese patient, or a patient who is unable to assume the ideal position), a 'winged' needle (e.g. the Weiss needle) may be useful (Figs 12.6, 12.7). The advantage in this case is that both hands can be used to advance the needle in slow, controlled steps, testing the resistance at the plunger after each millimeter of advancement. This technique is preferred for thoracic or cervical epidural placements, since any uncontrolled sudden advancement through ligamentum flavum can cause injury to the spinal cord with disastrous consequences.

Occasionally bone is contacted during insertion of the needle, which is probably the lamina of the lower vertebra. The needle is withdrawn 1 or 2 cm and redirected cephalad. Redirecting the needle deep into the interspinous ligament will result in curving of the proximal portion of the needle, but upon advancement the tip will still traverse the same path and hit bone again. Once the epidural space is presumably reached, the syringe is removed and any fluid leak is noted from the hub. If saline is used in the syringe, a slow drip of a few

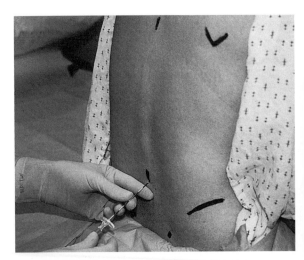

Fig. 12.6 Midline approach for lumbar epidural technique.

drops may be noticed, which would be the fluid injected in locating the space. This is why some anesthesiologists prefer not to use saline, so that any fluid dripping at the hub would be highly suggestive of dural puncture. If no fluid is noted, then the syringe is reattached and gentle aspiration is performed to reassure that no fluid or blood could be aspirated. If the aspiration is negative, the needle is presumed ready for injection of the drug of choice or placement of the epidural catheter.

Catheter placement

It is preferable to insert the catheter without giving any injections through the needle itself, and give both the test dose and the 'loading dose' through the catheter itself. However, some anesthesiologists prefer to dose the patient, so that the surgery can proceed, even if there is trouble passing the catheter. The catheter is advanced through the needle. Depending on the manufacturer, catheters have different markings to identify the point where the tip of the catheter is at the tip of the needle. The reader should be familiar with the details of the specific kits in use in his or her institution. At the point where the tip of the catheter is at the bevel, slight resistance is felt as the catheter emerges from the tip. 4–6 cm of catheter is pushed into the epidural space. The needle is then withdrawn, keeping constant pushing force on the catheter as the needle is being pulled out, to avoid pulling the catheter with it. One must not pull the catheter back out of the needle if there is trouble threading the catheter, as this may result in shearing off the catheter tip. Once the needle is out of the skin, the catheter is firmly grasped at the exit hole and the needle is removed from the catheter. A syringe connector, which usually comes with the kit, is then connected to the distal end of the catheter, where a syringe can be attached and injections made.

The catheter is tested for blood or CSF by aspiration. Then, a test dose is administered, watching the pulse rate for evidence of intravascular injection when epinephrine is used, and assessing the lower extremities for motor block. A rise in heart rate may occur with intravascular injection, and a rapid motor block will occur if the catheter is in the CSF. The catheter is secured by a sterile dressing, preferably one which is transparent in order to check the site daily for blood, discharge, leaks, etc.

Paramedian approach

Although this approach is the preferred approach for thoracic epidurals, it can be used for lumbar epidural catheter placement, especially when the spinous process and the interspinous ligament are to be avoided (Figs 12.8 & 12.9).

In this case the skin wheal is raised 1.5 cm from the midline either to the right or left, at the level of the upper border of the spinous process below the target interspace. The epidural needle is then inserted aiming towards the midline and slightly cephalad to contact and penetrate ligamentum flavum in the midline. Using the 'loss-of-resistance' technique the epidural space is identified as

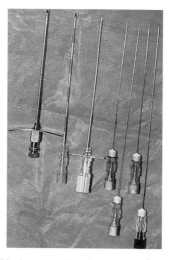

Fig. 12.7 Various needles for neuroaxial techniques. Note the needle tips and presence or absence of 'wings' and markings on the needles.

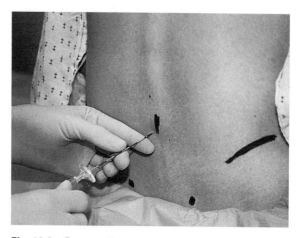

Fig. 12.8 Paramedian approach for lumbar epidural technique at L4–L5 interspace.

described above, and the catheter is inserted. It should be noted, however, that the ligamentum flavum is thickest at the midline, and tapers down to a thinner layer as it extends laterally, so that the initial tough resistance and the subsequent loss of resistance may not be as pronounced as with the midline approach.

Thoracic epidural techniques

Midline

Pertinent anatomic features of the thoracic vertebrae are relevant for the proper placement of needles and catheters at the thoracic level. The spinous processes of the T1, T2, T10, T11, and T12 are almost horizontal to the sagittal plane similar to those of the lumbar vertebrae and allow the needle to be inserted at around a 90° angle to the skin. The same midline approach for lumbar epidural catheterization can be applied for thoracic epidurals at these levels. The rest of the thoracic vertebrae, especially those from T3 through T7, are angulated caudally. The skin wheal is raised at the upper tip of the spinous process, which is below the chosen interspace, and the epidural needle is directed cephalad at an angle of 45–50°, advancing slowly by 'feeling' the way between the spinous processes. If bone is encountered, the needle is withdrawn 1–2 cm, angulated further, and then advanced. 'Loss-of-resistance' technique is applied as in lumbar epidurals once the increased resistance of the ligamentum flavum is felt. Occasionally it may be necessary to abandon a given level and

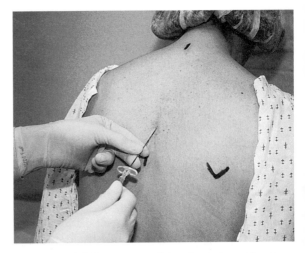

Fig. 12.10   Midline approach for thoracic epidural technique at T4–T5 interspace. Note the extreme angle that the needle makes with the skin.

change to one level up or down because of a 'tight' interspace (Figs 12.10 & 12.11).

Paramedian

The paramedian approach may be preferred in the midthoracic region, not only because the spinous processes are angulated, but also because the laminas tend to overlap each other. Although the spinous processes are avoided, the epidural needle still has to be at a relatively acute angle to negotiate the space between the laminas, which is occupied by the ligamentum flavum. The skin wheal is raised at 1–1.5 cm from the upper border of the spinous process below the chosen interspace and directed at an acute angle cephalad, aimed medially at an angle of 10–15° avoiding the spinous process. If bone is contacted, it must be the lamina, and then the needle is redirected to negotiate the space between the laminas. Angulation of the needle usually imparts protection to the dura, since the curved end of the Tuohy needle is the point of contact with the dura upon entry into the epidural space, therefore, puncturing of the dura is much less likely. In addition, insertion of the catheter is usually much easier than at the lumbar level, and will move cephalad without obstruction (Fig. 12.12).

Cervical epidural techniques

Cervical epidural block is primarily performed as one of the treatment modalities for complex

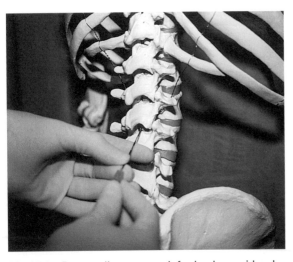

Fig. 12.9   Paramedian approach for lumbar epidural technique at L3–L4 interspace.

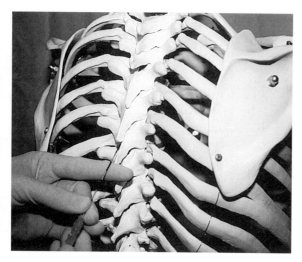

Fig. 12.11 Midline approach for thoracic epidural technique at T5–T6 interspace.

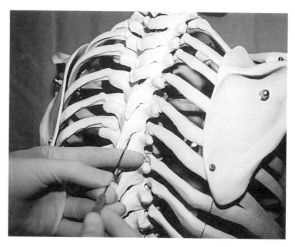

Fig. 12.12 Paramedian approach for thoracic epidural technique.

regional pain syndrome (CRPS), as an alternative for stellate ganglion block. It can also be used as postoperative analgesia for the upper extremity, especially if the patient is to have active physical therapy during the immediate postoperative period.

The cervical block is usually done with the patient in the sitting position; the head is flexed forward, although it can be done in the lateral position if the sitting position is inconvenient. The neck area is prepped as usual, and a surgical cap is worn by the patient to isolate the hair from the neck area. Midline approach is used, and the C6–C7 or C7–T1 interspace is identified (Figs 12.13, 12.14). The skin wheal is raised and the Tuohy needle is introduced at the midline into the interspace with the stylet in place. When the needle is engaged in the interspinous ligament the stylet is removed, and either a syringe is attached for 'loss-of-resistance' technique, or a drop of sterile saline is place at the needle hub for the 'hanging drop' technique. The 'hanging drop' is fairly dramatic at the cervical level. The needle is then advanced until the end-point is reached: either the resistance is lost, or the 'hanging drop' is sucked into the epidural space. Once in the epidural space, a gentle aspiration is done with a syringe to ascertain that the tip is not in the intravascular or subarachnoid space, and the catheter is advanced 2–4 cm into the space. The test dose is given and the catheter is secured.

Caudal epidural techniques

The main indications for caudal blocks are perineal operation, cystoscopies, urethral surgeries, cystocele and rectocele repairs, and inguinal herniorrhaphies, which require blockage of the sacral roots. Theoretically, if enough local anesthetic is injected, the drug can reach the lumbar and even the thoracic levels; in reality, however, it is often difficult to get the local anesthetic to spread high enough.

The sacral hiatus is the gap formed in the fifth sacral vertebra because of the absence of its lamina. A wide range of anatomic variations can occur, and occasionally the laminas of S4 and even S3 are also absent, creating an abnormally large hiatus. The hiatus is covered by the sacrococcygeal ligaments, which connect the coccyx to the sacrum. Caudal block is performed by entering the spinal canal through this hiatus.

The spinal cord ends at L1–2. The lower lumbar and sacral nerve roots traverse a long course within the spinal canal, forming the cauda equina. The nerves leave the subarachnoid space at the termination of the dura mater at S1 and enter the sacral epidural space. Various anatomical variations occur in this area, and the dura mater may end at a lower level than S1, in which case the subarachnoid space may be entered inadvertently.

The patient can be placed in the lateral decubitus position, or prone with a pillow under the pubis. The sacral cornua are palpated, and the sacral hiatus is localized. The skin is prepped as in lumbar epidural block, and a skin wheal is raised. A regular 21–23 gauge needle is used to perform the block, or a higher gauge needle is used if a catheter is to be placed. The needle is inserted at a 45° angle to the skin and the sacrococcygeal ligament is pierced. The needle then contacts the anterior wall of the sacral canal. The needle is redirected to a lower angle so it is in line with the sacral canal, and advanced 1–2 mm into the canal (Figs 12.15, 12.16 & 12.17). Injection of the local anesthetic is made, keeping a finger on the skin above the hiatus to feel any subcutaneous swelling, which means the needle placement is wrong (Fig. 12.17).

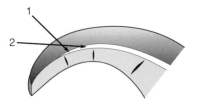

Fig. 12.15   Lateral view for needle placement in caudal technique: (1) shows initial needle trajectory; (2) shows final needle placement.

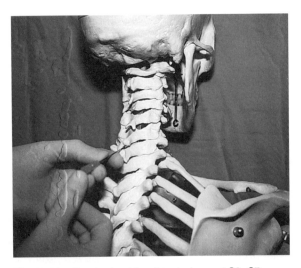

Fig. 12.13   Cervical epidural technique at C6–C7 interspace.

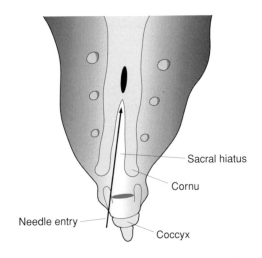

Fig. 12.16   Sacrum showing needle trajectory in caudal neuroaxial techniques.

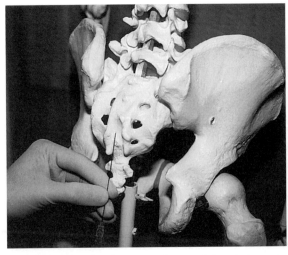

Fig. 12.14   Cervical epidural technique at C6–C7 interspace.

Fig. 12.17   Needle placement for caudal technique.

Spinal techniques

Spinal anesthesia is considered one of the oldest and most valuable techniques of regional anesthesia. It is the most efficient of blocks, since a small quantity of local anesthetic will cause widespread blockade of the spinal nerves and produce surgical anesthesia. Systemic toxicity is rarely a problem. Knowledge of the spinal anatomy is, however, essential for the safe administration of a subarachnoid block.

The spinal cord in adults ends at L1–L2; therefore, the spinal space is entered below that level to avoid injury to the cord. The subarachnoid space is situated between the pia and arachnoid maters and contains the CSF, the spinal cord, the spinal nerves, and the blood vessels supplying these structures. The arachnoid is closely applied, but not attached, to the dura mater. The subarachnoid space communicates superiorly with the pontine and cerebellomedullary cisterns, and ends caudally at the level of second sacral vertebra.

CSF is produced by the choroid plexuses in the cerebral ventricles, it circulates through the ventricular system and into the cerebral and spinal subarachnoid space, and is reabsorbed into the blood through the arachnoid villi in the superior sagittal sinus and some of the other venous sinuses. The CSF in the spinal canal has minimal circulation and drugs injected into it spread mainly by diffusion before being absorbed into the capillaries in the pia mater, the spinal nerves, and the spinal cord.

Midline spinal approach

The appropriate intervertebral space is identified, and the skin wheal is raised. The skin is held firmly against the adjacent spinous process while an introducer is placed (i.e. if a small gauge needle is utilized) equidistant between adjacent spinous processes in the midline, directed slightly cephalad. The bevel is pointed laterally. In thin patients, the increased resistance of the ligamentum flavum is often felt, the introducer should not be advanced further, to avoid piercing of the dura and causing post-dural puncture headache (PDPH). The spinal needle is then inserted through the introducer; the resistance of the ligamentum flavum is often felt. When it is thought that the spinal canal has been entered, the stylet is withdrawn and the needle hub inspected for CSF leakage. With fine spinal needles (25–27 gauge), CSF leakage is rather slow. A syringe is attached and an attempt at gentle aspiration may result in CSF being drawn into the syringe. Ideally CSF should continue to escape while the needle bevel is rotated through 360°.

If bone is contacted relatively superficially, probably the lamina or supraspinal process of the vertebra has been contacted. The needle and introducer are withdrawn and redirected cephalad.

Bone contacted deeply may mean the anterior wall of the spinal canal has been reached. In that case, the stylet is withdrawn, and the needle retracted slowly while looking for CSF leakage at the needle hub.

Paramedian spinal approach

This approach is used when ossification of the interspinous space hinders the advancement of the needle, or an adequate flexion of lumbar spine cannot be easily achieved. The skin wheal in this case is raised at a point 2 cm lateral to the spinous process below the selected interspace. The introducer is then directed cephalad and medial. If bone is contacted, it probably is the inferior surface of the lamina above the space. The needle is then withdrawn and redirected caudally.

Lumbosacral spinal approach

A related approach is the lumbosacral approach, where the needle is inserted 1 cm medial and 1 cm caudad to the posterior superior iliac spine, and directed medial and cephalad, roughly parallel to the dorsal surface of the sacrum. The needle tip reaches the lumbosacral interspace in the midline. If bone is contacted, it may be the posterior surface of the sacrum, in which case the needle is withdrawn and redirected more cephalad.

PEDIATRIC EPIDURALS (see also Ch. 17)

Most information is available about adult trauma patients chiefly because there is not much dealing specifically with pain management of pediatric trauma patients, especially epidural pain management of such patients. It is a well accepted fact that even infants do feel pain.[32] In this section, we focus our attention on children below 5 years of age. This is an age group where children are cognitively at a stage where they start to be able to interact with devices such as the PCA effectively. Therefore, they might be good candidates for modalities such as PCEA. For younger patients or those who have difficulty with the concept of PCA, a continuous infusion might be a better choice. Often, for children below 3 years, it is easier to place a caudal epidural catheter. This catheter, which may be used intraoperatively, can also be utilized postoperatively for pain relief. Epidural catheters have even been successfully used in situations where parenteral opioids were ineffective.[33] At our institution, these catheters are routinely placed for postoperative pain management of infants and the very young. One advantage of caudal insertion in these patients is that quite often the catheter can be advanced as high as the thoracic area.[34] That way, there can be dermatomal coverage of the thorax and the abdomen if, for example, local anesthetics are to be used. Furthermore, it has been shown that caudally-placed catheters can produce postoperative analgesia comparable to that afforded by a lumbar approach.[34] In terms of incidence of infections associated with short-term epidurals, Strafford et al showed a very low risk of infection in 1620 patients.[35]

The single-shot-dosing technique is another way of providing postoperative analgesia. This obviously does not provide long-lasting pain relief; however, at least it can provide better recovery room analgesia.[36] The dosages and protocols for management will be discussed later in this chapter.

PHARMACOLOGIC AGENTS

Local anesthetics (see Ch. 4)

Epidural use of local anesthetics plays a major role in management of pain in surgical patients. Once placed appropriately, they block the conduction of impulses from the affected site. This is achieved in a dermatomal fashion. Given adequate coverage of the painful area, the local anesthetic can be used as the sole agent in the epidural space for pain relief. However, in clinical practice, a combination of local anesthetics and opioids is used to take advantage of the synergy between the two. By using this technique, the amount of each agent is reduced leading to a better side effect profile for the combination solution. This is discussed in more detail below.

One should bear in mind that anesthetic and analgesic goals for trauma and postoperative patients are quite different at various points in the perioperative period. Whereas one may need significant motor block in an operative setting for a patient, this is not a quality that is needed for his or her pain management. In fact, the lowest amount of motor blockade is often desirable in the postoperative period. This translates into a situation in which the patient is comfortable enough to ambulate successfully, and for example, perform physical therapy maneuvers more effectively.

During the past decades, while a number of different local anesthetics have been used in the epidural space, the main two agents have been lidocaine and bupivacaine. Recently, a new agent, ropivacaine, has been introduced.

Lidocaine is one of the older local anesthetics which has been used extensively intrathecally and epidurally. Its use was first described in the 1940s.[37] It has a fairly rapid onset and a short-to-moderate duration of action. One disadvantage of lidocaine for postoperative epidural pain management is its low level of motor-sensory separation. In a comparative study, Columb & Lyons determined the effective concentration in 50% of patients (EC50) for bupivacaine and lidocaine in the first stage of labor and defined EC50 as the minimum local analgesic concentration (MLAC).[38] The results indicated that MLAC for bupivacaine was 0.065%, and for lidocaine it was 0.37% equivalent to 2 and 14 mmol solutions respectively. Thus, bupivacaine was 5.7 times more potent than lidocaine in weighted and 7 times more potent in molar ratios at analgesic EC50 in the volume of the local anesthetic studied. In trauma patients, as well as in any other surgical patients who need to ambulate quickly and without difficulty, an agent with higher sensory than motor blockade is desired. Obviously, if one deals with a patient who has sustained multiple lower extremity fractures who cannot leave the bed, the aforementioned issue does not bear much significance.

Traditionally, bupivacaine has been used as the local anaesthetic of choice for pain management of the postoperative patient. A moderately long duration of action and a preferential sensory rather than a motor block are two factors that make this agent particularly suitable. Of concern is the fact that potential toxicity with bupivacaine is a serious consideration as cardiac resuscitation can be extremely difficult if not impossible. One theory to explain the difficulty with resuscitation in bupivacaine toxicity is that while the bupivacaine molecules occupy the sodium channels in the myocardium as do lidocaine molecules, they dissociate from the channels very slowly.

Ropivacaine is a new local anesthetic, which exists almost entirely as the S-isomer form, whereas bupivacaine and other local anesthetics are a racemic mixture. The pK_a and the degree of protein binding of ropivacaine and bupivacaine are very similar.[39] The theoretical advantage of ropivacaine is its lower toxicity potential in case of overdose. This has been demonstrated in the animal model.[40] The central nervous system (CNS) toxicity profile of this local anesthetic also seems to be more favorable.[41] Successful use of ropivacaine has been demonstrated in a number of recent studies. It has also been shown to be effective in the obstetric population where a low level of motor block is desired for normal vaginal delivery.[42] Different concentrations of ropivacaine have been used in various protocols for postoperative pain management. Solutions of 0.1–0.2% seem to be the best concentrations, for balance between sensory and motor blockade.[43] This will be presented below in the section on protocols for infusions.

Another agent that needs to be mentioned here is epinephrine. This agent has been utilized in variety of combination protocols for management of pain or as an adjunct to subarachnoid injections in the operating room. It has been shown that addition of epinephrine to some local anesthetics prolongs the duration of their effect. This is more apparent for lidocaine,[44,45] while the results are not as consistent with bupivacaine.[46] It has also been used in the management of labor analgesia to improve the analgesic efficacy of epidurally-administered bupivacaine.[47] In addition, it has been noted that epinephrine may have some opioid-sparing effect when administered as an adjunct medicine in epidural solutions and infusions.[48,49] This could have significance since, theoretically by using less local anesthetic or opioid, one can reduce the amount of side effects associated with either of the two.

Opioids

Epidurally-injected opioids exert their effect by inhibiting neurotransmitter release at the presynaptic level in dorsal horn neurons of the spinal cord. They also cause hyperpolarization of the postsynaptic membrane in the dorsal horn neurons, making it more difficult for the neurotransmitters to depolarize.

Nociceptive signals reach the dorsal horn via C-fiber neurons, where neuropeptides such as neurokinin A, substance P (tachykinins) and other transmitters like glutamate, are released presynaptically. Tachykinins bind the postsynaptic neurokinin receptor (NK1 and NK2) leading to depolarization and changes in the second messengers (adenyl cyclase and CAMP), via guanosine triphosphate activation.

Glutamate, on the other hand, acts on both alpha-amino-3-hydroxy-5-methyl-4-isoxazolopropionic acid and N-methyl-D-aspartic acid- (NMDA) receptors on the postsynaptic membrane of the dorsal horn neurons. The ion channels linked to the NMDA-receptors are, under resting conditions, blocked by magnesium ions. Magnesium can be removed by depolarization of the cell, which leads to influx of calcium and sodium ions, causing further depolarization.

To exert its effect at the dorsal horn level of the spinal cord, a drug deposited in the epidural space must traverse a number of membranes and the CSF before reaching its site of action.[50] Lipophilic drugs, with their high octanol:buffer partition coefficient, can traverse lipid bilayer membranes readily because of their high lipid solubility, but find it difficult to dissolve in the interstitial and intracellular aqueous fluid environment of the membranes. This becomes the rate-limiting step in the onset of their action. Drugs with intermediate lipophilicity move readily between the lipid and the aqueous zones, with minimal limitations. The optimal octanol:buffer distribution coefficient that results in maximal meningeal permeability seems to be between 129 (for alfentanil) and 560 (for bupivacaine) (Table 12.1). These physicochemical properties of the opioids have practical clinical applications, which will be referred to in the appropriate sections below.

Epidurally-administered opioids produce analgesia without sympathetic or motor blockade, which presents an advantage in patients who are hemodynamically fragile or need to ambulate early in the postoperative period.[51]

Table 12.1 Octanol:buffer coefficients and meningeal permeability coefficients for selected opioids

Opioid	Octanol:buffer distribution coefficient	Meningeal permeability coefficient (cm/min × 0.001)
Morphine	1	0.6
Meperidine	525	n/a
Hydromorphone	525	n/a
Fentanyl	955	0.9
Sufentanil	1737	0.75
Alfentanil	129	2.3
Bupivacaine	560	1.6

n/a, not available.

Morphine

Morphine is the prototype opioid that was first used for epidural administration in the early 1970s, and was the first opioid approved by the FDA for intrathecal administration. Despite its low lipophilicity, which corresponds to its slow onset of action, morphine is a very useful drug for epidural administration because it is retained in the CSF longer; thus, providing a longer supply to the spinal cord, and consequently, a longer duration of analgesia after single dose administration.

Respiratory depression, somnolence, and pruritus are common side effects of all opioids, and appear to be associated with the degree of rostral migration of the opioid in the CSF. The timing for the appearance of these side effects after epidural administration varies between lipophilic and hydrophilic opioids. Following epidural administration, side effects follow a predictable time course and are dose dependent.

Respiratory depression may occur as a result of cephalad migration of morphine after single lumbar epidural administration, suggesting that the drug reaches the respiratory center in the brainstem in a significant amount.[52] Large-scale studies suggest that respiratory depression requiring treatment may be higher with intermittent bolusing than with continuous infusions. Mean doses between 7 and 13 mg/d given as intermittent bolus, compared to mean doses between 6 and 14 mg/d as continuous infusion, yielded different results for incidence respiratory depression: In the bolus-treated group, the incidence of respiratory depression was 1:500.[53] In contrast, in the continuous infusion group, the incidence was 1:1500.[54]

The results are reassuring that continuous epidural infusion method is safer than the intermittent bolusing method.

The quality of analgesia reported by a large variety of surgical patients appears to be superior when continuous infusion of epidural opioid is used compared to intermittent bolus dosing. This clinical impression is supported by a number of studies where patients reported a higher quality of analgesia and lower pain scores with continuous epidural infusion compared to intermittent boluses.[11,55] Among regional techniques, epidural analgesia with morphine (bolus of 70 microg/kg then infusion of 7 microg/kg/h for 72 h), has been found as effective as bupivacaine (0.5% in epinephrine 1:200 000; bolus of 0.3 mL/kg then infusion of 0.1 mL/kg/h for 72 h), when used as part of a continuous intercostal nerve block technique. The amount of IV supplemental morphine use was higher in the bupivacaine infusion group, and the serum concentration of bupivacaine had increased significantly, although not to toxic levels.[8] Thus, based on the apparent greater clinical efficacy, safety, and a lower incidence of respiratory depression compared to bolus regimen, continuous epidural infusion of opioids seems to be the best regimen available to provide safe and hemodynamically stable postoperative analgesia for the majority of surgical populations.

Hydromorphone

Structurally similar to morphine, hydromorphone seems to produce the same quality of analgesia as morphine. Its potency is at least seven times greater than morphine, a potency ratio of 7:1, so that 1.3 mg of hydromorphone (administered subcutaneously or intramuscularly) will produce the same degree of analgesia as 10 mg of morphine administered via the same route.[56] For continuous infusion of hydromorphone, the recommended potency equivalent to morphine is 3 (a ratio of 3:1), because of its shorter duration of action compared to morphine.[57]

Several characteristics of hydromorphone make it desirable for use in the clinical practice of postoperative pain management:

1. Hydromorphone is associated with much lower incidence of pruritus compared to morphine, and therefore, it can be used as an alternative in patients who develop pruritus. In one study,

hydromorphone infusion (50 microg/mL) at a rate of 0.15–0.30 mg/h was compared to morphine infusion (150 microg/mL) administered at a rate of 0.45–0.90 mg/h (3–6 mL/h). The incidence of pruritus was four times greater in the morphine group (44% vs 11%).[56]

2. Hydromorphone has a lipid solubility intermediate between morphine and fentanyl. Since the degree of spinal analgesia appears to be related, at least in part, to the degree of lipid solubility, patients receiving epidurally administered hydromorphone are expected to have a higher degree of analgesia (or require less hydromorphone) than those receiving it via the systemic route. Liu et al found that patients receiving IV hydromorphone required twice as much opioid to achieve the same degree of analgesia as those in the epidural group (3.5–11.5 vs 1.5–5 microg/kg/h, respectively; $P < 0.008$).[58]

3. Hydromorphone appears to have a faster onset and shorter duration of action than morphine.[59]

Fentanyl

Fentanyl is a synthetic opioid, which primarily acts on mu-receptors, and is estimated to be 80 times as potent as morphine as an analgesic. Its physicochemical properties impart certain characteristics that are relevant in epidural analgesia.

The concentration of fentanyl in the spinal cord is determined by the meningeal permeability, which is the difference between the amount deposited in the epidural space, and the amount that is reabsorbed from the epidural space into the adipose tissue and the vascular bed within that space. Being an opioid of high lipid solubility with high octanol:buffer distribution coefficient (Table 12.1), fentanyl seems to undergo vascular absorption readily, thus reaching systemic circulation fairly rapidly.[60] In fact, the use of fentanyl for epidural analgesia is controversial.

A number of investigators have demonstrated that the quality of analgesia, the incidence of side effects, and plasma levels after 24-hour of infusion are similar between patients receiving fentanyl via either epidural or intravenous routes.[61,62] Guinard et al concluded that, although patients receiving thoracic epidural fentanyl had better forced expiratory volume (FEV) and FEV_1 values and shorter hospital stays compared to patients receiving IV fentanyl during the postoperative period, the quality of analgesia, total amount of fentanyl use, and the incidence of morbidity were similar among IV and epidural groups (both thoracic and lumbar).[63] Other studies have suggested that epidural fentanyl does have a significant spinal effect, based upon the lower doses used, and lower plasma levels measured after epidural infusion.[64] Analysis of the other studies as well as our own experience demonstrates no significant clinical advantage to fentanyl administered alone via the epidural route when compared to the IV route. However, for an optimally-placed catheter close to the affected dermatomes, epidural use of fentanyl is more effective to obtain rapid pain relief.

Sufentanil

The potency of sufentanil is 5 to 10 times that of fentanyl, and its site of action is both spinal and supraspinal. The quality of analgesia produced, and the plasma levels measured after IV or epidural administration of sufentanil are similar.[65]

There are, however, at least two potential advantages of administering epidural sufentanil for postoperative analgesia. The more significant advantage of using epidural sufentanil, however, seems to be in patients who have developed tolerance to opioids, secondary to chronic use of morphine or equivalent. Patients with cancer pain who were on chronic oral morphine of > 250 mg experienced severe postoperative pain despite epidural bupivacaine 0.1% and morphine, up to 2 mg/h. Once switched to sufentanil, full pain control was achieved with smaller equianalgesic doses (14–17 microg/h).[66,67] One explanation for this effect is the high efficacy of sufentanil, which requires low receptor occupancy. In fact, when enough receptors were blocked by a noncompetitive antagonist (beta-funaltrexamine), morphine was converted into a partial agonist. Sufentanil, however, remained a full agonist, retaining full activity.[68] Moreover, in experimental animals made tolerant to opioid agonists with chronic opioid infusions, a marked right shift (increase in dose requirements to obtain the same effect) in the dose–response curve for morphine was demonstrated (more than 100-fold). In contrast, the infusion of sufentanil resulted in significantly smaller shift (less than 10-fold).[69]

Table 12.2 Equivalent doses of epidural opioids

Agent	Dosage
Morphine	5–10 mg
Meperidine	50–100 mg
Fentanyl	100–200 microg
Sufentanil	30–50 mg
Alfentanil	1000–1500 microg

Alfentanil

Although rapid intravascular absorption does not occur with alfentanil as seen with other lipophilic opioids, the duration of postoperative analgesia seems to be relatively short. Thus a continuous infusion is required for postoperative analgesia. The quality of analgesia and the incidence and severity of side effects observed is similar between the IV and epidural groups; therefore, there seems to be no advantage to administering it via the epidural versus the IV route.[70] One study reported, however, 39% lower alfentanil consumption in the group receiving it epidurally compared with the IV-PCA route. Since alfentanil is considerably more expensive than other opioids, one implication of this fact is that if the choice of opioid is limited in a particular patient because of side effects, allergy, etc., the epidural route is the more economical way to provide postoperative analgesia compared to the IV route.

Side effects of intrathecal and epidural opioids

Many side effects have been described in association with systemic, epidural, and intrathecal opioids. The most common side effects are pruritus, nausea and vomiting, urinary retention, and respiratory depression.

Pruritus. Pruritus is believed to be the most common side effect of intrathecal and epidural opioids, varying widely between 0 and 100%, and is often elicited only after direct questioning. Severe pruritus, however, is only about 1%. Typically it involves the face, neck, and upper thorax and is not associated with a rash, and starts within a few hours of the injection.

The mechanism of opioid-induced pruritus is not known. It does not seem to be related to systemic absorption of opioids. Although histamine release from mast cells is detected following opioid injection, reversal of pruritus with naloxone is not associated with a decrease in plasma histamine levels. Nonetheless most patients with mild-to-moderate pruritus do respond to antihistamines. In more severe and persistent cases, low dose naloxone infusion can be utilized (e.g. 3–5 microg/kg/h).

Nausea and vomiting. Approximately one-third of the patients experience nausea and vomiting following epidural or intrathecal administration of opioids, usually within 3 to 4 hours of injection. It has been explained on the basis of cephalad migration of the drug in the CSF and interaction with opioid receptors in the area postrema. Motion-induced nausea and vomiting produced by opioids is thought to be due to sensitization of the vestibular system.[71] This can be treated with dopamine antagonists such as droperidol and metoclopramide, or serotonin antagonists such as ondansetron.

Urinary retention. Wide variation in the incidence of urinary retention is reported following intrathecal and epidural injection of opioids, occurring most often in young male volunteers.[72] The incidence is reported to be much less after intravenous or intramuscular administration of equivalent doses of opioids.[73,74]

The mechanism of urinary retention following intrathecal and epidural administration of opioids is believed to be related to their effect on the opioid receptors in the sacral spinal cord, which promotes inhibition of sacral parasympathetic outflow, causing detrusor muscle relaxation and increase in bladder capacity. This effect of epidural morphine in humans has been reversed with naloxone.[75]

Respiratory depression. Clinically significant respiratory depression (defined as that requiring intervention) following intrathecal or epidural opioids is reported to be around 1%, which is similar to the incidence following conventional intravenous or intramuscular injections.[76,77] It has been reported to occur early (within 15 minutes) or late (after several hours) following administration of any opioid, either through the epidural or intrathecal route. High or repeated doses of opioids, advanced age, additional IV sedation, and thoracic placement are some of the factors that increase the risk of respiratory depression.

Early respiratory depression, defined as occurring within less than 2 hours after administration of an opioid, occurs mostly after epidural administration of fentanyl or sufentanil, and rarely after intrathecal fentanyl or sufentanil.[78,79,80,81] It is likely that respiratory depression after epidural fentanyl or sufentanil results from systemic absorption of these opioids, since their plasma concentration is proportional to the magnitude of respiratory depression.[82] Absorption into the CSF and cephalad migration of the opioid may be another explanation.

Delayed respiratory depression occurs more than 2 hours after injection of the opioid. This effect is seen with epidural and intrathecal morphine, but never reported with single injection of fentanyl or sufentanil, although continuous infusion of sufentanil has been associated with delayed respiratory effects.[83] Delayed respiratory depression is thought to result from cephalad migration of opioids in the CSF and interaction with opioid receptors in the ventral medulla.[84]

Other agents

Aside from conventional agents such as local anesthetics and opioids that have been used for epidural pain management, there has been intense research in discovering new medications, which could provide analgesia by themselves or could potentiate the effect of already existing agents. For the clinician in the trauma setting potentially useful medications are clonidine and tramadol.

Clonidine traditionally has been used as an antihypertensive medicine. It is an α_2-adrenergic agonist. It was recently approved for epidural use in the USA. Although it had been used in Europe and other places, it was not available in the USA in an injectable form which could be administered epidurally. Clonidine's mechanism of actions for analgesia seems to be mediated by cholinergic activation.[85] Intraspinal clonidine produces analgesia through α_2-stimulation causing spinal acetylcholine, norepinephrine, and nitric oxide release in various animals.[86] There have been a number of different human studies that have shown the analgesic property of clonidine once given epidurally. It has been used in a variety of situations such as in the management of intractable cancer and neuropathic pain, as well as in the operating room for anesthesia and analgesia.[87] De Kock et al showed that clonidine can even be used as the sole analgesic agent during and after abdominal surgery.[88]

Most studies, however, have shown its effect as an adjunct to either local anesthetics or opioids.[89,90] It is evident that clonidine can significantly potentiate the analgesic action of narcotics and can play an important role in combination with local anesthetics.

Conflicting reports exist concerning side effects; however, there seem to be more significant hemodynamic effects associated with clonidine than with opioids, and this appears to be a dose-dependent phenomenon.[90] This usually manifests as hypotension. Use of this agent in the acute perioperative setting still needs to be defined, especially in the acute trauma setting. Even though, it is an analgesic substance in the epidural space, its use in trauma patients may be troublesome. These patients often suffer from intravascular volume depletion secondary to hemorrhage and may remain hypovolemic even in the postoperative period; therefore, it should be used with caution. This same warning is true for local anesthetics as well, since they can also produce adverse hemodynamic effects.

Tramadol, at this date is still not approved by the FDA for epidural use, and is not yet available in injectable form in the USA. However, it has been used epidurally in Europe. Tramadol is a centrally-acting synthetic analgesic. Its mechanism of action appears to occur in two separate areas. It is a very weak μ-agonist, about 6000 times less than morphine, and at the same time, it inhibits reuptake of norepinephrine and serotonin leading to an increase in central synaptic levels of the above neurotransmitters.[91,92] There have been a number of studies in which tramadol was administered epidurally for abdominal and orthopedic procedures and postoperative pain management, but there are conflicting reports on the degree of analgesia achieved.[93,94] In at least one study, the incidence of nausea was higher in the tramadol patient group when 100 mg of tramadol was administered compared to the opioid group.[95]

DOSAGES

As with any other form of treatment, the goals for therapy should be established at the outset. These would include:

1. Providing adequate pain relief for increasing patient comfort and functionality
2. Avoiding side effects as much as possible.

The agents previously described can be utilized in combination or by themselves when indicated. The reason for administering various combinations or 'cocktails' is to maximize the advantages of the agents while at the same time decreasing possible side effects associated with these drugs. This can be achieved by taking advantage of the synergy of pain relief among these agents since the mechanism of action for each agent is different. Before administering any drugs, one must consider a number of very important parameters. Even though, a good number of patients can benefit from more or less the same dosing regimens, a 'cookbook' approach can be extremely hazardous. Many variables such as age, coexisting medical conditions, and drug interactions must be taken into account. The numbers and doses provided below and in other parts of this chapter are based on experiences in our institution, and the assumption that patients are otherwise healthy with no other specific contraindication unless otherwise stated.

In single-dosing regimens, local anesthetics are almost exclusively used for operating room analgesia and anesthesia. Therefore, only opioids are emphasized in the tables below (Tables 12.3, 12.4 & 12.5). Local anesthetics will be discussed in combination protocols.

OTHER AGENTS

Clonidine

Onset of action has been described in minutes and duration of action of 6 to 15 hours. Dosing is variable around 50–250 microg.[96,97]

Tramadol

Tramadol is not FDA-approved for use in neuroaxial injections in the USA. Doses of 50–150 mg with duration of action of 6 to 9 hours have been reported.[93,95]

CONTINUOUS EPIDURAL PROTOCOLS

Various medication solutions and protocols are employed for epidural pain control. We base these on our own experiences unless it is otherwise specified. These protocols are merely guidelines, and

Table 12.3 Common epidurally-administered opioids – lower doses should be selected for thoracic epidurals and elderly patients

	Morphine	Fentanyl	Sufentanil	Hydromorphone	Meperidine
Dose	1–5 mg	25–150 microg	10–40 microg	0.5–1.5 mg	25–100 mg
Onset (min)	30–60	5–15	5–15	15–30	10–30
Duration (h)	6–20	2–4	2–4	6–15	4–8

Table 12.4 Common spinally-administered opioids

	Morphine	Fentanyl	Sufentanil
Dose	0.1–0.6 mg	10–25 microg	5–15 microg
Onset (min)	10–30	2–5	2–5
Duration (h)	6–20	2–4	2–4

Table 12.5 Common pediatric single-shot dosing

	Morphine	Fentanyl	Bupivacaine (0.25% with epinephrine 1:200 000)
Dose	30–50 microg/kg	0.5–1.0 microg/kg	0.5–1.0 mL/kg or 0.05 mL/kg/dermatome

clinicians are encouraged to adapt these based on their specific patient population and the nature of their patients' injuries. Overall, the best side effect profile is achieved by combining local anesthetics and opioids in order to minimize the total dose of each drug and maximize their analgesic properties. In general, relatively higher concentrations of local anesthetics are utilized in thoracic catheters where the incidence of motor block interfering with patients' activity is minimal when compared with medications administered in the lumbar region. Placement of the catheter tip as close to the affected dermatomes as possible is of importance in decreasing the amount of drug required. This is especially helpful in thoracic surgery (e.g. pneumonectomy) where one is faced with a patient who could be very sensitive to the respiratory depressant effects of the opioids as well as to the sympathectomy generated by the local anesthetics.

For patients who are intolerant of the side effects of opioids or local anesthetics, we use single agent solutions. Usually, for thoracic catheters, morphine 0.05 mg/mL or bupivacaine 0.125% is used depending on the nature of the side effect, be it respiratory depression, intractable nausea, pruritus, or hypotension. For lumbar catheters, morphine 0.1 mg/mL is administered.

As is the case with IV-PCA, epidural application of this principle has been quite successful. The goal here is to empower the patient to control the pain by providing a programmable infusion pump. PCEA can be a very effective means of managing a patient's complex pain problems.

The values presented in these tables are only suggestions. Dosing regimens are to be chosen according to individual patient needs. We also recommend a loading bolus for these catheters. This should be based on the type of agent, dose,

Table 12.6 Common combinations for epidural analgesia in postoperative patients

Opioid	Morphine 0.05 mg/mL	Morphine 0.05 mg/mL	Fentanyl 3 microg/mL	Fentanyl 5 microg/mL	Sufentanil 2 microg/mL	Hydromorphone 20 microg/mL	Hydromorphone 40 microg/mL
Local anesthetic* (*bupivacaine*)	0.125%	0.0625%	0.125%	0.0625%	0.125%	0.125%	0.0625%

*Ropivacaine 0.1–0.2% can be substituted for bupivacaine 0.0625% and 0.125% respectively.

Table 12.7 Patient-controlled epidural analgesia guidelines

	Solution	Dose (mL)	Time interval (min)	Basal rate (mL)	Hourly limit (mL)
Thoracic	Morphine 0.05 mg/mL Bupivacaine 0.125%	2–3	15–30	3–5	7–11
	Fentanyl 3 microg/mL Bupivacaine 0.125%	2–3	10–15	3–5	7–11
	Sufentanil 2 microg/mL Bupivacaine 0.125%	2–3	10–15	3–5	7–11
	Hydromorphone 20 microg/mL Bupivacaine 0.125%	2–3	20–30	3–5	5–11
	Morphine 0.05 mg/mL*	2–3	15–30	3–6	5–12
	Bupivacaine 0.125%*	2–3	20–30	3–6	7–12
Lumbar	Morphine 0.05 mg/mL Bupivacaine 0.0625%	3–4	15–30	5–7	8–15
	Fentanyl 3–5 microg/mL Bupivacaine 0.0625%	3–4	10–15	5–7	8–15
	Hydromorphone 20 microg/mL Bupivacaine 0.0625%	3–4	15–20	5–7	8–15
	Morphine 0.1 mg/mL* *or* Hydromorphone 40 microg/mL*	1–2	20–30 15–20	1–4	2–4

*Single agent solutions for patients intolerant to side effects of opioids or local anesthetics.

Table 12.8 Pediatric caudal epidural infusion

Solution	Rate
Bupivacaine 0.1% Fentanyl 2 microg/kg	0.2–0.5 mL/kg/h
Bupivacaine 0.1% Morphine 0.02 mg/mL	0.2–0.5 mL/kg/h

and timing of anesthetics given in the operating room. Generally, we recommend a loading bolus of 1–1.5 mL per dermatome in the lumbar area and 0.5–1.0 mL per dermatome in the thoracic area, if the catheter had not been in use previously during surgery.

ADVANTAGES AND DISADVANTAGES OF EPIDURAL ANALGESIA

The following is a list of benefits of epidural techniques for pain control compared to other modalities. Epidural infusions can be managed safely in postsurgical general wards with minimal complications, provided appropriate monitoring proto-

cols are followed.[55,98] The disadvantages of epidural analgesia are related to its requirement of technical training and monitoring, which in many institutions may not be readily available (Table 12.9).

EFFECTS AND COMPLICATIONS OF EPIDURAL ANALGESIA

Respiratory effects

With high thoracic levels of epidural anesthesia, paralysis of intercostal and abdominal muscles are accompanied by a feeling of suffocation and breathing difficulty, loss of sensation, and even paralysis in the upper extremities. This can create significant anxiety in a patient, especially if the possibility is not explained beforehand. Occasionally the patient is unable to talk because of inability to move air adequately, and the combination of anxiety and the cardiovascular effects of the epidural anesthetic may cause loss of consciousness. If respiration is inadequate, mask ventilation or intubation may become necessary until the level of anesthesia recedes.

Table 12.9 Advantages and disadvantages of epidural analgesia

Advantages

Superior analgesia in sacral, lumbar, and thoracic dermatomes compared to other analgesic modalities[20,98]
Decreased ICU utilization, and potential for 'fast-tracking' because of decrease in pain-mediated stress response[7,125,126]
Aid in change of dressing for major open wounds, burns, etc.
Smoother transition between the OR and ICU (e.g. debridements, dressing changes, staged surgeries)
Aid in physical therapy and rehabilitation, and early restoration of function[94,127]
Improvement of the graft survival, decrease in intraoperative blood loss, and incidence of postoperative deep vein thrombosis[128]
Decrease in the incidence of postoperative ileus[18]
Shortening of hospitalization period[129]
Improved postoperative pulmonary outcome[10,14]
Slower onset of hemodynamic changes compared to spinal anesthesia
Decreased need for intubation and mechanical ventilation in thoracic wall injury (e.g. flail chest), especially in elderly patients

Disadvantages

Failure rate significant even after placement with good technique: catheter migration, partial analgesia coverage of the surgical area, etc.
Requirement for skilled anesthesiologist for insertion of catheter
Requirement for around-the-clock availability of skilled anesthesiology staff for trouble-shooting, maintenance: bolusing, running infusions, and management of side effects, etc.
Potential for side effects: delayed gastric emptying, nausea, vomiting, and urinary retention[75,130,131]
Potential for masking of serious surgical complications postoperatively because of superior pain control (e.g. pain of ischemia in the leg secondary to graft occlusion or compartment syndrome)[132]
Inability to provide adequate analgesia for head and neck injuries
Cost of expensive equipment, monitoring and personnel

ICU, intensive care unit; OR, operating room.

Circulatory effects

Hypotension is the most common circulatory effect of epidural anesthetics, and its magnitude is directly proportional to the level of sympathetic blockade. This effect is aggravated by reduced blood volume and upright posture.

Systemic vascular tone is maintained by the sympathetic nervous system, and interruption of the sympathetic outflow by epidural anesthesia accounts for the decrease in systemic vascular resistance. In addition, systemic venous dilatation and pooling decreases venous return to the right side of the heart, resulting in decrease in cardiac output and contractility. Interruption of sympathetic outflow functionally inactivates the baroreceptor reflex and cardiac accelerators, with resultant significant bradycardia. Paralysis of the intercostal muscles can result in shallow breathing, and a decrease in negative intrathoracic pressure, contributing to hypotension by decreasing venous return.

Urinary retention

Micturition is a result of coordinated action of the detrusor muscle, the trigone, and the urethral sphincter, which are controlled by a balance of sympathetic (relaxation of the detrusor and contraction of the sphincter) and parasympathetic (contraction of the detrusor and relaxation of the sphincter) nervous system. Neuroaxial block has frequently been associated with a high incidence of postoperative urinary retention.

Gastrointestinal effects

Interruption of the sympathetic outflow to the intestines favors parasympathetic tone with resultant hyperactive peristalsis and sphincter relaxation, frequently leading to bowel and colostomy movement. Theoretically, hyperactive peristalsis can lead to perforation in patients with intestinal obstruction. In fact, the incidence of colonic anastomotic dehiscence was reduced with epidural blockade, especially when epidural analgesia was continued postoperatively.[99] Although a welcome observation, the explanation for it is not clear.

Nausea and vomiting, on the other hand, have been reported to occur in 13–42% of patients during spinal anesthesia.[100]

The complications of the epidural blockade and catheter placement can be immediate or late, appearing hours or even days after the procedure. Fortunately, adverse effects are rare. The majority of the serious complications can be avoided by adhering to the safe techniques of performing the blockade, and when diagnosed promptly, can be quickly treated without permanent consequences.

Neurologic sequelae

Transient or permanent neurologic deficits are reported to be very rare (Table 12.10). The value of documenting any pre-existing neurologic deficits, especially in the trauma patient, cannot be overemphasized. In addition, any motor deficit that evolves while the patient has an indwelling epidural catheter should be investigated fully before attributing it to the epidural local anesthetic infusion.[101]

Mechanical trauma can be immediate, caused by the needle or catheter injuring a nerve root during placement. The patient immediately complains of a sharp, 'electric shock' type of shooting pain to the lower extremity, confined to a distinct dermatome, upon insertion of the catheter or injection of the drug. Depending on the extent of the trauma, the patient may complain of numbness or pain, which in the majority of the cases resolves within a few weeks.

Epidural hematoma formation with cord compromise is a complication with bleak outcome if not recognized and treated early. Although spontaneous hematoma formation has been reported in the literature, especially in patients on anticoag-

Table 12.10 Complications after lumbar and thoracic epidural block

	No. of cases	Complications (%)
Dural puncture	43152	1090 (2.5)
Accidental total spinal anesthesia	48297	102 (0.2)
Blood vessel puncture	6578	189 (2.8)
Toxic reaction	66366	144 (0.2)
Massive subdural anesthesia	16644	28 (0.1)
Severe hypotension	42900	797 (1.8)
Backache	9107	185 (2.0)
Transient paralysis	32718	48 (0.1)
Permanent paralysis	32718	7 (0.02)

Reproduced from Dawkins CJM[133]

ulation therapy, the presence of the epidural catheter can almost always be implicated as the cause.[102,103,104] Puncture of epidural vessels during placement of epidural catheters occurs in 3 to 12% of the cases with asymptomatic hematoma; symptomatic hematoma formation is a very rare event.[105] Symptoms develop relatively early, with progressive weakness and sensory deficits. Prompt recognition of the condition and diagnosis with computerized tomography (CT) or magnetic resonance imaging (MRI), followed by decompressive laminectomy is the key to avoiding permanent neurologic deficits and their sequelae.[103] Infections resulting from epidural catheters causing epidural abscess, on the other hand, may take several days to produce symptoms.[106] Diagnosis is by CT or MRI and the treatment involves laminectomy and decompression, drainage, and long-term IV antibiotics.[107]

Anterior spinal artery syndrome is a poorly understood and fortunately rare vascular complication, which causes a rapid, painless paralysis. Severe hypotension has been implicated as a significant contributing cause.

Local anesthetic toxicity

The epidural space contains large venous plexuses made up of fragile, thin-walled veins. Occasionally the epidural needle may puncture these veins, but more commonly they are entered by the epidural catheter, which can happen upon the initial threading of the catheter through the needle, or hours or days later during the course of epidural infusion. Failure of recovery of blood upon aspiration of the catheter does not necessarily mean that the catheter is extravascular, since aspiration may collapse the vein and fail to recover blood. Giving a test dose containing epinephrine is a reliable way to minimize the risk of intravascular injection of a large dose of local anesthetic.

Once in the epidural space, drugs are readily absorbed into the systemic circulation. This absorption is much slower than intravascular injection and the incidence of toxic reactions is rare. The addition of epinephrine makes the systemic absorption even slower. The earliest signs of toxicity after intravascular injection are related to the CNS. These include lightheadedness, dizziness, a metallic taste in the mouth, perioral numbness, slurred speech, and tinnitus. Higher doses will cause loss of consciousness and grand mal epilep-

tiform convulsions. Treatment consists of halting the injection, protecting the airway and, hyperventilating with 100% O_2. Diazepam and thiopental are indicated if the seizure episode persists.

Epidural infusions of relatively high concentrations of bupivacaine at the lumbar level are associated with high incidence (37–80%) of motor and autonomic blockade, including hypotension, urinary retention, pressure necrosis, and delayed ambulation.[108] Thoracic epidural catheters for postoperative analgesia have been associated with lower incidence of complications (2.5%) compared to lumbar catheters (20%).[109] This is presumably because of the segmental nature of the block that is limited to the thoracic area, with relatively little effect on the lumbar and sacral dermatomes, thus allowing compensatory vasoconstriction in these areas to maintain the blood pressure.

Accidental subarachnoid injection

Epidural block typically requires large doses of local anesthetics compared to subarachnoid block; therefore an accidental subarachnoid injection of a large dose will result in a total spinal block. Even properly-placed epidural catheters have been reported to 'migrate' intrathecally. A reliable way to avoid a massive intrathecal injection of local anesthetic is aspiration of the catheter each time an injection is made. The proper use of a test dose, and careful titration of the dose are also very important.

Signs and symptoms of total spinal block include paralysis of the diaphragm if the C3, C4, and C5 segments are affected. This, combined with the paralysis of the intercostal muscles, can result in respiratory arrest. Total sympathectomy and blockade of cardiac accelerator fibers can result in cardiovascular collapse. If the local anesthetic enters the cranium through the foramen magnum, cranial nerves are affected resulting in a 'total spinal' block.

Management includes endotracheal intubation and positive pressure ventilation as well as support of the cardiovascular system with pressors until the effect of the local anesthetic dissipates.

Post-dural puncture headache

Accidental dural puncture is the most common complication of epidural anesthesia occurring in 0.16 to 1.3% of attempted blockades. It is postulated that PDPH results from decreased CSF pressure when the dura is punctured and CSF leaks out. The decreased CSF pressure causes 'sagging' of the cranial nerves and stretching of the pain-sensitive structures in the cranium, which is made worse by erect posture. Compensatory vasodilatation of intracranial blood vessels to restore intracranial volume is also postulated, adding a vascular component to the PDPH.

The headache is frontal or occipital, and accompanied by other stigmata such as nausea, photophobia, diplopia, and tinnitus. A characteristic finding is that the headache is worsened by the erect position and lessened by the horizontal position. It can start immediately upon puncturing the dura, or may start 24 to 72 hours later. Some of the factors associated with PDPH are summarized in Table 12.11.

Treatment of PDPH includes:

- analgesics, hydration
- intravenous or oral caffeine
- epidural infusion of saline if the catheter is still in place
- oral or subcutaneous sumatriptan
- epidural blood patch.

Table 12.11 Relation of age, sex, and needle gauge used for lumbar puncture to incidence of post dural puncture headache[134]

Factors	No. of spinal anesthetics	No. of headaches	%
Sex			
Male	4063	302	7
Female	5214	709	14
Vaginal delivery	938	300	22
Other procedures	4276	489	12
Totals	9277	1011	11
Age (years)			
10–19	537	51	10
20–29	1994	321	16
30–39	1833	261	14
40–49	1759	192	11
50–59	1736	133	8
60–69	1094	45	4
70–79	297	7	2
80–89	27	1	3
Totals	9277	1011	11
Needle gauge			
16	839	151	18
19	154	16	10
20	2698	377	14
22	4952	430	9
24	634	37	6

Most of the PDPH cases resolve spontaneously within 2 weeks without therapy. In severe cases where patients are unable to sit in bed long enough to eat, therapy is indicated. Conservative therapy with intravenous infusion of 500 mg of caffeine sodium benzoate in 1 L of Ringer's lactate solution, followed by another liter has offered significant improvement in 80% of patients with PDPH.[110] Epidural infusion of saline requires infusion of 150–250 mL/h for at least 24 hours to be effective.[111] Subcutaneous sumatriptan is reported to be effective in aborting the PDPH. A dose of 6 mg given subcutaneously seems to have been effective in a small number of patients. Contraindications include angina and coronary artery disease since it may cause vasospasm in the coronary bed. Finally, epidural blood patch relieves PDPH in 96% of the patients on the first injection, but some may need a second or even a third injection. The epidural needle is placed a space above or below the presumed dural puncture level. In a sterile fashion, the skin is prepared aseptically and 15–20 mL of blood is drawn from the patient. This volume is injected over 20 to 30 seconds into the epidural space, and the needle is withdrawn. Most patients report immediate relief. Occasionally pressure sensation, back pain, neck pain, or radiculopathy is reported. The patient is kept in the supine position for an hour and in relative bed rest for an additional few hours. Prophylactic blood patching after unintentional dural puncture has been evaluated, but the available data concerning the efficacy of this approach are mixed.[112]

COMPLICATIONS OF SPINAL ANESTHESIA

Most of the complications of spinal anesthesia result from its exaggerated physiologic effects; chemical effects of the local anesthetics used, and isolated nerve injuries.

Hypotension

This is the most common complication of spinal anesthesia, resulting from widespread sympathetic blockade. It is due to decreased venous return because of vasodilatation and venous pooling, with secondary decrease in heart rate and cardiac output. This complication can be minimized or avoided by prehydrating the patient with

500–1000 mL of crystalloid prior to induction of spinal anesthesia, and positioning the patient supine with the lower extremities elevated slightly to increase the venous return and cardiac output.

When fluid resuscitation does not maintain the blood pressure at an acceptable level, a vasoconstrictor is used. A mixed α- and β-receptor agonist like ephedrine is preferred over a pure α-agonist like phenylephrine, because the latter can cause reflex bradycardia secondary to vasoconstriction, whereas the mixed agonist can also increase the heart rate by its beta action. Also, in most cases, the problem is not a significant reduction of the systemic vascular resistance, but it is decreased venous return.

Extensive spread of spinal anesthesia – the 'total' spinal

This occurs shortly after induction of spinal anesthesia. The signs and symptoms include apprehension, anxiety, agitation, hypotension, nausea and vomiting, respiratory depression leading to apnea (phrenic nerve paralysis), and loss of consciousness. Treatment includes control of the airway, oxygenation, ventilation, and support of blood pressure. Intubation may be necessary to prevent aspiration. Usually, the period of 'total' spinal is brief, and the respiration returns quickly to normal.

Nausea and vomiting

Nausea and vomiting are reported to occur frequently in patients undergoing spinal anesthesia. It may be the warning sign of a significant hypotension causing cerebral hypoxia; therefore, while starting O_2 therapy, hypotension should be treated. Other causes of nausea and vomiting such as vasovagal reflex and opioids should be sought and treated.

Backache

Backache after spinal anesthesia could result from periosteal trauma, muscular hematoma, ligamental strain because of profound muscle relaxation, or reflex muscle spasm. Although the overall incidence is reported to be up to 50%, only 3% of patients characterize the pain as severe.[113] It usually resolves within a few days with conservative therapy. Neurologic exam is performed to rule out

neurologic damage. Therapy includes reassurance, rest, oral muscle relaxants, or trigger point injections if necessary.

The 'failed' spinal

When the spinal anesthesia fails to provide adequate operating conditions for the planned surgical procedure, the anesthetic is labeled 'failed'. Even with adequate sensory block, some patients are unable to tolerate the procedure, in which case a little sedation may provide adequate relief. Occasionally, the anesthetic agent fails to provide a dermatomal level high enough for the planned procedure despite adequate dose of anesthetic used. Finally, the anesthetic agents may be injected into the subdural space thus resulting in a failed block. Admittedly, despite free flow of CSF prior to and after injection of the anesthetic, sometimes the block never sets. The reason for this is not totally clear.

The anesthetic choices at that point depend on the procedure planned. Options vary between repeating the spinal block, supplementing it with sedation (propofol, midazolam, ketamine), or to switch to general anesthesia.

Major neurologic sequelae

Major neurologic sequelae following spinal anesthesia are extremely rare. A review of neurologic sequelae after spinal anesthesia in 65 000 patients revealed 31 cases of neurologic deficit, 12 of which were exacerbations of pre-existing neurologic disease.[114] Some of the causes of neurologic damage after spinal anesthesia include:

- Trauma from lumbar puncture especially when multiple attempts are made
- Chemical or bacterial contamination of the injectate: with the use of disposable kits and following strict asepsis, this is virtually eliminated
- Toxic reactions to the local anesthetic: the only local anesthetic currently implicated as possibly neurotoxic is 5% preparation of lidocaine in 7.5% dextrose – cases ranging from transient monoradiculopathy to cauda equina syndrome have been reported, both with single and continuous injections
- Subarachnoid hemorrhage and expanding hematoma in patients on anticoagulants are exceedingly rare.[115]
- Spinal cord ischemia: extremely rare.

SPECIAL SITUATIONS

Patients on anticoagulation therapy

A patient who is fully anticoagulated is a contraindication to epidural catheter placement, because of the significant risk of epidural hematoma after a traumatic placement or migration of the catheter. Permanent paraplegia from epidural hematomas has occurred as a result of epidural catheter placement.[116] There are no well-controlled, randomized, prospective studies that have been performed to find an association or quantitate the incidence of epidural hematoma in anticoagulated patients. There are reports of epidural hematomas in patients with epidural catheters not receiving anticoagulation,[105] as well as reports of spontaneous hematomas in anticoagulated patients but without epidural catheters.[117] Epidural blockade has been performed in patients who were previously anticoagulated for vascular surgery without neurologic sequelae. Conversely, patients with epidural catheters who were subsequently anticoagulated intraoperatively did not produce any epidural hematoma postoperatively.[118] No epidural hematoma was detected in a group of 459 patients on oral anticoagulant and antiplatelet medications with a mean prothrombin time (PT) value of 14.1 ± 3.2 sec on the day of epidural catheter removal.[119] The decision to place an epidural catheter in a specific patient should therefore take into consideration the possible risks and benefits for that patient. In general, for postoperative epidural catheter placement, any PT value of less then 14 sec, activated partial thromboplastin time (aPTT) value of less than 36 sec, with a platelet count of $80\,000/mm^3$ would be acceptable. This is true as long as these values are not part of a downward trend (i.e. PT, aPTT increasing, and platelets decreasing) because of a variety of pathological conditions, such as leukemias, circulating antibodies against coagulation factors, disseminated intravascular coagulation etc.

Another situation where epidural catheter placement poses a potential problem is postoperative low dose heparin or low molecular weight heparin (LMWH) for prophylaxis of deep vein thrombosis and pulmonary embolism.

Wildsmith & McClure suggested some sensible guidelines for the use of epidural analgesia in these situations:[120]

- Epidural anesthesia is to be avoided in patients who are fully anticoagulated with warfarin or heparin, or who have had thrombolytic therapy.
- Avoid placement of epidural catheters in patients on low-dose heparin within 4 to 6 hours of subcutaneous administration, because high blood levels of heparin can be seen within 2 hours of subcutaneous administration.
- Intraoperative anticoagulation has been safely done in a large number of patients after epidural catheter placement, but it is advisable to wait 1 hour to initiate heparin therapy after placement of the catheter.
- The timing of epidural catheter removal should be carefully chosen. The catheter should be removed before full anticoagulation with warfarin (1 or 2 days), 3 to 4 hours after discontinuance of heparin infusion, or 1 hour before the next subcutaneous dose.

Since the introduction of the first LMWH – enoxaparin (Lovenox) – into the USA in May 1993, at least 40 cases of spinal hematomas causing neurologic injury were reported, which were associated with LMWH and neuroaxial blocks.[121] In December 1997 the FDA issued a public health advisory about the concurrent use of LMWH and neuroaxial block (US FDA Advisory, December 15, 1997).

Although LMWH has been in clinical use in Europe since 1987, only 11 cases of spinal hematomas associated with neuroaxial block and its use have been reported in the European literature. This low incidence can be attributed in part to the dose and scheduling of LMWH (40 mg once a day compared to 30 mg twice a day as approved by the FDA) and in part to the practice guidelines that have evolved in Europe and are consistently followed.

It is extremely difficult to list detailed and generalized recommendations for the safe placement of epidural catheters in every patient on LMWH and anticoagulation therapy – reviews by Horlocker et al and Vandermeulen et al cover the subject thoroughly.[122,123] The following points are meant to serve as practical guidelines to consider, before exposing the patient to undue risk of spinal hematoma and neurologic injury.

- Patients on LMWH are at risk of developing spinal hematomas and permanent neurologic injuries when they receive spinal or epidural anesthesia, or an epidural catheter for postoperative analgesia.

- The risk of spinal hematoma appears to be higher when nonsteroidal anti-inflammatory drugs or other anticoagulants and antiplatelets are used in conjunction with LMWH, or when the epidural technique is traumatic or repeated.
- Administration of enoxaparin does not result in a true trough in anticoagulant activity when the dosing schedule is twice a day.
- When using for thromboprophylaxis, the smaller dose (40 mg once daily) should be administered, which results in a true trough. This regimen was recently approved by the FDA as an alternate regimen for thromboprophylaxis after total hip arthroplasty.
- If an indwelling epidural catheter must stay, treatment with LMWH should be delayed at least 12 to 24 hours postoperatively.
- Removal of the epidural catheter should be done at the trough of the anticoagulant activity. When following a twice-daily dosing schedule, skipping the evening dose and removing the catheter in the morning should provide a safe condition, without significantly increasing the risk of a thromboembolic event.

Patients with known or suspected history of substance abuse

The patients with a known or suspected history of substance abuse comprise a special population with higher incidence of trauma-related injuries compared to the general population. After the initial resuscitation attempt to salvage life and organ function is successful, the pain management team is consulted for postoperative analgesia issues. This includes withdrawal symptoms, opioid tolerance, or drug-seeking behavior.

Early clinical manifestations of withdrawal are anxiety, irritability, insomnia, sweating, rhinorrhea, lacrimation, yawning, and sneezing, which progress into dilated pupils, tremors, chills, and muscle cramps. After 18 to 24 hours hypertension, tachycardia, tachypnea, fever, nausea, and vomiting become apparent. Treatment of withdrawal is administration of sufficient opioids to reverse the withdrawal. Taking a drug abuse history is necessary, but most of the time it is unreliable.

Although history of substance abuse is a relative contraindication to opioid administration because of the high rate of relapse, when there is a clear origin of acute pain (postoperative, post-traumatic), adequate analgesia is warranted regardless of the patient's history. Priority should be given to non-opioid drugs that can provide the best analgesia. Epidural analgesia can provide superb postoperative pain control without reinforcing drug-seeking behavior.

Epidural infusion of bupivacaine 0.1% with morphine sulfate 0.01% can usually provide adequate postoperative analgesia for thoracic or lumbar regions, at a rate proportional to the number of dermatomes covered. In opioid-tolerant patients, doubling the concentration of morphine will achieve adequate pain control. In patients with severe opioid dependency, replacing morphine with sufentanil 0.002% (2 microg/mL) has achieved successful pain control.[124] If the patient is in a methadone-maintenance program, the same dosage regimen can be continued separately.

Every effort is made to switch to non-opioid analgesics once the epidural and the opioids are discontinued. Drug-seeking behavior should be watched for and dealt with dispassionately. Long-term management of these patients is best handled by multidisciplinary team approach.

CONCLUSION

In this chapter, we have attempted to provide the reader with fundamentals of pain control through neuroaxial interventions. Epidural and spinal techniques have been extensively used for anesthesia purposes worldwide. They also remain as an effective means of pain control in a variety of patients from routine postoperative to the critically ill. As with any other interventional modality, a thorough understanding of the technique, patient selection, indications, contraindications, and complications is mandatory.

Proper use of these pain management techniques could provide superior pain control and patient comfort. It could also increase functionality and decrease morbidity in selected patients. The doses and protocols given throughout the chapter are guidelines only since every patient and treatment situation are unique.

REFERENCES

1. Whipple JK, Lewis KS, Quebbeman EJ, et al. Analysis of pain management in critically ill patients. Pharmacotherapy 1995; 15: 592–599.

2. Follin SL, Charland SL. Acute pain management: operative or medical procedures and trauma. Ann Pharmacothe 1997; 31: 1068–1076.

3. Moller IW, Rem J, Brandt MR, Kehlet H. Effect of posttraumatic epidural analgesia on the cortisol and hyperglycemic response to surgery. Acta Anesth Scand 1982; 26: 56.

4. Ferguson M, Luchette FA. Management of blunt chest injury. Respir Care Clin N Am 1996; 2: 449–466.

5. Mayberry JC, Trunkey DD. The fractured rib in chest wall trauma. Chest Surg Clin N Am 1997; 7: 239–261.

6. Gabram SG, Schwartz RJ, Jacobs LM, et al. Clinical management of blunt trauma patients with unilateral rib fractures. A randomized trial. World J Surg 1995; 19: 388–393.

7. Gaeta RR, Macario A, Brodsky JB, Brock-Utne JG, Mark JB. Pain outcomes after thoracotomy: lumbar epidural hydromorphone versus intrapleural bupivacaine. J Cardiothorac Vasc Anesth 1995; 9: 534–537.

8. Dauphin A, Lubanska-Hubert E, Young JE, Miller JD, Bennett WF, Fuller HD. Comparative study of continuous extrapleural nerve block and lumbar epidural morphine in post-thoracotomy pain. Can J Surg 1997; 40: 431–436.

9. Slinger P, Shennib H, Wilson S. Post-thoracotomy pulmonary function: a comparison of epidural versus intravenous meperidine infusions. J Cardiothorac Vasc Anesth 1995; 9: 128–134.

10. Schultz AM, Werba A, Ulbing S, Gollmann G, Lehofer F. Perioperative thoracic epidural analgesia for thoracotomy. Eur J Anesthesiol 1997; 14: 600–603.

11. Tsui SL, Lee DK, Ng KF, Chan TY, Chan WS, Lo JW. Epidural infusion of bupivacaine 0.0625% plus fentanyl 3.3 mcg/ml provides better postoperative analgesia than patient-controlled analgesia with intravenous morphine after gynecological laparotomy. Anesth Intensive Care 1997; 25: 476–481.

12. Frank E, Sood OP, Torjman M, Mulholland SG, Gomella LG. Postoperative epidural analgesia following retropubic prostatectomy: outcome assessment. J Surg Oncol 1998; 67: 117–120.

13. Jayr C, Thomas H, Rey A. Postoperative pulmonary complications: Epidural analgesia using bupivacaine and opioids versus parenteral opioids. Anesthesiology 1993; 78:666–676.

14. Bellantyne JC, Carr DB, deFerranti S, et al. The comparative effects of postoperative analgesic therapies on pulmonary outcome: cumulative meta-analyses of randomized, controlled trials. Anesth Analg 1998; 86: 598–612.

15. Rawal N, Sjostrand U, Christoffersson E. Comparison of intramuscular and epidural morphine for postoperative analgesia in the grossly obese: Influence on postoperative ambulation and pulmonary function. Anesth Analg 1984; 63: 583–592.

16. de Leon-Casasola OA, Lema MJ, Karabella D, Harrison P. Postoperative myocardial ischemia: epidural versus intravenous patient-controlled analgesia. A pilot project. Reg Anesth 1995; 20: 105–112.

17. Major CP Jr, Greer MS, Russell WL, Roe SM. Postoperative pulmonary complications and morbidity after abdominal aneurysmectomy: a comparison of postoperative epidural versus parenteral opioid analgesia. Am Surg 1996; 62: 45–51.

18. de Leon-Casasola OA, Karabella D, Lema MJ. Bowel function recovery after radical hysterectomies: thoracic epidural bupivacaine–morphine versus intravenous patient-controlled analgesia with morphine. A pilot study. J Clin Anesth 1996; 8: 87–92.

19. Tan PH, Chia YY, Perng JS, Chou AK, Chung HC, Lee CC. Intermittent bolus versus patient-controlled epidural morphine for post-operative analgesia. Acta Anesthesiol Sin 1997; 35: 149–154.

20. Rockemann MG, Seeling W, Goertz AW, Konietzko I, Steffen P, Georgieff M. Effectiveness, side effects, and costs of postoperative pain therapy: intravenous and epidural patient-controlled analgesia. Anasthesiol Intesivmed Notfallmed Schmerzther 1997; 32: 414–419.

21. St Pierre DM. Rehabilitation following arthroscopic surgery. Sports Med 1995; 20: 338–347.

22. Lovstad RZ, Halvorsen P, Raeder JC, Steen PA. Post-operative epidural analgesia with low dose fentanyl, adrenaline and bupivacaine in children after major orthopaedic surgery. A prospective evaluation and side effects. Eur J Anesthesiol 1997; 14: 583–589.

23. Bach S, Noreng MF, Tjellden NU. Phantom limb pain in amputees during the first 12 months following limb amputation, after preoperative lumbar epidural blockade. Pain 1988; 33: 297–301.

24. Nikolajsen L, Ilkjaer S, Christensen JH, Kroner K, Jensen TS. Randomised trial of epidural bupivacaine and morphine in prevention of stump and phantom pain in lower-limb amputation. Lancet 1997; 350(9088): 1353–1357.

25. Bengtsson M, Nettelblad H, Sjoberg F. Extradural catheter-related infections in patients with infected cutaneous wounds. Br J Anesth 1997; 79: 668–670.

26. Grocott HP, Mutch WA. Epidural anesthesia and acutely increased intracranial pressure.

Lumbar epidural space hemodynamics in a porcine model. Anesthesiology 1996; 85: 1086–1091.

27. Kariya N, Oda Y, Yukioka H, Fujimori M. Effective treatment of a man with head injury and multiple rib fractures with epidural analgesia. Masui 1996; 45: 223–226.

28. Bromage PR. Spread of analgesic solution in the epidural space and their site of action: a statistical study. Br J Anesth 1962; 34: 161.

29. Kitahara LM, Kosaka Y, Taub A, et al. Lamina specific suppression of dorsal horn activity by morphine sulfate. Anesthesiology 1974; 41: 39.

30. Duggan AW, Hall JG, Headley PM. Suppression of transmission of nociceptive impulses by morphine: selective effects of morphine administered in the region of substantia gelatinosa. Br J Pharmacol 1977; 61: 65.

31. Yaksh TL, Jessell TM, Gamse R, et al. Intrathecal morphine inhibits substance P release in vivo from mamallian spinal cord. Nature 1980; 286: 155.

32. Lederhaas G. Pediatric pain management. J Fla Med Assoc 1997; 84: 37–40.

33. Tobias JD. Indications and application of epidural anesthesia in pediatric population outside the perioperative period. Clin Pediatr (Phila) 1993; 32: 81–85.

34. Blanco DE, et al. Thoracic epidural anesthesia by the caudal route in pediatric anesthesia: age is a limiting factor. Rev Esp Anestesiol Reanim 1994; 41: 216.

35. Strafford MA, Wilder RT, Berde CB. The risk of infection from epidural analgesia in children: a review of 1620 cases. Anesth Analg 1995; 80: 234–238.

36. Payne KA, Hendrix MR, Wade WJ. Caudal bupivacaine for postoperative analgesia in pediatric lower limb surgery. J Pediatr Surg 1993; 28: 155–157.

37. Lofgren N. Studies on local anesthetics. Xylocaine. A new synthetic drug. Stockholm: Haegggstoms; 1948.

38. Columb MO, Lyons G. Determination of the minimal local analgesic concentrations of epidural bupivacaine and lidocaine in labor. Anesth Analg 1995; 81: 833–837.

39. Rosenberg PH, Kytta J, Alila A. Absorption of bupivacaine, etidocaine, lignocaine, and ropivacaine into n-heptane, rat sciatic nerve, and human extradural and subcutaneous fat. Br J Anaesth 1986; 58: 310–314.

40. Reiz S, Haggmark S, Johansson G, Nath S. Cardiotoxicity of ropivacaine–a new amide local anesthetic agent. Acta Anaesthesiol Scand 1989; 33: 93–98.

41. Scott DB, Lee A, Fagan D, Bowler GMR,

Bloomfield P, Lundh R. Acute toxicity of ropivacaine compared with that of bupivacaine. Anesth Analg 1989; 69: 563–569.

42. Gaiser RR, Venkateswaren P, Cheek TG, et al. Comparison of 0.25% ropivacaine and bupivacaine for epidural analgesia for labor and vaginal delivery. J Clin Anesth 1997; 9: 564–568.

43. Muir H, Writer D, Douglas J, Weeks S, Gambling D, Macarthur A. Double-blind comparison of epidural ropivacaine 0.25% and bupivacaine 0.25% for the relief of childbirth pain. Can J Anaesth 1997; 44: 599–604.

44. Swerdlow M, Jones R. The duration of action of bupivacaine, prilocaine, and lignocaine. Br J Anaesth 1970; 42: 335.

45. Bromage PR. A comparison of the hydrochloride salts of lignocaine and prilocaine for epidural analgesia. Br J Anaesth 1965; 37: 753.

46. Keir L. Continuous epidural analgesia in prostatectomy: comparison of bupivacaine with or without adrenaline. Acta Anesthesiol Scand 1974; 18: 1.

47. Eisenach JC, Grice SC, Dewan DM. Epinephrine enhances analgesia produced by epidural bupivacaine during labor. Anesth Analg 1987; 66: 447–451.

48. Baron CM, et al. Epinephrine decreases postoperative requirements for continuous thoracic epidural fentanyl. Anesth Analg 1996; 82: 760–765.

49. Huang KS, et al. Influence of epinephrine as an adjuvant to epidural morphine for postoperative analgesia. Ma Tsui Hsueh Tsa Chi 1993; 31: 245–248.

50. Bernards CM, Hill HF. Physical and chemical properties of drug molecules governing their diffusion through the spinal meninges. Anesthesiology 1992; 77: 750–756.

51. Torda TA, Pybus DA. A comparison of four opiates for epidural analgesia. Br J Anesth 1982; 54: 291–295.

52. Bromage PR, Camporesi EM, Durant PAC, Nielsen CH. Rostral spread of epidural morphine. Anesthesiology 1982; 56: 431–436.

53. Ready LB, Loper KA, Nessly M, Wild L. Postoperative epidural morphine is safe in the surgical ward. Anesthesiology 1991; 75: 452–456.

54. de Leon-Casasola OA, Parker B, Lema MJ, et al. Postoperative epidural bupivacaine–morphine therapy. Experience with 4227 surgical cancer patients. Anesthesiology 1994; 81: 368–371.

55. Scott DA, Beilby DS, McClymont C. Postoperative analgesia using epidural infusions of fentanyl with bupivacaine. A prospective analysis of 1014 patients. Anesthesiology 1995; 83: 727–737.

56. Chaplan SR, Duncan SR, Brodsky JB, Brose W.

Morphine and hydromorphone epidural analgesia. Anesthesiology 1992; 77: 1090–1094.

57. Reisine T, Pasternak G. Opioid analgesics and antagonists. In: Hardman JG, Limbird LE, eds. Goodman and Gilman's The pharmacological basis of therapeutics. 9th ed. New York: McGraw-Hill; 1996: 521–555.

58. Liu S, Carpenter RL, Mulroy MF, et al. Intravenous versus epidural administration of hydromorphone. Effects on analgesia and recovery after radical retropubic prostatectomy. Anesthesiology 1995; 82: 682–688.

59. Brose WG, Tanelian DL, Brodsky JB, et al. CSF and blood pharmacokinetics of hydromorphone and morphine following lumbar epidural administration. Pain 1991; 45: 11–15.

60. Mather LE. Clinical pharmacokinetics of fentanyl and its newer derivatives. Clin Pharmacokinet 1983; 8: 422–446.

61. Glass PSA, Estok P, Ginsberg B, et al. Use of patient-controlled analgesia to compare the efficacy of epidural to intravenous fentanyl administration. Anesth Analg 1992; 74: 345–351.

62. Sandler AN, Stringer D, Panos L, et al. A randomized double blind comparison of lumbar epidural and intravenous fentanyl infusions for post thoracotomy pain relief. Anesthesiology 1992; 77: 626–634.

63. Guinard J-P, Mavrocordatos P, Chiolero R, Carpenter RL. A randomized comparsion of intravenous versus lumbar and thoracic epidural fentanyl for analgesia after thoracotomy. Anesthesiology 1992; 77: 1108–1115.

64. Salomaki TE, Laitinen JO, Nuutinen LS. A randomized double blind comparison of epidural versus intravenous fentanyl infusion for analgesia after thoracotomy. Anesthesiology 1991; 75: 790–795.

65. Geller E, Chrubasik J, Graf R, et al. A randomized double-blind comparison of epidural sufentanil versus intravenous sufentanil or epidural fentanyl analgesia after major abdominal surgery. Anesth Analg 1993; 76: 1243–1250.

66. de Leon-Casasola OA, Lema MJ. Epidural sufentanil for acute pain control in a patient with extreme opioid dependency. Anesthesiology 1992; 76: 853–856.

67. de Leon-Casasola OA, Lema MJ. Epidural bupivacaine/sufentanil therapy for postoperative pain control in patients tolerant and unresponsive to epidural bupivacaine/morphine. Anesthesiology 1993; 80: 303–309.

68. Mjaneger E, Yaksh TL. Characteristics of dose-dependent antagonism by beta-funaltrexamine of the antinociceptive effect of intrathecal mu agonists. J Pharmacol Exp Ther 1991; 258: 544–550.

69. Stevens CW, Yaksh TL. Potency of spinal antinociceptive agents is inversely related to magnitude of tolerance after continuous infusion. J Pharmacol Exp Ther 1989; 250: 1–8.

70. Camu F, Debucquoy F. Alfentanil infusion for postoperative pain: a comparison of epidural and intravenous routes. Anesthesiology 1991; 75: 171–178.

71. Loper KA, Ready LB, Dorman BH. Prophylactic transdermal scopolamine patches reduce nausea in postoperative patients receiving epidural morphine. Anesth Analg 1989; 68: 144–146.

72. Bromage PR, Camporesi EM, Durant PAC, Nielsen CH. Nonrespiratory side effects of epidural morphine. Anesth Analg 1982; 61: 490–495.

73. Lanz E, Theiss D, Riess W, Sommer U. Epidural morphine for postoperative analgesia: a double-blind study. Anesth Analg 1982; 61: 236–240.

74. Peterson TK, Husted SE, Rybro L, Shurizek BA, Wernberg M. Urinary retention during IM and extradural morphine analgesia. Br J Anesth 1982; 54: 1175–1178.

75. Rawal N, Möllefors K, Axelsson K, Lingårdh G, Widman B. An experimental study of urodynamic effects of epidural morphine and of naloxone reversal. Anesth Analg 1983; 62: 641–647.

76. Gustafsson LL, Schildt B, Jacobsen K. Adverse effects of extradural and intrathecal opiates: report of a nationwide survey in Sweden. Br J Anaesth 1982; 54: 479–486.

77. Stenseth R, Sellevold O, Breivik H. Epidural morphine for postoperative pain: experience with 1085 patients. Acta Anesthesiol Scand 1985; 29: 148–156.

78. Brockway MS, Noble DW, Sharwood-Smith GH, McClur JH. Profound respiratory depression after extradural fentanyl. Br J Anaesth 1990; 64: 243–245.

79. Hays RL, Palmer CM. Respiratory depression after intrathecal sufentanil during labor. Anesthesiology 1994; 81: 511–512.

80. Palmer CM. Early respiratory depression following intrathecal fentanyl–morphine combination. Anesthesiology 1991; 74: 1153–1155.

81. Steinstra R, Pannekoek BJM. Respiratory arrest following extradural sufentanil. Anesthesia 1993; 48: 1055–1056.

82. Koren G, Sandler AN, Klein J, et al. Relationship between the pharmacokinetics and the analgesic and respiratory pharmacodynamics of epidural sufentanil. Clin Pharmacol Ther 1989; 46: 458–462.

83. Whiting WC, Sandler AN, Lau LC, et al. Analgesic and respiratory effects of epidural sufentanil in patients following thoracotomy. Anesthesiology 1988; 69: 36–43.

84. Shook JE, Watkins WD, Camporesi EM.

Differential roles of opioid receptors in respiration, respiratory disease, and opiate-induced respiratory depression. Am Rev Respir Dis 1990; 142: 895–909.

85. Klimscha W, Tong C, Eisenach JC. Intrathecal alpha 2-adrenergic agonists stimulate acetylcholine and norepinephrine release from the spinal cord dorsal horn in sheep. An in vivo microdialysis study. Anesthesiology 1997; 87: 110–116.

86. Bouaziz H, Hewitt C, Eisenach JC. Subarachnoid neostigmine potentiation of alpha 2-adrenergic agonist analgesia. Reg Anesth 1995; 20: 121–127.

87. Eisenach JC, et al. Epidural clonidine analgesia for intractable cancer pain. The Epidural Clonidine Study Group. Pain 1995; 61: 391–399.

88. De Kock M, et al. Epidural clonidine used as the sole analgesic agent during and after abdominal surgery. A dose-response study. Anesthesiology 1997; 86: 285–292.

89. Capogna G, Celleno D, Zangrillo A, Costantino P, Foresta S. Addition of clonidine to epidural morphine enhances postoperative analgesia after cesarean delivery. Reg Anesth 1995; 20: 57–61.

90. Paech MJ, et al. Postoperative epidural infusion: a randomized 'double-blind' dose-finding trial of clonidine in combination with bupivacaine and fentanyl. Anesth Analg 1997; 84: 1323–1328.

91. Raffa RB. A novel approach to the pharmacology of analgesics. Am J Med 1996; 101: 40S–46S.

92. Dayer P, Desmeules J, Collart L. Pharmacology of tramadol. Drugs 1997; 53 Suppl 2: 18–24.

93. Baraka A, et al. A comparison of epidural tramadol and epidural morphine for postoperative analgesia. Can J Anaesth 1993; 40: 308–313.

94. Grace D, Fee JP. Ineffective analgesia after extradural tramadol hydrochloride in patients undergoing total knee replacement. Anaesthesia 1995; 50: 555–558.

95. Delilkan AE, ViJayan R. Epidural tramadol for postoperative pain relief. Anaesthesia 1993; 48: 328–331.

96. Filos KS, Goudas LC, Patroni O, Polyzou V. Hemodynamic and analgesic profile after intrathecal clonidine in humans. A dose-response study. Anesthesiology 1994; 81: 591–601 (discussion 27A–28A).

97. De Kock M, Famenne F, Deckers G, Scholtes JL. Epidural clonidine or sufentanil for intraoperative and postoperative analgesia. Anesth Analg 1995; 81: 1154–1162.

98. Rygnestad T, Borchgrevink PC, Eide E. Postoperative epidural infusion of morphine and bupivacaine is safe on surgical wards. Organisation of the treatment, effects and side effects in 2000 consecutive patients. Acta Anesthesiol Scand 1997; 41(7): 868–876.

99. Liu SS, Carpenter RC, Mackey DC, et al. Effect of perioperative analgesia technique on rate of recovery after colon surgery. Anesthesiology 1995; 83: 757.

100. Crocker JS, Vandam LD. Concerning nausea and vomiting during spinal anesthesia. Anesthesiology 1959; 20: 578.

101. Kahn L. Neuropathies masquerading as an epidural complication. Can J Anesth 1997; 44: 313–316.

102. Badenhorst CH. Epidural hematoma after epidural pain control and concomitant postoperative anticoagulation. (Letter) Reg Anesth 1996; 21: 272–273.

103. Lovblad KO, Baumgartner RW, Zambaz BD, Remonda L, Ozdoba C, Schroth G. Nontraumatic spinal epidural hematomas. MR features. Acta Radiol 1997 38(1): 8–13.

104. Maingi M, Glynn MF, Scully HE, Graham AF, Floras JS. Spontaneous spinal epidural hematoma in a patient with a mechanical aortic valve taking warfarin. Can J Cardiol 1995; 11: 429–432.

105. Sage DJ. Epidurals, spinals and bleeding disorders in pregnancy: A review. Anaesth Intensive Care 1990; 18: 319–326.

106. Holt HM, Andersen SS, Andersen O, Gahren-Hansen B, Siboni K. Infections following epidural catheterization. J Hosp Infect 1995; 30: 253–260.

107. Danner RL, Hartman BJ. Update on spinal epidural abscess: 35 cases and review of literature. Review of Infectious Disease 1987; 9: 265–274.

108. Conacher ID, Paers MI, Jacobsen L, Philips PD, Heaviside DW. Epidural analgesia following thoracic surgery. Anesthesia 1983; 38: 546–551.

109. Hopf H-B, Weibach B, Peters J. High thoracic segmental epidural anesthesia diminished sympathetic outflow to the legs, despite restriction of sensory blockade to the upper thorax. Anesthesiology 1990; 73: 882–889.

110. Jarvis AP, Greenwalt JW, Fagraeus L. Intravenous caffeine for post dural puncture headache. Reg Anesth 1986; 11: 42.

111. Crawford JS. Prevention of headache consequent on dural puncture. Br J Anesth 1972; 44: 598.

111a. Schwander D, Bachmann F. Heparin and spinal or epidural anesthesia: Decision analysis. Ann Fr Anesth Reanim 1991; 10: 284–296.

112. Neal JM. Management of postdural puncture headache. Anesthesiol Clin North Am 1992; 10: 163.

113. Perz RR, Johnson DL, Shinozaki T. Spinal anesthesia for outpatient surgery. Anesth Analg 1988; 67: S168.

114. Vandam LD, Dripps RD. Exacerbation of pre-existing neurologic disease after spinal anesthesia. N Engl J Med 1956; 255: 843.

115. Eddie L, et al. Spinal subarachnoid hematoma after lumbar puncture and heparinization: a case report, review of literature, and discussion of anesthetic complications. Anesth Analg 1986; 65: 1201.

116. Wille-Jorgensen P, Jorgensen LS, Rasmussen LS. Lumbar regional anesthesia and prophylactic anticoagulant therapy: is the combination safe? Anesthesia 1991; 46: 623–627.

117. Odoom JA, Sih L. Epidural analgesia and antico-agulant therapy. Anesthesia 1983; 38: 254–259.

118. Rao TLK, El-Etr AA. Anticoagulation following placement of epidural and subarachnoid catheters: an evaluation of neurologic sequelae. Anesthesiology 1981; 55: 618–620.

119. Wu CL, Perkins FM. Oral anticoagulant prophy-laxis and epidural catheter removal. Reg Anesth 1996; 21: 517–524.

120. Wildsmith J, McClure JH. Anticoagulant drugs and central nerve blockade. Anesthesia 1991 46: 613–614.

121. Horlocker TT, Wedel DJ. Spinal and epidural blockade and perioperative low molecular weight heparin: Smooth sailing on the Titanic. Anesth Analg 1998; 86: 1153–1156.

122. Horlocker TT, Heit JA. Low molecular weight heparin: Biochemistry, pharmacology, periopera-tive prophylaxis regimens, and guidelines for regional anesthetic management. Anesth Analg 1997; 85: 874–885.

123. Vandermeulen EP, Aken HV, Vermylen J. Anticoagulants and spinal-epidural anesthesia. Anesth Analg 1994; 79: 1165–1177.

124. de Leon-Casasola OA. Postoperative pain man-agement in opioid-tolerant patients. Reg Anesth 1996; 21(6S): 114–116.

125. Kehlet H, Brandt MR, Rem J. Role of neurogenic stimuli in mediating the endocrine-metabolic response to surgery. JPEN 1980; 4: 152.

126. Kehlet H. The endocrine metabolic response to postoperative pain. Acta Anesthesiol Scand Suppl 1982; 74: 173.

127. Bertini L, Tagariello V, Molino FM, Posteraro CM, Mancini S, Rossignoli L. Patient-controlled postoperative analgesia in orthopedic surgery: epidural PCA versus intravenous PCA. Minerva Anesthesiol 1995; 61: 319–328.

128. Cousins MJ, Wright CFJ. Graft, muscle, skin blood flow after epidural block in vascular surgi-cal procedures. Surg Gynec Obstet 1971; 133: 59.

129. Bridenbaugh PO. Anesthesia and influence on hospitalization time. Reg Anesth 1982; 7(suppl): 5151.

130. Pertek JP, Haberer JP. Effects of anesthesia on postoperative micturition and urinary retention. Ann Fr Anesth Reanim 1995; 14(4): 340–351.

131. Thorn SE, Wickbom G, Philipson L, Leissner P, Wattwil M. Myoelectric activity in the stomach and duodenum after epidural administration of morphine or bupivacaine. Acta Anesthesiol Scand 1996; 40:773–778.

132. Price C, Ribeiro J, Kinebrew T. Compartment syndromes associated with epidural analgesia. A case report. J Bone Joint Surg Am 1996; 78: 597–599.

133. Dawkins CJM. Analysis of the complications of extradural and caudal block. Anesthesia 1969; 24: 554.

134. Vandam LD, Dripps RD. Long term follow up of patients who received 10,098 spinal anesthetics, III. Syndrome of decreased intracranial pressure (headache and ocular and auditory difficulties). JAMA 1956; 161: 586.

13

Continuous plexus blocks for the management of trauma to the extremities

Alon P Winnie, Kenneth D Candido and Maria L Torres

Introduction

**The rationale for continuous peripheral nerve
  blocks**
  Technological considerations: peripheral nerve
    stimulators and 'sheathed needles'

**Continuous plexus blocks for trauma of the upper
  extremity**
  Anatomical considerations: the brachial plexus
  Continuous axillary perivascular brachial plexus
    block
  Continuous infraclavicular brachial plexus block
  Continuous subclavian perivascular brachial
    plexus block

Continuous interscalene brachial plexus block
Clinical considerations

**Continuous plexus blocks for trauma of the lower
  extremity**
  Anatomical considerations: the lumbar plexus
  Continuous inguinal paravascular lumbar plexus
    block: the '3-in-1' block
  Continuous sciatic block
  Continuous lumbosacral plexus block
  Continuous psoas compartment block
  Clinical considerations

Summary/conclusion

INTRODUCTION

Much has been learned over the past several decades concerning the pathophysiologic responses to the stress of surgery and the many modalities that can modulate or even abolish them. It is beyond the scope of the present chapter to enumerate and delineate these responses (see Chs 3, 4, and 5), except to indicate that the stress response is a neuroendocrine and metabolic response mediated by the peripheral and central nervous systems.[1] The nociceptive signals to the central nervous system are transmitted primarily by small myelinated (A-δ) and unmyelinated (C) sensory afferent fibers to the substantia gelatinosa in the dorsal horn, with further rostral spread to the ventral-posterior nucleus of the thalamus.[2] Modulation of pain, thus, may occur at many

levels, including midbrain, medulla, and spinal cord, by means of powerful descending inhibitory systems; but the importance of afferent neural stimuli in mediating the stress response has been most widely evaluated in clinical studies using various techniques of neural blockade. Since the endocrine–metabolic response to surgery is initiated primarily by afferent stimuli traveling via somatic and sympathetic pathways, neural blockade with local anesthetic agents should abolish both pain and the stress response by interrupting these pathways,[3–8] and in fact, epidural analgesia with local anesthetic agents has been shown to be particularly effective in abolishing the stress response during and after lower abdominal surgery,[5–8] though it is less effective in upper abdominal surgery, the difference in efficacy presumably being due to the inadequacy of the level of analgesia to inhibit the release of cate-cholamines from the adrenal glands.[9,10] Interestingly, although spinally-administered nar-cotics are effective in eliminating pain after surgi-cal and accidental trauma,[10–12] neither epidural nor intrathecal opiates have been effective in blocking the stress response during and after surgery.[13–17] However, although local anesthetics administered epidurally suppress endocrine and metabolic responses to surgery more than epidu-rally (or even intrathecally) administered nar-cotics, they cannot *completely* reverse the moderate rise of plasma cortisol levels seen immediately after the initiation of surgery.[4,10,18,19]

The vast majority of the studies on the stress response have been carried out during and after elective surgery, and it is well known that the stress response after acute trauma and burn injuries is far greater than that observed after elec-tive surgery. Since many severely traumatized patients are also in much more severe pain than postoperative patients, analgesia itself may pro-vide a greater amelioration of the stress response and a better outcome in the trauma patient than in the postoperative patient. Unfortunately, the available data in trauma patients are insufficient to allow quantitative conclusions to be made; but certainly one can presume that, just as in postop-erative patients, adequate pain control in severely traumatized patients can modify the stress response significantly and undoubtedly improve outcome.

However, there are significant differences in the role of and need for regional analgesia in the severely traumatized patient. Firstly, unlike post-operative patients, severely traumatized patients often need pain relief *prior* to surgery (if surgery is necessary) or definitive treatment of their injuries immediately upon admission to the hospital (or ideally, even before admission), simply to tolerate the diagnostic work-up, i.e. X-rays, computed tomography (CT) scans, MRIs, etc., during which transfer, transportation, and positioning to allow the tests to be performed may be exquisitely painful. Secondly, following certain injuries, anal-gesia may form the basis of the treatment itself, such as in the reduction of a dislocated shoulder or manipulation of a fractured femur. Thirdly, regional anesthesia may allow surgery to be car-ried out for one of a patient's injuries (and mini-mize or abolish the stress response to that surgery) *without* the need for general anesthesia and the

depression of other traumatized vital organ sys-tems, such as a contused heart, lungs, or brain. And finally, regional analgesia and/or anesthesia needs to be continued for a longer period of time in the severely traumatized patient than in the postoperative patient to continue to inhibit stress, to facilitate mobilization, to allow restoration of function, and hopefully, by maintaining sympa-thetic blockade to improve blood flow and pro-mote healing and to prevent the development of post-traumatic pain syndromes. Obviously, anal-gesic therapy of a severely traumatized patient is not a major priority until primary resuscitative measures have been carried out; but all too fre-quently analgesia is ignored completely, even when the patient has been adequately stabilized. It is important for an optimal outcome that as soon as resuscitative measures have been accomplished, attention must focus on pain relief, using tech-niques that are individualized for each patient, depending on the site(s) of injury, so that analge-sia can be accomplished **without** producing side effects which might jeopardize the already impaired function of vital organ systems.

THE RATIONALE FOR CONTINUOUS PERIPHERAL NERVE BLOCKS

The vast majority of experience using regional anesthesia as a modality of pain relief in the post-operative and post-trauma patient has been with epidural and intrathecal local anesthetics, opioids, and adjuncts; but peripheral nerve blocks, partic-ularly **continuous** peripheral nerve blocks, have obvious advantages when appropriate in a given patient: While the use of regional anesthesia in trauma patients avoids the systemic effects of nar-cotics (sedation, nausea and vomiting, etc.), diminishes the stress response, and avoids the problems of a full stomach, hypovolemia is a rela-tive contraindication to the central neural block-ade provided by subarachnoid[20] or epidural anesthesia.[21] Although aggressive volume replen-ishment is mandatory for any trauma patient requiring it, peripheral nerve blocks have the advantage of producing a unilateral, postgan-glionic sympathetic block instead of a bilateral, preganglionic block, thus minimizing the inci-dence of hypotension, even if the patient is not severely hypovolemic (Table 13.1). Similarly, the fact that the sensory and motor blocks are unilat-

Table 13.1 Advantages and benefits of peripheral nerve blocks over spinal and epidural blocks

Advantages	Benefits
Unilateral sensory and motor block	Earlier mobilization and ambulation
Unilateral postganglionic sympathetic block	Lower incidence of hypotension
No parasympathetic block	No urinary retention

eral allows earlier mobilization, ambulation, and restoration of function. And finally, unlike spinal and epidural anesthesia, peripheral blocks do not interfere with bladder control and function. However, in spite of the benefits of peripheral nerve blocks to trauma patients, they are not often fully exploited, either because of the inexperience of those anesthesiologists who participate in the management of trauma patients, or because of the lack of participation of anesthesiologists at all on the trauma team. These techniques certainly deserve wider utilization, since when properly implemented, they usually produce total and long-lasting analgesia with only minimal side effects. Obviously, as with any other analgesic technique, the anesthesiologist administering peripheral blocks to the trauma patient has to limit the total dose of the local anesthetics employed, particularly in patients with compromised cardio-vascular function; and he or she must be aware of the possible serious complications related to some of the techniques and know how to avoid and/or manage them.

The trauma patient usually requires analgesia for a prolonged period of time, yet under certain circumstances, peripheral nerve blocks performed with long-acting local anesthetics may be inappro-priate, e.g. when assessment of limb function (and of pain) is important for diagnostic purposes, such as in compartment syndromes, appropriate appli-cation and/or placement of plaster casts, etc. Thus, for many years a major advantage of spinal or epidural analgesia has been the possibility of uti-lizing continuous techniques by placing a catheter within the epidural or subarachnoid spaces: with a catheter in place short-acting local anesthetics can be utilized by intermittent injections or by contin-uous infusions; but whenever necessary, they can be discontinued long enough to allow necessary diagnostic procedures to be carried out and/or to allow evaluation of possible complications.

Over the past several decades anesthesiologists have come to realize that, at some point in their development and/or distribution, all of the major plexuses (and the nerves derived from them) travel within fascial compartments formed by the fascia of the surrounding muscles. This concept allows placement of catheters within these peri-neural compartments in a manner similar to the placement of epidural and intrathecal catheters. Thus, continuous peripheral blocks are not only possible, **they are frequently the preferred technique for the management of pain in the postoperative and in the severely trauma-tized patient**. Once such a catheter has been placed, analgesia may be maintained either by repeated intermittent injections, if block-free intervals are necessary as described above, or by continuous infusions of local anesthetics. The use of continuous infusions carries with it an advan-tage: by adjusting the concentration of the local anesthetic and the rate of infusion, one can alter the intensity and the extent of the blockade; and once the block has been established, it is often possible to maintain analgesia with a relatively weak anesthetic solution, particularly if dilute solutions of narcotics are added to the infusate. However, it should be emphasized that while there is extensive experience with continuous regional techniques in the management of postop-erative pain after elective surgery, only a few stud-ies have investigated the efficacy of these techniques in **traumatized** patients before and after surgery. Furthermore, most of the studies, even in postoperative patients, have been carried out utilizing continuous epidural and/or continu-ous spinal anesthesia and analgesia, and many fewer studies have been carried out utilizing con-tinuous plexus blocks or continuous peripheral nerve blocks. Nonetheless, while the discussion in this chapter is for the most part based on intraop-erative and postoperative data obtained from elec-tively operated patients, the mechanisms subserving postoperative and post-traumatic pain are similar, so these techniques of pain manage-ment should have similar, if not identical effects.

Technological considerations: peripheral nerve stimulators and 'sheathed needles'

A significant technological development that has facilitated the use of peripheral nerve blocks, par-ticularly in the trauma patient, is the development of the modern peripheral nerve stimulator and specialized 'sheathed needles'.[22,23] While not essential for all nerve blocks under all clinical conditions, the peripheral nerve stimulator is especially useful in traumatized patients who may not be able to cooperate because of head injury and/or because of the effects of alcohol or drugs, regardless of whether the latter were self-administered or were administered therapeutically following the injury. This technology has made peripheral nerve blocks possible in situations where they were previously impossible. Although uninsulated needles can be used in emergencies to locate the nerve or plexus to be blocked, insulated needles with only the tip uncovered localize the neural target more precisely.[24,25] It is frequently useful when placing an 'extracath' mounted on a needle with a metal hub for a continuous block (or when placing a plastic introducer cannula to allow insertion of an 'intracath'), that the plastic catheter around the needle (or introducer cannula) converts that needle (or cannula) into a 'sheathed needle electrode' that can be used to place the needle or cannula within the appropriate sheath using a nerve stimulator. The usual minimum current by which proximity of the needle to the nerve is insured is about 0.3 mA.[23] Much smaller currents (0.09 mA) have been described,[26] but these values were probably obtained by using a long pulse width (5 ms).

The advantages afforded by the use of the nerve stimulator in placing a needle or catheter for a nerve block, particularly in a traumatized patient include the following: The use of a nerve stimulator requires little or no patient cooperation. Since motor fibers have a lower threshold to electric stimulation than sensory fibers, painless muscle twitch is the end-point sought, not a painful paresthesia. Furthermore, since the needle does not contact the nerve, the possibility of nerve damage is avoided; and finally, the stimulation of a motor nerve results in a characteristic twitch of the innervated muscle groups, precisely identifying the nerve stimulated.

CONTINUOUS PLEXUS BLOCKS FOR TRAUMA OF THE UPPER EXTREMITY

Anatomical considerations: the brachial plexus

The fact that the brachial plexus is enveloped by fascia from the point where the roots emerge from the intervertebral foramina to the point where the peripheral nerves are distributed in the axilla (Fig. 13.1) allows continuous brachial plexus anesthesia to be approached in a manner similar to continuous epidural anesthesia, i.e. the space surrounding the plexus and its derivatives can be entered at any level, and an injection of local anesthetic at that level will provide anesthesia, the extent of which depends on the level of the injection and the volume of local anesthetic injected. With this concept in mind, a continuous axillary

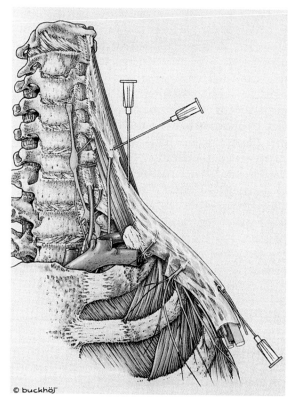

© buckhöj

Fig. 13.1 The fascial investment of the brachial plexus is derived from the surrounding muscles and forms a continuous perineural compartment which extends from the transverse process to the distal axilla. Thus, just as with peridural techniques, the space can be entered at any level to allow the injection of a local anesthetic. The extent of the anesthesia resulting from such an injection will depend on the volume of local anesthetic utilized and the level at which it is injected. Placement of a catheter within the space allows the intermittent re-injection or continuous infusion of local anesthetics. (Reproduced from Winnie AP. Perivascular techniques of brachial plexus blocks. With permission of the publisher)

perivascular brachial block becomes analogous to a continuous caudal, a continuous subclavian perivascular brachial block analogous to a continuous lumbar epidural, a continuous interscalene brachial block to a continuous thoracic epidural, and for that matter, a continuous interscalene cervical block to a continuous cervical epidural. The advantage of these continuous plexus blocks over the continuous peridural techniques results from the fact that the blocks are unilateral instead of bilateral, and this difference provides the patient with the advantages outlined in Table 13.1. In the patient with severe trauma to the upper extremity and/or shoulder girdle, as in the patient undergoing upper extremity surgery, the technique to be utilized depends primarily on the site of the injury and/or surgical intervention. Thus, usually an axillary block (or infraclavicular block) will be utilized for hand and forearm injuries or surgery, a subclavian perivascular block for injuries or surgery anywhere on the entire extremity up to the shoulder, and an interscalene block for injuries to or surgery on the upper arm and shoulder.

However, the choice of technique must always be individualized so that it is appropriate for the specific injury; for example, if the patient has an overt or potential infection of the hand with significant axillary lymphadenopathy, one would certainly choose an alternative to an axillary and/or infraclavicular block to avoid the possibility of encountering purulent lymph nodes with the needle and/or catheter. Furthermore, since catheters placed in the axillary perivascular space tend to be dislodged by changes in the position of the arm and shoulder, an infraclavicular catheter would be more stable and less likely to be dislodged if the catheter is to be left in for a prolonged period of time. Similarly, since interscalene catheters leave the interscalene space at right angles to the skin, they are difficult to immobilize and can also easily be dislodged by movement of the head and neck unless sutured into place.[27] Subclavian perivascular catheters, on the other hand, lie flat against the neck, move very little with movement of the patient's head and neck, and tend not to be easily dislodged.

Continuous axillary perivascular brachial plexus block

The axillary perivascular technique of brachial plexus block is appropriate for trauma and/or for surgical procedures involving the hand and forearm, though if necessary, analgesia and anesthesia of the elbow and upper arm can be provided by using large volumes of local anesthetic. Choosing either this technique or the infraclavicular technique obviates the possibility, albeit small, of complications associated with those blocks performed above the clavicle, namely, epidural or subarachnoid anesthesia, pneumothorax, or block of the phrenic nerve, recurrent laryngeal nerve, or stellate ganglion.

Musculocutaneous nerve block

One of the disadvantages of the axillary perivascular technique, however, is the occasional failure to block the musculocutaneous nerve, which exits from the axillary perivascular space high in the axilla. If the musculocutaneous nerve is not blocked, the powerful flexors of the forearm are not immobilized; and there is no anesthesia of the entire lateral aspect of the forearm. The possibility of failing to block this nerve can be minimized by increasing the volume of the local anesthetic injected, by depositing 5–7 mL of local anesthetic into the substance of the coracobrachialis muscle immediately superior to the axillary artery, or by threading a catheter high enough in the axillary sheath to block the musculocutaneous nerve. In any case, the presence of a catheter in the perivascular compartment allows repeated additional increments of local anesthetic to be added until the volume is sufficient to reach the musculocutaneous and even the axillary nerve.

Many techniques of carrying out a continuous axillary block have been described in the literature. Selander[28] described the earliest catheter technique using a Venflon catheter (AB Viggo, Helsingborg, Sweden), a Swedish extracath which was a flexible, 'over the needle', Teflon cannula designed for intravenous use. While the technique was introduced to avoid nerve damage from a needle and to prevent dislodgement of the needle during the injection, Selander did suggest that an advantage of the use of a catheter was that it offered the possibility of a continuous block and prolonged anesthesia and analgesia. Two years later Rosenblatt[29] in the USA described the insertion of a 5 cm Teflon-coated, intravenous catheter mounted on an 8.75 cm spinal needle, using a nerve stimulator to place the catheter to provide a continuous axillary block for the surgery and postoperative analgesia for 2 days in a 15-year-old boy with severe trauma to the hand. Six years later in Japan, Sada et al[30] reported 597 patients undergoing prolonged hand surgery under continuous axillary block carried out with an intravenous extracath, which consisted of an inner 23 gauge, 5.2 cm needle and an outer 19 gauge, 5.0 cm Teflon catheter.

The following year, in France Ang et al[31] described a continuous axillary block using a Seldinger technique, wherein a 5 cm, 19 gauge needle was inserted into the axillary sheath and through it a flexible guide wire was inserted 10–15 cm until resistance was felt. At that point the needle was removed, and an 8 cm, 18 gauge catheter was threaded over the guidewire and advanced into the axillary sheath, after which the guidewire was removed. A year later Haynsworth et al[32] described a continuous axillary block carried out in a patient with vascular insufficiency secondary to an inadvertent intra-arterial injection of methylphenidate, and they inserted an epidural catheter into the axillary sheath through a Crawford epidural needle. Plancarte et al[33] in Mexico reported a series of 50 patients in whom an epidural catheter was placed in the axillary sheath for a continuous block, but amazingly, they introduced the catheter through a 17 gauge Tuohy needle! And finally, a year later Büttner et al[34] in Germany described their technique, which consisted of placing an 18 gauge plastic cannula-introducer in the axillary sheath, inserting and advancing a longer, more flexible catheter far beyond the tip of the plastic introducer, and then removing the 18 gauge cannula, and injecting 40 mL of local anesthetic every 2 hours to maintain anesthesia. They utilized this technique in 1133 patients, both for prolonged surgical anesthesia and for postoperative pain relief with no serious complications. While all of these techniques are interesting and a tribute to the creativity of anesthesiologists in trying to fill a need, only the two most frequently employed techniques will be described in each approach, those using an 'extracath' (catheter over the needle) or an 'intracath' (catheter through the needle).

The authors' preferred technique of continuous axillary perivascular brachial plexus block is performed using a Teflon 'extracath'. Like the single injection technique,[35] it is performed with the patient supine, with the arm abducted approximately 90°, and with the elbow flexed 90° so that the dorsum of the hand lies on the table and the forearm is parallel to the long axis of the patient's body. Obviously, not all victims with traumatic injuries to the upper extremity will be able to assume or to tolerate this position; and these individuals will be more suitable candidates for the infraclavicular technique or one of the supraclavicular techniques, since these techniques can be carried out with the arm at the side. In any case, in positioning the arm for an axillary block, **hyper-**abduction of the arm should be avoided, as with the arm in this position, the head of the humerus may obliterate the brachial artery pulse, the single most important landmark. The arterial pulse is now palpated and is followed as far proximally as possible, ideally to the point where it disappears beneath the pectoralis major muscle. With the palpating finger on the pulse, a 22 gauge, short-beveled needle with a Teflon 'extracath' mounted on it is inserted immediately superior to the fingertip in the long axis of (actually, at a 10–20° angle with) the neurovascular bundle, i.e. toward the apex of the axilla. It may be necessary to raise a skin wheal with local anesthetic and make a 'stab wound' in the skin with an 18 gauge needle to facilitate passage of the 'extracath' through the skin. The entire unit is then slowly advanced until one of several end-points indicates proper placement of the tip of the needle within the axillary perivascular space: (1) A short-beveled or blunt needle will invariably produce a definite 'click' as it penetrates the fascial sheath surrounding the neurovascular bundle. When the 'click' is perceived, confirmatory evidence is provided by pulsation of the needle hub, but pulsation **alone** (without a 'fascial click') is insufficient evidence of proper placement; (2) if the advancing needle encounters the mantle fibers of one of the nerves lying within the axillary perivascular compartment, the resultant paresthesia provides indisputable evidence that the needle tip is within the sheath; or (3) a nerve stimulator may be utilized if the 'extracath' has a metal hub: if so, the 'alligator clip' is fastened to the metal hub, and the plastic cannula provides insulation except at the tip of the needle, so the 'extracath' functions as 'sheathed needle'. When the advancing needle produces contraction of an appropriate muscle group using only 0.3 mA, the needle is within 1 mm of a motor nerve and presumably lies within the sheath.[36,37]

Regardless of the end-point utilized, once the axillary sheath has been penetrated, the tip of the needle should lie close to the artery in the axillary perivascular space. At this point, after careful aspiration, 5–10 mL of local anesthetic are injected to distend the perivascular space, the 'extracath' is advanced several centimeters beyond the tip of the needle, and the needle is removed. Now, after again aspirating for blood, 20–40 mL of local anesthetic is injected in 3–5 mL increments, with aspiration for blood between each increment, until the desired volume of local anesthetic has been injected. Firm digital pressure should be applied behind the needle and maintained throughout the injection to enhance proximal spread (and minimize distal spread) of the local anesthetic. Following the injection, the catheter should be fitted with an injection port if intermittent injections are to be given or connected to an infusion if a continuous infusion is to be utilized. In either case, the catheter should be carefully taped or sutured in place and, if possible, the arm immobilized to prevent accidental displacement of the catheter when the arm is moved. If anesthesia of the medial brachial cutaneous and/or intercostobrachial nerves is essential, for example, to allow the use of a tourniquet for surgery, 3–5 mL of local anesthetic is deposited subcutaneously over the arterial pulse immediately distal to the catheter's point of entry. If the patient is alert and capable, a patient-controlled analgesia (PCA) infusion pump can be connected to allow the patient controlled plexus analgesia.

Continuous techniques of brachial plexus block were originally introduced to allow prolonged surgical procedures such as reimplantation of digits with nerve and/or vascular reapproximation.[38,62] Subsequent experience (and the introduction of plastic catheters) indicated that these techniques are useful, not only to provide prolonged surgical anesthesia and immobilization of the extremity, but also to provide profound postoperative sympathetic blockade and pain relief.[29–31,34,39]

As stated earlier, one of the earliest proponents of continuous axillary block with a catheter was Selander,[28] who was one of the first to propose placing a plastic catheter mounted on a needle into the axillary sheath; but his stated purpose in doing so was to minimize neural injury, since a plastic catheter, should it encounter a nerve, should not traumatize the nerve the way a needle would. The problem, of course, is that the catheter is introduced on a large needle, which could still produce nerve damage during the intro-

duction of the catheter; so even the 'extracaths' in use today must be inserted and advanced carefully. Nonetheless, in their report of 597 continuous axillary blocks using a deliberate paresthesia technique, Sada et al[30] found only three patients with postoperative nerve damage; and in only one did the damage involve the nerve in which the paresthesia had been elicited. Similarly, in an even larger series of 1133 cases, Büttner et al[34] reported that paresthesias were provoked by the needle itself in 41 cases (3.6%); but there were no postoperative neuropathies in their series. So it would appear that, used carefully, the 'extracath' technique does not increase the risk of nerve damage.

To minimize even further the possibility of nerve damage by the needle tip during insertion, Finucane[40,41] introduced a special 18 gauge, 2.5 inch catheter mounted on a 3.5 inch, 25 gauge needle (Arrow Single-shot or Continuous Brachial Plexus Set, Arrow® International, Inc., Reading, PA) (Fig. 13.2). The distal end of the needle is smooth and round ('bullet-tipped') without a cutting edge, the opening is on the side of the distal end of the needle (Fig. 13.3), and the hub of the needle is metal to allow attachment of an 'alligator clip' from a nerve stimulator. To use this needle the skin is infiltrated with local anesthetic and a small incision is made at the point of intended entry, using the cutting edge of a 17 gauge needle. The needle/catheter unit is advanced parallel to the axillary artery at an angle of about 60° until a distinct 'give' indicates penetration of the sheath (Fig. 13.4). At that point the negative lead from a nerve stimulator is connected to the metal hub, and the needle is advanced until an appropriate twitch response indicates proper placement of the needle without neural contact.

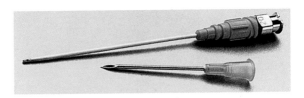

Fig. 13.2 Arrow Single-Shot or Continuous Brachial Plexus set consists of a 20 gauge atraumatic needle with a blunt distal end and side aperture aligned to the hub notch, and an 18 gauge sharp needle to prepuncture the skin to facilitate the insertion of the needle-catheter unit. (Courtesy of Arrow® International, Inc., Reading, PA.)

After aspiration and injection of 5–10 mL of local anesthetic, the catheter is advanced off the needle; and after removal of the needle, it is taped securely (or sutured) in place. Although this technique is certainly atraumatic, many anesthesiologists find the needle difficult to insert, and there are no data indicating that this technique improves the success rate over other techniques.

A popular alternative to the 'extracath' technique is the so-called 'intracath' technique, first introduced by Büttner[34,42–45] in Germany and popularized in the USA at the Mayo Clinic.[46–48] As with Finucane's 'extracath' technique, this technique

has the advantage of using equipment designed and marketed specifically for use in brachial plexus anesthesia, the Contiplex® Continuous Brachial Plexus Anesthesia kit marketed in both Europe (B. Braun Melsungen AG, Melsungen, Germany) and in the USA (B. Braun Medical, Inc., Bethlehem, PA) (Fig. 13.5). With the patient in the usual axillary block position, the skin is infiltrated with local anesthetic, and a sharp 18 gauge needle is used to make the initial skin puncture to facilitate insertion of the blunt 45° bevel, insulated needle. The insulated needle is inserted through the puncture site adjacent to the axillary artery at an angle of 30° to the skin. The insulated needle is connected to a nerve stimulator and is advanced until an appropriate twitch response at 0.3 mA indicates proper placement of the tip of the needle within the axillary sheath. Following aspiration and the injection of a few milliliters of local anesthetic, the plastic cannula is advanced over the needle (Fig. 13.6) and the needle withdrawn, leaving the plastic cannula in place. The flexible axillary catheter is now inserted through the cannula (Fig. 13.7) and advanced up to 12 cm or until resistance is encountered. Passing the catheter more than 12 cm offers no advantage and usually results in coiling or kinking of the catheter within the sheath.[46] On the other hand, the catheter should be advanced a minimum

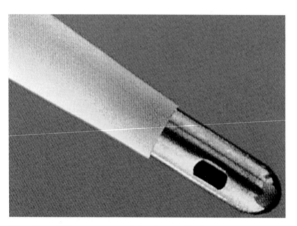

Fig. 13.3 Enlargement of the blunt 'bullet-tipped' needle designed to reduce the risk of neurovascular damage. (Courtesy of Arrow® International, Inc., Reading, PA.)

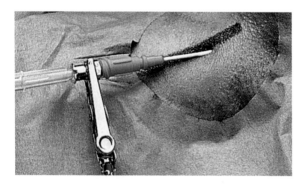

Fig. 13.4 After pre-puncture of the skin with the 18 gauge needle, the blunt needle and catheter are advanced until a tactile 'pop' indicates penetration of the axillary sheath. The metal hub of the needle facilitates the use of a nerve stimulator to confirm proper placement of the needle and catheter prior to removal of the needle. (Courtesy of Arrow® International, Inc., Reading, PA.)

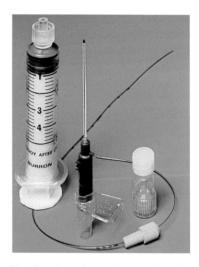

Fig. 13.5 The Contiplex® Continuous Brachial Plexus Anesthesia Tray consists of an 18 gauge plastic introducer cannula mounted on a short-bevel needle which can be connected to a nerve stimulator, a 400 mm flexible polyamide catheter, and an injection port. (Courtesy of B. Braun Medical, Inc., Bethlehem, PA.)

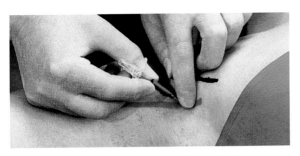

Fig. 13.6 After proper placement of the tip of the needle within the axillary sheath, the plastic cannula is advanced over the needle, and the needle is withdrawn, leaving the plastic cannula in place. (Courtesy of B. Braun Medical, Inc., Bethlehem, PA.)

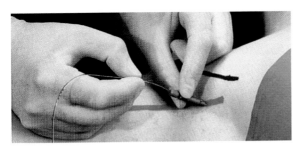

Fig. 13.7 The flexible polyamide catheter is inserted through the cannula and advanced the desired distance beyond the tip of the cannula, after which the cannula is withdrawn. (Courtesy of B. Braun Medical, Inc., Bethlehem, PA.)

of 5 cm to avoid retrograde leakage of injected local anesthetic[46].

After placement of the catheter the cannula is withdrawn, an adapter is attached to the distal end, the catheter is sutured in place, and a transparent drape is applied. Following negative aspiration, a test dose of 3 ml of 0.5% bupivacaine with 1:200,000 epinephrine is injected; and if there are no signs or symptoms of intravascular injection, 3–5 ml increments of local anesthetic are given up to the desired dose, usually about 40 ml. Approximately 45–60 minutes after anesthesia is established (to avoid toxic plasma levels), an infusion of 0.25% bupivacaine can be started at a rate of 8–10 ml/hr. When utilized for postoperative analgesia during constant passive motion (for postoperative rehabilitation, see Ch. 11), breakthrough pain may occur, which can be alleviated by a 5–10 ml 'rescue dose' of 0.5% bupivacaine or by increasing the infusion rate 2–6 ml/hr. If sympatholysis is the primary goal of the infusion, 0.125% bupiva-

caine will suffice; and in fact, this concentration will be adequate for post-traumatic and/or postoperative pain if 2–3 μg/ml of fentanyl is added.

Although the risk of serious complications from continuous axillary block is low, those that have been reported include *incorrect catheter placement* with *incomplete or absent anesthesia* and *subcutaneous or intrafascial kinking or coiling of the catheter*. With the intracath technique, this has not interfered with the injection or infusion of local anesthetic, or even with removal of the catheter[46]; but with the extracath technique, kinking requires removal and replacement.[28] *Penetration of the axillary artery or vein(s)* or *migration of the catheter* can result in a *hematoma*[30]; and of course, *intravenous and even intra-arterial injections of local anesthetic* are possible, but these can be minimized by careful frequent aspiration and the use of test doses. *Displacement of the catheter* is probably greatest with the axillary approach, but this is still infrequent; and it can be virtually abolished by suturing the catheter in place.[48] As with any approach, *nerve injury by needle or catheter* can occur,[30] but even when paresthesias have been elicited inadvertently, the incidence of nerve damage has been low or non-existent;[30,34] and *systemic toxic reactions* are possible if inappropriate doses or infusion rates are utilized. *Infection* is also possible, though in one study where infusions of 0.125% bupivacaine were administered for up to 11.5 days, routine cultures of catheter tips after withdrawal showed positive cultures only from catheters remaining in place more than 4 days, but none of the catheters with positive cultures caused signs or symptoms of local or systemic infection.[49]

Continuous infraclavicular brachial plexus block

Because the axillary approach to brachial plexus block is easy to perform and free from the serious side effects that can occur above the clavicle, it is undoubtedly the most widely used single injection technique for upper extremity surgery. Because of their familiarity with the single injection technique, many (if not most) anesthesiologists also utilize the axillary approach when a continuous technique is indicated. However, of all of the techniques of continuous brachial plexus block, the axillary technique probably has the highest rate of accidental displacement of the catheter owing to movement of the upper extremity (either active or passive), which tends to dislodge the catheter. In addition, hair and moisture in the axilla can make it difficult to maintain a sterile environment.[50] The infraclavicular approach, according to its advocates, allows easy threading of catheters; and once placed, the catheters are not affected by patient movement and have been kept in place for as long as 3 weeks.[50] On the other hand, the infraclavicular technique requires the use of long needles and catheters, and insertion of the catheter is more painful to the patient than with the other techniques; so it has not found great popularity and acceptance in many centers. In addition, the technique as described by Raj[51] requires locating the brachial plexus at a site far removed from easily identified landmarks or easily palpable arterial pulsations, and it requires penetration of the thick pectoral muscles; and these problems have resulted in several variations in technique.[52–54] Nevertheless, the technique of Raj can provide anesthesia and analgesia of the entire arm without the complications possible above the clavicle; and it does lend itself to continuous catheter placement and long-term catheter maintenance without the incidence of catheter displacement seen with the continuous axillary technique.[55] Furthermore, continuous infraclavicular brachial plexus block is particularly useful in those trauma patients who cannot abduct or rotate the upper extremity because of fracture, dislocation, or pain, making the axillary technique impossible; and in such patients the infraclavicular approach provides a logical alternative.

The procedure is performed with the operator standing on the side opposite the arm to be blocked. While the block, if necessary, may be successfully performed with the patient's head and arm in almost any position, usually the arm is abducted and the head turned to the opposite side. A skin wheal is raised at the anticipated point of needle insertion, which is approximately 1 inch below the mid-point of the clavicle. Again, it may be advantageous to make a 'stab wound' through the skin wheal to facilitate insertion of the needle and catheter. In any case, a 3½ inch 'extracath' with a metal hub is inserted through the 'stab wound' with the negative lead of a nerve stimulator clipped to the needle hub and the positive (ground) electrode placed on the opposite shoulder or anterior chest wall. The needle is advanced in a lateral direction (toward the axillary artery) at a 45° angle to the skin. As the needle tip pene-

trates the pectoralis muscle group, the shoulder will adduct; but this must not be misinterpreted to indicate that the unsheathed needle tip has arrived at its destination. As the needle passes through the pectoralis major and minor muscles and approaches the brachial plexus, those muscles innervated by the median, ulnar, or radial nerves will contract, so the desired end-point is indicated by extension of the elbow or flexion or extension of the wrist and/or fingers, with a good response evoked by no more than a 0.3 mA current. *Stimulation of the musculocutaneous nerve with flexion of the elbow is probably not a satisfactory end-point, since this nerve may be stimulated after it has exited the sheath and is traveling in the coracobrachialis muscle. Injection of local anesthetic at this point will produce isolated block of the musculocutaneous nerve.*[56]

After an appropriate motor response and after negative aspiration for blood in several quadrants, 5–10 mL of local anesthetic are injected to open the heretofore potential perivascular compartment. This volume will cause the muscular twitching to stop, after which the catheter is advanced several centimeters beyond the tip of the needle and the needle is withdrawn. The catheter is taped or sutured in place, and after repeated aspiration, 20–40 mL of local anesthetic is injected in 3–5 cc increments with repeated aspiration between increments. Following the injection an injection port is attached to the hub if intermittent injections are to be utilized or an infusion is attached if continuous infusion is desired.

A theoretical advantage of the infraclavicular approach is that with this technique the local anesthetic is deposited at the level of the cords above the level at which the musculocutaneous and axillary nerves leave the sheath. Thus, with the infraclavicular technique, all of the nerves derived from the plexus should be blocked with a smaller volume of local anesthetic than is required with the axillary technique. In reality, the lateral direction of the needle and catheter may place the needle tip distal to the level at which the musculocutaneous and axillary nerves leave the sheath; and advancement of the catheter will place it even more distally; so that the initial injection through the needle and subsequent injections through the catheter may fail to block these nerves.

Because of the lateral direction of the needle and the plastic introducer cannula mounted on it, the authors do not use an 'intracath' for the infraclavicular technique, since the farther the flexible catheter is advanced beyond the introducer cannula, the greater is the likelihood that the local anesthetic will be injected at a point where several of the major derivatives will have left the sheath.

Continuous subclavian perivascular brachial plexus block

The subclavian perivascular technique of brachial plexus block is ideal for upper extremity trauma or surgical procedures involving any part of the upper extremity from the shoulder to the hand. Unlike the axillary perivascular technique, with this technique the arm does not have to be abducted or externally rotated for its successful completion, an obvious advantage in the patient with severe, painful trauma to the hand, arm, or shoulder. The technique, as originally described,[57] used paresthesias to place the needle properly; but in patients who are impaired or obtunded by trauma or by drugs or by the administration of analgesics and/or preoperative medications, a peripheral nerve stimulator may be essential to ensure correct placement of the needle. This technique does, perhaps, provide the greatest ease of placement and maintenance of a continuous brachial plexus catheter for trauma, for prolonged operations, or for postoperative pain relief *without displacement of the catheter*.

A continuous subclavian perivascular brachial plexus block is performed as follows.[57] With the patient in the dorsal recumbent position and with the head turned slightly towards the opposite side, the patient is asked to elevate his or her head to bring the sternocleidomastoid muscle into prominence. The anesthesiologist places his finger posterior to the lateral (clavicular) head of this muscle at the level of C6 (the level of the cricoid cartilage) and tells the patient to relax. As the sternocleidomastoid muscle relaxes, the palpating finger moves medially behind it, after which the palpating finger is rolled laterally across the belly of the anterior scalene muscle until the interscalene groove is encountered at its lateral border. A skin wheal is raised in the groove at C6, and a 'stab wound' is made using a 16 gauge needle. An 'extracath' is then inserted through the 'stab wound' slightly closer to the middle scalene than to the anterior scalene muscle. This point of insertion is higher than that used when carrying out a single injection technique, since a higher point of insertion allows

more of the catheter to be subcutaneous; so that the catheter, once placed, lies flat against the neck. The 'extracath' is now advanced directly caudad with the hub of the needle against the skin of the neck until a paresthesia, preferably below the shoulder, indicates contact with one of the three trunks. If a nerve stimulator is utilized, it is advanced until an appropriate twitch response occurs at no more than 0.3 mA current. In either case, at this point careful aspiration is carried out in several quadrants, after which 5–10 mL of local anesthetic are injected to open up the space. The catheter is then advanced several centimeters beyond the tip of the needle, the needle is removed, and 20–40 mL of local anesthetic are injected. The catheter is now immobilized by tape or suture, and an injection port is inserted into the catheter hub to allow intermittent injections, or an infusion is connected if a continuous infusion is desirable.

Continuous subclavian perivascular brachial plexus block has two distinct advantages over all other techniques: The first is that at this level of injection, the plexus is reduced to its fewest components, the three trunks; and thus the volume of the cylinder formed by the fascia surrounding them is smaller; and as a result, blockade of the entire plexus can be achieved with a smaller volume of local anesthetic. The second advantage is that the catheter placed with this technique lies flat against the patient's neck and is affected very little by movement of the patient; so the chance of displacement is probably less than with any of the other techniques. Continuous subclavian perivascular block has been utilized by Hilgier[58] in 100 consecutive, prolonged, microsurgical procedures requiring nerve grafting; and in every case this technique provided excellent surgical anesthesia for an average of 10 hours. In addition, postoperative analgesia was provided by repeated doses of bupivacaine for an average of 2 days without any complications whatsoever.

As with the continuous infraclavicular technique, there have been no reports of continuous subclavian brachial block using an 'intracath' technique, except for a single case report where intractable, terminal cancer pain was controlled by inserting an epidural catheter through a Tuohy needle which was placed using a nerve stimulator.[59]

If carried out properly, complications are extremely rare with the subclavian perivascular technique. *Pneumothorax* is possible, but because the course of the 'extracath' is directly caudad, if all of the trunks are missed by the advancing 'extracath', the first rib, not the lung, will be encountered. However, it is rarely necessary to advance the 'extracath' that far. Blockade of the roots of the phrenic nerve with consequent *diaphragmatic paresis* is probably not uncommon,[60–62] but this is usually without adverse signs or symptoms unless the patient has pulmonary disease and/or damage.[63] *Epidural and subarachnoid injections* are extremely rare complications of continuous subclavian perivascular brachial block, but this possibility should always be kept in mind. As with all techniques, *intravenous injections* are possible with resultant systemic reactions, but frequent, intermittent aspiration during catheter placement and local anesthetic injection can minimize these. The possibility, though rare, of *injection of local anesthetic into the nearby vertebral artery* is something that should also be kept in mind. Though never reported with this technique, such an injection causes almost instantaneous though transient convulsions following the injection of even minute quantities of local anesthetic because of the proximity of the injection to the brain. Finally, as with any regional anesthetic technique, *nerve damage* is a possible but unlikely complication. The development of *Horner's syndrome* is not an infrequent side effect of this technique, and while harmless, the relationship to the block should be noted, so it is not misinterpreted as an indication of neurological injury. Similarly, *recurrent laryngeal block* and resultant hoarseness is a side effect that is usually without sequelae, though the patient should receive nothing by mouth until the hoarseness disappears, lest he or she aspirate ingested fluids. However, again, the relationship to the block should be noted (if it occurs) so that the hoarseness is not mistaken to be a sign of airway trauma.

Continuous interscalene brachial plexus block

Perhaps, the continuous technique that has become the most widely utilized regional anesthetic for upper extremity and shoulder surgery and postoperative pain management is continuous interscalene brachial plexus block. Its popularity is due to the ease with which the landmarks can be identified, the technical simplicity of carrying out the block, and the inherent safety of a technique that, while supraclavicular, is performed well above both the subclavian artery and the cupola of the

lung. Nonetheless, as with any technique, complications can occur if the anesthesiologist is not completely familiar with the anatomy, and if the technique of needle and catheter insertion is not carried out with careful attention to the landmarks.

The continuous catheter technique of interscalene brachial plexus block was first published in 1970 by Winnie,[64] who suggested its use for prolonged surgical procedures on the upper extremity. In 1978 Manriquez & Pallares[65] described its use for postoperative pain management; and a few years later Kirkpatrick et al[66] demonstrated the safety of the blood levels resulting from constant infusions of bupivacaine for this purpose for as long as 4 days. As originally described, the technique is carried out, if possible, with the patient supine and with the head turned slightly to the side opposite that to be blocked. The level of C6 is determined by dropping a line laterally from the cricoid cartilage. The patient is then asked to elevate his or her head (if possible) to bring the sternocleidomastoid into prominence, the anesthesiologist's index and middle fingers are placed behind the taut sternocleidomastoid muscle, and the patient is told to relax. The palpating fingers now lie on the belly of the anterior scalene muscle, and as the patient's sternocleidomastoid muscle relaxes, the fingers move toward the medial edge of that muscle. The fingers are now rolled laterally across the anterior scalene muscle until the interscalene groove is encountered. If the palpating fingers are separated slightly, the skin between them will actually be indented into the interscalene groove, minimizing the distance between the skin and transverse process. A skin wheal is raised between the palpating fingers at the level of C6, a 'stab wound' is made with a 16 gauge needle, and a 22 gauge 'intracath' is inserted in a direction described as directly perpendicular to the skin in every plane, i.e. mostly mesiad, slightly caudad, and slightly dorsad. The slightly caudad direction is critical to the safety of the technique, since the needle or catheter which is advanced too far will be stopped by a bony transverse process, so that it cannot continue to be advanced and enter a vertebral vessel, the epidural space, or the spinal canal. The needle is now advanced very slowly and carefully until a paresthesia is elicited, preferably below the shoulder, or if a nerve stimulator is used, a twitch response in appropriate muscles in the hand or arm is produced at a setting of 0.3 mA or less. Obviously, a nerve stimulator is not only a great advantage, it is essential in patients who are inebriated, heavily sedated, or obtunded from their trauma. At that point 5–10 ml of local anesthetic are injected to 'open up' the space, after which the needle is fixed, the catheter is carefully advanced 1–2 cm beyond the needle tip, and the needle is removed.

While the authors prefer to utilize a standard Teflon intravenous 'extracath', Haas[67] recently described the use of the Arrow, bullet-tipped needle/catheter device (Arrow Single Shot or Continuous Brachial Plexus Set, Arrow® International, Inc., Reading, PA), presumably to minimize the chance of nerve damage. Because of the blunt 'bullet tip', this 'extracath' can only be inserted through a 'stab wound' made at the injection site with a 16 gauge needle and advanced with the aid of a nerve stimulator. But whatever device is used, because the catheter with this technique emerges from the skin at right angles to it, it is difficult to immobilize. If taped to the skin, the catheter tends to kink, it tends to leak, and usually, it falls out.[67] All of these problems are avoided by suturing the catheter in place.[27] Once the catheter has been immobilized, 20–40 ml of local anesthetic are injected in 3–5 ml increments with repeated aspiration between increments, after which an injection port or an infusion is connected to the hub of the catheter, depending on whether intermittent injections or a continuous infusion is to be utilized.

As with the other approaches, there are investigators who prefer to utilize an 'intracath' to provide continuous interscalene blocks. Using a nerve stimulator connected to the metal hub of the plexus block introducer cannula (Contiplex®, B. Braun Medical, Inc., Bethlehem, PA), the plexus is identified, and after negative aspiration, an initial dose of 20–25 ml of local anesthetic is injected in increments after which the needle is withdrawn and a flexible catheter is introduced through the cannula into the interscalene space. The plastic cannula is then removed, the catheter is fixed to the skin, and an infusion of dilute local anesthetic begun.[27,68,69] A Finnish group of anesthesiologists has published extensively on the use of this technique for shoulder surgery, both for intraoperative and for postoperative pain; and it was this group that found that when the catheter was immobilized with tape, it tended to loosen and become dislodged with patient movement. When they sutured the catheter in place, none of them were dislodged accidentally.[27]

Regardless of whether an 'extracath' or 'intracath' is utilized, the *potential* complications associated with continuous interscalene brachial block are similar to those associated with the single injection interscalene technique. However, the published incidence is very low. There have been no reports of *infection, bleeding,* or *hematoma* caused by the catheter, though there is a single case report of *unintentional arterial catheterization* with resultant bupivacaine toxicity[70] and another report of *unsuspected extradural catheterization* with resultant cervical epidural block.[71] In both of these cases the 'intracath' technique was utilized, with a catheter inserted through an introducer needle or cannula. In the first case, the flexible catheter was advanced further than usual through the introducer cannula (12 cm from the skin), and it penetrated the vertebral artery as it was advanced, making a 90° angle at the point of entry (as demonstrated on X-ray). The right angle 'kink' in the catheter did not allow the aspiration of blood, and the injection of 45 mg of bupivacaine resulted in instantaneous coma without convulsions. In the second case the catheter was also inserted 12 cm through the introducer cannula, but in this case the initial injection of 10 mL of 0.25% bupivacaine produced the expected anesthesia in the left hand and forearm, as did the second 10 mL dose. However, the third 10 mL not only produced the expected anesthesia in the left upper extremity, but also warmth and numbness of the **right** arm and shoulder, so the catheter was withdrawn 3 cm. The following day, another 10 mL of 0.25% bupivacaine resulted in bilateral anesthesia of the upper extremities and postural hypotension. A subsequent X-ray taken after 2 mL of non-ionic contrast medium had been injected through the catheter showed the catheter entering the extradural space at C6–7, with the dye moving cephalad to outline the whole cervical extradural space. Both of these patients responded to appropriate supportive treatment with no serious sequelae; but clearly the lessons to be learned from these two cases are that when using the 'intracath' technique for continuous interscalene block (1) the catheter should be advanced only 1–2 cm beyond the tip of the introducer cannula; (2) even the soft, pliable Contiplex® catheter can penetrate a blood vessel; (3) catheters can migrate with time and enter the epidural or subarachnoid spaces; and (4) failure to aspirate blood (or cerebrospinal fluid (CSF) could be a 'false negative' because of kinking of the catheter. Nonetheless, the *incidence* of serious complications appears to be very low.

Since Urmey has shown that *hemidiaphragmatic paresis* occurs after virtually all single-injection interscalene brachial plexus blocks,[72–74] it would not be surprising to find that continuous blocks, whether maintained by intermittent injections or by infusions, also affect pulmonary function. The Finnish group studied the effect of continuous interscalene block on diaphragmatic motion and on ventilatory function in 10 patients using double-exposure radiography and pulmonary function tests.[75] An initial dose of 20–28 mL of bupivacaine 0.75% with epinephrine was injected for surgery, followed by an infusion of 5–9 mL/h of bupivacaine 0.25% for the next 24 hours to provide postoperative pain relief. Three hours after the initial block, all 10 patients had an ipsilateral paresis of the diaphragm on X-ray, with the amplitude of the diaphragmatic motion being a mean of 12% (5 to 32%) of the preoperative value. After 24 hours of the continuous infusion of bupivacaine 0.25%, there was partial recovery in 5 patients to 65 to 84% of the preoperative values, but the diaphragmatic paresis persisted in 5 patients at 4 to 37% of preoperative values. Spirometric studies were done at 3 hours, 8 hours, and 24 hours postoperatively and showed significant reductions in forced vital capacity (FVC), forced expiratory volume in 1 second (FEV_1), and peak expiratory flow rate (PEFR) at 3 and 8 hours, but all returned to levels that were not statistically significantly reduced from preoperative levels by 24 hours. Although all patients had good surgical anesthesia and postoperative analgesia, none of them had any symptoms of respiratory distress. Nonetheless, these patients had no respiratory disease, and these data indicate that continuous interscalene blocks should be performed with great caution in patients with significant respiratory dysfunction, whether due to disease or trauma.

Side effects of continuous (and single injection) interscalene block include *Horner's syndrome* and hoarseness due to *recurrent laryngeal nerve block*: The incidence of Horner's syndrome is apparently related to the volume of local anesthetic injected, being low (12.5%) if the volume is small[27] and high (75%) if the volume is large.[76] The 20% incidence of hoarseness reported by the Finnish group[27] might also be higher following the injection of a larger volume of local anesthetic. While none of these side effects had any adverse clinical sequelae,

as mentioned earlier, when they occur in the patient with head and/or neck trauma, their relationship to the block should be noted so their presence is not misinterpreted as being related to the trauma.

Clinical considerations

As stated in the introductory section of this chapter, most of the experience with continuous peripheral blocks of both the upper and lower extremity has been gained using these techniques for surgical anesthesia and postoperative analgesia. There are well over 3000 cases of continuous brachial plexus blocks reported in the literature, of which less than 3% were stated to be utilized for trauma, although clearly, many of the surgical procedures reported were the result of trauma. However, the use of continuous techniques as an integral part of the management of trauma is rapidly increasing, as is the use of externalized and implanted catheters and ports for post-traumatic CRPS I and II[77–79] (see Chs 5 and 24). As a matter of fact, as anesthesiologists have become more experienced with these techniques, they have come to appreciate the fact that they are *particularly* useful in the patient with trauma involving the extremities, where pain relief is required during the preoperative, intraoperative, and postoperative periods without further *insult* to the patient's hemodynamic status.

To be sure, the choice of the appropriate technique will depend primarily on the level and/or extent of injury, though the decision may be modified by other injuries or disease states, i.e. serious contralateral pulmonary injury or disease may contraindicate continuous interscalene block, etc. Interestingly, though a continuous technique may be carried out using any local anesthetic, short- or long-acting, the vast majority of the cases reported in the literature involve the use of bupivacaine, a long-acting agent. With any continuous technique, one must be cognizant of the possibility of cumulative toxicity, whether one is utilizing a continuous infusion or intermittent boluses. Fortunately, as with continuous epidural blocks, once the steady state has been reached, the drugs being infused do not accumulate if the rate of administration is not increased. For example, Tuominen et al have reported that an initial dose of 3 mg/kg of bupivacaine in a continuous axillary block followed 30 minutes later with a second dose of 1.5–2.4 mg/kg resulted in a venous concentration of 1.2–2.4 µg/ml 30 to 60 minutes later without any clinical evidence of toxicity.[80] The same group injected a large initial dose (150–210 mg) of 0.75% bupivacaine into an interscalene catheter followed by a continuous infusion of 12.5–22.5 mg/h for 24 and 48 hours, and though this resulted in marked accumulation of bupivacaine and its metabolites in the plasma, there were no toxic concentrations or clinical symptoms.[69] These authors concluded that a 48-hour continuous interscalene plexus infusion is safe, but that prolonging the infusion beyond 48 hours may eventually give rise to toxicity. However, elsewhere they point out that bupivacaine is bound to α_1-acid glycoprotein and that as part of the stress reponse (to trauma surgery) the plasma concentration of α_1-acid glycoprotein increases progressively for at least 5 days,[69] by which time its concentration has doubled.[68] Therefore, during this time a greater percentage of bupivacaine becomes bound to this acute phase protein with the result that the levels of free bupivacaine may not increase (and may even decrease) with the passage of time.

Mezzatesta et al compared the efficacy and safety of continuous axillary block with 0.25% bupivacaine by intermittent bolus and by continuous infusion in the management of postoperative pain, and they found no difference in the sensory or motor block or in the need for supplemental narcotics; and while the infusions resulted in statistically significantly higher plasma levels after 26 hours than the intermittent injections, neither group showed clinical signs of toxicity.[81] While the 0.25% of concentration bupivacaine has been used most frequently for continuous brachial block, under certain circumstances it is advantageous to vary the concentration. Obviously, if complete anesthesia and/or motor block is required, the concentration should be increased to 0.5%, at least for the period of time when these conditions are required. However, reducing the concentrations of the infusion (or dose) to 0.125% has been shown to provide excellent pain relief but has allowed clinical assessment of motor function and maintenance of the sympathetic block, features of great importance in certain types of trauma.[49] However, when considering the use of these lower concentrations of bupivacaine, it may be important to remember that while 0.25% and 0.5% bupivacaine have been shown to significantly inhibit bacterial growth, 0.125% bupivacaine exhibits no antimicrobial activity.[49] Though the use of 0.125% bupivacaine has been used for prolonged periods

without serious infection, positive cultures have been reported when infusions were utilized for more than 4 days.[49]

While it is obvious that the vast majority of reports of continuous brachial block have involved the use of bupivacaine, one could legitimately ask why such a long-lasting, relatively toxic agent has been used for continuous techniques which allow shorter-acting, less toxic agents to be used effectively. There are very few reports of such a practice, but Büttner, in one of the largest series of continuous axillary blocks in the literature (1133 cases),[34] utilized mepivacaine, the drug reported to be the safest of all of the amide local anesthetics in terms of systemic toxicity.[82,83] Büttner utilized an initial dose of 40 mL of plain 1% mepivacaine and repeated the same dose every 2 hours for 16 hours. Using this intermittent injection technique, he found that within the first 8 hours (during which the patients received four 400 mg doses) the serum levels of all 17 patients remained below the level of 5–6 µg/ml, which is said to be the lower level for central toxic reactions in venous blood.[84] Although as much as 3600 mg of mepivacaine were given over 16 hours, only one of the patients exceeded this level by 1 µg/ml, and none of the patients exhibited signs of serious systemic toxicity. Clearly, these are higher doses than necessary in most cases, but this study does demonstrate the clinical safety of this agent; and perhaps more studies should be carried out using it.

Over the past few decades many adjuvant agents have been added to local anesthetics in an effort to enhance their effectiveness. Bicarbonate has been added to shorten the onset and prolong the duration of local anesthetics,[85] but it would appear that these effects may only be significant when bicarbonate is added to local anesthetics containing epinephrine (added at the time of their manufacture).[86,87] Alpha-agonists[88] added to local anesthetics have been shown to prolong the duration of brachial plexus anesthesia, and the addition of certain narcotics can provide postoperative analgesia for 24–48 hours.[89] However, when continuous peripheral blocks are used *in trauma patients*, the authors feel that the addition of these adjunctive agents is unnecessary and may serve only to complicate the pharmacologic management of the patient. With a catheter in place, the duration of anesthesia and/or analgesia can be extended indefinitely; and by varying the concentration of the local anesthetic the intensity of the block can be modified to provide motor block, if muscle relaxation is desirable, sensory block if only analgesia is necessary, or even just a sympathetic block if that is what is indicated.

In any case, continuous brachial block is an extremely useful procedure for pain management in patients with trauma to the upper extremity and shoulder girdle and can also be utilized for intraoperative and postoperative pain relief if indicated, obviating the need for general anesthesia, endotracheal intubation, and mechanical ventilation. In addition, the accompanying sympatholysis provides increased extremity blood flow promoting healing, graft or anastomosis survival and, hopefully, preventing the development of sympathetically maintained pain.

CONTINUOUS PLEXUS BLOCKS FOR TRAUMA OF THE LOWER EXTREMITY

Anatomical considerations: the lumbar plexus

As stated earlier, continuous plexus blocks of the upper extremity are possible because the brachial plexus is invested in fascia from the intervertebral foramina to the distal axilla; so the plexus and its derivatives pass sequentially through the interscalene, subclavian perivascular, and axillary perivascular spaces. Thus, just as with continuous epidural techniques, a catheter can be placed in this space at any level, and the injection of a local anesthetic will produce analgesia and/or anesthesia, the extent and intensity of which will depend on the volume and concentration of the local anesthetic and the level at which it is injected.

However, the fascia surrounding the brachial plexus confines the plexus progressively; and as the plexus passes over the first rib, it enters the axilla through a 'fascial funnel', with most (though not all) of the nerves entering the arm in close proximity to one another. At first glance it would appear that the situation is totally different in the lower extremity, with all of the nerves derived from the lumbar and sacral plexuses taking widely disparate courses to the leg and entering the thigh widely separated from each other and at differing depths beneath the skin. A closer look, on the other hand, reveals that the lumbar plexus either forms within or passes through the space between the quadratus lumborum and psoas major muscle (after leaving the latter muscle), so at this point the nerves lie within the compartment formed by

the fascia of these muscles. Whereas the *lateral femoral cutaneous* nerve, once formed, leaves the lateral border of the psoas major muscle at about its mid-point and enters the lateral thigh at a very superficial level (Fig. 13.8) and the *obturator nerve* leaves the medial border of the psoas major muscle and enters the medial thigh at a very deep level, the *femoral nerve*, the largest branch of the lumbar plexus, appears at the lateral margin of the psoas major muscle at the junction of its middle and lower thirds and remains in the groove between the psoas major and iliacus muscles throughout its course to the thigh. Thus, above the inguinal ligament (Fig. 13.9) the femoral nerve is bounded laterally and posteriorly by the iliac fascia, medially by the psoas fascia, and anteriorly by the transversalis fascia; so in its descent to the thigh the femoral nerve is enveloped in a fascial compartment which is continuous proximally with the fascial compartment between the psoas major and quadratus lumborum muscles. Distally, below the inguinal ligament, the fused iliopsoas fascia continues to provide the posterolateral wall of this perineural compartment, the iliopectineal fascia the medial wall, and the fascia lata the anterior wall.

From these anatomical considerations it would appear that there *are* similarities between the lumbar and brachial plexuses, at least in terms of fascial investments: Because the femoral nerve carries with it a tubular fascial sheath which forms

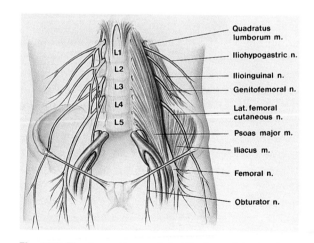

Fig. 13.8 The formation and distribution of the lumbar plexus and its relationship to the quadratus lumborum, psoas major, and iliacus muscles. (Reproduced from Anesth Analg 1973; 52: 990, with permission of the publisher.)

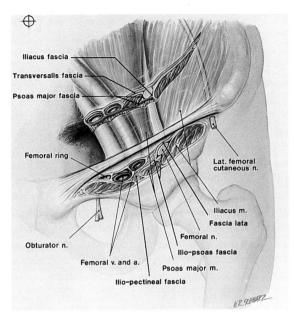

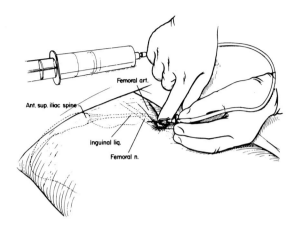

Fig. 13.9 A cross-section above and below the inguinal ligament in Figure 13.8, illustrating the perineural compartment surrounding the femoral nerve throughout its course to the leg. (Reproduced from Anesth Analg 1973; 52: 991, with permission of the publisher.)

Fig. 13.10 The inguinal paravascular technique of lumbar plexus block ('3-in-1' block). With a finger palpating the femoral artery, a needle is inserted just lateral to this point and advanced until an appropriate paresthesia (or appropriate muscular response to a nerve stimulator) indicates the tip of the needle is in the perineural compartment. (Reproduced from Anesth Analg 1973; 52: 992, with permission of the publisher.)

a perineural compartment that is an extension of the more proximal compartment surrounding much of the plexus, an injection of local anesthetic can be made into the sheath below the inguinal ligament and forced cephalad to the level where all three nerves exist within a common fascial envelope. Unlike the close neurovascular relationship of the terminal brachial plexus in the axilla, where the axillary sheath envelops the whole neurovascular bundle, in the inguinal region the neural and vascular elements are spatially separated, and their separation is reinforced structurally by the femoral sheath. Because of this difference, the technique by which the nerves derived from the lumbar plexus are blocked in the inguinal area is properly termed, 'the inguinal paravascular technique of lumbar plexus block',[90] although its more popular designation is the '3-in-1' block.

The technique, as originally described, is performed with the patient supine and the anesthesiologist standing beside the patient on the side opposite that about to be blocked. With the index finger palpating the femoral artery pulse (Fig. 13.10), a 22 gauge, 'immobile needle' is inserted just lateral to the artery and is advanced in a cephalad direction until a paresthesia of the

femoral nerve indicates penetration of the 'sheath'. At that point, following aspiration for blood, 20–30 ml of local anesthetic are injected in increments with firm digital pressure applied behind the needle (Fig. 13.11) to prevent retrograde flow caudad and to enhance cephalad flow of the local anesthetic. Alternatively, the needle can be placed utilizing a nerve stimulator; but with

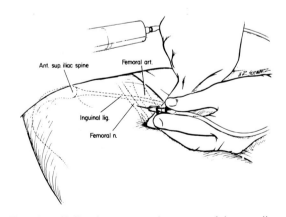

Fig. 13.11 Following proper placement of the needle, the palpating finger is placed just distal to the needle and firm digital pressure is applied to prevent the retrograde flow of the local anesthetic during the injection. (Reproduced from Anesth Analg 1973; 52: 993, with permission of the publisher.)

this technique the anesthesiologist needs to be cognizant of the fact that it is possible to evoke a motor response through the fascia, in which case, the local anesthetic might be deposited outside the sheath. Therefore, the twitch response should be obtained at no more than 0.2 mA to ensure that the needle tip is within the sheath.

In addition to the femoral nerve, the lumbar plexus gives rise to the lateral femoral cutaneous and obturator nerves, so the lumbar plexus provides the sensory innervation of the entire anterior, medial, and lateral surfaces of the lower extremity, i.e. all but the area innervated by the sciatic and posterior femoral cutaneous nerves. Therefore, since the '3-in-1' block also produces motor block of the powerful quadriceps muscles, it has been utilized effectively alone in the management of femoral fractures.[91] More frequently, however, the '3-in-1' block is combined with a sciatic block to provide anesthesia for surgery on the entire lower extremity, though Sprotte did suggest the use of this block alone to provide analgesia for traumatic and/or postoperative pain.[92]

Continuous inguinal paravascular lumbar plexus block: the '3-in-1' block

It was Rosenblatt[93] who first demonstrated the utility of a continuous catheter technique for postoperative pain relief. Concerned about the use of opiates for postoperative pain control in a 13-year-old boy with cystic fibrosis undergoing knee surgery, Rosenblatt threaded a 5 cm, 18 gauge, Teflon intravenous catheter over a 22 gauge, 3½ inch spinal needle and introduced the needle and catheter in a cephalad direction through a small incision just lateral to the femoral artery. Using a nerve stimulator, the needle and catheter were advanced until the appropriate motor response indicated the tip of the needle to be properly placed, following which 15 mL of 0.75% bupivacaine was injected and the catheter was advanced up the distended sheath. Following surgery under general anesthesia, it was determined that anesthesia was present in the distribution of the femoral, obturator, and lateral femoral cutaneous nerves; so the catheter was utilized to maintain postoperative analgesia for 2 days, first by repeated injections of bupivacaine at 6-hour intervals and then by a continuous infusion of bupivacaine. Actually, Rosenblatt had expected to provide analgesia in the distribution of the femoral nerve only,

so he was surprised that all three nerves were blocked following the injection of local anesthetic. He concluded that the "fact that satisfactory postoperative analgesia was produced using a femoral approach indicates that a '3-in-1' block similar to that described by Winnie et al[90] was obtained".[93]

As with continuous brachial plexus block, there are basically two techniques for carrying out a continuous lumbar plexus block, one using an 'extracath' (catheter over the needle) technique, and the other using an 'intracath' (catheter through the needle) technique. The technique utilized by the authors is almost identical to the original single injection '3-in-1' technique and similar to the technique of Rosenblatt except that a standard 20–22 gauge, Teflon intravenous 'extracath' is used instead of an intravenous catheter mounted on a spinal needle. The area lateral to the femoral artery pulse is prepared with an antiseptic solution and draped. The anesthesiologist, standing beside the patient on the side opposite that to be blocked, palpates the femoral artery pulse and raises a skin wheal 1–2 cm below the inguinal ligament and just 1 cm lateral to the pulse. An 18 gauge needle is used to puncture the skin, and through this wound a 20–22 gauge Teflon 'extracath' is inserted. The 'extracath' is advanced in a cephalad direction (at an angle of approximately 45° with the skin) with the bevel in the long axis of the nerve (to minimize the possibility of nerve damage) until a paresthesia indicates that the tip of the needle is in the perineural sheath. After careful aspiration for blood, 5–10 mL of local anesthetic are injected to open and distend the sheath, after which the catheter is advanced off the needle several centimeters and immobilized with tape or a suture. An additional 10–20 mL of local anesthetic is then injected in increments through the catheter (with frequent aspiration) to complete the initial injection. At this point an injection port or infusion can be connected to the catheter hub. Placement of the catheter can be carried out using a nerve stimulator, but the needle must have a metal hub to allow the 'extracath' to function as a sheathed needle. Contraction of the quadriceps muscle indicates proper placement of the needle tip with this technique and assures good anesthesia and/or analgesia.[94,95] However, if utilizing a peripheral nerve stimulator in patients with a femoral fracture, the search for the femoral nerve twitch should be carried out using a very low current, since vigorous contractions of the quadriceps muscle can be very painful. Whichever technique is utilized, firm digital pressure should be applied just distal to the injection site to promote cephalad and prevent caudad spread of the local anesthetic.

The limitation of the 'extracath' technique as described above and as reported by Rosenblatt is the inability to advance the catheter much beyond the level of the inguinal ligament. As the '3-in-1' block became more widely utilized and the continuous technique evolved, to allow higher placement of the catheter a larger 'extracath' was utilized so that after removing the needle, a smaller but much longer catheter could be inserted through the larger catheter and advanced as far as desired, after which the original catheter was removed. This, then, is the 'intracath technique' described above in the techniques of continuous brachial plexus block. Because of the greater distance between the entry site and the plexus in the inguinal approach to lumbar plexus block than in the axillary approach to brachial plexus block, the 'intracath technique' has become more popular. As a matter of fact, in 1984 Postel & Marz[96] reported 76 patients and in 1988 Nebler & Schwippel[97] reported 104 patients whose perioperative pain management was provided by continuous '3-in-1' block using a 'lumbar plexus block kit' (Alphaplex®, Firma Sterimed, Saarbrücken) available commercially in Germany. These investigators located the femoral nerve using a nerve stimulator and a small-lumen cannula. Then the indwelling catheter was inserted through the cannula using the Seldinger technique, and advanced to the desired level. Postel & Marz emphasized the special utility of this technique in patients with femoral fractures, facilitating their preoperative work-up and management as well as their postoperative mobilization without the need for narcotics.[96] The catheters were left in place an average of 6 days, with the longest being 44 days in the report of Nebler & Schwippel.[97]

There is no question that the group in Århus, Denmark has studied the continuous lumbar plexus block most extensively, and in doing so has answered many questions concerning its use. First of all, because several reports in the literature had indicated that perineural morphine could provide analgesia,[98–101] Dahl et al[102] compared the analgesia provided by '3-in-1' blocks carried out using morphine with the analgesia provided by epidural morphine in a double-blind, randomized, crossover study in patients after knee surgery. This study

showed that good relief was provided by morphine injected into the epidural space, while virtually no relief followed morphine injected into the femoral sheath, casting doubt on the theory of neuroaxonal transport of morphine from the periphery to the spinal cord.[98,99] Clinically, this study invalidates the addition of opiates to local anesthetics peripherally, a common practice in pain management. Next, Dahl et al[103] established the therapeutic benefit of continuous lumbar plexus block for postoperative pain relief by comparing infusions of bupivacaine with infusions of sodium chloride in a double-blind, randomized, controlled investigation. Both infusions were given through catheters inserted into the patients' femoral nerve sheath using the '3-in-1' block technique; and not surprisingly, the patients treated with bupivacaine had significantly less pain and a significantly reduced demand for morphine. Blood levels of bupivacaine were also determined to be below toxic levels, and there were no signs or symptoms of toxicity.

The above study was carried out using 0.5% bupivacaine for the initial dose followed by an infusion of 0.25% bupivacaine. To determine the minimal effective concentration of bupivacaine. Anker-Moller et al[104] compared the analgesic effect and plasma concentrations produced by 0.25% and 0.125% bupivacaine after knee surgery; and they found that 0.125% infusions of bupivacaine offer the same pain relief when used for continuous lumbar plexus block as 0.25% infusions. In addition, the resultant plasma levels of bupivacaine were significantly lower in the patients receiving the lower concentration, thus significantly reducing the possibility of toxic signs and/or symptoms.

Finally, since the standard postoperative alternative to this new therapy had been the use of epidural narcotics, Schultz et al[105] compared the efficacy of continuous lumbar plexus block using bupivacaine with continuous epidural morphine in a prospective, randomized, double-blind study. The results of this study indicated that, while there were no significant differences between the two methods with respect to analgesia, lumbar plexus block produced a statistically-significant reduction in the incidence of nausea, vomiting, pruritus, and urinary retention, which the investigators felt made lumbar plexus block the preferable modality for postoperative pain relief after open knee surgery.

In all of these studies by the group in Århus[102–105] most of the catheters were advanced 15–20 cm into the femoral sheath, and the results were uniformly good. Recently, however, Singelyn[106] looked at the significance of the level of catheter placement in 80 patients receiving continuous lumbar plexus blocks for pain relief after hip or knee surgery. In 40 of the patients the catheters were inserted 'blindly' using the Seldinger technique described above and advanced a mean of 13 ± 2 cm, while in the other 40 patients the catheter was inserted and advanced under X-ray control as far as possible to 'a lumbar paravertebral position', a mean distance of 26 ± 3 cm from the skin. Following aspiration for blood or CSF, 40 mL of 0.25% bupivacaine with epinephrine 1:200 000 were injected followed by a continuous infusion of 0.125% bupivacaine at 10 mL/h; and what is impressive is that in the group of patients with the catheter tip at the higher level, *complete '3-in-1' block* was obtained 2.5 times more frequently than in the group where the tip of the catheter was lower. Clearly, the level to which the catheter is inserted is important in terms of the *extent* of blockade. Furthermore, it would appear that injecting a larger volume at a lower level is not as effective, since Seeberger & Urwyler found that doubling the volume from 20 mL to 40 mL did not appear to influence the extent of blockade.[95] However, the catheter can be advanced too far, as Singelyn & Gouverneur[107] reported a patient in whom the catheter was advanced 'as cephalad as possible' and produced epidural anesthesia following the injection of 40 mL of 0.25% bupivacaine. As a result of this case Singelyn advised not only aspiration for blood or CSF prior to injection, but also verification of the position of the catheter tip with a radio-opaque contrast medium to rule out epidural placement.

Several authors have advanced epidural catheters through Tuohy needles placed in the femoral sheath: Edwards & Wright[108] placed the needle with the 'double loss-of-resistance' technique described by Khoo and Brown.[91] Hirst et al[109] utilized a nerve stimulator and an 18 gauge insulated Tuohy needle; and Mansour & Bennetts[110] utilized both endpoints to confirm correct placement of an unsheathed Tuohy needle, i.e. the two 'fascial clicks' *and* the contraction of one of the components of the quadriceps muscle in response to nerve stimulation. While all of these investigators reported successful pain relief, most investigators have continued to use the 'intracath' technique as described, with[111] or without the Seldinger introducer,[112] though some continue to use an 'extracath'.[113]

In summary, all of the above studies would seem to indicate the following: (1) the 'intracath' technique is preferable to the 'extracath' technique for the lumbar plexus block, as it allows advancement of the indwelling catheter to a much higher level, and a high level of injection significantly increases the incidence of *complete '3-in-1' block*; (2) bupivacaine 0.125% is as effective as the 0.25%, so use of this lower concentration enhances the safety of the technique by reducing the blood level without decreasing the efficacy; and (3) the addition of opioids to the local anesthetic does **not** enhance the efficacy of lumbar plexus block, it simply results in the unwanted side effects of opiates.

Of course, no technique is completely devoid of complications; and lumbar plexus block is no exception. However, there have really been only two **major** complications reported, one a *severe postoperative femoral neuropathy*[114] and the other an *acute compression syndrome of the femoral nerve caused by a subfascial hematoma*.[115] A *systemic toxic reaction* to bupivacaine has been reported, but only when an inadvertent overdose was given.[116] Lesser complications have included *inadvertent arterial puncture, intravascular catheter placement*, and *redness of the puncture site*.[116]

Nonetheless, while continuous lumbar plexus block is an effective means of managing pain following trauma involving the hip, thigh, and/or knee or pain following surgical procedures performed on them, it is obviously inadequate to provide *complete* analgesic for injuries to or surgery on those parts of the leg innervated by the sciatic nerve. Even following major trauma to or surgery on the hip, femur, and/or knee, the '3-in-1' block alone provides incomplete analgesia.[117] Because of the greater efficacy of *combined sciatic and '3-in-1' blocks* for open knee surgery.[118,119] Mansour & Bennetts added a single-shot sciatic block to continuous lumbar plexus block to provide the greater extent of analgesia necessary after knee surgery.[110] Obviously, while the single-shot sciatic block would supplement the continuous '3-in-1' block for the duration of surgery and the immediate postoperative period, the duration would be insufficient to provide the prolonged analgesia required for the continuing pain of major trauma.

Continuous sciatic block

A continuous sciatic block was utilized by Smith et al[120] to provide prolonged analgesia for 4 days and in combination with a continuous inguinal paravascular block to provide *complete* surgical and postoperative analgesia. However, this technique attempts to place a catheter near the sciatic nerve after it has exited the pelvis via the greater sciatic foramen, an area where dense connective tissue and poorly defined fascial planes make it difficult to thread a catheter and to prevent catheter migration and/or dislodgement.[121] Morris & Lang[122] have recently combined a continuous parasacral sciatic nerve block with a lumbar plexus block to provide several days of analgesia in two patients, using the landmarks and technique described by Mansour.[123] This technique actually places the needle tip (and hence the catheter) within the pelvis in close proximity to the sacral plexus. These investigators found that with this technique the catheters are easy to place, there is little resistance to advancement, and they remained functional for 48 hours in spite of ambulation. While this technique deserves further investigation as a companion block to continuous lumbar plexus block, a continuous technique capable of providing anesthesia and analgesia of both the lumbar and sacral plexuses through a single catheter is certainly more desirable.

Continuous lumbosacral plexus block

It was pointed out earlier that the lumbar plexus either forms within or passes through the space between the quadratus lumborum and psoas major muscles (after emerging from the latter muscle); so at this point the lumbar plexus lies within the potential space formed by these muscles. The iliac fascia and the psoas fascia continue to invest the femoral nerve as it descends to the leg, and the lateral femoral cutaneous nerve travels beneath the iliacus fascia as it descends to the leg. The sacral plexus is ensheathed by an expansion of the fascia of the piriformis muscle, which is continuous with that covering the obturator internus muscle;[124] and because of the continuity of these fasciae and the potential spaces they form, one should not be surprised to find that a sufficient volume of local anesthetic injected in the fascial compartment around the lumbar plexus finds its way to the sacral plexus as well.

The combined lumbosacral block as originally described in 1974[125] utilizes these interconnected fascial compartments and is carried out in a manner that is almost identical to that which would be used to perform a paravertebral block of L4 except

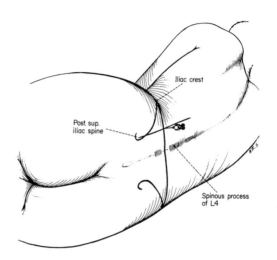

Fig. 13.12 Combined lumbosacral plexus block. With the patient in the lateral position, a 3½ inch spinal needle is inserted at the intersection of the intercristal line and a line drawn parallel to the spine through the posterior superior iliac spine. (Reproduced from Anesthesiology Review 1974; 1: 15, with permission of the publisher.)

for the large volume of local anesthetic injected. The patient is placed in the lateral position, lying on the side opposite that to be blocked. While the lateral position may be uncomfortable or painful for the patient with trauma to the lower extremity, it is usually tolerable if the patient is helped to assume that position, particularly if the traumatized leg is uppermost. A line is drawn between the superior margins of both iliac crests, indicating the approximate level of the L4–L5 interspace; and a second line is drawn parallel to the spine but passing through the posterior, superior iliac spine (Fig. 13.12). At the point where the intercristal line crosses the paraspinous line, a 3½ inch, 22 gauge spinal needle is inserted perpendicular to the skin, but with a very slight mesiad direction. As the needle is advanced, it may encounter the transverse process of L4; and if so, the needle is withdrawn and re-directed slightly more caudally until the advancing needle no longer encounters the transverse process. It is now advanced until a paresthesia (usually in the distribution of the femoral nerve) is produced, indicating that the tip of the needle lies in the potential space between the quadratus lumborum and the psoas major muscle (Fig. 13.13). An injection of 40 mL of local anesthetic into this interfascial space dissects caudad to

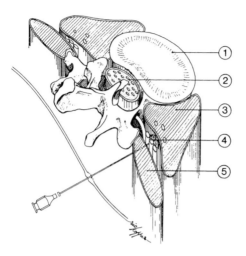

Fig. 13.13 The needle is advanced perpendicular to the skin until an appropriate paresthesia (or appropriate muscular response to a nerve stimulator) indicates appropriate placement of the tip of the needle within the space between the quadratus lumborum and the psoas major muscle. (1) vertebral body of L4; (2) subarachnoid space containing cauda equina; (3) psoas major muscle; (4) lumbar plexus; (5) quadratus lumborum (Reproduced from Miller RD. Anesthesia, 2nd ed. New York: Churchill Livingstone, with permission of the publisher.)

bathe both the lumbar and sacral plexuses and usually provides anesthesia of both. If the anesthesiologist has difficulty in obtaining a paresthesia, the use of a nerve stimulator can identify the proper position of the needle tip as that point at which contraction of the quadriceps muscle occurs in response to a current of 0.3 mA or less.

Using the same landmarks, Vaghadia et al described *continuous* lumbosacral plexus block using a Tuohy needle and an epidural catheter.[126] The technique was identical to the single-injection technique described above except that after the Tuohy needle had been advanced deep to the transverse process of L4, a 5 mL glass syringe containing saline was attached and a 'loss-of-resistance' technique was used during needle advancement. Using this technique, the authors stated that 'entry of the needle tip into the potential space between the quadratus lumborum and psoas muscle was accompanied by a slight click, as well as loss of resistance.' They did not elicit paresthesias or utilize a nerve stimulator to confirm the position of the needle, but simply, after

the loss of resistance, advanced a radio-opaque epidural catheter 8 cm beyond the tip of the needle and taped it in place. The authors indicated that the catheter advanced easily; and after a test dose, 40 mL of local anesthetic were injected. In all of the 12 patients they reported effective anesthesia of both the lumbar and sacral plexuses during surgery and postoperative analgesia thereafter.

Continuous psoas compartment block

Two years after the introduction of *the combined lumbosacral plexus block* by Winnie et al,[125] a technique termed *the psoas compartment block* was described by Chayen et al,[127] and these two techniques have subsequently either been used interchangeably or have been confused with each other. The terminology of Chayen et al is based on the statement by the authors that the lumbar plexus 'is located deep in the substance of the psoas major muscle in a kind of compartment formed by the muscle and its fascia anteriorly, the bodies of the lumbar vertebrae medially, the transverse processes of the same vertebrae, the intertransverse ligaments and muscles, and the quadratus lumborum muscle posteriorly.' It is not readily apparent whether the difference between the 'psoas compartment' of Chayen and the potential space between the quadratus lumborum and psoas major muscles described by Winnie, is an anatomical difference or a semantic one; but the technique of blocking the lumbar plexus described by Chayen would seem to place the injection of local anesthetic in a different area than that described by Winnie. First of all, in carrying out the technique described by Chayen, a 6 inch, 20 gauge needle is inserted at a point 3 cm caudad to the intercristal line and 5 cm from the midline until it encounters the fifth lumbar transverse process, at which point the needle is withdrawn and re-directed in a more cephalad direction until it glides above the transverse process. A 20 mL syringe containing air is then attached, and the needle is advanced 1–2 cm until it enters the quadratus lumborum muscle. Light tapping on the plunger of the syringe indicates resistance produced by the muscle or fascia. The needle is advanced 1 cm at a time until a loss of resistance indicates the tip of the needle to be in the psoas compartment, the depth of penetration usually being about 5 inches. *This is 1½ inches greater than the length of the needle used for a combined lum-*

bosacral block! At this point 20 mL of air is injected to dilate the compartment, after which 30 mL of local anesthetic is injected. The anesthesia provided in 90 of the 100 cases they reported only included the lumbar plexus.

Nicholls[128] subsequently carried out a CT study of Chayen's technique in patients and found that the point at which the local anesthetic is injected (5 inches below the skin) lies almost 2 inches anterior to the plexus in all cases, and in 50% of patients it was within viscera. This would probably explain why the resultant anesthesia was inadequate for surgery in 50% of the six cases where it was utilized clinically in the same report.[128] Another significant finding in the CT study was that when a needle is inserted at the point 5 cm from the midline and 3 cm below the intercristal line, the wing of the ilium is encountered in 55% of the patients, rather than the transverse process of L5.

A clinical comparison of the two techniques by Dalens et al,[129] though carried out in children, is revealing, to say the least; but in reviewing their findings, one must remember that because the techniques were carried out in children, a nerve stimulator was used to place the needle **with both techniques**. Nonetheless, they found that the combined lumbosacral block technique produced anesthesia of both the lumbar and sacral plexuses *in the blocked leg* in 92% of the patients and anesthesia of the lumbar plexus only in the other 8%, with no failures. Interestingly, the psoas compartment block produced epidural anesthesia that included both legs and the lower trunk in 88% of the patients, and lumbar plexus anesthesia only in 8%, with complete failure in the other 4%. An additional interesting finding was that the depth at which the injection was made was greater (by 6–10 mm) in the group receiving the combined lumbosacral block than in the group receiving the psoas compartment block. In the original description of the psoas compartment block, the depth at which the injection was made was 1½ inches greater than the depth at which the injection is made using the combined lumbosacral block technique. It may very well be that the use of the nerve stimulator is the reason for the success of the psoas compartment block in Dalen's study (albeit epidural anesthesia) and more importantly, the lack of complications (other than unexpected epidural anesthesia).

Nonetheless, only 2 years after the publication of the psoas compartment block, Brands & Callanan[130] reported the first continuous technique based on Chayen's article. These authors reported their experience in 21 patients with femoral neck fractures: They placed an 18 gauge needle according to the technique described by Chayen, except that instead of the needle being advanced above the fifth lumbar transverse process, it was directed so as to pass above the fourth and advanced until loss of resistance was appreciated, usually 2–3 cm beyond the transverse process. Following aspiration, 30 mL of air was injected to open the space, after which a radio-opaque catheter was threaded through the needle and advanced until 5 cm of the catheter lay within the compartment. After aspiration 30 mL of bupivacaine 0.5% with epinephrine 1:200 000 were injected. In 21 patients the catheters were placed on admission to the hospital and kept in place for 48 hours postoperatively. While the actual extent of anesthesia was not reported, 17 of the 21 patients obtained sufficient pain relief to make narcotic analgesic administration unnecessary. Ten of these patients obtained complete analgesia, and the other seven complained of mild pain only during nursing procedures.

In subsequent publications concerning continuous techniques that attempt to approach the lumbar and/or sacral plexuses posteriorly,[131–134] it is unclear as to which technique is actually utilized – combined lumbosacral plexus block technique or the psoas compartment block technique – as the term 'psoas compartment' is used interchangeably with 'the space between the psoas major and quadratus muscles'. However, whether these two spaces are the same or not (or whether the injections are actually made into the substance of the psoas major muscle and confined by its fascia),[135,136] the use of a nerve stimulator seems to maximize success, since it definitely identifies the compartment within which the nerves lie, whatever it is. Therefore, until the anatomical relationships of the lumbar and sacral plexuses (and the fascia surrounding them) are more clearly delineated, the use of a nerve stimulator is certainly desirable for posterior approaches, regardless of technique.

Complications following posterior approaches are rare, and the total number of reports concerning these techniques are few. However, as stated earlier, *epidural anesthesia*[129] is not uncommon, and *subcapsular hematoma*[137] and *intravascular injection*,[127] have been described after the psoas compartment block, while *spinal*[138] *and epidural*[139] *anesthesia* have been reported after continuous lumbosacral plexus block.

Clinical considerations

As with the upper extremity, most of the experience to date with continuous plexus blocks has been gained in providing surgical anesthesia and postoperative analgesia, though their use for trauma is increasing as anesthesiologists become increasingly involved in the management of trauma patients. Because of the role of the lower extremities in weight-bearing and ambulation, continuous peripheral blocks can play a unique role in the trauma patient, since unlike continuous spinal and epidural, if the trauma is confined to one extremity, unilateral block can provide pain relief *and* preserve the ability to ambulate. Admittedly, the matter is complicated by the fact that unlike the upper extremity, the lower extremity is innervated by two plexuses; but knowledge of the innervation of the area of the trauma will indicate if a block of one plexus will suffice or if blockade of both is necessary.

Thus, the choice of technique will depend on the site, extent, and type of injury. While the Danish group has demonstrated that the *analgesia* provided by 0.125% bupivacaine is equal to that provided by 0.25% bupivacaine, if severe muscle spasm is present (as is so often the case following trauma) motor block is essential to provide relaxation, so a higher concentration may be preferable. However, there is obviously a wide margin of safety with bupivacaine in lower extremity blocks: Even when the '3-in-1' block was combined with a sciatic block using 0.5% bupivacaine, the plasma concentration of bupivacaine associated with toxicity[140] was not reached, with or without epinephrine, even though the dose exceeded the manufacturer's recommended dose by 50%;[141] nor were there any clinical signs of toxicity. While the addition of epinephrine did not reduce plasma levels significantly in this study, in another study using 0.25% bupivacaine with and without epinephrine for psoas compartment block, the addition of epinephrine did decrease the plasma levels significantly; and though one patient receiving plain bupivacaine achieved a peak concentration of 4.54 µg/ml, none of the patients in either group showed signs of systemic toxicity.[142]

Farny et al[143] studied the blood levels resulting from the use of lidocaine 2% with epinephrine for combined lumbosacral plexus block *and* sciatic block in 45 patients; and in spite of the fact that they utilized a total of 680 mg of lidocaine, the plasma concentrations were all within 'safe limits', except for one patient who had a level of 9.54 µg/ml. None of the patients showed any signs of systemic toxicity. Similarly, Atanassoff[144] used 650 mg of lidocaine (65 mL of 1% lidocaine with epinephrine) for combined sciatic and '3-in-1' blocks, and he found that none of the patients approached toxic plasma levels of lidocaine; and none of the patients showed clinical signs of toxicity, though the dose again exceeded the manufacturer's recommended dose by 30%.

Simon et al[145] studied the plasma concentration of mepivacaine resulting from the combination of psoas compartment block and sciatic block using 55 mL of 1.33% mepivacaine with epinephrine 1:600 000, a total dose of 731.5 mg of mepivacaine; and even with this high dose (almost 50% greater than that recommended by the manufacturer), the maximal concentration of mepivacaine in the plasma stayed well below 6.0 µg/ml, (the threshold for toxicity)[146] in 19 of the 20 patients; and though the other patients achieved a plasma level of 7.07 µg/ml, none of the patients exhibited signs of systemic toxicity.

An interesting, rational, and perhaps safer approach to continuous block anesthesia and/or analgesia was proposed by Rung,[147] who abandoned the use of intermittent injections of long-acting amide-type local anesthetics in managing continuous lumbar plexus blocks in favor of a continuous infusion of 1% chloroprocaine. He listed the following reasons for this change in his practice:

1. the ester-type local anesthetics may pose a lower risk of systemic toxicity, because they are rapidly metabolized in the plasma;
2. the high peak plasma concentrations attained after intermittent boluses of local anesthetics (and the attendant risk of toxicity) are avoided;
3. a continuous infusion of local anesthetic provides continuous analgesia;
4. the use of a short-acting local anesthetic permits quick reversal of drug effect should neurologic or other examination of the extremity be required (this reason is particularly important in the trauma patient).

In using continuous nerve blocks for pain management *in trauma patients*, the present authors do not advocate the addition of adjunctive agents such as sodium bicarbonate, α agonists, or opioids, to enhance local anesthetic activity as their benefit is minimal, if not controversial; and their use simply complicates the pharmacologic management of the patient, particularly in patients with severe and extensive injuries. Whether intermittent injections or a continuous infusion is chosen, there is a wide variety of local anesthetics from which one can choose that will provide the desired duration; and by using the proper concentration one can modify the intensity of blockade and, to a certain degree, the modalities blocked.

Perhaps even more important for successful analgesia in the lower extremity than in the upper extremity is selection of the proper technique: If the hip alone is involved, or even if the hip and thigh are all that is involved, a continuous '3-in-1' block almost always is sufficient. If the knee is also involved, advancing the catheter to a high level may render the analgesia adequate;[106] but the obturator nerve may still be missed by this technique alone.[148,149] However, the addition of a sciatic nerve block to a continuous '3-in-1' block has been shown to provide complete analgesia of the knee in the vast majority of cases;[110] so the inadequate analgesia observed by some investigators[150,151] who used the '3-in-1' block for knee surgery may be due to the unblocked sciatic rather than obturator nerve.

For trauma and/or surgery involving the knee or below (or for that matter, the entire lower extremity), while one can select continuous '3-in-1' *and* continuous sciatic block, it is simpler and probably more effective to utilize a continuous combined lumbosacral plexus block. Though it is possible to obtain good anesthesia of both the sacral and lumbar plexuses with this technique, especially if an adequate volume of local anesthetic is injected,[125,126,129] several investigators have added a sciatic block to this technique to ensure anesthesia and/or analgesia of the sacral plexus.[134,136,138] Obviously, the single-injection technique is simpler, whether anesthesia of the lumbar plexus only is desired, as for femoral fractures, or if anesthesia of both plexuses is needed, as for injuries to the knee or below.

SUMMARY/CONCLUSION

Whatever the level of the trauma, continuous peripheral plexus blocks can provide complete anesthesia and/or analgesia of an extremity and avoid the unwanted effects of opioids. In those cases where continuous epidural and/or intrathecal analgesia might be considered, continuous plexus blocks allow the same improvement in blood flow to the extremity, but because the sympathetic block is unilateral and postganglionic, the plexus block avoids the hypotension and tachycardia that may result from the bilateral, preganglionic sympathetic block produced by epidural or spinal, an event that can be disastrous in the trauma patient. Continuous peripheral blocks, unlike central blocks, do not interfere with bladder and rectal control and/or function; and being unilateral, they allow earlier mobilization and ambulation. Placed early, continuous peripheral blocks can provide pain relief and reduce muscle spasm for painful diagnostic and therapeutic procedures, for surgery, and for the postoperative period; and the analgesia can be interrupted periodically to allow evaluation of possible complications or of neurological function, and then be reinstituted to facilitate recovery. And finally, the use of continuous plexus blocks to manage the acute pain following trauma and/or surgery may prevent the development of the complex regional pain syndromes that can result from traumatic injuries to the extremities.

REFERENCES

1. Wilmore DW, Long JM, Mason AD, Pruitt BA. Stress in surgical patients as a neurophysiologic reflex response. Surg Gynecol Obstet 1976; 142: 257.
2. Yaksh TL, Hammond DL. Peripheral and central substrates involved in the rostrad transmission of nociceptive information. Pain 1982; 13: 1–85.
3. Kehlet H. Does regional anesthesia reduce postoperative morbidity? Intens Care Med 1984; 10: 165–167.
4. Moller IW, Rem J, Brandt MR, Kehlet H. Effect of posttraumatic epidural analgesia on the cortisol and hyperglycemic response to surgery. Acta Anaesthesiol Scand 1982; 26: 56–58.
5. Beran DR. Modification of the metabolic response to trauma under extradural analgesia. Anaesthesia 1971; 26: 188–191.
6. Brandt MR, Fernades A, Mordhorst R, Kehlet H. Epidural analgesia improves postoperative nitrogen balance. Br Med J 1978; 1: 1106–1108.
7. Kehlet H. The endocrine-metabolic response to postoperative pain. Acta Anaesthesiol Scand 1982; 74(Suppl): 173–175.

8. Kehlet H, Brandt MR, Rem J. Role of neurogenic stimuli in mediating the endocrine-metabolic response to surgery. JPEN 1980; 4: 152–156.

9. Bromage PR, Schibata HR, Wiloughby HW. Influence of prolonged epidural blockade on blood sugar and cortisol responses to operations upon the upper part of the abdomen and the thorax. Surg Gynecol Obstet 1971; 132: 1051–1056.

10. Rutberg H, Hakanson E, Anderberg B, et al. Effects of the extradural administration of morphine or bupivacaine on the endocrine response to upper abdominal surgery. Br J Anaesth 1984; 56: 233–238.

11. Christensen P, Brandt MR, Rem J, et al. Influence of extradural morphine on the adrenocortical and hyperglycemic response to surgery. Br J Anaesth 1982; 54: 23–27.

12. Solimen IE, Safwat A. Successful management of an elderly patient with multiple trauma. J Trauma 1985; 25: 806–807.

13. Child CS, Kaufman L. Effect of intrathecal diamorphine on the adrenocortical, hyperglycemic and cardiovascular responses to major colonic surgery. Br J Anaesth 1985; 57: 389–393.

14. Downing B, Davis J, Black J, Windsor CWO. Effect of intrathecal morphine on the adrenocortical and hyperglycaemic responses to upper abdominal surgery. Br J Anaesth 1986; 58: 858–861.

15. Hjortso NC, Christensen NJ, Andersen T, et al. Effects of the extradural administration of local anesthetic agents and morphine on the urinary excretion of cortisol, catecholamines and nitrogen following abdominal surgery. Br J Anaesth 1985; 57: 400–406.

16. Jorgensen BC, Anderson HB, Engquist A. Influence of epidural morphine on postoperative pain, endocrine-metabolic and renal responses to surgery: A controlled study. Acta Anaesthesiol Scand 1982; 26: 63–68.

17. Sebel PS, Aun C, Fiolet J, et al. Endocrinological effects of intrathecal morphine. Eur J Anaesthesiol 1985; 2: 291–296.

18. Asoh T, Tsuji H, Shirasaka C, Takeuchi Y. Effect of epidural analgesia on metabolic response to major upper abdominal surgery. Acta Anaesthesiol Scand 1983; 27: 233–237.

19. Hakanson E, Rutberg H, Jorfeldt L, Martensson J. Effects of the extradural administration of morphine or bupivacaine on the metabolic response to upper abdominal surgery. Br J Anaesth 1985; 57: 394–399.

20. Kennedy WF, Bonica JJ, Akamatsu TJ, et al. Cardiovascular and respiratory effects of subarachnoid block in the presence of acute blood loss. Anesthesiology 1968; 29: 29–35.

21. Bonica JJ, Kennedy WF, Akamatsu TJ, et al. Circulatory effects of peridural blocks III. Effects of acute blood loss. Anesthesiology 1972; 36: 219–227.

22. Raj PP, Rosenblatt R, Montgomery SJ. Use of the nerve stimulator for peripheral blocks. Reg Anes 1980; 5: 14–21.

23. Pither CE, Raj PP, Ford DJ. The use of peripheral nerve stimulators for regional anesthesia. A review of experimental characteristics, technique, and clinical applications. Reg Anes 1985; 10: 49–58.

24. Ford DJ, Pither CE, Raj PP. Comparison of insulated and uninsulated needles for locating peripheral nerves with a peripheral nerve stimulator. Anesth Analg 1984; 63: 925–928.

25. Basheim G, Haschke RH, Ready LB. Electrical nerve location: Numerical and electrophoretic comparison of insulated vs uninsulated needles. Anesth Analg 1984; 63: 919–924.

26. Yasuda I, Hirano T, Ojima T, et al. Supraclavicular brachial plexus block using a nerve stimulator and an insulated needle. Br J Anaesth 1980; 52: 409–411.

27. Tuominen MK, Haasio J, Hekali R, Rosenberg PH. Continuous interscalene brachial plexus block: Clinical efficacy, technical problems and bupivacaine plasma concentrations. Acta Anaesthesiol Scand 1989; 33: 84–88.

28. Selander D. Catheter technique in axillary plexus block. Acta Anaesthesiol Scand 1977; 21: 324–329.

29. Rosenblatt R, Pepitone-Rockwell F, McKillop MJ. Continuous axillary analgesia for traumatic hand injury. Anesthesiology 1979; 51: 565–566.

30. Sada T, Kobayashi T, Murakami S. Continuous axillary brachial plexus block. Can Anaesth Soc J 1983; 30: 201–205.

31. Ang EG, Lassale B, Goldfarb G. Continuous axillary brachial plexus block–a clinical and anatomical study. Anesth Analg 1984; 63: 680–684.

32. Haynsworth RF, Heavner JE, Racz GB. Continuous brachial plexus blockade using an axillary catheter for treatment of accidental intraarterial injections. Reg Anes 1985; 10: 187–190.

33. Plancarte R, Amescua C, Marron M, et al. Continuous brachial block introducing catheters through a Tuohy needle in the axilla. Anesthesiology 1987; 67: A287.

34. Büttner J, Klose R, Argo A. Continuous axillary plexus block: A prospective evaluation of 1133 cases. Reg Anes 1988; 13(Suppl 2): 60.

35. Winnie AP. Plexus anesthesia I: The perivascular techniques of brachial plexus block. Philadephia: WB Saunders; 1993.

36. Baranowski AP, Pither CE. A comparison of three methods of axillary brachial plexus anaesthesia. Anaesthesia 1990; 45: 362–365.

37. Albrecht RF, Lennon RL. Description of an evoked motor response guided, single dose axillary block. Anesth Analg 1995; 80: S5.

38. Ansbro FP. A method of continuous brachial plexus block. Am J Surg 1946; 71: 716–722.

39. Lee VC, Abram SE. Continuous brachial plexus anesthesia; axillary sheath cannulation using a spinal needle–intravenous catheter combination. Reg Anes 1987; 12: 139–142.

40. Finucane BT, Yilling F, Santora A. Single shot or continuous axillary block: A refinement of technique. Reg Anes 1987; 12: 99–100.

41. Finucane BT, Yilling F. Safety of supplementing axillary brachial plexus blocks. Anesthesiology 1989; 70: 401–403.

42. Büttner J, Kemmer A, Argo A, Klose R, Forst R. Axillary block of the brachial plexus (German). Reg Anaesth 1988; 11: 7–11.

43. Büttner J, Klose R. Serum concentrations of mepivacaine-HCl in continuous axillary brachial plexus block for prolonged operations of the hand. Reg Anes 1988; 13(Suppl 2): 59.

44. Büttner J, Klose R, Hoppe U, Wresch P. Serum levels of mepivacaine-HCl during continuous axillary brachial plexus block. Reg Anes 1989; 14: 124–127.

45. Büttner J, Klose R, Hammer H. Continuous axillary catheter plexus anesthesia: A method for postoperative analgesia and sympathetic block after hand surgery (German). Handchir Mikorochir Plastchir 1989; 21: 29–32.

46. Hall JA, Wedel DJ, Lennon RL. Axillary catheter technique for brachial plexus blockade in upper extremity surgery. Reg Anes 1990; 15: S–46.

47. Hall JA, Lennon RL, Wedel DJ. Continuous bupivacaine infusion for postoperative pain relief via an axillary catheter. Reg Anes 1990; 15: S–58.

48. Lennon RL, Stinson LW Jr. Continuous axillary brachial plexus catheters. In: Morrey BF, ed. The elbow and its disorders. 2nd ed. Philadelphia: WB Saunders; 1993: ch 11.

49. Gauman DM, Lennon RL, Wedel DJ. Continuous axillary block for postoperative pain management. Reg Anes 1988; 13: 77–82.

50. Raj PP. Infraclavicular approaches to brachial plexus anesthesia techniques. Techniques in Regional Anesthesia and Pain Management 1997; 1: 169–177.

51. Raj PP, Denson DD. Prolonged analgesia technique with local anesthetics. In: Raj PP, ed. Practical management of pain. Chicago: Year Book Medical; 1986: 687–700.

52. Sims TK. A modification of landmarks for infraclavicular approach to brachial plexus blocks. Anesth Analg 1977; 56: 554–555.

53. Whiffler K. Coracoid block–a safe and easy technique. Br J Anaesth 1981; 53: 845–848.

54. Pippa P, Aito S, Commeli E, et al. Brachial plexus block using the transcoracobrachial approach. Eur J Anaesth 1992; 3: 235–239.

55. Bridenbaugh LD. The upper extremity: somatic blockade. In: Cousins MJ, Bridenbaugh PO, eds. Neural blockade in clinical anesthesia and management of pain. 2nd ed. Philadelphia: JB Lippincott; 1988: 387–416.

56. Fitzgibbon DR, Debs AD, Erjavec MK. Selective musculocutaneous nerve block and infraclavicular brachial plexus anesthesia. Reg Anes 1995; 20: 239–241.

57. Winnie AP, Collins VJ. The subclavian perivascular technique of brachial plexus anesthesia. Anesthesiology 1964; 25: 353–363.

58. Hilgier M. Continuous brachial block. Personal communication.

59. Fischer HBJ, Peters TM, Fleming IM, et al. Peripheral nerve catheterization in the management of terminal cancer pain. Reg Anes 1996; 21: 482–485.

60. Dhuner KG, Moberg E, Onne L. Paresis of the phrenic nerve during brachial plexus block analgesia and its importance. Acta Chir Scand 1955; 109: 53–57.

61. Shaw WM. Paralysis of the phrenic nerve during brachial plexus anesthesia. Anesthesiology 1949; 10: 627–628.

62. Farar MD, Scheybani M, Nolte H. Upper extremity blocks: Effectiveness and complications. Reg Anes 1981; 6: 133–134.

63. Hood J, Knoblanche G. Respiratory failure following brachial plexus block. Anaesth Intensive Care 1979; 7: 285–286.

64. Winnie AP. Interscalene brachial plexus block. Anesth Analg 1970; 49: 455–466.

65. Manriquez RG, Pallares V. Continuous brachial plexus block for prolonged sympathectomy and control of pain. Anesth Analg 1978; 57: 128–130.

66. Kirkpatrick AF, Bednarczyk LR, Hime GW, et al. Bupivacaine blood levels during continuous interscalene block. Anesthesiology 1985; 62: 65–67.

67. Haas DG, McDonnell FJ. Interscalene brachial plexus block. A convenient and cost-effective method of catheter insertion for continuous infusion. International Monitor on Regional Anesthesia 1993; 5(No. 3): 1.

68. Haasio J, Tuominen MK, Rosenberg PH. Continuous interscalene brachial plexus block during and after shoulder surgery. Ann Chir Gynaecol 1990; 79: 103–107.

69. Rosenberg PH, Pere P, Hekali R, Tuominen MK. Plasma concentrations of bupivacaine and two of its metabolites during continuous interscalene brachial plexus block. Br J Anaesth 1991; 66: 25–30.

70. Tuominen MK, Pere P, Rosenberg PH. Unintentional arterial catheterization and bupivacaine toxicity associated with continuous interscalene brachial plexus block. Anesthesiology 1991; 75: 356–358.

71. Cook LB. Unsuspected extradural catheterization in an interscalene block. Br J Anaesth 1991; 67: 473–475.

72. Urmey WF, McDonald M. Hemidiaphragmatic paresis during interscalene brachial plexus block: Effects on pulmonary function and chest wall mechanics. Anesth Analg 1992; 74: 352–357.

73. Urmey WF, Talts KH, Sharrock NE. One-hundred percent incidence of hemidiaphragmatic paresis associated with interscalene brachial plexus anesthesia as diagnosed by ultrasonography. Anesth Analg 1991; 72: 498–503.

74. Urmey WF, Gleoggler RJ. Pulmonary function changes during interscalene block: Effects of decreasing local anesthetic injection volume. Reg Anes 1993; 18: 244–249.

75. Pere P, Pitkanen M, Rosenberg PH, et al. Effect of continuous interscalene brachial plexus block on diaphragm motion and on ventilatory function. Acta Anaesthesiol Scand 1992; 36: 53–57.

76. Vester-Andersen T, Christiansen C, Hansen A, et al. Interscalene brachial plexus block: Area of analgesia, complications and blood concentrations of local anesthetics. Acta Anaesthesiol Scand 1981; 25: 81.

77. Aguilar JL, Domingo V, Samper D, et al. Long-term brachial plexus anesthesia using a subcutaneous implantable injection system. Reg Anes 1995; 20(3): 242–245.

78. Canovas M, Dominquez M, Martin M, et al. Axillary continuous blockade in patients with complex regional pain syndrome I. Br J Anaesth 1997; 78(Suppl 1): 124.

79. Borgeat A, Schappi B, Biasca N, Gerber C. Patient-controlled analgesia after major shoulder surgery. Anesthesiology 1997; 87: 1343–1347.

80. Tuominen MK, Rosenberg PH, Kalso E. Blood levels of bupivacaine after single dose, supplementary dose and during continuous infusion in axillary plexus block. Acta Anaesth Scand 1983; 27: 303–306.

81. Mezzatesta JP, Scott DA, Schweitzes SA, Selander DE. Continuous axillary brachial plexus block for postoperative pain relief. Reg Anes 1997; 22: 357–362.

82. Feldman HS. Toxicity of local anesthetic agents. In: Rice S, Fish K, eds. Anesthetic toxicity. New York: Raven Press; 1994; 109–133.

83. Feldman HS, Arthur GR, Covino BG. Toxicity of intravenously administered local anesthetic agents in dog: Cardiovascular and central nervous system effects. In: Roth SH, Miller KW, eds. Molecular and cellular mechanisms of anesthetics. New York: Plenum; 1986: 395–404.

84. Tucker GT, Mather LE. Pharmacokinetics of local anesthetic agents. Br J Anaesth 1975; 47: 213–224.

85. Hilgier M. Alkalinization of marcaine for prolongation of brachial block. Reg Anes 1985; 10: 59–61.

86. Bedder MD, Kozody R, Craig DB. Comparison of bupivacaine and alkalinized bupivacaine in brachial plexus anesthesia. Anesth Analg 1988; 67: 48–52.

87. Candido KD, Winnie AP, Covino BG, Raza SM, Vasireddy AP, Masters RW. Addition of bicarbonate to plain bupivacaine does not significantly alter the onset or duration of plexus anesthesia. Reg Anes 1995; 20: 133–138.

88. Singelyn FJ, Gouverneur JM. Duration of block and analgesia after brachial plexus anesthesia with mepivacaine: Effect of clonidine added to the anesthetic solution. Reg Anes 1992; 17: 148–150.

89. Viel EJ, Eledjam JJ, de la Coussaye JE, D'Athis F. Brachial plexus block with opioids for postoperative pain relief: Comparison between buprenorphine and morphine. Reg Anes 1989; 14: 274–278.

90. Winnie AP, Ramamurthy S, Durrani Z. The inguinal paravascular technic of lumbar plexus anesthesia: The 3-in-1 block. Anesth Analg 1973; 52: 989–996.

91. Khoo ST, Brown TCK. Femoral nerve block–The anatomical basis for a single injection technique. Anaesth Intensive Care 1983; 11: 40–42.

92. Sprotte G. The inguinal technique of lumbar plexus blockade for pre- and post-operative analgesia for trauma and orthopaedic surgery (German). Reg Anaesth 1981; 4: 39–41.

93. Rosenblatt RM. Continuous femoral anesthesia for lower extremity surgery. Anesth Analg 1980; 59: 631–632.

94. Kaiser H, Niesel HC, Klimpel L, Bodenmueller M. Prilocaine in lumbosacral plexus block–general efficacy and comparison of nerve stimulation amplitude. Acta Anaesth Scand 1992; 36: 692–697.

95. Seeberger MD, Urwyler A. Paravascular lumbar plexus block: Block extension after femoral nerve stimulation and injection of 20 vs. 40 ml mepivacaine 10 mg/ml. Acta Anaesth Scand 1995; 39: 769–773.

96. Postel J, Marz P. Continuous block of the lumbar plexus ('3-in-1 Block') in pre- and post-operative pain therapy (German). Reg Anaesth 1984; 7: 140–143.

97. Nebler R, Schwippel U. Continuous lumbar

plexus blockade with the '3-in-1' block catheter technique in pain therapy (German). Reg Anaesth 1988; 11: 54–57.

98. Mocavero G. Selective analgesia with perineural morphine (Italian). Rianimazione e Scienze Affini 1981; 16: 1–3.

99. Sanchez R, Nielsen H, Heslet L, Iverson AD. Neuronal blockade with morphine: A hypothesis. Anaesthesia 1984; 39: 788–789.

100. Nielsen H, Sanchez R, Knudsen F. Perineuronal morphine for pain relief of chronic pain. Anaesthesia 1986; 41: 768–769.

101. Mays KS, Lipman JJ, Schnapp M. Local analgesia without anesthesia using peripheral perineural morphine injections. Anesth Analg 1987; 66: 417–420.

102. Dahl JB, Daughard JJ, Kristoffersen E, et al. Perineuronal morphine: A comparison with epidural morphine. Anaesthesia 1988; 43: 463–465.

103. Dahl JB, Christiansen CL, Daughard JJ, et al. Continuous blockade of the lumbar plexus after knee surgery–postoperative analgesia and bupivacaine plasma concentration. Anaesthesia 1988; 43: 1015–1018.

104. Anker-Möller E, Spangsberg N, Dahl JB, et al. Continuous blockade of the lumbar plexus after knee surgery: A comparison of the plasma concentration and analgesic effect of bupivacaine 0.25% and 0.125%. Acta Anaesthesiol Scand 1990; 34: 468–472.

105. Schultz P, Christensen EF, Anker-Möller E, et al. Postoperative pain treatment after open knee surgery: Continuous lumbar plexus block with bupivacaine versus epidural morphine. Reg Anes 1991; 16: 34–37.

106. Singelyn FJ, Van Roy C, Goossens F, Gouverneur JM. A high position of the catheter increases the success rate of continuous '3-in-1' block. Anesthesiology 1996; 85: A723.

107. Singelyn FJ, Gouverneur JM. Epidural anesthesia complicating continuous 3-in-1 lumbar plexus blockade. Anesthesiology 1995; 83: 217–219.

108. Edwards ND, Wright EM. Continuous low-dose 3-in-1 nerve blockade for postoperative pain relief after total knee replacement. Anesth Analg 1992; 75: 265–267.

109. Hirst GC, Lang SA, Dust WN, et al. Femoral nerve block: Single injection versus continuous infusion for total knee arthroplasty. Reg Anes 1996; 21: 292–297.

110. Mansour NY, Bennetts FE. An observational study of combined continuous lumbar plexus single-shot sciatic nerve blocks for post-knee surgery analgesia. Reg Anes 1996; 21: 287–291.

111. Singelyn FJ. Continuous femoral and popliteal sciatic nerve blockades. Techniques in Regional Anesthesia and Pain Management 1998; 2: 90–95.

112. De Andres J, Bellver J, Barrera L, et al. A comparative study of analgesia after knee surgery with intraarticular bupivacaine, intraarticular morphine, and lumbar plexus block. Anesth Analg 1993; 77: 727–730.

113. Serpell MG, Millar FA, Thomson MF. Comparison of lumbar plexus block versus conventional opioid analgesia after total knee replacement. Anaesthesia 1991; 46: 275–277.

114. Uhrbrand AB, Jensen TT. Iatrogenic femoral neuropathy after blockade of the lumbar plexus (3-in-1 block) (German). Ugeskrift for Laeger 1988; 150: 428–429.

115. Johr M. A complication of continuous femoral nerve block (German). Reg Anaesth 1987; 10: 37–38.

116. Lynch T, Arhelger S, Krings-Ernst I. Repeated femoral nerve block following open knee surgery. Reg Anes 1990; 15:5.

117. Singelyn FJ, Gouverneur JM. The continuous '3-in-1' block as postoperative pain treatment after hip, femoral shaft, or knee surgery: A large scale study of efficacy and side effects. Anesthesiology 1994; 81: A1064.

118. Misra U, Pridie AK, McClymont C, et al. Plasma concentrations of bupivacaine following combined sciatic and femoral 3-in-1 nerve blocks in open knee surgery. Br J Anaesth 1991; 66: 310–313.

119. Elmas C, Atanassoff PG. Combined inguinal paravascular (3-in-1) and sciatic nerve blocks for lower limb surgery. Reg Anes 1993; 18: 88–92.

120. Smith BE, Fischer HBJ, Scott PV. Continuous sciatic nerve block. Anaesthesia 1984; 39: 155–157.

121. Berde C. Regional anesthesia in children: What have we learned? Anesth Analg 1996; 83: 897–900.

122. Morris GF, Lang SA. Continuous parasacral nerve block: Two case reports. Reg Anes 1997; 22: 469–472.

123. Mansour NY. Re-evaluating the sciatic nerve block: Another landmark for consideration. Reg Anes 1993; 18: 322–323.

124. Williams PL, Warwick R. The fasciae and muscles of the lower limb. In: Williams PL, Warwick R, eds. Gray's anatomy. 36th ed. Churchill Livingstone, Edinburgh; 1980: 593–604.

125. Winnie AP, Ramamurthy S, Durrani Z, Radonjic R. Plexus blocks for lower extremity surgery. Anesthesiol Rev 1974; 1: 11–16.

126. Vaghadia H, Kapnoudhis P, Jenkins LC, Taylor D. Continuous lumbosacral block using a Tuohy needle and catheter technique. Can J Anaesth 1992; 39: 75–78.

127. Chayen D, Nathan H, Chayen M. The psoas compartment block. Anesthesiology 1976; 45: 95–99.

128. Nicholls BJ. Psoas compartment block: A study using computerized tomography and clinical comparison with lumbar paravertebral block. Reg Anes 1988; 13: 77.

129. Dalens B, Tanguy A, Vanneuville G. Lumbar plexus block in children: A comparison of two procedures in 50 patients. Anesth Analg 1988; 67: 750–758.

130. Brands E, Callanan VI. Continuous lumbar plexus block–analgesia for femoral neck fractures. Anaesth Intensive Care 1978; 6: 256–258.

131. Ben-David B, Lee E, Croitoru M. Psoas block for surgical repair of hip fracture: A case report and description of a catheter technique. Anesth Analg 1990; 71: 298–301.

132. Rung GU, Hanks G, Kalenak A, Satterfield J. Continuous lumbar plexus block after anterior cruciate ligament repair. Reg Anes 1990; 15: S–53.

133. Rung GU. A safer continuous lumbar plexus block technique. Anesth Analg 1991; 72: 564–565.

134. Bolt SL, Teiken PJ, Pitcher D, et al. Use of psoas compartment catheter and sciatic nerve block during femur reconstruction. Anesth Analg 1995; 80: 547.

135. Hanna MA, Peat SJ, D'Costa F. Lumbar plexus block: An anatomical study. Anaesthesia 1993; 48: 675–678.

136. Farny J, Drolet P, Girard M. Anatomy of the posterior approach to the lumbar plexus. Can J Anaesth 1994; 41: 480–485.

137. Aida S, Takahashi H, Shimoji K. Renal subcapsular hematoma after lumbar plexus block. Anesthesiology 1996; 84: 452–455.

138. Ezri T, Szmuk P, Priscu V, Soroker D. Combined lumbosacral plexus block. Can J Anaesth 1993; 40: 189–190.

139. Muravchick S, Owens WD. An unusual complication of lumbosacral plexus block: A case report. Anesth Analg 1976; 55: 350–352.

140. Reynolds FA. Comparison of the potential toxicity of bupivacaine, lignocaine, and mepivacaine during epidural blockade for surgery. Br J Anaesth 1971; 43: 567–571.

141. Misra U, Pridie AK, McClymont C, Bower S. Plasma concentrations of bupivacaine following combined sciatic and femoral 3-in-1 nerve blocks in open knee surgery. Br J Anaesth 1991; 66: 310–313.

142. Odoom JA, Zuurmond WWA, Sih IL, et al. Plasma bupivacaine concentrations following psoas compartment block. Anaesthesia 1986; 41: 155–158.

143. Farny J, Girard M, Drolet P. Posterior approach to the lumbar plexus combined with a sciatic nerve block using lidocaine. Can J Anaesth 1994; 41: 486–491.

144. Atanassoff PG, Elmas C. Increased dosage of lidocaine 1% in combined sciatic-femoral 3-in-1 block for lower limb surgery. Reg Anes 1992; 17: 48.

145. Simon MAM, Gielen MJM, Lagerwarf AJ, Vree TB. Plasma concentrations after high doses of mepivacaine with epinephrine in the combined psoas compartment/sciatic nerve block. Reg Anes 1990; 15: 256–260.

146. Jorfeldt L, Lofstrom B, Pernow B, et al. The effect of local anesthetics on the central circulation and respiration in man and dog. Acta Anaesthesiol Scand 1968; 12: 153–169.

147. Rung GW. A safer continuous lumbar plexus block technique? (Letter to the Editor) Anesth Analg 1991; 72: 564–565.

148. Parkinson SK, Mueller JB, Little WL, Bailey SL. Extent of blockade with various approaches to the lumbar plexus. Anesth Analg 1989; 68: 243–248.

149. Dalens B, Tanguy A, Vanneuville G. Lumbar plexus blocks and lumbar plexus nerve blocks. (Letter to the Editor) Anesth Analg 1989; 69: 852–854.

150. Tierney E, Lewis G, Hurtig JB, Johnson D. Femoral nerve block with bupivacaine 0.25% for postoperative analgesia after open knee surgery. Can J Anaesth 1987; 34: 455–458.

151. Ringrose NH, Cross MJ. Femoral nerve block in knee joint surgery. Am J Sports Med 1984; 12: 398–402.

14

Thoracic blocks

Gilles Orliaguet and Pierre Carli

Introduction

Techniques
Epidural analgesia
Intercostal nerves block
Intrapleural analgesia
Patient-controlled analgesia

Analgesia for the thoracic trauma patient
Epidural analgesia
Intercostal nerves block and related techniques
Intrapleural analgesia
Intravenous analgesia

Critical analysis of the literature
Strategy of management of locoregional
    analgesia after thoracic trauma

Analgesia post-thoracotomy
Epidural analgesia
Intercostal nerves block and related techniques
Intrapleural analgesia
Intravenous analgesia
Strategy of management of locoregional
    analgesia after thoracotomy

Conclusion

INTRODUCTION

In order to perfectly understand the role occupied by thoracic blocks in the management of thoracic trauma, it is very important to remember the evolution of the pathophysiological theory as well as the evolution of the strategy of management of thoracic trauma during the last 30 years. Schematically, in the 1960s the pathophysiology of the respiratory failure seen in thoracic trauma patients with flail chest relied mainly upon 'paradoxical respiration' and 'pendelluft'. In the pendelleluft theory, it was postulated that the pendulum-like movement of air from one lung to the next during inspiration and expiration explained the inefficient ventilation seen in patients with flail chest.[1] This pathophysiologic theory had led, in a very logical manner, to several forms of therapy directed primarily at stabilizing the chest wall by external fixation, internal fixation, or internal pneumatic stabilization, which requires tracheal intubation and mechanical ventilation. However, the elegant studies of Maloney et al[2] and Duff et al[3] suggested that in the presence of flail chest, pendelluft does not occur. Moreover, some years later, Dahan demonstrated that the phenomenon of paradoxical respiration

had a less important impact on respiratory failure than previously believed.[4] This criticism of the old classical pathophysiological theory has led to a new hypothesis for explaining the respiratory failure seen in thoracic trauma (Fig. 14.1).

In this new hypothesis, the respiratory failure is related not only to the chest wall instability, but more importantly to the pain created by the excessive mobility of the flail segment, as well as to the underlying pulmonary contusion, nearly always associated with flail chest.[5,6] In fact, on the one hand, the excessive mobility of the flail segment creates pain, which affects chest wall movement as a whole, producing shallow respiration and decreasing ventilation. Coughing is almost a mechanical impossibility in these patients because of the major pain it induces, and because the entire expulsive force of the cough is dissipated in the paradoxic motion of the chest wall. Consequently, bronchial secretions cannot be effectively removed, therefore accumulation of secretions may occur with resultant atelectasis and pneumonitis. On the other hand, the combination of paradoxic respiration produced by the flail segment and the associated pulmonary contusion result in intrapulmonary shunting and hypoxemia with respiratory distress.[7,8,9]

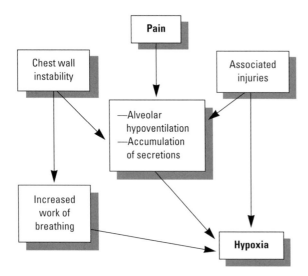

Fig. 14.1 Pathophysiology of the respiratory failure seen in thoracic trauma patients.

In the new theory, a prominent feature of the chest wall lesion is pain, which interferes with efficient ventilation and coughing, therefore pain relief is paramount. Indeed, analgesia plays a major role in the management of thoracic trauma, especially because it is thought that control of pain may improve ventilation and obviate the need for mechanical ventilation, particularly for patients without any other cause of respiratory failure. So, as early as 1973, Gibbons[10] then Trinkle[11], as well as other authors like Shackford[12] and Richardson[13] proposed to perform a locoregional thoracic analgesia in association with a physiotherapy regimen, and have shown that this management significantly decreased the complications associated with thoracic trauma.

Thus, Trinkle[11] has compared two groups of thoracic trauma patients. One group of patients, breathing spontaneously, was treated by an intercostal nerve block, and the other group of patients was mechanically ventilated. It was observed that the patients breathing spontaneously developed far fewer infectious diseases (pneumonia), and demonstrated a decrease in mortality as compared to the patients who were mechanically ventilated. More recently, Bolliger,[14] comparing ventilatory to nonventilatory management (mask-continuous positive airway pressure and locoregional analgesia) for the treatment of multiple ribs fractures, observed that the 'nonventilatory management' enabled a decrease in the overall duration of hos-

pital stay and in the duration of stay in the intensive care unit (ICU). Moreover, there was a clear decrease in morbidity and mortality in the group of patients treated by nonventilatory management. Of specific interest was the decrease of nosocomial pneumonia from 50% in the ventilatory management group to 15% in the nonventilatory management group.

Different methods of analgesia have been proposed for pain relief after thoracic trauma, all of which have their own advantages and drawbacks. It should also be noted that there is a major difference between 'analgesia for thoracic trauma' and 'postperative pain management', even if the surgical procedure was related to a thoracic injury. So, the different methods of thoracic analgesia will be discussed, including their advantages and drawbacks, with special attention to the specific indication for thoracic trauma or postperative pain management.

TECHNIQUES

Epidural analgesia

Epidural analgesia may be performed either at the thoracic or lumbar level, and the two approaches will be described. However, whichever approach is adopted, before an epidural catheter is inserted, the possibility of a coagulation defect or sepsis, complications that occur commonly in trauma victims, should be considered. Clotting abnormalities, if present, should be corrected before a needle is inserted into the epidural space. Sepsis is only a relative contraindication; most clinicians will perform the procedure if proper antibiotic coverage is provided. Of course, strict asepsis should be maintained for the duration of the procedure.

Thoracic epidural block (paramedian approach)

The patient is positioned on the least painful side, and sometimes a small roll is placed between the bed and the midthorax to provide slight scoliosis, thus facilitating the procedure. Some practitioners prefer the paramedian approach, because flexion of the thoracic spine is often impossible and because the epidural space presents a larger target from the lateral direction because of the alignment of the thoracic spinous processes.

The following variation will be discussed here: the needle should be inserted 1 cm lateral to the spinous process, at a 10° angle to the saggital plane and directed cephalad with a 30° angle. The needle is advanced until it contacts the lamina of the vertebra. It is withdrawn and then directed further cephalad until it enters the epidural space. Once the space has been identified, the catheter should be inserted with the bevel of the Tuohy needle facing cephalad or caudad. Once the catheter has been inserted, it is secured. After negative aspiration, a test dose may be given.

The use of a test dose to ensure proper placement of the catheter tip depends on local preference; in fact, some authors claim that the use of a test dose is a custom rather than a necessity. The choice of the solution for infusion is discussed below.

Lumbar epidural block

The technique for inserting a lumbar epidural catheter is similar to that for thoracic epidural catheters, with several notable differences. The spinous processes of the lumbar vertebrae are more horizontally inclined and thus offer a larger target to the anesthesiologist using a midline approach. In addition, the epidural space is slightly deeper to the skin in the lumbar region and has less negative pressure than the thoracic epidural space.

Even if the technique of paramedian approach remains possible, the midline approach is more often used at this level (see also Ch. 12). This latter approach requires that the patient be positioned in the sitting or, more often, in the fetal position. The Tuohy needle is advanced in the longitudinal plane with slight cephalad inclination until loss of resistance identifies the epidural space. The average depth from skin to space is 4.6 cm in the majority of the cases, with a range of 3.5–6.3 cm.[15] Once the catheter has been inserted, it is secured. After negative aspiration, a test dose may be given.

Intercostal nerves block (also see Ch. 19)

Intercostal nerves block (ICNB) has been widely used to perform a regional technique either to provide analgesia after thoracic surgery or thoracic trauma. The technique is quite different in the case of chest trauma and in the case of thoraco-tomy. After thoracotomy, and according to the classical technique, the ICNBs are performed 7 cm from the midline posteriorly, with 5 mL of bupivacaine (bupivacaine 0.5% with adrenaline 5 microg/mL) injected into each of the 6th to 12th intercostal spaces. In case of chest trauma, it is required that the intercostal blocks be performed on several (usually 2 or 3) intercostal nerves above and below the traumatized zone. Because of the rapid vascular absorption of local anesthetics injected into the intercostal space, there is a clear risk of occurrence of local anesthetic-induced toxicity, especially if more than 6 to 8 intercostal spaces are blocked. In fact, ICNBs are associated with higher blood concentrations of local anesthetic than most other types of nerve block.[16] Finally, repetitive injections of local anesthetics increase the risk of inducing an iatrogenic pneumothorax and are painful for the patient, making it awkward for the patient as well as the hospital personnel.

More recently, the technique of ICNB has been modified, and successful maintenance of widespread ICNB over a prolonged period by insertion of a catheter to an intercostal space with repeated 'top-up' doses or continuous infusion of local anesthetic has been reported. Again, there is a big difference between post-thoracotomy and chest trauma patients. In fact, in case of thoracic surgery the catheter may be inserted by the surgeon while the thorax is open, with correct placement of the catheter ensured visually and by palpation. Conversely, for the chest trauma patient, the catheter is inserted using a 'blind' technique, while the patient is awake.

For this method, using an aseptic technique, an appropriate intercostal space is selected. Following local infiltration of the skin with lidocaine, and following skin puncture, a Tuohy needle is introduced at the angle of the rib (approximately 7 cm from the midline posteriorly). The needle is advanced until contact is made with the upper rib, then it is 'walked' down the rib and advanced 3 mm under the lower border of the uppermost rib. In most cases a slight 'give' can be felt as the intercostal muscles are pierced. Following a negative aspiration, and with the bevel of the needle pointed medially, a catheter is advanced 3–4 cm into the intercostal space, and the needle is withdrawn. Following a negative aspiration, the catheter is secured in position and taped to the back, with a micropore filter attached.

Intrapleural analgesia

This technique of regional analgesia involves injecting a local anesthetic solution into the intrapleural space, using either an epidural catheter or a chest tube (introduced in the intrapleural space for the drainage of a hemo- or pneumothorax) (also see Ch. 19).

In fact, different methods have been proposed to perform intrapleural analgesia (IPA). They are all derived from the method described by Reiestadt & Stromskag.[17] The procedure is similar to the method used to perform epidural analgesia, using similar equipment. The patient is positioned the affected side up. The area of skin over the intercostal space chosen is prepared aseptically and draped. The level of puncture may vary according to different authors, from 6–10 cm from the spinous processes and between the 5th and 8th intercostal spaces. After infiltration with subcutaneous and intradermal local anesthetic, a Tuohy epidural needle is inserted. The location of the pleural space, performed initially using the 'loss-of-resistance' technique, is now performed by the 'hanging-drop' technique, because of a lesser risk of pneumothorax. Once the space has

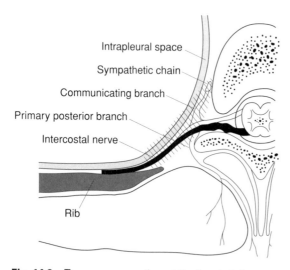

Fig. 14.2 Transverse section at the level of the intervertebral foramen. The gray triangle represents the paravertebral space. The anatomical position of the intercostal nerve, enables a clear understanding of its retrograde blockade by diffusion of the local anesthetic, injected in the intrapleural space. The same explanation applies to the retrograde blockade of the sympathetic chain.

been located, an epidural catheter is advanced into the space, and after negative aspiration the catheter is secured.

The mechanism of action of IPA is not perfectly understood, but it has been suggested that the local anesthetic solution diffuses from the pleural space through the parietal pleura and the innermost intercostal muscle to reach the intercostal space, where blockade of the intercostal nerves occurs unilaterally[18] (Fig. 14.2).

Patient-controlled analgesia

Traditional therapy for post-traumatic chest pain or post-thoracotomy analgesia consists of intramuscular or intravenous administration of opioid analgesics. However, the major clinical problem is the narrow therapeutic window. Low dose ranges result in failure to control pain, while moderate dose ranges result in adverse effects including nausea and vomiting, somnolence, and respiratory depression. These problems have led to the introduction of new modalities of administration of opioid analgesics, like nurse- or patient-controlled analgesia (PCA). But recently reported respiratory depression associated with the use of opioids by PCA systems is cause for considerable concern.[19]

It should be noted that systemic opioids are generally considered to be the usual control against which all other treatment modalities are compared, and it has even been claimed that alternative analgesic regimens are opioid-sparing but not substitutes.[20] Therefore, few studies have documented the usefulness of systemic opioids alone, and there are very few data evaluating the safety and efficiency of systemic opioids alone. On the other hand, the IV route is the most practical and convenient method of administering opioids, and the important side effects are predictable and require close monitoring. In practice PCA devices have proved popular as they also relieve the patient from some of the anxieties related to a sudden, almost total dependence on a busy staff.

ANALGESIA FOR THE THORACIC TRAUMA PATIENT

Epidural analgesia

Epidural analgesia was one of the first techniques of locoregional analgesia used for pain relief in thoracic trauma. Epidural analgesia may be performed either at the thoracic level, using opioids or local anesthetics; or at the lumbar level, using opioids. Until now, all the studies published demonstrate that this method of analgesia is very effective, enabling the control of spontaneous pain, facilitating effective physiotherapy, improving ventilation, and decreasing infectious complications.[21–23] Ulmann[24] has demonstrated that thoracic epidural analgesia with morphine was more effective than intravenous administration of morphine. Comparing patients suffering from at least six rib fractures, matched for injury severity, he observed that patients treated by epidural morphine administration had a significantly better increase in tidal volume (during spontaneous ventilation) than those receiving morphine by the intravenous route. Moreover, only one patient treated by epidural morphine required mechanical ventilation and tracheostomy, compared to five patients in the group treated by intravenous morphine. Mackersie[23] has shown that continuous epidural fentanyl analgesia was also very effective in this circumstance. In a group of 40 patients, treated by a thoracic or lumbar epidural infusion of fentanyl (75 microg/h), the author observed 95% effective analgesia, as well as significant increases in vital capacity (VC) and maximal inspiratory force. In this study, there were few complications, and except for pruritus, transient somnolence, or urinary retention, no severe adverse effects were noted.

It should be noted that when one wants to perform opioid lumbar epidural analgesia, it is perhaps more advantageous to use a hydrosoluble opioid, like morphine, rather than a lipid-soluble one like fentanyl. In fact, a highly lipophilic opioid, such as fentanyl, passes rapidly from the dural space through the dura and thus has a rapid onset of action; but a less lipophilic drug, such as morphine, tends to have a longer duration of action, because of reduced clearance by the epidural blood supply.

Epidural analgesia with local anesthetics is also a therapeutic possibility which has been studied. Bupivacaine (0.0625%–0.167%) appears to be the ideal local anesthetic for continuous epidural infusion. The use of this low concentration of bupivacaine rarely results in motor block, and so allows early mobilization and comfort for the patient. Cicala et al have compared thoracic bupivacaine with lumbar morphine in thoracic trauma.[25] Thoracic epidural administration of bupivacaine was associated with a greater increase in VC, tidal volume, and better pain relief than lumbar morphine. Nevertheless, it should be emphasized that in this study the thoracic epidural administration of bupivacaine was associated with severe arterial hypotension in two patients, compared to minor adverse effects in the lumbar epidural morphine group. These results confirmed those of Worthley et al,[22] who observed very good analgesia after the thoracic epidural administration of bupivacaine in 161 patients, but also several severe mishaps: 1 epidural abscess, 27 episodes of arterial hypotension, and 2 cardiac arrests. Combined, these results confirmed the efficiency of epidural analgesia with local anesthetics, but also the possibility of severe adverse effects with this technique, especially in hypovolemic traumatized patients. Consequently, it must be appreciated that epidural analgesia is not without drawbacks, even though it is a very efficient method of analgesia.

Additionally, there are also complications directly related to the territory which is blocked. An issue that is not particular to epidural infusions, but applies to all regional techniques in trauma patients, is the risk of obscuring the clinical signs and symptoms of early neurovascular injury and/or of associated lesions. In fact, epidural analgesia may be responsible for unrecognized associated lesions, like liver or spleen hematoma, with a risk of secondary rupture. In the case of mobile flail chest, the increase of the chest wall movement during cough or physiotherapy may be responsible for a worsening of the parietal injury secondary to bruising of the underlying lung by the induced excessive mobility of the flail segment.

Further, it is important to consider the inherent difficulty of performing a thoracic epidural block in an emergency, in a dyspneic patient in tremendous pain, as well as the absolute necessity to monitor these patients in an ICU in order to closely observe for a secondary complication or an initially unrecognized injury.

Finally, current evidence suggests that the most satisfactory analgesia is obtained with a combination of local anesthetics and opioid analgesics given by continuous infusion. Several therapeutic regimens have been proposed, and one possibility is to use the following formula: fentanyl (2 microg/kg) and bupivacaine 0.125%, administered at a rate of 4–12 mL/h. At present, studies are evaluating the use of patient-controlled epidural analgesia, with the aim of being able to provide better analgesia during the typical peaks of pain, as can occur during physiotherapy and mobilization (also see Chs 12 & 19).

Intercostal nerves block and related techniques

ICNBs have also been widely used to perform a regional analgesic technique in thoracic trauma. They are particularly useful in cases of unilateral multiple-dermatome rib injuries, but when these blocks are performed with the conventional technique, they carry the disadvantage of multiple and painful injections, and increase the risk of pneumothorax. More recently, the technique of ICNB has been modified, and successful maintenance of widespread ICNB over a prolonged period by insertion of a catheter to an intercostal space with repeated 'top-up' doses of local anesthetic has been reported in patients with multiple rib fractures. Indeed, O'Kelly[26] has demonstrated that it was possible to introduce a catheter into an intercostal space and to perform repetitive injections of local anesthetics (15–20 mL), after thoracic trauma.

However, contrary to the situation of thoracic surgery, where this technique has been widely used, there are very few studies of continuous ICNB in thoracic trauma. Haenel et al[27], in 1995, delivered bupivacaine to the intercostal nerves of 15 thoracic trauma patients by means of an extrapleural catheter, and observed an improvement in pain scores and ventilatory parameters as compared to PCA. So, even though this new method of ICNB seems to be interesting in thoracic trauma patients, with the possibility of repetitive injection without making it cumbersome to the patients as well as to hospital personnel, more studies are needed before performing it routinely (also see Ch. 19).

Intrapleural analgesia

First applied to thoracic trauma by Rocco et al[28] and Carli et al[29], IPA provides unilateral analgesia, but the quality and intensity can be variable. Sometimes, when there is a hemothorax, which has not been fully evacuated, authentic failures have been reported. In fact, it appears that the more fluid present in the pleural space to dilute

the local anesthetic, the less likely it is to obtain good analgesia. Nevertheless, IPA improves the ventilatory pattern of thoracic trauma patients, without inducing any significant adverse effects. However, the intrapleural injection of local anesthetics is associated with rapid intravascular absorption, with a bioavailability of approximately 1.[30] Therefore high peak serum concentrations of local anesthetics are often obtained, and may sometimes reach the toxic level. This is the reason why some authors, like Carli et al, recommend the exclusive use of lidocaine. Indeed, lidocaine provides a greater margin of security than bupivacaine, which is the local anesthetic of choice for IPA after abdominal surgery (post-cholecystectomy). The optimum concentration and dosing regimen remain to be defined; however the injection of 100 mg bupivacaine with epinephrine or of 1 mg/kg of 2% lidocaine has been reported and has achieved satisfactory results.[28–30] It has been suggested that continuous pleural infusion of local anesthetic offered better pain relief than did bolus administration.[31,32]

The efficiency of IPA for thoracic trauma, compared with other techniques of analgesia, remains a controversial issue. Luchette et al[33] studied thoracic trauma patients suffering from at least three unilateral fractured ribs, and compared continuous thoracic epidural analgesia with bupivacaine with intrapleural bupivacaine (Fig. 14.3). During the 72 hours of the study, the authors observed that epidural bupivacaine provided better pain relief than intrapleural bupivacaine. Moreover, the pulmonary function was significantly improved by epidural bupivacaine as compared to intrapleural bupivacaine. On the other hand, it should be noted that in this study, epidural bupivacaine was associated with several episodes of arterial hypotension, requiring vascular loading or the injection of ephedrine, which is not without potential drawbacks in this context. In contrast, IPA was not associated with any adverse effects. These results are consistent with the literature regarding the lack of deleterious hemodynamic effects of IPA. However, Stromskag et al[34] note the possibility of pneumothorax (2% of the cases), of displacement of the catheter, or of toxicity of local anesthetics. One other possible drawback of IPA, already noted with other methods of locoregional analgesia, was reported by Pond et al[35] who described the case of a patient in whom the pain of delayed splenic rupture was masked by IPA,

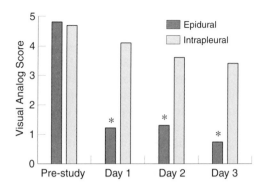

Fig. 14.3   Pain induced by movement or coughing in the epidural and intrapleural bupivacaine groups. Pain was significantly less throughout the study in the epidural group ($P < 0.05$). (From Luchette FA, et al.[33].)

which had been performed to provide pain relief after traumatic unilateral multiple rib fractures. IPA is nevertheless a useful method for short-term control of unilateral chest injuries (also see Ch. 19).

Intravenous analgesia

Intravenous analgesia for thoracic trauma, although less effective than locoregional analgesia, may have some interesting indications. Except for the injection of minor analgesic drugs, which should be considered only as a complementary technique associated with a more potent method, the injection of opioids (either a mixed agonist–antagonist or a pure agonist opioid) could initially provide good pain relief on an emergency basis, especially in healthy young patients without associated injuries. So, one may consider in an emergency the injection of a titrated bolus dose of a pure agonist opioid, enabling the performance of complementary examinations (clinical and radiological) to search for associated lesions. Then, after a brief time lapse, an intravenous PCA may be started. However, this method is not commonly used for thoracic trauma, and even if some trials seem to have been conclusive, there are no large studies of patients comparing these techniques to other emergency analgesic methods.[27] Nevertheless, this method presents the advantage of treating both the thoracic trauma pain and the pain of potentially-associated lesions. However,

from a practical point of view, the use of PCA is limited in the emergency setting because of the difficulty in learning the correct operation of the apparatus and the restricted availability of the equipment.

Critical analysis of the literature

It should be noted, that despite the studies published in favor of locoregional analgesia, like epidural analgesia with opioids, this technique could prove cumbersome from a practical point of view, especially for patients without any medical history. Regardless of the results of studies published to date, the numbers of patients studied have been relatively small, and the studies have involved selected patients, and may include several types of bias. Perhaps a frequent bias which may exist is the comparison of two methods of analgesia of different potency. So, for example, when Ulmann[24] compared the efficiency of intravenous and thoracic epidural morphine, the dose received by the patients of each group was the same, while it should have been different to obtain an equipotent analgesia. The specific time at which analgesia was administered differs from one study to another, and sometimes the time differs in the same study between two methods of analgesia. This specific point deserves attention, because pain after injury is a dynamic phenomenon, with important variations in the intensity of pain over time, and because there are typical peaks of pain. Finally, it is to be noted that the possibility of performing a proper randomized, double blind study is very limited in this setting.

One factor to be considered regarding the discussion of the relative importance of the different methods of analgesia is, in particular, the evolution of the analgesic requirements of the thoracic trauma patient. It is clear that early and potent analgesia is mandatory in emergency, and that this analgesia must necessarily be maintained at least over 2 to 4 days. On the other hand, the majority of authors come to an agreement about the possibility to decrease the doses of analgesia at the end of the first week after trauma. Anyway, within the context of thoracic trauma, analgesia is particularly intended to overcome a difficult initial phase and is mandatory in emergency, while the problem of the duration of a potent analgesia should be assessed later on, on a case-by-case basis.

Strategy of management of locoregional analgesia after thoracic trauma

Several factors should be carefully considered in the strategy of management of a thoracic trauma patient, because some of them may influence either the intensity or the method of analgesia. For example, the existence of associated injuries, especially of a significant pulmonary contusion, hypoxemia, or head trauma with altered levels of consciousness, may indicate emergency mechanical ventilation with intravenous analgesia.

In the same way, even in the case of isolated thoracic parietal trauma, a defective health status (old age, chronic respiratory insufficiency) may suggest a very potent method of analgesia, like epidural analgesia.

The type and topography of thoracic lesions may also influence the selection of the method of analgesia, which will be different for a relatively stable posterior flail chest versus that required for an anterior flail chest associated with excessive mobility of the flail segment which can be particularly painful. Finally, one should consider the potential difficulty of the technical aspects of administering locoregional analgesia in an emergency, and that the technique must be adapted to the skill of the health provider, as well as to the basic requirements for monitoring to be anticipated for the patient. Studying the factors related to mortality and morbidity in a group of old patients, Wissner[36] observed that mortality was directly related to old age and injury severity. Within this context, epidural analgesia decreases mortality and the incidence of severe complications, like pneumonia. This consideration frames the balance of costs affected by epidural analgesia, in an overall assessment of the costs of medical care of these patients. Finally, one may schematically suggest the following management:

- When there are *severe associated injuries*, mechanical ventilation, internal pneumatic stabilization, and intravenous analgesia are the treatment of choice. Ideally, this combination shall lead to a weaning from mechanical ventilation as early as possible, as a function of the associated injuries.
- When the *thoracic trauma is isolated*, the main issue is to avoid tracheal intubation if possible (but that should not be interpreted to mean postponing a mandatory tracheal intubation if indicated). So, one may use the classical criteria of Barone[37] to decide if tracheal intubation is necessary on an emergency basis. These criteria are: (1) an elevated heart rate and respiratory rate, associated with (2) arterial hypotension and (3) hypoxemia. This combination is important if there are other associated injuries.
- When the patient has a *severe pre-existing physical illness*, like chronic respiratory insufficiency, old age, pulmonary history, or other risk factors, the best choice seems to be a locoregional analgesia. In the same way, when there are extensive thoracic parietal defects, epidural analgesia represents the method of choice, and lumbar epidural morphine seems to be the easiest to use in emergency. However, in this case, close monitoring in the ICU is mandatory, especially as the patient may quickly develop complications.
- Conversely, thoracic trauma occurring in an *ASA 1 physical status patient* may benefit from different management. So, in the case of unilateral injuries, ICNB, or IPA may be performed, and will be further facilitated if a chest tube is required. This method will enable the provision of a rapid analgesia, even if the effectiveness is less than epidural analgesia. On the other hand, in case of bilateral injuries, one may select intravenous analgesia, either classical or using PCA. Moreover, in this latter situation, the use of adjuvant therapeutic, like a transient fixing of the flail segment, may be interesting.

ANALGESIA POST-THORACOTOMY

Thoracotomy has been suggested to produce the most intense clinical postoperative pain experiences known, and successful analgesia is one of the hallmarks of optimal post-surgical and anesthetic management.[38] The pathophysiology of pain after thoracic surgery is quite different from the pain after chest trauma, explaining why some therapeutic options effective for chest trauma fail to provide an effective analgesia after thoracotomy. In fact, after thoracic surgery, pain from both somatic and visceral origin, corresponding to different levels of innervation, are involved. This fact explains why locoregional analgesia, usually of segmental efficiency, does sometimes fail to provide sufficient pain relief.

Somatic pains constitute the main source of postoperative pain. Bone pain, related to a rib fracture, may be associated. The nociceptive out-it generated by all of these components is conducted centrally via the intercostal nerves. The stretch, by the surgical retractor, of the costotransverse and costovertebral ligaments and of the paravertebral muscles may be responsible for severe dorsal pain. The cutting of the muscles, e.g. latissimus dorsi, serratus anterior, pectoralis major, and intercostal muscles, induces pain when the arm or the shoulder are moved.

Visceral pains correspond to the pleural irritation, related to surgical manipulations, chest tubes, or to a pleural effusion of blood. These pains, of which nociceptive output passes through the pleural branch of the intercostal nerves (except for the diaphragmatic pleura which track with the phrenic nerve), are increased by cough and respiratory movements. The nociceptive output generated by stimuli from lung and mediastinum, including the mediastinal pleura, are carried by the vagus nerve.

Finally, two types of projected pain, shoulder pain and pain of the anterior side of the thorax, may be found after thoracic surgery. The shoulder pain is commonly attributed to a pleural or diaphragmatic irritation, while the pain of the anterior side of the thorax may be due to the irritation of the bronchial mucosa.

So, considerable pain may follow such a procedure, generated from several sources, both during and after operation; these include soft tissue injury and inflammation, bone and joint trauma, and visceral damage. Moreover, pain is exacerbated by movement, especially by the obligatory movement of ventilation. These postoperative pains, generally rated as severe, represent one of many factors involved in the postoperative reduction of pulmonary reserve, responsible for producing a restrictive pattern of ventilation with reduced lung compliance and resulting hypoxemia.

Epidural analgesia

Epidural analgesia techniques that have been described for post-thoracotomy analgesia include thoracic local anesthetics, epidural opioids (including opioid agonist–antagonists), thoracic epidural local anesthetics combined with opioids, and thoracic epidural adrenergic agonists. Infrequent, but sometimes serious, adverse effects have been reported and include: significant systemic toxicity of local anesthetics, respiratory depression after epidural opioids, spinal cord or

nerve trauma, hematoma, and infection or inflammatory reaction associated with introduction of the catheter or needle.[38] Less serious, but troublesome problems include nausea, pruritus, and urinary retention after epidural opioids; hypotension, temporary paralysis, urinary retention, and paresthesia after epidural local anesthetics; and a low incidence of post-dural headache after instrumentation for both modes of treatment.

Thoracic epidural local anesthetics

Studies of epidural local anesthetics alone have been limited to intermittent (and occasionally toxic) bolus administration; or, have examined continuous infusions with either concomitant administration of systemic opioids, epidural opioids, or systemic nonsteroidal anti-inflammatory analgesics (see Chs 12 & 19).[38] Therefore, the true efficacy of thoracic epidural local anesthetics alone for post-thoracotomy analgesia remains to be documented in appropriately conducted studies.

Thoracic or lumbar epidural opioids

Epidural opioids have been administered by the thoracic or lumbar routes to provide analgesia after thoracic surgery (see Chs 12 & 19). In a study by El-Baz et al comparing continuous infusions or intermittent bolus doses of thoracic epidural morphine with intermittent thoracic epidural bupivacaine, the continuous thoracic epidural morphine regimen resulted in comparable analgesia to that provided by the two other regimens.[39] In addition, the continuous infusion was associated with fewer adverse effects than the other regimens.

The results regarding lumbar epidural sufentanil, administered as bolus-doses, show that sufentanil provides rapid and effective analgesia, but with a short duration of action.[37,38] Furthermore, increasing the doses fails to improve analgesia but results in an increased incidence of respiratory depression.

Studies of epidural fentanyl have shown that thoracic and lumbar epidural resulted in comparable pain relief; lumbar epidural fentanyl resulted in similar analgesic and respiratory effects compared with intravenous administration; thoracic epidural fentanyl produced similar analgesia to the intravenous route but with fewer adverse effects and lower infusion, when fentanyl infusions were titrated to patient Visual Analog Scale

(VAS) pain ratings. In a review of analgesic techniques for pain control after thoracic surgery,[38] Kavanagh et al concluded the chapter regarding epidural opioids by stating that:

> the optimal methods for administering epidural morphine include lumbar epidural bolus doses and low-dose continuous thoracic infusion with intravenous supplementation as required; … the role, level of administration and optimal dose of epidural sufentanil remain to be defined; … 'there was little justification for the lumbar epidural administration of fentanyl, but thoracic epidural administration may have advantages; … there did not appear to be beneficial effects associated with the concomitant administration of epidural or intravenous opioids agonoist-antagonists with epidural opioids in the treatment of post-thoracotomy pain.

Combined thoracic epidural local anesthetics and opioids

The strategy underlying the combination of thoracic epidural local anesthetics and opioids is to synergistically block spinal nociceptive pathways while reducing the dose-related adverse effects of either class of agent alone. Several studies have examined the effectiveness of this technique after thoracotomy. The addition of bupivacaine (0.2%) to a continuous thoracic epidural infusion of fentanyl (50 microg/h) has been shown to result in reduced pain scores on the first postoperative day (also see Ch. 12).[40]

Thoracic epidural adrenergic agonists

Epidural adrenergic agonists seem to have the potential for effective pain relief after epidural administration. The mechanism of action appears to be modulation of the endogenous postsynaptic adrenergic receptors in the dorsal horn cells.[41] However, until now only preliminary clinical results have been available, and dose-response data are required to define the efficacy and complications associated with epidural clonidine and other α_2-agonists in post-thoracotomy analgesia.

Lumbar intrathecal opioids

Lumbar intrathecal opioids have been used for post-thoracotomy analgesia in published studies.[38] This technique has several advantages, including simplicity, reliability, and because of the sm doses used, potentially fewer adverse effects fro systemic opioid absorption.[38] Thus, the intrathec injection of a small dose of morphine (0.25–C mg) seems to permit very good pain relief, exten ing from 18 to 30 hours. However, there are n enough clinical data in the available literature comment further on the clinical utility of this tec nique for post-thoracotomy analgesia.

Intercostal nerves block and related techniques

ICNB has been used extensively for analgesia aft thoracic surgery. Agents may be administered a single treatment under direct vision, before ch closure, as single preoperative percutaneous tre ment, as multiple percutaneous serial injectior or via an indwelling intercostal catheter.[38] T main concern with ICNB is a high level of sy temic absorption, although clinical studies ha documented safe plasma levels of local anesth ics.[38] The results of a study comparing the inje tion of bolus doses of either 0.5% bupivacaine normal saline via indwelling intercostal cathete every 6 hours, for 24 hours after surgery, ha shown that bupivacaine caused a significa decrease, although transient, in VAS pain scor and the consumption of opioid analgesics.[42] another study, similar results were observed wit comparable design, but with a continuous inf sion of bupivacaine instead of intermittent bol doses.[43] More recently, Dryden et al have doc mented the efficiency of the infusion of 0.25 bupivacaine through paired indwelling intercos catheters.[44] Finally, in the review by Kavanagh al,[38] the authors concluded that ICNB by inte mittent or continuous infusion of 0.5% bupiv caine with epinephrine was an effective meth as was continuous infusion of 0.25% bupivacai through indwelling intercostal catheters, for su plementing systemic opioid analgesia for post-th racotomy pain.

Intrapleural analgesia

Since the publication of Rosenberg et al,[45] IPA h been increasingly used after thoracic surge Before then, the results of the different stud published suggested that intrapleural bupivacai (0.25–0.5%) might improve analgesia in patier after thoracic surgery.[38] However, the benefits short duration and there does not appear to be significant overall opioid-sparing effect. Moreover, the optimum concentration and dosing regimen remain to be defined.

avenous analgesia

pioids are classically considered as the traditional therapy for post-thoracotomy analgesia. Moreover, it has been claimed that alternative analgesic regimens are opioid-sparing, but not substitutes. However, the major clinical problem is the narrow therapeutic window; on the one hand, the risk of inadequate pain relief in case of low dose ages; on the other hand, the risk of respiratory depression in case of overdosage. Because, opioid administration based on patient request (i.e. 'RN') is considered as poorly structured (too much delay between request and injection, fixed dose range usually insufficient, etc.), systematic morphine administration at short intervals (5–10 g every 4 hours) has been sometimes preferred. However, the risk of respiratory depression is increased with this latter method, especially because patient requirements may vary and increase with time. Therefore, PCA devices have become popular, enabling a quasi-instantaneous adaptation of the dosage regimen to the patient requirements. But, it has been claimed that baseline VAS scores become less than 30 mm only after 4 to 6 hours. Moreover, pain induced by cough and mobilization may remain severe (VAS score: 50–60 mm), thus limiting the beneficial effects of physiotherapy. Accordingly, other drugs, like nonsteroidal anti-inflammatory drugs (NSAIDs), have been used as therapeutic adjuncts to opioid analgesics. From a clinical perspective, potential problems with NSAIDs include gastrointestinal bleeding, acute reversible renal dysfunction, and systemic bleeding associated with platelet dysfunction. But, these effects are unlikely to cause significant clinical problems with short-term use. Finally, these products are thought to be potent and safe adjuncts to systemic opioid analgesia after thoracic surgery, resulting in clear benefits in terms of pain and analgesic consumption.

rategy of management of locoregional analgesia after thoracotomy

summary, systemic opioids form the cornerstone of post-thoracotomy analgesia therapy, and

have constituted the control group in the majority of clinical studies. Pain or analgesic consumption is reduced significantly with the following techniques: indwelling intercostal catheter with bupivacaine, interpleural catheters with bupivacaine, epidural morphine (with an infusion in the thoracic route or bolus administration in the lumbar route), combined infusions of thoracic epidural bupivacaine with either thoracic epidural or intravenous sufentanil, thoracic epidural fentanyl, and systemic NSAIDs as adjuncts to systemic opioids.

Thus, several therapeutic regimens are available and effective for post-thoracotomy analgesia, but when choosing one of the different methods, the physician must consider several factors, which include:

1. the physician's experience, familiarity, and complication rate with specific techniques
2. the specific clinical circumstances, including the presence of contraindications to various analgesic methods and medications
3. availability of an appropriate surrounding for the safe and effective initiation and maintenance of the technique
4. availability of adequate facilities for patient assessment and monitoring
5. the informed consent of the patient, especially the acceptance that the technique falls within reasonable risk–benefit and cost–benefit constraints.

CONCLUSION

In conclusion, analgesia for thoracic trauma and after thoracic surgery has taken its course, largely as a result of a better understanding of the pathophysiology. The respective place of the different therapeutic methods is best determined. However, the literature reveals a lack of studies of large series of patients to confirm the current results. Moreover, different factors must be considered when choosing a method for analgesia in this context, without forgetting that most of these factors are a function of the physician's training, experience and competence, and ongoing education of hospital anesthetic and perioperative surgical support staff. Therefore, rather than proposing rigid and universal recommendations, it seems more logical, from a practical point of view, to suggest that each practitioner determines the strategy which is best adapted for his or her own institution, with special consideration given to reasonable risk–benefit and cost–benefit constraints.

REFERENCES

1. Bauer L. Erfahrungen and uberlegungen zur lungenkollapstherapie. Bietr Klan Tuberk 1909; 12: 49–54.
2. Maloney JV, Schmutzer KJ, Raschke E. Paradoxical respiration and 'pendelluft'. J Thorac Cardiovasc Surg 1961; 41: 291–298.
3. Duff JH, Goldstein APH, McLean MD, Agrawal SN, Munro DD, Gatelius JR. Flail chest: a clinical review and pathophysiological study. J Trauma 1968; 8: 63–74.
4. Dahan M, Vanche J, Chauveau N. Etude expérimentale de la respiration paradoxale. Rev Med Toulouse 1982; 15–18.
5. Alfano GS, Hale HW. Pulmonary contusion. J Trauma 1965; 5: 647–658.
6. Williams JR, Stenbridge VA. Pulmonary contusion secondary to non-penetrating chest trauma. AJR 1964; 91: 284–290.
7. Garson AA, Gourin A, Seltzer B, Chiu C, Karlson AE. Severe blunt chest trauma. Ann Thorac Surg 1996; 2: 629–639.
8. Reid JM, Baird WLM. Crushed chest injury: some physiological disturbances and their correction. BMJ 1965; 1: 1105–1109.
9. Craven KD, Oppenheimer L, Wood LDH. Effects of contusion and the flail chest on pulmonary perfusion and oxygen exchange. J Appl Physiol 1979; 47: 729–737.
10. Gibbons J, James O, Quail A. Relief of pain in chest injury. Br J Anaesth 1973; 45: 1136–1138.
11. Trinkle J, Richardson J, Franz J, et al. Management of flail chest without mechanical ventilation. Ann Thorac Surg 1975; 19: 355–363.
12. Shackford S, Virgilio R, Peters R. Selective use of ventilatory therapy in flail chest injury. J Thorac Cardiovasc Surg 1981; 81: 194–201.
13. Richardson J, Adams L, Flint L. Selective management of flail chest and pulmonary contusion. Ann Surg 1982; 196: 481–486.
14. Bolliger CT, Van Eeden SF. Treatment of multiple rib fractures. Randomized controlled trial comparing ventilatory to nonventilatory management. Chest 1990; 97: 943–948.
15. Dow AC. Regional anesthesia. In: Grande CM, ed. Textbook of trauma anesthesia and critical care, St Louis: Mosby–Yearbook; 1993: 485–500.
16. Covino BG, Vassalo HG. Local anesthetics: Mechanisms of action and clinical use. New York: Grune & Stratton; 1976: 97.
17. Reiestadt F, Stromskag KE. Interpleural cathe in the management of postoperative pain, prelir nary report. Reg Anesth 1986; 11: 89–91.
18. Orliaguet G, Carli P. Analgésie interpleurale. A Fr Anesth Réanim 1994; 13: 233–247.
19. Baxter AD. Respiratory depression with pati controlled analgesia. (Editorial) Can J Anae 1994; 41: 87–90.
20. Conacher ID. Pain relief after thoracotomy. B Anaesth 1990; 65: 806–812.
21. Dittmann M, Ferstl A, Wolff G. Epidural anal sia for the treatment of multiple rib fractures. E Intensive Care Med 1975; 1: 71–75.
22. Worthley LIG. Thoracic epidural in the mana ment of chest trauma. A study of 161 cases. Int Care Med 1985; 11: 312–315.
23. Mackersie RC, Shackford SR, Hoyt D Karagianes TG. Continuous epidural fenta analgesia: ventilatory function improvement w routine use in treatment of blunt chest injury Trauma 1987; 27: 1207–1212.
24. Ulmann D, Wimpy R, Fortune J, Kennedy T. T treatment of patients with multiple rib fractu using continous epidural infusion. Reg Anae 1989; 14: 43–47.
25. Cicala RS, Voeller GR, Fox T, Fabian TC, Kuo K, Mangiante EC. Epidural analgesia in thora trauma: effects of lumbar morphine and thora bupivacaine on pulmonary function. Crit Ca Med 1990; 18: 229–231.
26. O'Kelly E, Garry B. Continuous pain relief multiple fractured ribs. Br J Anaesth 1981; 989–991.
27. Haenel JB, Moore FA, Moore EE, Savaia A, Re AR, Burch JM. Extrapleural bupivacaine amelioration of multiple rib fracture pa J Trauma Inj 1995; 38: 22–27.
28. Rocco A, Reiestad F, Gudman J, McKay Intrapleural administration of local anesthetics pain relief in patients with multiple rib fractu Reg Anesth 1987; 12: 10–14.
29. Carli P, Lambert Y, Mazoit X. Analgésie int pleurale par la lidocaine pour le traitement di gence des traumatismes thoraciques. Cahi d'Anesthèsiologie 1989; 6: 425–427.
30. Carli P, Duranteau J, Mazoit X, Gaupin Eccofey C. Pharmocokinetics of interpleural li caine administration in trauma patients. Anes Analg 1990; 70: 448–453.
31. Aguilar JL, Montero A, Llamazares JF, Montes Vidal F, Pastor C. Continuous pleural infusion bupivacaine offers better pain relief than do bolus administration. Reg Anesth 1992; 1 12–14.
32. Hudes ET. Continuous infusion interpleural an gesia for multiple fractured ribs. Can J Anaes 1990; 37: 705–714.

33. Luchette FA, Radafshar SM, Kaiser R, Flynn W, Hassett JM. Prospective evaluation of epidural versus intrapleural catheters for analgesia in chest wall trauma. J Trauma 1994; 36: 865–870.

34. Stromskag KE, Minor B, Steen PA. Side effects and complications related to interpleural analgesia: an update. Acta Anaesthesiol Scand 1990; 34: 473–477.

35. Pond W, Somerville GM, Thong SH, Ranochak JA, Weaver GA. Pain of delayed traumatic splenic rupture masked by intrapleural lidocaine. Anesthesiology 1989; 70: 154–155.

36. Wissner DH. A stepwise logistic regression analysis of factors affecting morbidity and mortality after thoracic trauma: effect of epidural analgesia. J Trauma 1990; 30: 799–805.

37. Barone J, Pizzi W, Nealon T, Richman H. Indications for intubation in blunt chest trauma. J Trauma 1986; 334–337.

38. Kavanagh BP, Katz J, Sandler AN. Pain control after thoracic surgery. A review of current techniques. Anesthesiology 1994; 81: 737–759.

39. El-Baz NM, Faber LP, Jensik RJ. Continuous epidural infusions of morphine for treatment of pain after thoracic surgery: A new technique. Anesth Analg 1984; 63: 757–764.

40. George KA, Wright PMC, Chisakuta A. Continuous thoracic epidural fentanyl for post thoracotomy pain relief: With or without bupivacaine? Anaesthesia 1991; 46: 732–736.

41. Howe JR, Wang IY, Yaksh TL. Selective antagonism of the antinociceptive effect of intrathecally applied alpha-adrenergic agonists by intrathecal prazosin and intrathecal yohimbine. J Pharmacol Exp Ther 1983; 224: 552–558.

42. Chan VWS, Chung F, Cheng DCH, et al. Analgesic and pulmonary effects of continuous intercostal nerve block following thoracotomy. Can J Anaesth 1991; 38: 733–739.

43. Sabanathan S, Mearns AJ, Bickford Smith PJ, et al. Efficacy of continuous extrapleural intercostal nerve block on post-thoracotomy pain and pulmonary mechanics. Br J Surg 1990; 77: 221–225.

44. Dryden CM, McMenemin I, Duthie DJR. Efficacy of continuous intercostal bupivacaine for pain relief after thoracotomy. Br J Anaesth 1993; 70: 508–510.

45. Rosenberg Ph, Scheinin BMA, Lepantalo MJA, Lindfors O. Continuous intrapleural infusion of bupivacaine for analgesia after thoracotomy. Anesthesiology 1987; 67: 811–813.

15

Non-pharmacologic techniques for pain management

Barry R Snow and Paul Gusmorino

Introduction

Factors influencing pain control
  Beliefs
  Information
  Social support
  Under-reporting and under-medicating for pain

Behavioral strategies for pain control

Physical emphasis
  Tense–release
Cognitive emphasis
  Imagery
  Hypnosis
  Psychotherapy

Biofeedback and combined techniques

Modalities
  Transcutaneous electrical nerve stimulation
  Acupuncture
  Therapeutic cold
  Mobilization techniques
  Therapeutic heat

Energy-based approaches
  Qigong and Reiki

Advisory for pain consultants

INTRODUCTION

The past decade has seen an increased interest in non-pharmacologic techniques for pain management. This interest arises from a number of causes. A growing trend currently exists for patients to become full partners in their own care rather than passive recipients of pharmacologic treatment. This trend is accompanied by a growing cultural and philosophical acceptance of behavioral and complementary techniques in medicine. Additionally, health professionals are becoming more aware of the role of social and psychological factors in determining pain and pain relief. Clinicians are already recognizing that just as tension and negative belief can interfere with the effect of medication, so too can relaxation and positive expectancy enhance the effects of medication. Finally, some medical procedures are unable to provide sufficient relief to the patient or avoid producing side effects. These factors encourage attention to non-pharmacologic approaches to pain relief.

This chapter reviews some of the personality and situational factors that influence acute pain management in the trauma patient. Behavioral and modality-based non-pharmacologic strategies that have been proven to be useful for the clinical setting are then outlined. Finally, specific questions that should be used by the clinician for the evaluation of pain and interest in non-pharmacologic pain control techniques are presented.

FACTORS INFLUENCING PAIN CONTROL

The idea that psychological as well as physical factors can influence pain is intrinsic to the gate control theory proposed by Melzack and his colleagues.[1,2] This interpretive model of pain proposes three systems related to the processing of nociceptive stimulation – sensory discriminative, motivational-affective and cognitive-evaluative. This theory thus represents a major shift from pain being explained solely by focusing on peripheral factors. Rather, the role of past experience and beliefs, information obtained, and anxiety can play a significant role in influencing pain processing at the level of the spinal cord and brain.

Beliefs

The beliefs that a patient brings to the situation can have a profound influence on pain experience and recovery. In an intriguing study of patient hospitalization for acute brain injuries, Kiecolt-Glaser & Williams[3] showed that the belief that responsibility for the injury lay with the individual was significantly associated with increased depression and pain behavior, and poorer adherence to treatment guidelines. An additional strong negative factor was the perception that the pain would be for the rest of one's life rather than a discrete, time-limited experience.[4] Cognitive techniques that specifically focused on addressing the patient's expectations regarding pain can have a beneficial impact on reducing pain level.

Information

The amount of information that patients have about their condition and treatment can also affect level of perceived pain. Numerous studies have shown that educating patients about the sensory experiences they will have and coping skills they should use can have a significant effect on coping with pain in dental and non-surgical procedures.[5] These findings arise from the fact that anxiety concerning the future reduces the pain threshold. This anxiety is especially heightened in the trauma patient for whom the pain onset typically was in an unexpected and frightening way. Information that is tailored to the needs of the person can also help minimize non-compliance with medical procedures and recovery.[6]

Social support

The role of family support in reducing procedural pain and length of recovery is also significant. Supportive familial environments, as well as interactive patterns that emphasize the use of pre-arranged coping strategies, have consistently shown decreased procedural pain and enhanced pain-coping ability.[7,8] This influence is especially important as hospital length of stay becomes shorter and the burden of post-surgical care and recovery shifts to family and friends. The use of behavioral non-pharmacologic techniques that emphasize the role of patients and family as active partners in recovery is thus of special importance.

Under-reporting and under-medicating for pain

Perhaps one of the most significant factors in influencing levels of relief from pain through pharmacological techniques is the level of medication that the individual is actually receiving. Despite the early identification of the extent of under-medicating for pain and the low risk of addiction in patients with active disease, clinicians persist in this practice.[9,10] This practice is often unintentionally reinforced by patients who share the same fear of becoming addicted or do not wish to bother the staff by repeatedly asking for pain medications. Even when patients are offered the use of patient-controlled analgesia (PCA) pumps, they often fail to deliver adequate blood concentrations of analgesia.[11] This tendency may be especially heightened by the post-surgical state of dependency that interferes with the proactive response that PCA requires for adequate pain relief. The use of behavioral techniques may offer patients alternatives to their unsuccessful quest for pharmacologic pain relief.

BEHAVIORAL STRATEGIES FOR PAIN CONTROL

The key to adequate non-pharmacologic control of pain using behavioral techniques is to match the skill and strategy being taught to the patient's personality and lifestyle. Patients who, for example, have a primarily action-oriented personality will do better with skills such as progressive muscle relaxation that allows them to feel that they are actually doing something. The same preference may be true for patients who are more biologically-oriented. In contrast, patients, who are more dependent, may need to talk first or engage in brief psychotherapy before learning self-control skills. The imagery choices these patients respond to may be more escape- than control-oriented.

The next section of this chapter describes a variety of procedures that are useful for these different groups.

PHYSICAL EMPHASIS

Breathing

The most basic physical technique – the one that also underlies other more cognitive relaxation techniques – is slow-paced breathing. Patients are taught to close their eyes and concentrate on breathing from the diaphragm (expanding the

Table 15.1 Relaxation breathing (diaphragmatic/abdominal breathing)

1. Initially it is easier to practice relaxed breathing while lying on your back in a bed, a recliner chair, or on a well-padded floor. (Once you can breathe easily in this position, practice while sitting and, later, while standing.)
2. Loosen any tight clothing, especially around your abdomen and waist.
3. Place your feet slightly apart and close your eyes. (Rest one hand comfortably on your abdomen near your navel. Place the other hand on your chest.)
4. Inhale through your nose while mentally counting slowly to four, about 1 second per count. As you inhale gently, slightly extend your abdomen, causing it to rise about 1 inch. You should be able to feel the movement with your hand. Remember, do not pull your shoulder up or move your chest. (As you breathe in, become aware of your breathing and imagine the warmed and relaxing air flowing in.)
5. Pause for 1 second after inhaling.
6. Slowly exhale to the count of four. While you exhale, your abdomen will slowly recede as the diaphragm relaxes upward against your lungs. (As air flows out, imagine that tension is also flowing out.) (You may also say or think the word "one" to yourself.)
7. Repeat Steps 4, 5 and 6 – the slow inhaling, pausing, slow exhaling and pausing – about 5 to 10 times. As you practice, remember that initially every breath will not reach the lower parts of the lungs. This will improve with practice. The idea is to passively concentrate on slow, even, easy breathing.
8. When you finish, sit quietly for several minutes, at first with your eyes closed and later with your eyes opened. Do not stand up for a few minutes.
9. Do not worry about whether you are successful in achieving a deep level of relaxation. *Maintain a passive attitude and permit relaxation to occur at its own pace.* When distracting thoughts occur, try to ignore them by not dwelling upon them and return to your breathing. With practice, the response should come with little effort.

From Snow.[22]

Table 15.2 Sample muscles to be included in progressive tense–release exercises

Forehead	Neck	Thighs
Jaw	Shoulders	Legs
Eyes	Chest	Arms
Lips	Stomach	

lungs fully while keeping the chest and shoulders relaxed and allowing the abdomen to expand). They are taught to slow the pace of their breathing to no more than 12 breaths a minute, preferably slower. Patients are instructed to use this technique to counteract the rapid-paced breathing induced by pain and anxiety experienced by them and they are encouraged to practice on a regular schedule, slow deep breathing. Table 15.1 shows a sample handout that patients receive to instruct them in this procedure.

Tense–release

Other patients prefer to relax by an even more physical technique that emphasizes progressive tensing and releasing (relaxing) of different muscle groups. This procedure provides the distraction of a repetitive physical focus as well as the actual physical sensation of relaxation following muscular tension. Depending on the nature of the pain problem, progressive tense–release exercise may start from the forehead and proceed to the legs, or vice versa. Patients, however, need to be cautioned not to overly clamp down on a muscle group that could exacerbate their current pain problem. Table 15.2 gives an example of the muscle groups used in these exercises.

COGNITIVE EMPHASIS

Cognitive approaches to pain control emphasize the goal of shifting the patient awareness from pain to more relaxing alternatives.[12] When properly used, however, imagery can go beyond distraction to creating actual physical changes. The common experience of salivating when imagining eating a lemon points to the ability of the nervous system to create physical change with sufficient cues. With proper training, physical changes incompatible with pain can be an effective tool in pain relief.

Imagery

The most basic form of cognitive techniques involves the use of repetitive thoughts to block out pain signals. These thoughts can be neutral or relaxing phrases or images. Autogenic phrases, which are brief phrases focusing on thermal regulation and relaxation, have been found to be helpful. A more elaborate use of the strategy is for the patient to focus on changing numbers or patterns that interfere with the reception of their pain signals.

The use of relaxation imagery whereby the patient imagines a pleasant scene such as lying on the beach, feeling the warm sunshine, and listening to the waves, or imagines strolling through the woods on a brisk winter evening is a next step in the cognitive approach. Patients are encouraged to use all their senses and feel as if they are actively in the scene as a way of capturing their interest as well as occupying all data-processing channels and pain gates in an attempt to block out pain messages. Patients can also be helped by using tapes with appropriate background sounds and music or detailed tapes with relaxation imagery scenes of their choosing. As with other behavioral techniques, it is important to select a scene and image that fits the individual person's image of relaxation (e.g. warm beach versus cold forest stream) to ensure that it can be personally involving.

Hypnosis

A more formal, structured approach to imagery and suggestion is the use of hypnosis.[12,13] An intriguing view of the traumatized patient is that of an individual who is already in a highly focused state of attention as he or she is concerned for survival of life and limb.[14] Using this definition, many clinicians have spoken of the natural state of hypnosis that these patients assume and the advisability of using hypnotic techniques with them. Hypnosis can involve basic suggestions for relaxation that just attempt to distract the person from the pain. More detailed suggestions that focus on change in the image of pain the person is experiencing or to numb a part of the body can also be taught to receptive individuals. Hypnosis is also a useful treatment if the pain began in a life-threatening traumatic accident that is now producing nightmares that aggravate the patient's pain. It

should be borne in mind that people differ in their susceptibility to hypnotic suggestion and in their culturally-bred fear of hypnosis. The clinician will take this problem into account when developing treatment plans. Tables 15.3 and 15.4 show a variety of hypnotic imagery and suggestion that can be used. Table 15.5 reviews the steps of self-hypnosis training.

An interesting use of hypnosis during the postoperative period should be mentioned. A growing literature attests to the presence of intraoperative awareness in some patients with adequate muscu-

Table 15.3   Hypnotic suggestions

1. As the days go by, I am finding that I can remain comfortable for a longer time.
2. My concentration is improving as I become more relaxed. I can begin to work steadily and calmly.
3. Very soon I can let go of these troubling thoughts.
4. Each time I relax, my body feels healthier and becomes stronger.
5. In an hour, I can feel even more relaxed than I am now.
6. I can feel more relaxed and confident in myself.
7. I am taking more and more pride in my assets.
8. My sleeping is becoming sounder and deeper.
9. In just a few minutes I will be able to fall asleep and sleep peacefully all night.
10. I can awaken refreshed and rested.
11. I am developing more energy and vitality every day. I am making progress towards returning to work.

From Snow.[22]

Table 15.4   Hypnotic imagery

1. Suggestion for **change** in symptom (pain, energy level, feared object):
   A. Direct increase or reduction (pain locked up, deep sleep)
   B. Dissociation/separation (protective bubble)
   C. Anesthesia/numbing of painful area (dental)
   D. Displacement/transfer to other part of body (fingers)
   E. Transformation/manipulation/substitution (change color, temp of pain, knitting of muscles)
2. **Changes in self-image/awareness** age regression (to past), age progression (to future) [thru bridge, river][1]
3. **Exploration for self-discovery** (trusted friend, animal)[2]

[1]*Process* Imagery where the image of travelling on these structures is used to facilitate patient's progress in recovery.
[2]*Safe place* Imagery where the patient imagines being accompanied by a trusted entity.
From Snow.[22]

Table 15.5

1. Find a time of day when you have 10 minutes of uninterrupted time.
2. Get into a comfortable position in a softly-lit room in a place as far as possible from noise and distraction. (Set a timer for 10 minutes.)
3. Pick some point at eye level or a little above it. Stare steadily at that spot. Count to yourself from 1 to 100.
4. As you count, let yourself remember the feelings of hypnosis and deep relaxation. Think to yourself I am going deeper with each number that I count. Take three deep relaxing breaths and think to yourself 'I'm taking three deep relaxing breaths and letting the relaxed feeling spread throughout my body.'
5. Let your eyes flutter and close and your head fall forward gently.
6. You may deepen your state of hypnosis by imagining yourself getting on an escalator (elevator) that's moving down and feeling yourself slowly sinking to the next floor where it is quieter, the lights are softer and no-one else is around. You may go as deep as you want.
7. Say to yourself 'I'm now experiencing a peaceful, pleasant, relaxing time, just like I was at the beach/mountains/lake.' Picture the blue sky, the clear blue water, the white fluffy clouds, etc. Stay at the beach for a while.
8. You may also deepen your state of hypnosis by concentrating on the different parts of your body and feeling them go limp or feeling the wave of warmth from the beach spread through your body. Begin relaxing your feet, and slowly continue upwards to your ankles, calves, thighs, buttocks, abdomen, chest, hands, arms, shoulders, neck, face.
9. During the hypnotic state, you can make suggestions to yourself by repeating goals that you have or telling yourself things that you know are true, 'As the days go by, I am finding that I can remain comfortable for a longer time'; 'I am taking more and more pride in my assets and sense of increased self-control and well-being'; 'My sleeping is becoming sounder and deeper'; etc.
10. During the hypnotic state, you may use the various visualizations that affect the nature of your pain. These images can include the control room image, color, shape and distance exercise, and/or the garbage disposal exercise.
11. Let yourself enjoy the relaxed experience until you hear the sound of the tone.
12. Say to yourself, 'Now I'm going to end the experience by counting backwards slowly from 5 to 1 and coming out refreshed, alert, and able to do what I want to do. *five*, I begin to feel more alert; *four*, I feel my body beginning to regain muscle tone; *three*, I'm becoming more aware of sounds around me; *two*, I'm feeling more and more alert; *one*, I'm opening my eyes and feeling fine, alert, and refreshed.'
13. Flex and relax your muscles a few times before standing up. You may want to take a deep breath to reorient yourself.
14. Set a time for your next hypnotic session.

From Snow.[22]

lar paralysis but insufficient level of anesthetics.[15,16,17] Those patients will have a more troubled postoperative recovery period with increased pain and nightmares. Hypnotic examination of these patients has often revealed a heightened awareness of negative comments regarding their prognosis that were inadvertently made by authority figures during their surgery and were subconsciously processed by the patient. Hypnotic suggestion emphasizing security and survival can be efficiently used for these patients in the postoperative period to complete the recovery process.

Psychotherapy

The use of psychotherapy with the traumatized patient can significantly improve the patient's coping skills. At its most basic level, psychotherapy can provide a supportive context during which the patient may face the challenges of hospitalization and recovery. This support is especially important as hospitalization represents a threat to an individual's sense of autonomy. Issues faced by the patient may include guilt and the nature of the injury, fear of the future, and the overall meaning of the pain to the patient.[18]

Psychotherapy strategies that emphasize cognition and behavioral principles can be especially valuable for alleviating the meaning of the pain to the individual, changing it from a life-threatening insult to a challenge with which the person is actively coping. 'Stress inoculation' programs, for example, help build 'psychological antibodies' through a systematic program of preparatory information, skills acquisition, and rehearsal so that the stressful stimuli may be strong enough to arouse defenses but not strong enough to overwhelm them. These kinds of programs have been extensively used for pain associated with invasive medical procedures such as biopsies, dental treatment, and burn dressing changes.[5,19,20]

BIOFEEDBACK AND COMBINED TECHNIQUES

Biofeedback techniques utilize instruments to monitor the physiological response of individuals and then feedback the information to themselves so they can train themselves to effect change. These procedures can convince patients of the efficacy of their relaxation techniques on a physiological level long before the degree of pain relief has changed. This 'window' into their own physiology can be very helpful to patients who are not sure if they should persist in the practice of the coping skills.

Biofeedback training can be used in conjunction with the cognitive and physical techniques described earlier. Thus, patients can practice breathing and imagery skills while attached to biofeedback devices. These ambulatory devices provide meaningful physiologic end-points such as:

1. temperature that measures peripheral vasoconstriction
2. sEMG that measure surface muscle activity
3. electrodermal response that measures autonomic nervous system response
4. electroencephalogram that measures brain wave activity during the relaxed and more agitated state.

Patients are often encouraged by the significant feedback they receive in the effort towards relaxation as pain control.

MODALITIES

Behavioral techniques may be combined with physical and energy-based modalities in a more comprehensive non-pharmacologic approach. A brief review of these techniques follows.

Transcutaneous electrical nerve stimulation – TENS

TENS is a commonly-used modality for the treatment of a wide variety of acute, chronic, and postoperative pain syndromes. It involves the application of electrical stimulation to the skin for pain reduction. When effective, the ease of use, safety, and portability make a preferred treatment. Active and intelligent participation by the patient is needed, however, to achieve a good result.

The origin of TENS in Western medical society dates back to Roman times when the use of electric fish was ascribed analgesic properties. The modern basis for the widespread use of TENS for pain control is the previously described gate control theory proposed by Melzack & Wall.[2] This theory suggests that hypothetical 'gates' in lamina V of the substantia gelatinosa could be closed to block pain stimuli traveling from A-δ and C afferent fibers in the peripheral nervous system where they synapse into the central nervous system.

In principle, TENS applies an electrical force that stimulates pain-suppressing A-β afferent nerve fibers which compete against pain-carrying A-δ and C fibers. Basebaum & Fields[21] proposed a model of endogenous pain control to explain the effects of TENS. Their data support the existence of supraspinal descending pain control systems that use inhibitory neurotransmitters and endorphins. They propose that neurons in either the brain stem or periaqueductal gray matter of the medulla send inhibitory messages down to the dorsal horn of the spinal cord. One of several relay connections between the afferent sensory system and the endogenous pain control system might be activated by TENS. Related to this mechanism is the fact that naloxone has been shown to reduce the effects of TENS. Besides reducing pain perceptions, there are other physiologic and psychologic effects of TENS – it increases skin blood flow, modulates sympathetic and reflex tone, acts as a placebo, and as an external device may satisfy unfulfilled dependency needs.

The use of TENS has mixed results clinically because of several factors, including waveform, frequency, pulse repetition rate, intensity, alternating versus direct current, electrode placement, and treatment time. TENS devices must be tried at a variety of settings and electrode placements to achieve optimal pain relief for a given patient. Stimulation should feel pleasant and permit the patient to improve his or her functional status. Most TENS units work with maximum currents around the 60 milliampere range, delivered for about 250 microseconds. The most common output is biphasic to avoid the side effects of polarization.

In general, alkaline batteries are preferred for constant stimulation, because they have a relatively slow linear power decay. Initially, dry pads were provided that required the use of a gel. This was messy, provided uneven conductivity, and caused minor skin burns at high currents. At present, self-adhesive, carbon-based electrodes are available that are semi-disposable and generally affordable. Electrode placement is perhaps the greatest variable in eliciting successful results with TENS. Electrodes are usually placed 'between the pain and the brain', along nerve roots, dermatomes of the respective nerve levels, following the referred pain pathway, or on trigger points. The electrodes must not touch, nor should the conductive gel be spread across the skin between them. This will short-circuit the electrodes, and patients will report little sensation at full-amplitude settings. Several combinations of pulse repetition rate, pulse width, intensity, electrode placement, and time and frequency of stimulation may have to be attempted before desirable results from TENS are obtained. When the electrodes are over a superficial sensory nerve, the user will note a paresthesia in that nerve distribution. If muscle twitches are noted, patients should be instructed to reduce stimulus intensity or move the electrodes.

TENS is advantageous over other forms of analgesia for variable pain because it can be adjusted frequently. An associated disadvantage, however, is the tinkering required for the average pain patient to find the best combination of variables for effective relief. There are very few contraindications with TENS. All electrical modalities are contraindicated for pregnant women and patients with demand-type pacemakers. Electrodes should not be placed on broken or insensate skin. Also it is essential that milliampere TENS electrodes are not placed on the head or neck. This is especially true regarding treatment directly over the carotid sinuses, as stimulation of the baroreceptors may result in a vasovagal syncope.

Acupuncture

Although acupuncture originated some 4000 years ago in China, it has recently become an acceptable therapeutic modality in the Western world. This recent acceptance occurred after studies of neurochemical mechanisms became available, providing scientific explanations for its effects. Acupuncture analgesia uses stimulation of designated body sites by manual rotation of needles to produce a sensation known as *teh chi*. Classical acupuncture stimulation has been modernized more recently by the application of slow frequency (<5 Hz) stimulation of needles, which also produces powerful muscle contractions. Acupuncture produces a high-intensity stimulation that is believed to induce a chemical modulation of pain, which explains why relief is not confined to a local segmental distribution.

Therapeutic cold

Ice cubes in plastic bags and massage with ice cubes mounted on a wooden stick are the most common ways of applying cold to affected areas. This is a relatively safe, inexpensive, and simple-to-use modality. Cold is especially indicated after trauma where the goal is to reduce the inflammatory reaction.

Mobilization techniques

These are passive exercises directed toward restoration of tissue extensibility, perfusion, and joint mobility.

Massage

Although only temporary, massage has a definite soothing and relaxing effect. It is believed that its effects include stretching of shortened soft tissues, resolution of edema, improved tissue perfusion, and removal of metabolic waste products.

Manipulation

Manipulation, which often relieves muscle spasm, involves a forced passive movement of the articular elements beyond the usual physiological range of motion.

Traction

Traction involves a force applied to stretch the soft tissues or to distract articulating surfaces. It is believed that pain relief results from stretching muscles which leads to their relaxation and improved local circulation.

Therapeutic heat

Heat increases the metabolic rate, nerve conduction velocity, and muscle contractility. The therapeutic effects of heat may be local or distant. If pain occurs as a result of accumulated metabolites in a poorly perfused area, applied heat will cause vasodilatation and rapid removal of the pain-producing substances.

Heating a stiff joint decreases the viscosity of the synovial fluid, thereby facilitating therapeutic stretching. The optimal therapeutic effect of heat is achieved when the tissue temperature during the treatment session is between 41°C and 45°C. The relaxing and sedating effect of heat, in addition to reflexive vasodilatation, provides a distant therapeutic effect. In patients with mental confusion or grossly impaired sensation a risk of a burn exists. Heat should not be used on ischemic areas, acutely inflamed areas, and fresh bleeds. There is concern that heat will increase metabolic activity in tissues overlying malignant growths.

Deep-heating devices

Chronic or acute inflammatory conditions and soft-tissue shortening are the most common indications for the use of deep-heating modalities. Here a primary form of energy is converted into heat resulting in a temperature rise in muscles, bones, and deep joints.

Ultrasound. The mechanical effect of ultrasound is used to loosen adhesions and help resolve edema in inflammatory tissue. Ultrasound is applied using a sound head or applicator that is rhythmically moved over the treatment area, which is either immersed in water or covered with a gel. Sonic energy is converted into heat.

Microwave diathermy. Uses the conversion of electromagnetic waves into heat.

Short-wave diathermy. Here radio waves are converted into electrical current. Patients with metallic implants may need to avoid this modality as these implants may be selectively heated and thus cause deep burns.

Superficial devices

These include the heating pad, hot water bottle, hydrocollator pack, paraffin wax bath, and heating lamp. Superficial heat results in a temperature rise of the skin, subcutaneous tissue, and in some instances, superficial musculature.

ENERGY-BASED APPROACHES

Recently renewed interest in energy-based approaches to pain control and healing necessitates a brief mention of these approaches. Energy-based techniques have been discussed under a variety of names including 'laying on of hands',

'chakra balancing', 'therapeutic touch', 'bioenergy', and 'spiritual healing'.

Qigong and Reiki

These techniques involve the scanning and manipulation of energy fields that surround the individual and may play a role in pain control and healing. Increasing research is being conducted as to the efficacy of these procedures. Interested healers may wish to offer these options to their patients.

ADVISORY FOR PAIN CONSULTANTS

The significance of behavioral factors in pain control presented in this chapter points to the importance of having pain consultants included in the initial intake interview so that specific questions on pain can be asked and preference for behavioral and modality-based pain management techniques established. These questions are of course determined to an important degree by how readily the patient will admit to pain. As discussed elsewhere, some individuals will, for example, attempt a stoic ignorance of the pain, while others will show exaggerated and/or highly emotional responses. The attitude of the patients and their family about pain also needs to be investigated. Patients or significant family members who believe such myths that one should always 'tough out' pain, or that pain medication will always cause addiction or even that behavioral and/or modality techniques are ineffective can place difficult demands on professional staff caring for them. Identification of the individual concerns and their inclusion in a comprehensive managed plan can be an important aid in healing and recovery.

REFERENCES

1. Melzack R, Casey KL. Sensory, motivational and central control determinants of pain. A new conceptual model. In: Kenshalo D, ed. The skin sense. Springfield: Charles C. Thomas; 1968: 423–443.
2. Melzack R, Wall PD. Pain mechanisms: A new theory. Science 1965; 50: 71–97.
3. Kiecolt-Glaser J, Williams DA. Self-blame, compliance, and distress among burn patients. J Pers Soc Psychol 1987; 53: 187–193.

4. James LD, Thorn BE, Williams DA. Goal specification in cognitive–behavioral therapy for chronic headache pain. Behav Ther 1993; 24: 305–320.
5. Wardle J. Psychological management of anxiety and pain during dental treatments. J Psychosom Res 1983; 27: 299–402.
6. Snow BR. Compliance with therapeutic regimens: assessment and treatment issues. In: Finkel J, ed. Consultation/liaison psychiatry: Current trends and new perspectives. New York: Grune & Stratton; 1983: 97–113.
7. Blount RL, Corbin SM, Sturges JW, Wolfe VV, Prater JM, James LD. The relationship between adults' behavior and child coping and distress during BMA/LP procedures: A sequential analysis. Behav Ther 1989; 20: 585–601.
8. Gil KM, Ginsberg B, Muir M, Sullivan F, Williams DA. Patient controlled analgesia: The relationship of psychological factors to pain and analgesic use in adolescents with postoperative pain. Clin J Pain 1992; 8: 215–221.
9. Marks RM, Sachar EJ. Undertreatment of medical inpatients with narcotic analgesics. Ann Intern Med 1973; 78: 173–181.
10. Agency for Health Care Policy and Research (AHCPR). Acute pain management: Operative or medical procedures and trauma. (Clinical Practice Guideline No. 1, AHCPR Publication no. 92-0032.) Rockville: U.S. Department of Health and Human Services; 1992.
11. Welchew EA. On demand analgesia: A double blind comparison of on demand intravenous fentanyl with regular intramuscular morphine. Anaesthesia 1983; 38: 19–25.
12. Blankfield RP. Suggestion, relaxation and hypnosis as adjuncts in the care of surgery patients: A review of the literature. Am J Clin Hypn 1991; 33: 172–186.
13. Snow BR. The use of hypnosis in the management of preoperative anxiety and postoperative pain in a patient undergoing laminectomy: A case report. Bull Hosp Jt Dis 1985; 46: 22–30.
14. Mutter CB. Posttraumatic stress disorder. In: Dowd ET, Healy JM Case studies in hypnotherapy. New York: Guilford Press; 1986.
15. Bennett JL. Perception and memory for events during adequate general anesthesia. In: Pettinati HM, ed. Hypnosis and memory. New York: Guilford Press; 1988: 193–231.
16. Blacher RS. On awakening paralyzed during surgery. A syndrome of traumatic neurosis. JAMA 1975; 234: 67–68.
17. Peebles MJ. Through a glass darkly: The psychoanalytic use of hypnosis with post traumatic stress disorder. Int J Clin Exp Hypn 1989; 192–206.
18. Grozesch RC, Ury GM, Dworkin RH. Psychodynamic psychotherapy with chronic pain patients, 1988. In: Gothel RJ, Turk DC, eds. Psychological approaches to pain management: A practitioners handbook. New York: Guilford Press; 1996.
19. Turk DC, Meichenbaum D, Genest M. Pain and behavioral medicine: A cognitive–behavioral perspective. New York: Guilford Press; 1983.
20. Varni JW, Jay SM, Masek BJ, Thompson KL. Cognitive–behavioral assessment and management of pediatric pain. In: Holzner AP, Turk DC, eds. Pain management: A flashback of psychological treatment approaches. Elmsford: Pergamon Press; 1986.
21. Basebaum AT, Fields HL. Endogenous pain control systems: brain stem spinal pathways and endorphin circuitry. Ann Rev Neurosci. 1984; 7: 309.
22. Snow BR. Stress management workshop booklets. 1985.

PAIN MANAGEMENT FOR SPECIFIC TRAUMA PATIENT POPULATIONS AND INJURED ORGAN SYSTEMS

16

Regional anesthesia for pediatric trauma

Lynn M Broadman and Nancy L Glass

Introduction

General guidelines
Regional anesthesia in the acute trauma setting
Scheduled procedures in the post-trauma
    period
Nerve stimulators
Needle selection
Selection of local anesthetic agents
Avoiding complications

Pediatric upper extremity blocks
Brachial plexus blocks
    Axillary approach
    Interscalene approach
    Parascalene approach
Distal upper extremity blocks
Intravenous regional anesthesia

Pediatric lower extremity blocks
Sciatic nerve block
Posterior approach to the sciatic nerve
Anterior approach to the sciatic nerve

Lateral approach to the sciatic nerve
Comparison of sciatic nerve blocks

Lumbar plexus and component nerve blocks
Femoral nerve block
'3-in-1' block
Fascia iliaca block
Lumbar plexus block
Block of the lateral femoral cutaneous nerve
Nerve blocks at the knee
Common peroneal nerve block

Caudal and epidural blocks
Introduction
Needle selection for caudal block
Technique for caudal block
Dosage, drug selection, and duration of caudal
    anesthesia

**Continuous caudal and epidural catheter
    techniques**

Summary

INTRODUCTION

Trauma is the number one cause of death in children over 1 year of age. Trauma and the resultant disabilities are major pediatric health care issues. All children and young adults are at risk for death and disability from trauma, since traumatic injuries occur irrespective of age, gender, ethnicity, religion, or socio-economic status.

During 1996, 27% (330 of the 1272) of the admissions to The Jon Michael Moore Trauma Center were younger than 20 years of age.[1] Since such a large percentage of trauma patients being admitted are in the pediatric age range, it is inter-

esting to note that fewer than a dozen of the more than 300 articles published on pediatric regional anesthesia deal specifically with pediatric trauma.

This chapter will cover regional anesthetic techniques and indications for their use in the care of pediatric trauma victims.

GENERAL GUIDELINES

Regional anesthesia in the acute trauma setting

Ideally, children with acute injuries for whom regional anesthesia is recommended should not receive intravenous sedation or general anesthesia with a mask during placement of the regional block. The blocks should be performed on awake, unsedated children, should be limited to extremity blocks and should be performed only on cooperative children with whom one can communicate. Having the parent present to calm and console the child may be very helpful during placement of the block.

To facilitate comfort during placement of the block, EMLA cream may be applied to the area 1 hour prior to the anticipated time of injection. When performing a nerve block on an awake child, it is important **not** to seek a paresthesia since the child may be distressed by the sensation and become uncooperative. A nerve stimulator will be invaluable in locating the ideal needle placement for the block.

After administering the block, some type of diversion is necessary to keep the child relaxed. Avoiding or minimizing visual and auditory cues from the surgical field is crucial. Talking with the child about sports, TV programs, and school may be effective distracters. Listening to music through headphones or reading a story aloud are other ways to provide a calming atmosphere.

In the event that a regional block has been performed and does not appear to be working, one should resist the urge to 'supplement' the block with large doses of sedatives or narcotics. Likewise, one should not administer general anesthesia by mask or laryngeal mask airway (LMA) to such a child in the presence of a full stomach. A safer approach would be to induce general anesthesia with a rapid sequence technique and tracheal intubation. This caveat also applies to the child in whom the block is working but who becomes unable to lie quietly in the operating room.

Sometimes, however, regional anesthesia alone in an awake child is neither advisable nor practical. Age of the child, level of cooperation, the presence of multiple injuries, and the expected duration of surgery may preclude the use of the regional block alone. For example, the child who has suffered a mild head injury in addition to a broken arm may be too incoherent or uncooperative to tolerate an axillary block. Combining general anesthesia with a regional block in situations such as this one may be ideal, but will require the practitioner to balance the advantages of the regional technique with the added time, risks, and disadvantages of the block. One obvious advantage to the use of regional techniques is the opportunity to provide excellent postoperative analgesia without using large doses of systemic opioids.

Scheduled procedures in the post-trauma period

The post-trauma patient presenting for additional reconstructive surgery may be an ideal candidate for regional anesthetic techniques. Following the induction of general anesthesia by inhalation or intravenous methods, regional nerve blocks may be performed. In this manner, the advantages of regional anesthesia can be achieved while the patient is lightly anesthetized under general anesthesia. Since the block provides surgical anesthesia, the inspired concentration of the volatile anesthetic can be markedly reduced.

Prior to the introduction of the LMA, it was usually necessary to have two anesthesiologists available during placement of a regional block; one to hold the mask and maintain a patent airway, while the other colleague performed the nerve block. However, using the LMA, a single practitioner can induce anesthesia, place the LMA in the spontaneously breathing patient, and then perform the nerve block. When employing this technique, it is imperative that all monitors and alarms are operational and that the anesthesiologist is constantly vigilant and responsive to any change in the vital signs or oxygen saturation level.

If intravenous access is available, anesthesia can be induced with propofol 1.0–1.5 mg/kg, and maintained with an infusion of 50–100 microg/kg/min. While the patient is anesthetized with propofol, the regional block can be performed. Once the surgical procedure is underway, the infusion rate of the propofol may be decreased. A similar technique can be designed for the child who presents without intravenous access after an inhalation induction.

Nerve stimulators

Wright[2] found a new and exciting use for the devices used to monitor the effects of skeletal muscle relaxants. He noted that motor fibers are stimulated at a lower milliamperage than sensory fibers. At low current levels, depolarization of muscle fibers causes a visible contraction; however, there may be little to no perception of the electrical stimulus because the sensory fibers have not been depolarized. Therefore, at low milli-amperage levels, a muscle twitch can be obtained without discomfort to the patient. Montgomery et al[3] extended the description of this technique to the use of unsheathed needles.

The nerve stimulator makes it possible to place the block needle in close proximity to the nerve in order to maximize the chances of achieving an effective block. When preparing to perform the block, the negative electrode of the nerve stimulator is attached to the block needle by means of an alligator clamp, the positive electrode is attached to the skin of the trunk a short distance away, and the current is set at 1–3 mA. Detection of a muscle twitch at the surgical site using the lowest possible current confirms that the needle is very close to the nerve to be blocked. This technique simplifies the process of locating the nerve, and increases the clinical applicability of peripheral nerve blocks in infants and children.

Needle selection

The short, 'B'-bevel needle may be safer for performing nerve blocks than a long-bevel needle. Selander et al[4] demonstrated in 1977 that long-bevel needles caused more injury to rabbit nerves when pierced than when the same procedure was performed with a short-bevel needle. Based on this work it has been recommended that short-bevel needles are used for all peripheral nerve blocks.

Selection of local anesthetic agents

Several choices of local anesthetics for peripheral nerve blocks are available. One option for extremity blocks is the combination of lidocaine plus tetracaine with epinephrine. Lidocaine, in a concentration of 0.5 to 1.5%, provides rapid onset of anesthesia. Tetracaine 0.1% with epinephrine 1:200 000 is useful for sensory block. Increasing the concentration of tetracaine to 0.2% results in both sensory and motor blockade. When these local anesthetics are combined, the lidocaine offers rapid onset of surgical anesthesia while the tetracaine ensures good postoperative pain relief.

The toxic plasma level for tetracaine or for the combination of lidocaine plus tetracaine has not been established for children. When lidocaine and tetracaine are combined their toxic effects are additive. However, Scott & Cousins have successfully utilized this combination of lidocaine plus tetracaine in adults.[5] The author (LMB) has not noted a toxic reaction in more than 750 nerve blocks in pediatric patients when this combination is used for extremity anesthesia.

In Wedel's series, 15 children received chloroprocaine in a dose of 11 mg/kg along with bupivacaine 2.25 mg/kg. Others received mepivacaine or bupivacaine separately. No child showed any signs of toxicity from the use of the local anesthetic agent.[6]

Campbell et al injected bupivacaine 3.0 mg/kg for axillary blocks in children. Measurements of venous plasma levels were found to be only 1.84 microg/ml.[7] Eyres studied plasma levels following caudal and lumbar epidural anesthesia using bupivacaine 3.0 mg/kg, and found no toxic levels when the dose did not exceed 3.0 mg/kg.[8,9] Because it is easy to obtain plasma lidocaine levels in most hospital laboratories, Yaster has suggested that lidocaine may be the local anesthetic of choice for pediatric regional anesthesia.[10]

Avoiding complications

Intravascular injections

Gentle aspiration should always be performed prior to injecting local anesthetic to decrease the risk of an intravascular injection. Periodic aspiration should be performed if large volumes of local anesthetic agent are to be injected since the needle may move during injection. This safety habit is especially important when performing nerve blocks in the area of the head and neck since intravascular injections may demonstrate retrograde flow, reaching the brain.

Systemic toxic reactions

It is essential that the body weight of the child is known prior to the administration of the local anesthetic agent. In order to avoid local anesthetic overdose, the total dose in mg/kg to be used must be calculated based on the child's body weight. As a further safety precaution, only that amount of drug planned for injection should be drawn into the syringe, and the concentration of the agent should be rechecked at the time of preparation.

Neural damage

Injuries to nerves may be avoided by the use of short-'B'-bevel needles and by using a nerve stimulator so that paresthesias need not be sought.

PEDIATRIC UPPER EXTREMITY BLOCKS

Brachial plexus blocks

Brachial plexus blocks can be used in the trauma setting for the repair of lacerations and for the reduction of both open and closed fractures. These blocks in combination with a light general anesthetic may be particularly advantageous during microvascular surgery for the reattachment of digits, since sympathetic blockade improves blood flow to the anesthetized extremity. Brachial plexus blocks are also effective in upper extremity surgical procedures performed on an elective basis.

Agents most commonly used for brachial plexus blocks include lidocaine 1%, bupivacaine 0.5%, and etidocaine 1%, with or without epinephrine. Combinations of lidocaine and bupivacaine, or bupivacaine and etiodocaine are often used. Volumes and doses are related to the patient's weight. Dalens uses 0.75 ml/kg for the first 20 kg, 15 ml for children between 21 and 30 kg, 20 ml for those between 31 and 55 kg, and 25 ml for those whose weight exceeds 55 kg.[11]

Doses described for the axillary approach are generally lower than for the more proximal blocks. A mixture of lidocaine and tetracaine (0.5% lidocaine and 0.2% tetracaine) may be used for this block in a dose of 0.33 ml/kg. Others have described successful use of different concentrations and agents: Eather[12] used 0.57–0.75 ml/kg; Tryba et al[13] used 0.7–1.1 ml/kg of prilocaine; Campbell et al[7] reported the use of 0.6 ml/kg of 0.33% bupivacaine. Winnie's dose is based on height.[14]

Axillary approach

Accardo & Adriani[15] described the axillary approach to the brachial plexus in children in 1949. A single-injection 'sheath' technique was introduced by Eriksson[16] in 1965. He used a distal tourniquet in conjunction with this block for reduction of fractures in unsedated children. Niesel et al[17] in 1974 described the use of a nerve stimulator to perform axillary blocks for the

reduction of humeral and forearm fractures; 94% of the children in this series required no supplemental anesthesia.

The axillary approach to the brachial plexus is appropriate for procedures distal to the elbow. Proper positioning for the axillary block requires that the child is able to abduct and externally rotate the arm. In contrast to the landmarks for the administration of the block in adults, this block is performed more distally in children. The musculocutaneous nerve is not blocked by the axillary block, and therefore requires a separate injection of local anesthetic into the coracobrachialis muscle.

Wedel et al[6] analyzed the records of 109 patients who received 142 blocks. These children were all under 18 years of age (mean age of 14.8 years). All four children less than 7 years of age had the block administered under general anesthesia. Of the older children, 11.6% (16 of 138) received general anesthesia prior to their block. In the remaining patients (88.4%), intravenous sedation was used in conjunction with the regional block. The medications used to provide sedation for block placement included fentanyl (1.0 microg/kg) in 78% and midazolam (30.0 microg/kg) in 46% of cases. Of the children who had a brachial plexus block performed under intravenous sedation, 92% did not require any additional anesthesia.

This study demonstrated that most adolescents tolerate surgery of the upper extremity under regional anesthesia with only minimal doses of intravenous fentanyl and/or midazolam. In addition, very few of the children who received a regional block experienced nausea and vomiting, unlike those children undergoing general anesthesia, who experienced a much higher incidence of postoperative nausea and/or vomiting. Fewer children who received a brachial plexus block required narcotic analgesia prior to discharge (12%) compared with those who received a general anesthetic (31%), which was significant at $P < 0.05$.

Technique

With the arm abducted to 90°, the pulsations in the axillary artery are identified 1–2 cm below the pectoralis muscle (see Fig. 16.1). The nerve sheath can be palpated in this position distal to the pectoralis muscle. A nerve stimulator and a 22 gauge

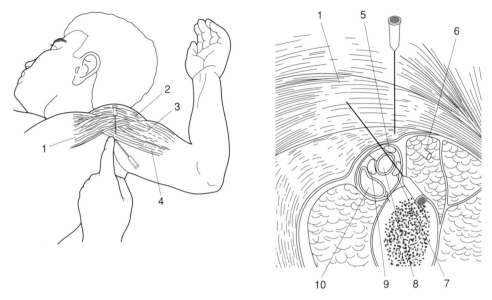

Fig. 16.1 Axillary block. 1, pectoralis major; 2, deltoid; 3, biceps; 4, coracobrachialis; 5, median nerve; 6, musculocutaneous nerve; 7, radial nerve; 8, axillary artery; 9, ulnar nerve; 10, axillary vein.

1½ inch 'B'-bevel needle are used to perform the block. The needle is advanced at a 45° angle and a 'pop' is noted when the sheath is penetrated. At this point the electrical impulses generated from the nerve stimulator and needle should show motor activity in the distal arm. When the best twitch is identified at the lowest possible current, one should aspirate to ensure that the needle is not intravascular before injecting 1–2 ml of anesthetic. This small dose of local anesthetic should eliminate the twitch response and serves as confirmation that the needle is in the correct position. With injection and intermittent aspiration, the total dose of 0.33 ml/kg is then injected.

Dalens suggests a slight variant on this approach, with needle insertion somewhat distal to that described above.[18] He describes a perpendicular insertion of the needle at the point where the pectoralis major muscle crosses the coracobrachialis muscle, easily palpated superficially in most children (Fig. 16.1). A similar 'pop' is felt when the needle enters the sheath. Distal pressure will again facilitate proximal spread of the local anesthetic solution after nerve stimulation confirms muscle twitch in the hand.

The author (LMB) prefers to locate separate branches of the brachial plexus with the nerve stimulator and inject 2–5 ml of local anesthetic close to each nerve. The median nerve is identified on the lateral side of the artery as noted by flexion of the wrist or fingers. Advancing the needle slightly elicits triceps muscle activity, indicating radial nerve stimulation. Finally, inserting the needle on the ulnar side of the artery should make it possible to demonstrate ulnar nerve activity, as indicated by flexion of the little and ring fingers.

To complete the block, the musculocutaneous nerve should be identified by advancing the needle into the coracobrachialis muscle located caudad to the biceps and cephalad to the artery. As the needle is advanced toward the shoulder, contraction is noted in the biceps. 3–5 ml of local anesthetic are administered and the contractions should stop, indicating that the musculocutaneous nerve has been successfully located.

If bright red blood is obtained prior to obtaining a twitch response, a 'through and through' technique is substituted. The needle is advanced until blood is no longer aspirated. One-half of the anesthetic dose is administered posterior to the artery and the remainder after the needle is withdrawn back through the artery and no more blood is aspirated. In order to prevent formation of a hematoma, firm pressure is held over the axillary artery for 5 to 7 minutes.

Since children may not describe or recognize the feeling of a paresthesia, another technique which does not require patient cooperation is the 'bounce' technique. This method was described by Winnie,[14] who first identifies the pulsation of the axillary artery as a primary landmark. The needle is then inserted at an angle of 45° to the skin parallel to the artery. A 'pop' is noted when the needle enters the sheath surrounding the neurovascular bundle. In this position, the pulsations of the artery will be noted from the movement of the needle and the needle will 'bounce' in synchrony with the tone from the electrocardiogram or pulse oximeter.

The needle is fixed in position and the local anesthetic is injected from a syringe connected to the needle with extension tubing. Using a needle that is remote from the syringe decreases the likelihood of movement of the needle with pressure on the syringe plunger. It is very important to aspirate frequently during the injection to be certain that the needle has not entered the vessel. Because the plexus is deeper in adults than in children, there is a tendency for adult anesthesiologists to insert the needle deeper than necessary. This will result in a failed block, and is another reason to suggest the use of the nerve stimulator.

Interscalene approach

Winnie described the interscalene block in 1970.[19] Its use is indicated in infants and children for procedures of the shoulder and upper arm but not for those of the forearm or hand. It is not necessary to abduct the arm to 90° when performing the interscalene block; therefore, this approach is useful for the child with a painful injury who will become very uncomfortable and uncooperative if the injured arm is moved.

Insertion of the needle for this block is generally carried out after the induction of general anesthesia. If the procedure is elective, and the patient has had nothing by mouth (NPO), then the block may be performed either with IV sedation or under general anesthesia.

Technique

The interscalene block is performed in children just as in adults, but the interscalene groove is only a space (Fig. 16.2). The posterior border of the sternocleidomastoid muscle is palpated at the level of the cricoid cartilage, the finger is then lifted off to palpate the anterior scalene muscle and then the groove between the anterior and middle scalene muscles. It is at this point that the needle is inserted perpendicular to the skin. With the use of a nerve stimulator, maximal twitch at the lowest possible current is sought in the shoulder and upper arm. Aspiration prior to injection of the local anesthetic should be performed to make

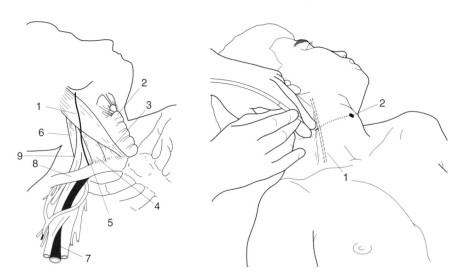

Fig. 16.2 Interscalene block. 1, external jugular vein; 2, cricoid cartilage; 3, sternocleidomastoid–sternal head; 4, sternocleidomastoid–clavicular head; 5, anterior scalene muscle; 6, middle scalene muscle; 7, axillary artery; 8, clavicle; 9, bracheal plexus.

certain that the needle is not in a blood vessel or in the subarachnoid space.

Parascalene approach

The parascalene approach to the brachial plexus is another option for providing anesthesia to the upper extremity. Dalens et al[20] compared the results of supraclavicular and parascalene approaches in 120 children aged 8 months to 17 years; one-third of these children were awake for both the block and the surgery. 97% of children who had a parascalene approach experienced complete analgesia, compared with 88% in the supraclavicular group.

Dalens et al also noted that it was easier to obtain muscle twitches on the first attempt with the parascalene approach, and that the parascalene approach provided better blockade to those areas supplied by the lower branches of the cervical plexus. Finally, they were able to demonstrate in this study that the incidence of puncture of the subclavian vessels and the incidence of Horner's syndrome were both lower using the parascalene approach. There were no clinically evident pneumothoraces with either approach in this series. If the axillary approach is not appropriate for a particular child, Dalens et al recommend the parascalene approach for regional anesthesia of the proximal upper extremity.

Technique

The child is placed in the supine position with the head turned away from the side to be blocked (Fig. 16.3). A rolled towel is placed behind the shoulders. The landmarks are outlined: the midpoint of the clavicle, the cricothyroid membrane, and the posterior border of the clavicular head of the sternocleidomastoid muscle. A line is drawn laterally from the cricothyroid membrane to a line demarcating the posterior border of the sternocleidomastoid muscle. Deep to the muscle in this location is Chassignac's tubercle, which is easily palpated in most children. The needle insertion point is located at the lower third of the line between the midpoint of the clavicle and Chassignac's tubercle.

An insulated needle connected to a nerve stimulator is advanced at a 90° angle to the skin in an anterior–posterior direction through the anterior scalene muscle until twitches are demonstrated emanating from the brachial plexus. If an adequate twitch response is not obtained with the first pass, the needle should be inserted at a point slightly lateral to the initial insertion. Following aspiration, a small dose of local anesthetic should be injected to abolish the twitch response. After proper needle position is confirmed, the remainder of the dose of local anesthetic is injected incrementally with repeated aspiration.

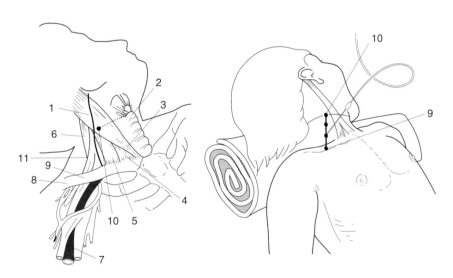

Fig. 16.3 Parascalene block. 1, sternocleidomastoid muscle; 2, cricoid cartilage; 3, sternocleidomastoid–sternal head; 4, sternocleidomastoid–clavicular head; 5, anterior scalene muscle; 6, middle scalene muscle; 7, axillary artery; 8, clavicle; 9, midpoint of the clavicle; 10, Chassignac's tubercle; 11, bracheal plexus.

Distal upper extremity blocks

For surgical procedures on the hand, the radial, median, and ulnar nerves can be blocked at the wrist utilizing from 0.5–1.0 ml of local anesthetic solution. The ulnar nerve is blocked at the level of the ulnar styloid process under the flexor carrpi ulnaris tendon where the pulsation of the ulnar artery can be felt. The median nerve is blocked by inserting the needle at the same level on the lateral side of the palmaris longus tendon. To block the radial nerve, superficial infiltration with local anesthetic is performed along the dorsum and volar aspect of the wrist. Solutions containing epinephrine are contraindicated when performing peripheral nerve blocks in the hand. These blocks can also be used to supplement or improve an incomplete block of one or more branches of the brachial plexus.

Intravenous regional anesthesia

August Bier introduced intravenous regional anesthesia in 1908, and the block is commonly called Bier's block in his honor.[21] Its use was more recently popularized by Holmes in 1963.[22] Intravenous regional anesthesia in pediatric patients is generally limited to the upper extremity for the management of fractures, dislocations, and other simple procedures.[23–29] Many children will require sedation when this technique is performed.

Technique

It is helpful to apply EMLA cream 1 hour prior to the time of anesthesia at the site where the intravenous cannula is to be inserted. A double-cuffed tourniquet is placed as high in the axilla as possible after adequate padding has been applied to the arm. An intravenous catheter flushed with heparin or saline is placed into a vein on the dorsum of the hand to be operated, and capped off. If a butterfly-style needle is chosen, it should be flushed with saline so that the blood does not clot in the tubing. The catheter or needle is then secured so that it cannot be dislodged during exsanguination of the arm.

Exsanguination is accomplished by wrapping an Esmarch bandage tightly around the raised arm; this may be poorly tolerated in children with acute or painful injuries. Alternatively, 'exsanguination'

can be accomplished by raising the arm for approximately 3 minutes and allowing gravity drainage to minimize the blood volume remaining in the arm. Following exsanguination, the proximal tourniquet is inflated to a pressure 50 mmHg higher than the child's systolic blood pressure. Confirm successful tourniquet inflation before injection of anesthetic agent by palpating for the radial pulse, which should be absent.

Lidocaine 3.0 mg/kg of 0.5% lidocaine without epinephrine or preservative is injected into the arm. Injection should be done slowly since very high pressures during injection may push local anesthetic under the inflated tourniquet and into the circulation.[30] The needle in the vein is then removed and a gauze is held over the injection site for approximately 2 minutes. Elevation of the arm is helpful in preventing leakage of solution from the injection site.

If the surgical procedure lasts less than 20 minutes, it has been recommended that the cuff is not deflated until a minimum of 20 minutes has elapsed since the injection of local anesthetic. This will prevent local anesthetic solution from entering the general circulation with possible toxic effects. If the procedure lasts longer than 20 minutes, the distal cuff should be inflated over the anesthetized area and the proximal cuff deflated. It is preferable to change cuffs after 20 minutes rather than waiting for the patient to complain of tourniquet pain. Some investigators recommend that, at the end of the procedure, the tourniquet should be deflated in a staged or cyclical fashion with deflation, inflation, deflation, inflation and deflation; others believe that this step is not necessary.

Several authors have reported seizure activity following the administration of lidocaine for an intravenous regional block. Dawkins et al[31] reported two cases of toxicity upon release of the tourniquet; however, in both cases, the tourniquet was released only 3 to 5 minutes after the injection of the lidocaine bolus. In another case, Finsterbush et al reported seizure activity following the administration of 8.0 mg/kg of lidocaine resulting from a dose miscalculation.[32] Both reports highlight the need for meticulous attention to technique in the safe performance of intravenous regional anesthesia, as well as the potential for considerable toxicity.

Even when the tourniquet is deflated after an appropriate interval, local anesthetic agent may enter the circulation and cause toxic affects. Some protection may be afforded by the use of benzodi-azepines for sedation. Another technique that may be protective is to administer a small dose of propofol just prior to release of the tourniquet. Acute administration of propofol or benzodi-azepines would not be appropriate if the patient has a full stomach.

PEDIATRIC LOWER EXTREMITY BLOCKS

Occasions may arise when regional anesthesia is preferable for surgery on the lower extremity but central neuraxial blockade with spinal or epidural anesthesia is contraindicated. Alternative techniques include blocking the sciatic, femoral, or lateral femoral cutaneous nerves, alone or in combination. Depending on the site of the surgery, other lower extremity blocks which may be helpful include the '3-in-1' block, the fascia iliaca block, or the lumbar plexus block.[33–35] In the trauma setting, one must be cognizant of those injuries likely to be associated with the development of a compartment syndrome, since the insensate limb may be difficult to assess for ischemic pain.

Sciatic nerve block

In addition to providing anesthesia for open or closed reductions of fractures of the tibia and fibula, the sciatic block provides good anesthesia for surgery on the foot and ankle. When the sciatic nerve block is combined with blocks of the femoral and lateral femoral cutaneous nerves, anesthesia will be adequate for any surgery on the lower extremity. Selection of long-acting, local

anesthetic agents offers the additional advantage of prolonged, postoperative pain relief.

There are any number of approaches to the sciatic nerve, including the posterior approach of Labat[36] and the anterior approach of Beck[37] which was adopted by McNicol[38] and reported for use in children. The lateral approach of Ichiyanaghi[39] was modified by Guardini et al[40] and was then described by Dalens et al[41] for pediatric patients. The lithotomy position is seldom used in pediatric patients. The author (LMB) favors the posterior approach, blocking the nerve between the greater trochanter and ischial tuberosity.

Regardless of which approach to the sciatic block is chosen, the use of the nerve stimulator is considered mandatory for successfully locating this nerve. In the trauma patient, the anterior and lateral approaches may be the preferred choices, since the patient does not have to be moved in order to perform the block. Some clinicians advocate performing a femoral block prior to the anterior approach to the sciatic in order to decrease the discomfort associated with this approach. In most pediatric patients, however, these blocks are performed after the induction of general anesthesia. One may expect 12 hours of analgesia in the blocked area from a single injection of bupivacaine.[42]

Posterior approach to the sciatic nerve

The classic approach to the sciatic nerve is the posterior approach described by Labat for adults; this technique can be used for children as well. However, a simpler approach has been described by Dalens[43] (Fig. 16.4). In the lateral position,

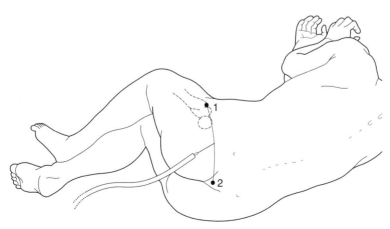

Fig. 16.4 Sciatic block: posterior approach. 1, greater trochanter of the femur; 2, coccyx.

with the injured extremity uppermost and flexed at the hip, a single line is drawn between the greater trochanter of the femur and the coccyx. The center of this line is the insertion site for the needle, which enters the skin at a 90° angle to the skin, oriented toward the ischial tuberosity. When a muscle twitch is demonstrated in the foot, the local anesthetic is injected.

Anterior approach to the sciatic nerve

The anterior approach to the sciatic nerve is indicated when the child cannot be moved from the supine position. The technique used is the approach described by Beck[37] for adults and then later described by Dalens et al[41] for children (Fig. 16.5).

A line is drawn from the anterior superior iliac crest to the pubic tubercle, corresponding to the inguinal ligament, and this line is further divided into three segments. A second line is drawn parallel with the first, crossing over the greater trochanter of the femur. A perpendicular line drawn between the medial and middle thirds of the first line meets the second line at the insertion site for the anterior sciatic block. The needle is inserted at a 90° angle to the skin; if the medial border of the femur is encountered, the needle is re-directed more medially. The point of greatest foot twitch at the lowest current is identified, and the local anesthetic injected at that site.

Dalens et al[41] reported an 89% success rate for the sciatic block in 60 infants and children when using the nerve stimulator. The anterior approach is more difficult than posterior or lateral approaches, and carries with it the additional risk of damage to femoral vessels.[44]

Lateral approach to the sciatic nerve

As was described by Guardini et al,[40] the patient is placed on the operating room table in the supine position (Fig. 16.6). The lateral prominence of the greater trochanter is identified. A point 2.0–3.0 cm distal and 2.0 cm posterior to this area is marked, and a skin wheal is raised. Then an insulated needle is passed through the wheal from lateral to medial where it may encounter the shaft of the femur. If that occurs, the needle is then re-directed so that it passes posterior to the femur and is directed more medially, toward the ischial tuberosity. When the maximum twitch is noted at the lowest milliamperage in the foot, local anesthetic agent is administered.

Dalens et al[41] used 0.5 ml/kg of local anesthetic with the volume not to exceed 25 ml in older children. With this dose he reported a 97% success rate for the sciatic block in 60 pediatric patients.

Comparision of sciatic nerve blocks

The posterior approach to the sciatic nerve may be the most commonly used, but it may be less applicable in the trauma patient than the lateral approach, since the patient does not have to be moved from the supine position. The anterior approach is more difficult and carries with it the additional hazard of damage to the femoral vessels, while the lateral approach may be the simplest for the beginner.[41] Regardless of approach, the use of the nerve stimulator is required.

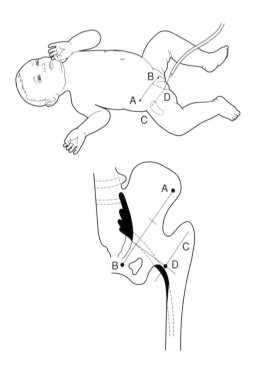

Fig. 16.5   Sciatic block: anterior approach. A, anterior superior iliac spine; B, pubic tubercle; C, parallel line through greater trochanter; D, needle insertion site.

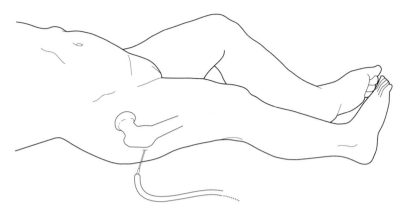

Fig. 16.6 Sciatic block: lateral approach.

LUMBAR PLEXUS AND COMPONENT NERVE BLOCKS

The lumbar plexus consists of the ventral rami of the first four lumbar spinal nerves.[45] It is enclosed within the psoas muscle. The upper plexus gives rise to the iliohypogastric, ilioinguinal, and genitofemoral nerves, as well as to the motor nerves supplying quadratus lumborum, psoas minor, and psoas major. The dorsal and ventral branches of the lower plexus form the femoral, lateral cutaneous, and obturator nerves.

Blocking individual components of the lumbar plexus has become common practice in pediatric anesthesia. The most superficial branches of the ilio-inguinal and ilio-hypogastric nerves are easily blocked on the anterior abdominal wall for hernia repair or other groin surgery. Likewise, the femoral nerve block is an easy block to perform for children with femur fractures.

Others have attempted to extend the usefulness of the femoral nerve block by also anesthetizing additional components of the lumbar plexus. Winnie et al[33] introduced 'The Inguinal Paravascular Technique of Lumbar Plexus Anesthesia' or '3-in-1' block as the technique for blocking all of the nerves of the lumbar plexus with a single injection. Rosen & Broadman[46] have described the use of the '3-in-1' block for muscle biopsies of the lateral thigh in children. However, Dalens et al[34] have questioned the efficacy of the '3-in-1' block as described by Winnie et al.[33]

They showed both in humans and in cadavers that the '3-in-1' block as originally described is unlikely to block all the components of the lumbar plexus. As an alternative, Dalens injects a large volume of local anesthetic solution deep to the fascia iliaca, to block the components of the plexus.

Femoral nerve block

The femoral nerve block is an ideal block for providing analgesia and muscle relaxation for children with fractures of the shaft of the femur.[47–49] This block can be performed preoperatively on children who are awaiting transfer to the operating room to minimize the discomfort of a 'bumpy ride'. Likewise, the femoral nerve may be blocked preoperatively for those children in traction prior to transfer to the operating table when it is not feasible to induce anesthesia in the bed. Remarkable pain relief is obtained and transfer to the operating room table is smooth.

Block of the femoral nerve using a continuous catheter technique was described by Malawar et al for use in children undergoing complex orthopedic surgical procedures expected to require prolonged pain relief.[50] McNicol[51] recommended combining femoral nerve and lateral femoral cutaneous nerve blocks of the thigh for muscle biopsies. In the trauma setting, this technique would also provide anesthesia for the harvesting of skin grafts from the anterior and lateral aspects of the thigh.

Technique

With the patient supine, a line is drawn from the anterior superior iliac spine to the pubic tubercle (Fig. 16.7). A needle is advanced at a 45° angle

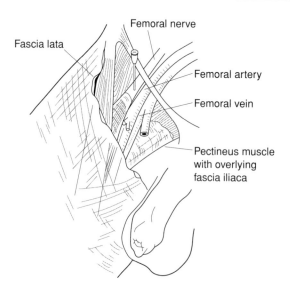

Fig. 16.7 Femoral nerve block.

toward the femoral nerve, which lies just laterally to the femoral artery. Using the nerve stimulator set at 1–2 mA, the twitch is demonstrated in the muscles on the anterior aspect of the thigh. After aspirating to ensure that the needle is not intravascular, 2 ml of local anesthetic is injected to abolish the twitch response. The remainder of the local anesthetic can then be incrementally injected with intermittent aspiration. Dosages in the range of 0.25–0.3 ml/kg of local anesthetic have been recommended, and distal pressure is not applied.

'3-in-1' block

The '3-in-1' block is a femoral block that also blocks the lateral cutaneous nerve and the obturator nerve. The surface landmarks and point of injection are the same as for the classical femoral nerve block (see Fig. 16.8). What is the difference between the femoral nerve block and a '3-in-1' block? The major difference between the two is the volume of local anesthetic solution injected. In a '3-in-1' block, a larger dose of 0.5 ml/kg of local anesthetic is required. In addition, distal digital pressure should be applied during the injection to maximize proximal spread and to increase the chances that the lateral femoral cutaneous and obturator nerves will be successfully blocked. Some have also recommended that the needle is angled toward the head for this block.[52]

Concern has been raised about toxicity of local anesthetics administered for '3-in-1' blocks. However, it has been shown by Ronchi et al[49] that bupivacaine 2.0 mg/kg used for femoral nerve blocks in children was associated with plasma levels that were substantially below the toxic range for adults.

Fascia iliaca block

The fascia iliaca block described by Dalens et al is yet another approach for blocking the combination of femoral, lateral femoral cutaneous, and obturator nerves.[53] This is one block that is performed **without** the use of a nerve stimulator. First, the inguinal ligament is identified by drawing a line from the anterior superior iliac spine to the pubic tubercle; this line is then divided into thirds (Fig. 16.8). Where the lateral and middle thirds meet, a skin wheal is raised 0.5 cm below the inguinal ligament.

The fascia iliaca block is then performed using a 'loss of resistance' technique. A short-bevel needle and syringe with local anesthetic are advanced at a 90° angle to the skin. The first 'loss of resistance'

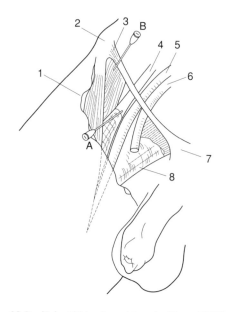

Fig. 16.8 '3-in-1' block and fascia iliaca block. A, '3-in-1' block; B, fascia iliaca block; 1, fascia lata; 2, anterior superior iliac spine; 3, inguinal ligament; 4, femoral nerve; 5, femoral artery; 6, femoral vein; 7, pubic tubercle; 8, pectineal muscle covered by fascia iliaca.

indicates that the fascia lata has been punctured. As the needle is advanced further, a second 'loss of resistance' is noted, indicating penetration of the fascia iliaca. While distal digital pressure is applied, 0.7 ml/kg of local anesthetic is injected. Cephalad spread is also enhanced by massage of the thigh. A swelling of the groin at the site of the injection can be expected. Dalens et al have also reported placement of a catheter beneath the fascia iliaca for continuous analgesia.

Comparison of '3-in-1' and fascia iliaca blocks

Dalens used a nerve stimulator to compare the '3-in-1' block and the fascia iliaca block in 60 pediatric patients. The children who received the '3-in-1' block showed good femoral nerve anesthesia but only about 15% obtained sensory analgesia of the other nerves of the lumbar plexus. In the fascia iliaca group, 90% obtained sensory analgesia in all the nerves of the lumbar plexus, including the genitofemoral nerve.

Lumbar plexus block

Direct proximal blockade of the lumbar plexus is uncommonly performed in pediatric patients, but it may be considered an alternative to the epidural block, if that technique is contraindicated. However, the approach described by Chayens et al does, in fact, result in an epidural block in many patients.[54] Using the technique described by Winnie et al,[55,56] the result is generally a unilateral block of the lumbar and sacral plexuses.

Indications for this block have not been firmly established for pediatric patients. The insertion and use of a continuous catheter in the psoas space have been described in adult patients,[57,58] but not in children. Because there is the possibility and risk of causing visceral damage with needle insertion, the authors suggest that the practitioner carefully weighs the risks and benefits prior to performing this block.

Technique

In Winnie's technique, the patient is placed in the lateral decubitus position with the side to be blocked uppermost (Fig. 16.9). A line is drawn along the lumbar spine. A second line, parallel to the first, is drawn crossing the posterior superior iliac spine. Finally, a third line is drawn across the two iliac crests. Where this third line and the line drawn through the posterior superior iliac crests intersect is the needle insertion site. A needle attached to the nerve stimulator is inserted perpendicular to the skin until the transverse process is encountered. Then the needle is slid off the transverse process inferiorly. Muscle twitching in the quadriceps muscle indicates optimal positioning of the needle. When the maximum twitch at the lowest current is achieved, 0.75 ml/kg of local anesthetic is administered with the volume not to exceed 25 ml.[35]

Dalens et al compared these two different

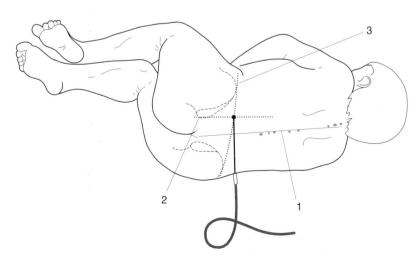

Fig. 16.9   Lumbar plexus block: Winnie's technique. 1, line along spinass processes; 2, posterior superior iliac spine; 3, line across the two iliac crests.

approaches to the lumbar plexus in a series of 50 children undergoing lower extremity surgery.[35] He noted that Winnie's technique was easy to perform and resulted in a successful unilateral lumbar plexus block in all cases. Moreover, in 23 of the 25 blocks, the sacral plexus was also blocked. The technique of Chayen was more difficult and resulted in bilateral blockade in 22 of 25 cases; he considered this block to be an alternate approach to the lumbar epidural space.

Block of the lateral femoral cutaneous nerve

Blocking the lateral femoral cutaneous nerve, in combination with a femoral nerve block, provides anesthesia for the anterior and lateral aspect of the thigh. This technique is useful for obtaining skin grafts or muscle biopsy specimens for the diagnosis of malignant hyperthermia.[59,60] In the trauma setting, blocking the lateral femoral cutaneous nerve will be helpful if a tourniquet will be used on the thigh.

Technique

The patient lies on the operating room table in the supine position. The needle is placed 1.5 cm medial and 1.5 cm inferior to the anterior superior iliac spine, and injection is made in a fanwise manner from lateral to medial with 2–3 cc of local anesthetic agent.

Dalens describes two alternative techniques for blocking the lateral femoral cutaneous nerve.[61] In the first, the point of injection is just below the inguinal ligament; in the other, the injection point is anterior and medial to the superior anterior iliac spine. Both techniques involve 'loss of resistance' to injection at fascial planes, which in the experience of these authors, is frequently difficult to detect in young children.

Nerve blocks at the knee

Kempthorne & Brown[62] described nerve blocks at the knee in children with head injuries to relieve muscular spasms so they could undergo physiotherapy and manipulation of the extremities prior to application of casts. These blocks may be considered alternatives to the proximal sciatic nerve block, and they are easier to perform.

The pertinent contents of the popliteal fossa include the common peroneal and tibial nerves, which are branches of the sciatic nerve, as well as the popliteal artery and vein. The popliteal fossa is delineated medially by the semitendinosus muscle, laterally by the biceps femerus muscle, and inferiorly by the two heads of gastrocnemius muscle. The tibial nerve traverses the superior aspect of the popliteal fossa just lateral to both the popliteal vein and the popliteal artery. Sensory branches of the tibial nerve include the medial sural cutaneous nerve. The common peroneal nerve, on the medial border of the biceps femerus muscle, passes caudad to the head of the fibula and enters the anterior aspect of the leg.

Technique

The patient is turned prone on the operating room table. The popliteal fossa is outlined (Fig. 16.10). The nerves to be blocked are found in the superior lateral aspect of the popliteal fossa. The needle is placed in the upper lateral aspect of the popliteal fossa and is directed perpendicular to the skin. As the needle is advanced, a 'loss of resistance' is noted with a 'pop' when piercing the fascia overlying the popliteal fossa. When the 'pop' is felt, aspirate for blood before injecting 0.25–0.5 ml/kg of local anesthetic solution, with the volume not to exceed 10 ml. Using a nerve stimulator, plantar flexion of the foot may be elicited to confirm that the needle is in close proximity to the tibial nerve.

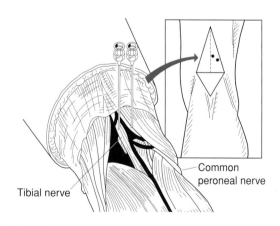

Fig. 16.10   Sciatic nerve blocks in the popliteal fossa.

Common peroneal nerve block

To supplement the tibial nerve block in the popliteal fossa, the common peroneal nerve can be easily blocked with infiltration of 3–5 ml of local anesthesia just below the head of the fibula. In the event that surface landmarks are difficult to palpate, use of the nerve stimulator to elicit ankle eversion will help to identify the correct location for infiltration.

CAUDAL AND EPIDURAL BLOCKS

Introduction

Caudal blocks have not been considered routine in the management of pediatric trauma victims, but this otherwise common technique deserves reconsideration in the setting of acute trauma care. One author (NLG) believes that caudal anesthesia and analgesia should be considered for a wide range of procedures below the level of the diaphragm. Caudal blocks may also be useful in the weeks following trauma when skin grafts or orthopedic surgical procedures are being performed.

A single caudal injection can be a helpful adjunct in the management of a wide variety of traumatic injuries, including bony or soft tissue injuries of the lower extremities, injuries to the groin or genitalia, and injuries requiring abdominal exploration. Although there may be few absolute contraindications to performing a caudal block in the trauma setting, the author (NLG) would advise against placement of the block if the patient shows evidence of lower back injuries or damage to the skin overlying the sacral hiatus, or if there is cardiovascular instability. One may reconsider the caudal block at the end of the case if the patient's condition has stabilized. Although delayed micturition has been observed following caudal blocks, intervention is almost never required. In the trauma setting, one would want to be particularly mindful of the patient's fluid status, and would consider the possibility of a renal or bladder injury following blunt trauma to the abdomen or back.

The common practice is to place the caudal block immediately following the induction of general anesthesia and prior to the beginning of surgery.[63–65] How the airway is secured and maintained during the procedure will be determined by the patient's condition and NPO status as well as by any special surgical requirements. Once the caudal block has been performed, a light plane of general anesthesia should be sufficient for the procedure. At the end of the procedure, the patient should awaken quickly, and should remain pain-free for several more hours, depending on the time elapsed since injection. In the post-anesthesia care unit the child should be relaxed and comfortable, and should not be moving about excessively, putting the surgical repair at risk.

Caudal blocks are easy to perform in children who are under 12 years of age, or less than 50 kg in body weight. Most of the complications ascribed to caudal anesthesia have been noted in infants younger than 6 months of age. The use of a caudal in conjunction with light anesthesia provides analgesia for the surgical procedure as well as postoperative pain relief for up to 6 hours.

Needle selection for caudal block

The 'B'-bevel needle is also the authors' choice for the single injection caudal block. Others have advocated the placement of intravenous catheters in the caudal space, with the assumption that these catheters would make it easier to identify intravascular placement. That assumption has not been borne out in the experience of one of the authors (NLG), in whose institution four infants developed ventricular tachycardia following presumed intravascular injection of bupivacaine. Three of the four infants had intravenous catheters placed in the caudal space, and all had negative aspirates prior to injection. In addition, numerous catheters have appeared frayed or kinked upon removal, raising the concern that foreign material could be left in the caudal or subcutaneous space. This observation has been made most commonly in instances where inexperienced practitioners required several attempts to place the catheter in the caudal space.

Another choice advocated for use in performing single shot caudal blocks is the butterfly-type needle with attached tubing. Although this needle offers the advantage of permitting re-injection during or following the procedure, it is wise to remember that the bevel of the butterfly needle is both long and cutting; a higher incidence of blood return may be noted. It is possible that part of the anesthetic dose may be injected into the subcutaneous space if the entire bevel has not been inserted through the sacral hiatus. The possibility that the cutting edge of the needle might move during surgery argues against its being left in place for re-injection.

Technique for caudal block

The child is placed into the lateral decubitus position after the induction of general anesthesia. Flexing the hips onto the abdomen stretches the skin overlying the sacral hiatus and facilitates palpation of the sacral hiatus, which is bounded on either side by the sacral cornua. Once the skin has been cleansed, a 'no touch' technique is used. The landmarks and positioning are shown in Figure 16.11.

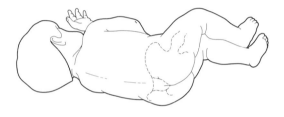

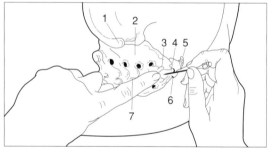

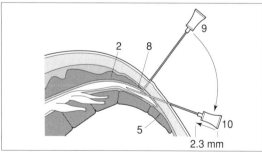

Fig. 16.11   Caudal block. 1, posterior superior iliac spine; 2, sacrum; 3, sacral cornu; 4, sacral hiatus; 5, coccyx; 6, sacrococcygeal joint; 7, median sacral crest; 8, sacrococcygeal membrane; 9, initial insertion angle; 10, re-direction of the needle into the caudal canal.

A 22 or 23 gauge 'B'-bevel needle is inserted at a 60° angle to the skin to pierce the sacrococcygeal membrane.[66] A 'pop' is generally felt as the needle enters the sacral canal. Once the needle has entered the canal, the needle is re-directed by depressing the hand as the needle is advanced another 2.0 mm in a plane parallel to the spinal axis.[66-69] After the needle is positioned in the sacral canal, aspiration is performed to detect cerebrospinal fluid or blood prior to administration of the local anesthetic.

Some would recommend abandoning the procedure if cerebrospinal fluid is aspirated. Unfortunately, even a gentle aspiration may not demonstrate penetration of the subarachnoid membrane; therefore, a negative aspiration is not a guarantee that the needle has not entered the subarachnoid space. Extreme vigilance in the depth of needle insertion is the best way to avoid a subarachnoid injection of local anesthetic agent, caused by inserting the needle too far into the canal. Desparmet[70] reported a case of total spinal anesthesia after caudal anesthesia in an infant.

If blood is aspirated during caudal epidural needle placement, the needle is repositioned and aspiration is repeated. If aspiration is negative on the second attempt, then 0.5 ml of bupivacaine is injected, with repeated aspiration until one is convinced that the needle is not in a vessel. If blood is aspirated after repositioning, begin again by inserting the needle at a different site at the sacral hiatus. The use of a test dose with epinephrine does not appear to be a valid test for an inadvertent intravascular injection.[71]

An inadvertent subarachnoid injection is much more likely to occur than an intravascular injection, especially in young infants. Early recognition and treatment are required to avoid further complications.[70,72] Notably, an inadvertent subarachnoid injection in a patient receiving general anesthesia with controlled ventilation may be very difficult to detect. Fixed and dilated pupils may be noted, but the vital signs may not change.[70,72] For those children breathing spontaneously with a mask, respiratory irregularity or paralysis may ensue, necessitating endotracheal intubation and mechanical ventilation until the block recedes. Although most children will demonstrate respiratory signs, a motor block that is higher or more intense than expected at the conclusion of the procedure may suggest that some or all of the intended caudal dose was injected into the subarachnoid space. The duration of the block will depend upon the agent and dose of local anesthetic agent administered.

Dosage, drug selection, and duration of caudal anesthesia

Dalens & Hasnaoui[73] recommend 0.75–1.0 ml/kg of local anesthetic, while Wolf[74] suggests a volume of 0.75 ml/kg. These doses will provide anesthesia to the T10 level. Wolf et al[74] showed that children who received caudal anesthesia with bupivacaine in a concentration of 0.125 to 0.25% had better pain relief and required significantly less supplementary analgesia for about 12 hours postoperatively than those who did not receive caudal anesthesia. The use of bupivacaine 0.125% produced good postoperative analgesia without the motor blockade noted when bupivacaine 0.25% was used. Earlier ambulation and discharge were also demonstrated following the use of the more dilute bupivacaine.[75]

Gunter et al[76] added epinephrine 1:200 000 to bupivacaine and was able to produce an increase in the duration of caudal blockade to 150 minutes from 120 minutes. However, there are a number of reports in the literature of cardiac dysrhythmias following the injection of bupivacaine with epinephrine, particularly following inhalation induction with halothane. Freid et al reported five instances of ST-T wave elevation and relative bradycardia following test doses containing epinephrine in five small infants.[77] In each case, the changes were transient, but three of the five infants had a negative aspirate for blood both before and after the test dose. Ved et al reported two infants who developed ventricular tachycardia and circulatory collapse following the injection of bupivacaine with epinephrine without a test dose; both recovered quickly but did not have evidence of a successful caudal block.[78] Although there may be advantages to the addition of epinephrine to the caudal bupivacaine, one could reasonably discourage its use in young infants based on these and other reports of cardiac toxicity.

Luckily, the new agent ropivacaine is now available for use in caudal analgesia, and it appears to have less cardiac depression and a lower risk of cardiac toxicity than bupivacaine.[79–82] In comparing the clinical effects of ropivacaine and bupivacaine, Brockway et al have demonstrated a similar duration of the sensory blockade, but a shorter duration of motor block with ropivacaine.[80] Ivani et al reported similar onset times and block intensity with ropivacaine 0.2% when compared with bupivacaine 0.25% in 245 children having minor surgery.[81,82] However, they found that the duration of the block was greater with ropivacaine than with bupivacaine by approximately 40 minutes,[81,82] which is different from the reports of ropivacaine block duration in adults.[80]

The addition of an opiate to caudal analgesia has become popular in recent years. Adding fentanyl 1–2 microg/kg to the local anesthetic prolongs the duration of caudal analgesia and permits the use of a more dilute concentration of local anesthetic, decreasing the risk of motor blockade and urinary retention.[83] Another choice is the addition of caudal morphine, which may provide analgesia for 12 to 24 hours following a single injection of 70–100 microg/kg.[84,85] Doses in the higher range do not prolong analgesia but have been associated with a higher incidence of late respiratory depression, pruritus, and somnolence. Since the respiratory depression following administration of caudal morphine may be delayed by many hours, one must weigh the advantages of this technique with the requirement for respiratory monitoring or higher levels of nursing observation. And just as with systemic administration, all epidural opioids have the potential to cause nausea and vomiting, so prophylactic administration of anti-emetics should be considered.

In the trauma setting, the addition of epidural opioids can provide excellent analgesia, while eliminating or minimizing the need for systemic opioids. One example of the usefulness of this technique might be the child who has sustained a head injury along with a significant orthopedic injury to a lower extremity. In this example, being able to provide good analgesia for the early hours after injury without systemic opioids makes it easier to follow the patient's neurologic exam. The use of caudal morphine also provides long-lasting pain relief to patients with rib fractures, who might otherwise require high doses of systemic opioids, further compromising respiratory function. Administering caudal opioids, with or without dilute local anesthetic, to the patient at risk for a lower extremity compartment syndrome provides analgesia without masking the signs of ischemia. And finally, the administration of either epidural fentanyl or morphine in addition to local anesthetic provides the opportunity to extend analgesia beyond the operative period in facilities that do not otherwise have the capability to manage continuous epidural infusions in children.

CONTINUOUS CAUDAL AND EPIDURAL CATHETER TECHNIQUES

Continuous techniques for both caudal and epidural catheters may be very helpful in pediatric trauma victims, as a further extension of anesthetic care into the postoperative phase. Appropriate patient selection is critical, as the management of epidural catheters is both time- and labor-intensive. Catheters may be placed in the caudal, lumbar, or thoracic epidural space. Threading the catheter from the sacral hiatus into the thoracic space has also been described, most commonly in infants.[86,87] In general, insertion of thoracic epidural catheters in anesthetized children should be done only by those with special training and expertise in this area. The site of insertion depends on the site of the injury, as well as on the practitioner's choice and experience.

The kind of injuries for which continuous epidural analgesia may be recommended is nearly unlimited. Orthopedic injuries lend themselves particularly well to this technique, in that the degree of both sensory and motor blockade may be adjusted depending on the degree and stage of injury. For those children with external fixators in place, the density of the epidural block can be increased prior to adjustment of the fixator, or prior to particularly painful muscle stretching or physical therapy. The same is true of degloving injuries to the lower extremity, which may require frequent debridement and dressing changes. Administering an extra bolus dose of local anesthetic through the catheter prior to a dressing change may make it possible to perform this procedure without returning to the operating room, avoiding additional NPO periods and caloric deprivation during the catabolic post-injury period.

Abdominal injuries also lend themselves well to epidural therapy, provided that intra-abdominal hemorrhage is controlled prior to the insertion and injection of the epidural catheter. Particularly for upper abdominal surgery, the use of epidural analgesia may prevent the decline in respiratory function postoperatively. In addition, numerous studies have demonstrated the advantages of epidural analgesia on the duration of postoperative ileus, particularly when the catheter is located above T12.[88] And finally, epidural analgesia should be highly recommended for children with injuries requiring thoracotomy tubes, since both comfort and respiratory function may be maintained without systemic opioids.

Reluctance to use epidural anesthesia and analgesia in the setting of acute trauma is centered around the risk of hypotension with sympathetic blockade, and the risk of infection of the epidural catheter. Injured patients who are hypotensive on arrival are not candidates for epidural therapy until blood loss has been stopped, and intravascular volume has been replaced. The possibility for ongoing blood loss should also be considered. It would be reasonable then to place an epidural catheter after the injuries have been assessed and surgically corrected.

Judging the risk of infection of the epidural catheter will require some assessment of the risk of systemic sepsis related to the injuries, i.e. the patient with bowel rupture and spillage of intestinal contents into the peritoneum might not be an appropriate candidate for early epidural therapy. Careful patient selection, meticulous attention to aseptic technique on insertion, daily inspection of the insertion site, and institutional policies regarding epidural catheter removal for fever will decrease the risk of epidural catheter infections. In a group of 210 children who had caudal and lumbar epidural catheters in place for 1 to 5 days, Kost-Byerly et al[89] reported that 35% of the catheters were colonized with bacteria, although none of the children had evidence of systemic infection. How long epidural catheters can remain in place remains unclear. It is the author's (NLG) practice to change or remove the catheter every 5 to 7 days even if the patient is afebrile and the site is clean; patients who need epidural analgesia for longer than 1 week usually require operative debridement, which allows catheter replacement under anesthesia.

Technique

The technique for placing catheters into the caudal or lumbar epidural space does not differ from those techniques used for adults. For entering the caudal space, either pediatric Tuohy or Crawford needles may be chosen; the author (NLG) prefers the Crawford needle. Although 24 gauge catheters have become commercially available, the larger 20 gauge catheter is easier to place, and less likely to kink or become obstructed; for this reason, the author recommends using the larger catheter. Securing the catheter in place with a transparent dressing allows for daily inspection of the insertion site; additional tape will be required to ensure that the active child does not remove the epidural catheter prematurely.

In most instances, continuous infusion of both local anesthetic and opioid is chosen, paying careful attention to the total hourly dose of local anesthetic. One popular combination is bupivacaine 0.1% plus fentanyl 2 microg/ml, infused at a rate not to exceed 0.4 mg/kg/h. For larger children, a higher concentration of fentanyl, 5 microg/ml, may be recommended. If pruritus is refractory to management, bupivacaine with hydromorphone may be substituted. Other agents have also been described.[90]

Side effects of epidural analgesia, including nausea and vomiting, pruritus, and urinary retention, occur in children just as they do in adults. Small doses of naloxone will reverse irritating side effects without reversing the analgesia. Symptomatic management of side effects is indicated, but one should be cautious in administering anti-emetics or anti-pruritics that will potentiate somnolence, as these agents will make it more difficult to assess level of consciousness related to opioid absorption. Somnolence may precede respiratory depression in children, and requires careful assessment and vigilance.

SUMMARY

In the last 20 years, there has been an explosion of interest and research related to the use of regional anesthesia techniques in children. Modifying the anatomical approaches for children, studying new agents and combinations of agents, and an increased acceptance of performing regional blocks in anesthetized patients have made these techniques more accessible to children. The next step is for practitioners to consider the advantages of regional anesthesia in the care of injured children, and to incorporate creative postoperative analgesia into the anesthetic plan.

REFERENCES

1. Trauma registry annual report. West Virginia University; 1996.

2. Wright B. A new use for the block-aid monitor. Anesthesiology 1969; 30: 236.

3. Montgomery SJ, Raj PP, Nettles D, et al. The use of the nerve stimulator with standard unsheathed needles in nerve blockade. Anesth Analg 1973; 52: 827.

4. Selander D, Dhuner KG, Lundborg G. Peripheral nerve injury due to injection needles used for regional anaesthesia. Acta Anaesthesiol Scand 1977; 21: 182–188.

5. Scott DB, Cousins MJ. Clinical pharmacology of local anesthetic agents. In: Cousins MJ, Bridenbaugh PO, eds. Neural blockade. Philadelphia: JB Lippincott; 1980.

6. Wedel DJ, Krohn JS, Hall JA. Brachial plexus anesthesia in pediatric patients. Mayo Clin Proc 1991; 66: 583–588.

7. Campbell RJ, Ilett KF, Dusci L. Plasma bupivacaine concentrations after axillary block in children. Anaes Intens Care 1986; 14: 343–346.

8. Eyres RL, Hastings C, Brown TCK, Oppenheim RC. Plasma bupivacaine concentrations following lumbar epidural anaesthesia in children. Anaesth Intens Care 1986; 14: 131.

9. Eyres RL, Bishop W, Oppenheim RC, Brown TCK. Plasma bupivacaine concentrations in children during caudal epidural analgesia. Anaesth Intens Care 1983; 11: 20–22.

10. Yaster M, Tobin JR, Billett C, et al. Epidural analgesia in the management of severe vaso-occlusive sickle cell crisis. Pediatrics 1994; 93: 310–315.

11. Dalens BJ. In: Dalens BJ, ed. Pediatric regional anesthesia. Boca Raton, FL: CRC Press; 1990:233.

12. Eather KF. Axillary brachial plexus block. Anesthesiology 1958; 19: 683–684.

13. Tryba M, Haensch K, Zenz M. Axillary brachial plexus block for emergency procedures in young children. Anesthesiology 1991; 75: A757.

14. Winnie AP. Plexus anesthesia, volume 1: Perivascular techniques of brachial plexus block. Edinburgh: Churchill Livingstone; 1983.

15. Accardo NJ, Adriani J. Brachial plexus block: A simplified technique using the axillary route. South Med J. 1949; 42: 920.

16. Eriksson E. Axillary brachial plexus anaesthesia in children with Citanest®. Acta Anaesth Scand 1965; 9 (suppl 16): 291–296.

17. Niesel HC, Rodriguez P, Wilsmann I. Regional analgesia of the upper extremity in children. Anaesthetist 1974; 23: 178–180.

18. Dalens B. In: Dalens B, ed. Regional anesthesia in infants, children, and adolescents. Baltimore: Williams & Wilkins; 1995; 305.

19. Winnie AP. Interscalene brachial plexus block. Anesth Analg 1970; 49: 455–466.

20. Dalens B, Vanneuville G, Tanguy A. A new approach to the brachial plexus in children:

Comparison with the supraclavicular approach. Anesth Analg 1987; 66: 1264–1271.

21. Bier A. Ueber einen neun Weg Lokalanasthesie an den Gliedmassen zu erzeugen. Arch Klin Chir 1908; 96: 1007–1016.

22. Holmes C. Intravenous regional anaesthesia. Lancet 1963; i: 245–247.

23. Carrel ED, Eyring EJ. Intravenous regional anesthesia for childhood fractures. J Trauma 1971; 11: 301–305.

24. Schiller MG. Intravenous regional anesthesia for closed treatment of fractures and dislocations of the upper extremities. Clin Orthop 1976; 118: 25–29.

25. Turner PL, Batten JB, Hjorth D, et al. Intravenous regional anaesthesia for the treatment of upper limb injuries in childhood. Aust NZ J Surg 1986; 56: 153.

26. Olney BW, Lugg PC, Turner PL, et al. Outpatient treatment of upper extremity injuries in childhood using intravenous regional anaesthesia. J Pediatr Orthopaed 1988; 8: 576.

27. Colizza WA, Said E. Intravenous regional anaesthesia in the treatment of forearm and wrist fractures and dislocations in children. Canad J Surg 1993; 36: 225.

28. Fitzgerald B. Intravenous regional anaesthesia in children. Br J Anaesth 1976; 48: 485.

29. Rudzinski JP, Ampel LL. Pediatric applications of intravenous regional anesthesia. Reg Anesth 1983; 8: 69–72.

30. Rosenberg PH, Kalso EA, Tuominen MK, Linden HB. Acute bupivacaine toxicity as a result of venous leakage under the tourniquet cuff during a Bier block. Anesthesiology 1983; 58: 95.

31. Dawkins OS, Russel ES, Adams AK et al. Intravenous regional anesthesia. Can Anaesth Soc J 1964; 11: 243–246.

32. Finsterbush A, Stein H, Robin G, et al. Recent experience with intravenous regional anesthesia in limbs. J Trauma 1972; 12: 81–84.

33. Winnie AP, Ramamurthy S, Durrani Z. The inguinal paravascular technique of lumbar plexus anesthesia: The '3-in-1 Block'. Anesth Analg 1973; 52: 989–996.

34. Dalens B, Vanneuville G, Tanguy A. Comparison of the fascia iliaca compartment block with the 3-in-1 block in children. Anesth Analg 1989; 69: 705–713.

35. Dalens B, Tanguy A, Vanneuville G. Lumbar plexus block in children: a comparison of two procedures in 50 patients. Anesth Analg 1988; 67: 750–758.

36. Labat G. Regional anesthesia, its technique and clinical application. 2nd ed. Philadelphia: WB Saunders; 1928.

37. Beck GP. Anterior approach to sciatic nerve block. Anesthesiology 1963; 24; 213–218.

38. McNicol LR. Sciatic nerve block for children–Sciatic nerve block by the anterior approach for postoperative pain relief. Anaesthesia 1985; 40: 410–414.

39. Ichiyanagi K. Sciatic nerve block: lateral approach with the patient supine. Anesthesiology 1959; 20: 601–604.

40. Guardini R, Waldron BA, Wallace WA. Sciatic nerve block: a new lateral approach. Acta Anaesth Scand 1985; 29: 515–519.

41. Dalens B, Tanguy A, Vanneuville G. Sciatic nerve blocks in children: Comparison of the posterior, anterior, and lateral approaches in 180 pediatric patients. Anesth Analg 1990; 70: 131–137.

42. Dalens B. Peripheral nerve blockade in the management of postoperative pain in children. In: Schechter NL, Berde CB, Yaster M, eds. Pain in infants, children and adolescents. Baltimore: Williams & Wilkins; 1993: 272.

43. Dalens B. Sacral plexus blocks. In: Dalens B, ed. Regional anesthesia in infants, children, and adolescents. Baltimore: Williams & Wilkins; 1995: 348–350.

44. Dalens B. Peripheral nerve blockade in the management of postoperative pain in children. In: Schechter NL, Berde CB, Yaster M, eds. Pain in infants, children and adolescents. Baltimore: Williams & Wilkins; 1993: 271.

45. Dalens B. Lumbar plexus blocks. In: Dalens B, ed. Regional anesthesia in infants, children, and adolescents. Baltimore: Williams & Wilkins; 1995: 313–340.

46. Rosen KR, Broadman LM. Anaesthesia for diagnostic muscle biopsy in an infant with Pompe's disease. Can Anaesth Soc 1986; 33: 790–794.

47. Berry FR. Analgesia in patients with fractured shaft of femur. Anaesthesia 1977; 32: 576.

48. Riou B, Barriot P, Viars P. Femoral nerve block in fractured shaft of femur. Anesthesiology 1988; 69: A375.

49. Ronchi L, Rosenbaum D, Athouel A, et al. Femoral nerve block in children using bupivacaine. Anesthesiology 1989; 70: 622.

50. Malawar MM, Buch R, Khurana JS, et al. Postoperative infusional continuous regional analgesia. Clin Orthopaed 1991; 266: 227.

51. McNicol LR. Lower limb blocks for children. Anaesthesia 1986; 41: 27.

52. Dalens B. Lumbar plexus blocks. In: Dalens B, ed. Regional anesthesia in infants, children, and adolescents. Baltimore: Williams & Wilkins; 1995: 328–329.

53. Dalens B. Lumbar plexus blocks. In: Dalens B, ed. Regional anesthesia in infants, children, and adolescents. Baltimore: Williams & Wilkins; 1995: 321–333.

54. Chayen D, Nathan H, Dhayen M. The psoas compartment block. Anesthesiology 1976; 45: 95–99.

55. Winnie AP, Ramamurthy S, Durrani Z, Radonjic R. Plexus blocks for lower extremity surgery. New answers to old problems. Anesthesiol Rev 1974; 1: 11–16.

56. Winnie AP. Regional anesthesia. Surg Clin North Am 1975; 55: 861–892.

57. Ben-David B, Lee E, Croitoru M. Psoas block for surgical repair of hip fracture: A case report and description of a catheter technique. Anesth Analg 1990; 71: 298–301.

58. Rung GW. A safer continuous lumbar plexus block technique? Anesth Analg 1991; 72: 564–565.

59. Berkowitz AR, Rosenberg H. Safety of femoral and lateral femoral cutaneous nerve block for muscle biopsy for malignant hyperthermia. Reg Anesth 1984; 9: 32.

60. Wedel DJ. Femoral and lateral femoral cutaneous nerve block for muscle biopsy in children. Reg Anesth 1989; 14: 63.

61. Dalens B. Lumbar plexus blocks. In: Dalens B, ed. Regional anesthesia in infants, children, and adolescents. Baltimore: Williams & Wilkins; 1995: 334–337.

62. Kempthorne PM, Brown TCK. Nerve blocks around the knee in children. Anes Intens Care 1984; 12: 14–17.

63. Hannallah RS, Broadman LM, Belman AB, Abramowitz MD, Epstein BS. Comparison of caudal and ilioinguinal/iliohypogastric nerve blocks for control of post-orchiopexy pain in pediatric ambulatory surgery. Anesthesiology 1987; 66: 832–834.

64. Rice LJ, Pudimat MA, Hannallah RS. Timing of caudal block placement in relation to surgery does not affect duration of postoperative analgesia in paediatric ambulatory patients. Can J Anaesth 1990; 37: 429–431.

65. Broadman LM, Hannallah RS, Norden JM, McGill WA. 'Kiddie caudals': experience with 1154 consecutive cases without complications. Anesth Analg 1987; 66: S18.

66. Broadman LM. Pediatric regional anesthesia and postoperative analgesia. In: Barash PG, ed. American Society of Anesthesiologists Refresher courses in anesthesiology, volume 14. Philadelphia: JB Lippincott; 1986: 42–60.

67. Broadman LM. Regional anesthesia for the pediatric outpatient. Anesthesiology Clin N Am 1987; 5: (1): 53–72.

68. Broadman LM, Rice LJ. Pediatric regional anesthesia and perioperative analgesia. In: Brown DL, ed. Problems in anesthesia. Philadelphia: JB Lippincott; 1988: 386–407.

69. Rice LJ, Broadman LM. Regional anesthesia in pediatric patients. In: Stoelting RK, ed. Advances in anesthesia, volume 6. Chicago: YearBook Medical Publishers; 1988: 291–321.

70. Desparmet J. Total spinal anesthesia after caudal anesthesia in an infant. Anesth Analg 1990; 70: 655–657.

71. Desparmet J, Mateo J, Ecoffey C, Mazoit X. Efficacy of an epidural test dose in children anesthetized with halothane. Anesthesiology 1990; 72: 249–251.

72. Lumb AB, Carli F. Respiratory arrest after a caudal injection of bupivacaine. Anaesthesia 1989; 44: 324–325.

73. Dalens B, Hasnaoui A. Caudal anesthesia in pediatric surgery: Success rate and adverse effects in 750 consecutive patients. Anesth Analg 1989; 68: 83–89.

74. Wolf AR, Valley RD, Fear DW, Roy WL, Lerman J. Bupivacaine for caudal analgesia in infants and children: the optimum effective concentration. Anesthesiology 1988; 69: 102–106.

75. Rice LJ, Binding RR, Vaughn GC, Thompson R, Newman K. Intraoperative and postoperative analgesia in children undergoing inguinal herniorrhaphy: A comparison of caudal bupivacaine 0.125 per cent and 0.25 per cent. Anesthesiology 1990; 73(3A): A3.

76. Gunter JB, Dunn CM, Bower RJ, Temberg JL. Epinephrine and caudal epidural anesthesia in infant: Onset, duration and hemodynamic effects. Anesthesiology 1990; 73(3A): A1098.

77. Freid EB, Bailey AG, Valley RD. Electrocardiographic and hemodynamic changes associated with unintentional intravascular injection of bupivacaine with epinephrine in infants. Anesthesiology 1993; 79: 394–398.

78. Ved SA, Pinosky M, Nicodemus H. Ventricular tachycardia and brief cardiovascular collapse in two infants after caudal anesthesia using a bupivacaine–epinephrine solution. Anesthesiology 1993; 79: 1121–1123.

79. Scott DB, Lee A, Fagan D, Bowler GMR, Bloomfield P, Lundth R. Acute toxicity of ropivacaine compared with that of bupivacaine. Anesth Analg 1989; 69: 563–569.

80. Brockway MS, Bannister J, McClure JH, McKeown D, Wildsmith JAW. Comparison of extradural ropivacaine and bupivacaine. Br J Anaesth 1991; 66: 31–37.

81. Ivani G, Mereto N, Lampugnani E, et al. Ropivacaine in paediatric surgery: preliminary results. Paediatr Anaesth 1998; 8: 127–129.

82. Ivani G, Lampugnani E, Torre MA. Comparison of ropivacaine with bupivacaine for paediatric caudal block. Br J Anaesth (in press).

83. Murat I. Pharmacology. In: Dalens B, ed. Regional anesthesia in infants, children, and adolescents. Baltimore: Williams & Wilkins; 1995: 114–118.

84. Valley RD, Bailey AG. Caudal morphine for postoperative analgesia in infants and children: A

report of 138 cases. Anesth Analg 1991; 72: 120–124.

85. Krane EJ, Tyler DC, Jacobson LE. The dose response of caudal morphine in children. Anesthesiology 1989; 71: 48–52.

86. Bosenberg AT, Bland BAR, Schulte-Steinberg O, Downing JW. Thoracic epidural anesthesia via caudal route in infants. Anesthesiology 1988; 69: 265–269.

87. Gunter JB, Eng C. Thoracic epidural anesthesia via the caudal approach in children. Anesthesiology 1992; 76: 935–938.

88. Steinbrook RA. Epidural anesthesia and gastrointestinal motility. Anesth Analg 1998; 86: 837–844.

89. Kost-Byerly S, Tobin JR, Greenberg RS, Billett C, et al. Bacterial colonization and infection rate of continuous epidural catheters in children. Anesth Analg 1998; 86: 712–716.

90. Desparmet J. Central blocks in children and adolescents. In: Schechter NL, Berde CB, Yaster M, eds. Pain in infants, children and adolescents. Baltimore: Williams & Wilkins; 1993: 245–260.

Volume of local anesthetic suggested for regional anesthesia

	<10 Kg	10–20 Kg	20–30 Kg	30–40 Kg	40–50 Kg	>50 Kg
Axillary block	.75 ml/Kg	.75 ml/Kg	10–12 ml	12–15 ml	15–18 ml	20–25 ml
Interscalene, Parascalene	1ml/Kg	.75 ml/Kg	15–20 ml	20–23 ml	23–25 ml	25–30 ml
Femoral n. block	0.7 ml/Kg	.5–.7 ml/Kg	.5 ml/Kg	.5 ml/Kg	.4 ml/Kg	.4 ml/Kg
Sciatic n. block	1ml/Kg	.75 ml/Kg[1]	.75 ml/Kg	.6 ml/Kg	.5 ml/Kg	.5 ml/Kg
Fascia iliaca, "3-in-one" block	.7 ml/Kg	.75 ml/Kg	.75 ml/Kg	.75 ml/Kg	.75 ml/Kg	.75 ml/Kg
Caudal block, single shot	1 ml/Kg	1 ml/Kg	15–20 ml	20 ml	30 ml	Infrequently performed

Important note: Physician *must* calculate maximum safe dose of local anesthetic in mg/Kg, as differing concentrations or combinations of agents may exceed safe doses in volumes described above.

17

Pregnant trauma patient

Patricia Dalby and Sivam Ramanathan

Introduction

Evaluation of the pregnant trauma patient
    Cardiovascular changes
    Pulmonary issues
    Airway changes
    Gastrointestinal changes
    Hematological issues
    Central nervous system changes
    Musculoskeletal changes
    Anesthetic issues

Teratology
    Local anesthetic agents
    Sedatives

Narcotics
Antibiotics

Anesthetic and perioperative management of the pregnant trauma patient
    General considerations
    Operative regional anesthesia techniques
    Perioperative pain management
    Postoperative regional techniques

Special considerations in regional anesthesia
    Ropivacaine

Summary

INTRODUCTION

Maternal trauma is the leading non-obstetric cause of fetal demise.[1] As recent improvements in obstetric and medical care have had a favorable impact on other causes of maternal mortality, trauma has assumed an increasingly important role in the etiology of maternal death.[2] Accidental injuries occur in 6 to 7% of all pregnancies.[3] Minor trauma is more common than severe trauma, and the incidence of injuries increases with increasing gestational age.[4] In late pregnancy a change in body stability or a shift in the body's center of gravity may be contributory to this problem.[5] Motor vehicle accidents account for the majority of serious traumatic injuries in pregnancy, with associated abdominal blunt trauma and placental abruption.[6] Other causes of serious traumatic injury during pregnancy are as listed in Table 17.1. Maternal mortality from trauma appears to approximate that of non-pregnant women if aggressive diagnosis and treatment are provided. However, the fetal death rate is disturbingly high in pregnant trauma victims even with minor injuries.[7,8] This is attributed to a higher incidence of placental abruption, preterm labor, direct fetal injury, and spontaneous abortion.[9] Anesthesiologists and other traumatologists must pay considerable attention to these factors during preoperative evaluation of pregnant trauma victims.

EVALUATION OF THE PREGNANT TRAUMA PATIENT

The evaluation of the pregnant trauma patient can present a dilemma for the subspecialists involved in her care. Many obstetricians are not familiar with new advances made in the management of critically ill trauma patients. Many trauma intensivists do not fully comprehend how maternal physiologic changes may complicate the manage-

Table 17.1 Traumatic injuries in pregnancy

Causes	Associations
Motor vehicle accidents	Head injury
	Cervical spine injury
	Whiplash injury
	Blunt abdominal trauma
	Placental separation
	Blunt chest trauma
	Pelvic fractures
	Vascular shearing injury
Domestic violence	Stab wounds
	Blunt abdominal trauma
	Gunshot wounds
	Direct uterine or fetal injury
Falls	Head and spine injury
	Multiple fractures
	Blunt trauma
	Ruptured spleen
Burns	Carbon monoxide poisoning
	Airway injury
	Sepsis
	Massive fluid requirements
Suicide	Poisoning
	Ante- and postpartum depression
	Drug abuse
Electrocution	Lightning
	Cardiac asystole
	Burns

Table 17.2 Physiologic and anatomical changes of pregnancy

Cardiovascular
Cardiac output increases 40%
Pulse rate increases 10–15 beats per minute
Blood volume increases 50%
Mild decrease in blood pressure
Peripheral vascular resistance decreases
Supine aortocaval compression
ECG: left axis shift

Respiratory
Minute ventilation increases 40%
Tidal volume increases
Respiratory rate slightly increased
Oxygen consumption increases 15%
Functional residual capacity decreases
Pa_{CO_2} decreases to low 30s
Diaphragm is raised 4 cm
Heart is pushed up and rotated to the left (C-X-ray)

Hematologic
Plasma volume increases
Leucocytosis to 18 000 cells/mm^3
Fibrinogen increases to 450 mg/dL
Coagulation factors VII, VIII, IX, X, and XII increase
Hematocrit decreases to low 30s

Gastrointestinal
Generalized hypomotility
Delayed gastric emptying
Frequent esophageal reflux
Increased gastric acid production

Genitourinary
Increased GFR and renal blood flow
Decreased BUN and creatinine
Ureteral hypomotility and dilatation
Bladder displaced into the abdominal cavity

Musculoskeletal
Pelvic joint separation
Generalized ligamentous loosening

Central nervous system
Pituitary gland doubles in size

ECG, electrocardiogram; Pa_{CO_2}, arterial carbon dioxide partial tension; C-X-ray, chest X-ray; GFR, glomerular filtration rate; BUN, blood urea nitrogen.

ment of the pregnant trauma victim. Many healthcare workers may be emotionally overwhelmed when presented with an unborn child. A coordinated approach that emphasizes maternal welfare provides the best possible means of ensuring an optimal outcome for both the mother and her fetus. All subspecialists should be involved early, but the initial evaluation and resuscitation should not differ from those of a non-gravid woman. The American College of Surgeons revised their formal guidelines embodied in the 'Advanced Trauma Life Support' program in 1997, for the initial care of the pregnant trauma victim.[10] The usual assessment of airway, breathing, and circulation should be made, with the provision of supplemental oxygen and adequate intravenous access even in less serious injuries. Left lateral uterine displacement with 20° right hip elevation must be provided after the mid-second trimester to optimize venous return.

The physiologic changes that occur in pregnancy are outlined in Table 17.2 and important key findings that have a bearing on managing pregnant trauma victims are discussed below.

Cardiovascular changes

Aortocaval compression occurs as early as 16 weeks of gestation and compression of the inferior vena cava occurs in over 90% pregnant women at term.[11] This compression may mimic hypovolemia and induce hypotension if the pregnant woman is left in the supine position. The high flow through the low-resistance uteroplacental vascular channels is dependent on the perfusion pressure and the flow through the circuit is not autoregulated. Left lateral uterine displacement of 20° must be provided by a displacement device or table tilt.

The progressive increase in both cardiac output and total blood volume may mask an undiagnosed hemorrhage. The gradual loss of 35% of the total blood volume has been shown to be tolerated by the pregnant woman without major hemodynamic consequences.[12] This blood loss may occur at the silent expense of uterine blood flow unless fetal monitoring is done.[13]

Cardiopulmonary collapse may be difficult to treat in advanced pregnancy. Treatment algorithms are different depending on gestational age and may involve perimortem cesarean delivery to eliminate aortocaval compression in the late second and third trimesters.[14] Similarly management of the unstable pregnant trauma victim calls for early delivery of the fetus, with the possible exception of very prolonged (hours) hypovolemic shock and subsequent arrest.[10] Figure 17.1 is a proposed algorithm for the management of an unstable trauma victim. Neonatal survival rates are poor if the gestational age is <26 weeks.[15]

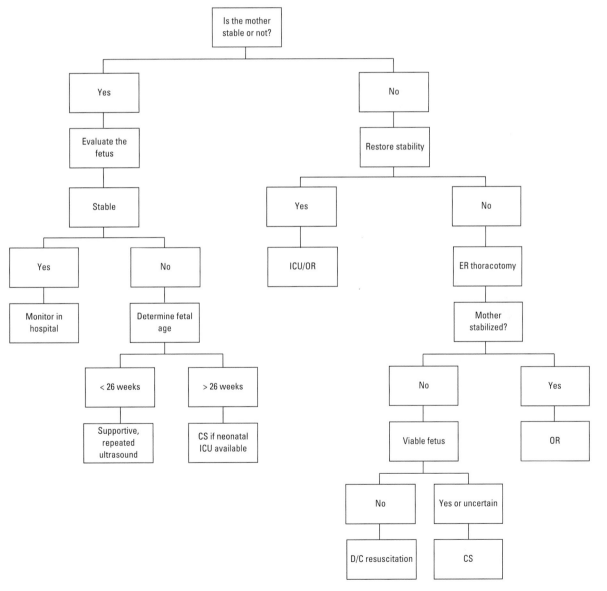

Fig. 17.1 Algorithm for initial evaluation and management of an injured pregnant patient. ER, emergency room; CS, cesarean section; D/C, discontinue; ICU, intensive care unit; OR, operating room. Based on references[10,14].

Pulmonary issues

Decreased functional residual capacity, and increased fetal–placental metabolic demands, among others, can lead to the development of hypoxia very rapidly if hypoventilation develops. Hypoxic damage to the fetus rapidly follows maternal hypoxia.

Airway changes

In addition, swollen and friable airway mucosa and enlarged breasts render the pregnant airway more difficult to manage.[16] Repeated attempts at the placement of an endotracheal tube may also lead to laryngeal edema. Profuse epistaxis may develop with the insertion of nasal airways or nasogastric tubes. Airway compromise must be managed judiciously and without delay.

Gastrointestinal changes

Gastrointestinal changes of pregnancy place every pregnant trauma victim at increased risk for aspiration of gastric contents, especially when she is obtunded. Aspiration prophylaxis either with non-particulate antacid and/or H_2 antagonists such as ranitidine should be instituted.

Hematological issues

Maternal blood is normally hypercoagulable during pregnancy owing to changes in coagulation factors and decreased clot lysis. However after maternal trauma, placental separation is a common complication and is the leading cause of fetal death.[17] Even with a small abruption, disseminated intravascular coagulation can develop that may preclude regional anesthesia techniques.[18] Fetal ultrasound evaluation is useful as a diagnostic tool for abruption (although unreliable for small blood accumulations). Placental abruption may cause the onset of uterine contractions. Therefore most centers will institute fetal heart rate and uterine contraction monitoring following maternal trauma.[19] Tocolysis of preterm labor is occasionally provided with ritodrine, terbutaline, or magnesium after ruling out the possibility of an abruption.

Fetal hemorrhage may occur and the detection of fetal red blood cells in the maternal blood is possible with a Kleishauer–Betke test which is sensitive for fetomaternal hemorrhage of > 30 mL. D(Rho[D]) immune globulin [300 microg Rhogam] is routinely to be administered to Rh-negative mothers who have sustained abdominal trauma, even in the absence of known fetal hemorrhage.[20]

Central nervous system changes

The most common cause of maternal death after trauma is due to head injury.[6] It is important to remember that some pregnancy-related conditions such as preeclampsia and eclampsia may result in changes in sensorium, headaches, and seizures and thus mimic head injury.

Musculoskeletal changes

Widening of the pelvic joint spaces by the 7th month of pregnancy has implications in the interpretation of pelvic X-rays of the traumatized pregnant woman. If pelvic fracture occurs, the engorged pelvic vessels can contribute to massive retroperitoneal bleeding.

Anesthetic issues

There are altered responses to anesthetics in pregnancy. Pregnancy decreases the MAC for inhaled anesthetics, and augments the effects of both depolarizing and non-depolarizing muscle relaxants.[13] Pregnancy reduces the local anesthetic requirement for spinal and epidural anesthesia and for peripheral nerve blockade.[21] Reports from the 1980s indicated that pregnancy may predispose to enhanced bupivacaine cardiac toxicity.[22] The recent introduction of ropivacaine into clinical practice may obviate some of these toxicity issues in pregnant patients. Pregnancy has not been shown to be associated with increased cardiac toxicity of ropivacaine.[23]

TERATOLOGY

Routine diagnostic or therapeutic modalities used within normal trauma care protocols may raise concerns for teratogenicity in pregnant patients. There are several reviews of this subject.[24,25] This chapter will consider only agents utilized for regional anesthetic techniques. The incidence of maternal drug abuse is increased in pregnant victims of violence, and many of these women may not have received prenatal care.[26] Adverse reproductive outcomes are associated with maternal substance abuse; maternal cocaine use is also associated with an increased incidence of placental abruption.[27]

Fetal gestational age at the time of exposure to the drug, together with extent and duration of exposure, are important determinants of teratogenicity. Morphologic teratogenicity (involving structural abnormality of an organ) is most likely to occur with drug maternal exposure during embryogenesis (from the 6th gestational day to the 9th gestational week). Prior to the 6th day, significant teratogenic exposures are likely to result in loss of the pregnancy. Exposure occurring beyond the period of organagenesis may lead to behavioral teratogenicity as evidenced by neurological dysfunction of varying severity including mental retardation in the baby.

In trauma victims two other factors have been associated with teratogenic fetal effects:

- Hypoglycemia (perhaps as a result of improper intravenous fluid therapy) has been associated with skeletal and neural tube defects[28]
- Traumatic stress and hospitalization stress have been associated with mental retardation and congenital malformations.[29]

Local anesthetic agents

There has been no evidence linking local anesthetics directly to morphologic teratogenicity. However, indirect harm to the fetus can occur if hypotension is produced secondary to profound sympathetic block; or respiratory compromise occurs from high spinal or epidural anesthesia; or, if acute systemic local anesthetic toxicity develops.

Early reports of adverse neonatal neurobehavioral outcomes with lidocaine have not been reproduced in later investigations.[30] The fetus cannot efficiently metabolize local anesthetics such as mepivacaine that require ring-hydroxylation, so other amide local anesthetics such as lidocaine, bupivacaine, and ropivacaine are safer. The ester local anesthetic 2-chloroprocaine is hydrolyzed rapidly by neonatal pseudocholinesterase and may be suitable for use for surgical procedures of short duration. Tetracaine is an ester local anesthetic that is available for intrathecal administration and of longer duration.

Sedatives

In the non-pregnant patient, sedatives are employed with regional anesthetic techniques to allay patient anxiety during institution of the regional block or during the operative procedure. However, the United States Food and Drug Administration (FDA) recommends that the benzodiazepines, diazepam and chlordiazepoxide, not be used during the period of embryogenesis because of possible association with fetal cleft lip and palate deformities.[31] The use of large dosages of the benzodiazepines in labor is associated with decreased neonatal muscle tone and ability to withstand cold stress.[32] Use of some of the phenothiazines (promethazine) during pregnancy has been associated with fetal cardiac anomalies.[33]

Narcotics

In the absence of respiratory depression or subsequent maternal blood acid–base abnormalities, the use of most narcotics for pain relief is safe, with the possible exceptions of codeine and propoxyphene[24] (Table 17.3). However, fetal growth retardation has been seen with chronic use of the narcotic agents.[34] Epidural or intrathecal use of narcotics usually produces lower maternal systemic concentrations of the narcotic than parental administration (especially with more hydrophilic narcotics such as morphine) and thus minimizes fetal narcotic exposure.

Antibiotics

Prophylactic or therapeutic antibiotics are commonly prescribed to trauma patients, and some of these do have known teratogenic effects. In addition, if the mother will soon deliver, some antibiotics are not advisable during the breast-feeding period. Reviews of this topic are available.[35] The penicillins, cephalosporins, ethambutol, and acyclovir are considered safe in pregnancy and their entry into breast milk is thought not to be associated with any neonatal problems. Erythromycin and metronidazole are used clinically during pregnancy and breast-feeding, but reproduction–toxicology studies are incomplete with these agents. The aminoglycosides and some antimalarials (cloroquine and hydroycloroquine) are known teratogenic agents. The sulfonamides, rifampin, and chloramphenicol can cause neonatal hemolytic

Table 17.3   FDA classification of pain medication use in pregnancy

FDA classification	Definition	Examples
Category A	Possibility of harm to fetus remote. Human studies show no fetal risk	Prenatal vitamins
Category B	Controlled human studies have shown no fetal risk. Animal studies show no risk or can not be reproduced in humans	Acetaminophen Ibuprofen Fentanyl Hydrocodone Methadone Meperidine Morphine Oxycodone Oxymorphone Nalbuphine Butorphanol Prednisone Prednisolone
Category C	No controlled human studies have been done. Animal studies indicate teratogenic or embryocidal risk; or have not been done.	Aspirin Ketorolac Propoxyphene Codeine
Category D	Positive evidence of human fetal risk, but in certain cases benefits may outweight risks of drug use	Phenobarbital Phenytoin Diazepam Amitriptyline Imipramine
Category X	Positive evidence of fetal risk. Risk outweighs benefit of use	Ergotamine

Adapted from Rothmell et al[24]

anemia and thrombocytopenia when administered close to the time of delivery.[36] Tetracycline can cause fetal bone deformities, and trimethoprim should be avoided because it may cause interference with folic acid metabolism.

ANESTHETIC AND PERIOPERATIVE MANAGEMENT OF THE PREGNANT TRAUMA PATIENT

General considerations

The initial management of the pregnant trauma patient does not differ from the initial triage of any trauma patient except that left uterine displacement must be provided. It must be remembered that concern for maternal welfare supercedes concern for fetal welfare, and that (in general) what is best for the mother is best for the fetus.

Fetal monitoring along with non-invasive monitoring of uterine contractions should be instituted early in the hospital course. An obstetrician, or a maternal–fetal medicine specialist (if available) should be consulted. The possibility of uterine

abruption or the onset of labor should always be entertained, even with minor falls or mild abdominal injuries.[9] Fetal heart rate is utilized to guide not only proper intrauterine resuscitative efforts (optimization of oxygenation and perfusion pressure) but to enable clinicians to decide if, and when, to perform a prompt cesarean delivery. The need for neonatal intensive care cannot be overemphasized, especially when a preterm delivery is anticipated. Head injuries, as well as injuries to the vertebral column, constitute important challenges for the clinician.

Maternal pelvic radiation shields should be used to minimize fetal radiation exposure. Guidelines for maximum permissible radiation for the fetus must be followed.[7]

Fluid resuscitation is performed aggressively to avoid decreases in fetal perfusion. When large volumes of crystalloid administration is necessary, lactated Ringer's solution is preferred because excessive amounts of normal saline solution may lead to maternal and fetal hyperchloremic acidosis.[37] Venous return is augmented by left uterine displacement. Fresh blood has been advocated in preference to stored, packed red blood cells because of its higher content of 2,3-diphospho-glycerate, but may not be readily available.[38]

Maternal ketosis can be avoided by the judicious administration of glucose solutions to maintain maternal blood sugar between 80 and 120 mg/dL.

Invasive hemodynamic monitoring is used as dictated by the maternal condition, with arterial blood gas determinations serving as a guide to avoid acidosis and maintain maternal $PaCO_2$ between 33 and 36 mmHg. Vasopressors such as ephedrine do not cause a reduction in uteroplacental blood flow and may be preferable to pure α-agonist agents in this setting.[6] Coagulation defects should be corrected before surgery, bearing in mind that pregnancy-induced changes affect certain coagulation parameters, such as fibrinogen.

Many pregnant trauma patients may not be candidates for regional anesthetic techniques because of the high incidence of occult head and/or vertebral column injury as well as visceral injuries. Increased abdominal girth and increased metabolic demands of pregnancy may actually hasten the development of occult or overt respiratory failure. Contraindications to regional anesthesia include maternal coagulopathy, septicemia, ongoing severe hemorrhage, the potential for infection at the site (as in burns), or patient refusal (Table 17.4). A full discussion of general anesthesia for non-obstetric surgery during pregnancy is beyond the scope of this chapter, and excellent reviews are found elsewhere.[35,39]

Regional anesthesia, when feasible, is the preferred anesthetic technique in pregnancy, for the simple reason that it minimizes the amount of systemic medication administered and consequently, the amount of placental transfer of medication to the fetus is minimized. Also, in the majority of cases regional anesthetic techniques avoid airway

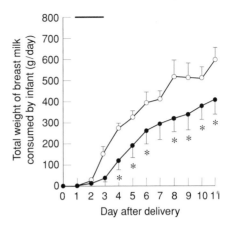

Fig. 17.2 Time course of amount of breast feeding after delivery in the S (●) and SE (○) groups. Solid bar represents the time period when epidural bupivacaine was used in the SE group. *$P<0.05$ versus the SE group. SE = group with spinal anesthesia and continuous postoperative epidural analgesia (n = 15). S = group with spinal anesthesia alone (n = 15).

manipulations. The data developed by Confidential Inquiries into Maternal Deaths in England and Wales and mortality statistics from the USA consistently point to airway problems as a leading cause of maternal death.[40,41] However, even if a regional technique is not feasible for surgery, it may be a possible modality to provide perioperative pain control. This could be accomplished utilizing combinations of intrathecal or epidural narcotics, dilute local anesthetic solutions, peripheral nerve blocks, or local infiltration techniques. Local anesthetics are associated with a low teratogenic potential. It has been recently shown that neonates whose mothers were given an epidural infusion for postoperative pain control gained more weight in the first week of life compared with those whose mothers were administered parental narcotics[42] (Fig. 17.2).

Operative regional anesthesia techniques
Spinal anesthesia

Spinal anesthesia for lower extremity and lower abdominal procedures is very common and has been investigated in trauma scenarios.[43] Lidocaine, bupivicaine, and tetracaine are available in commercial kits, generally in hyperbaric

Table 17.4 Contraindications to regional anesthesia in the pregnant trauma patient

Uncorrected absolute or relative hypovolemia
Sepsis
Infection or potential infection (burns) at insertion site
Vertebral or head trauma
Extensive abdominal trauma
Maternal coagulopathy
Impending respiratory failure
Absolute patient refusal

preparations. Both traditional and combined spinal epidural techniques can be used. The use of spinal microcatheters is currently not recommended in the USA because of reports implicating them in the development of cauda-equina syndrome.[44] We advise caution against using hyperbaric lidocaine for spinal anesthesia because of a possible association with residual neurologic sequelae, especially in trauma patients who already have a potential for trauma-related nerve damage.[45]

The onset of sympathectomy with spinal anesthesia can be precipitous (with subsequent systemic hypotension), and therefore prophylactic intravenous prehydration with crystalloid is advocated. Although the effectiveness of prophylactic hydration has been questioned in preventing spinal hypotension in pregnant patients,[46] we recommend prophylactic hydration in this setting because of the risk of added hemodynamic instability in injured patients. If systolic pressure falls 20% or more, it should be treated with 5–10 mg doses of ephedrine with additional hydration. If ephedrine is ineffective, then 50–100 microg increments of phenylephrine can be given safely.[47] Adjunctive intraoperative pain control is achieved with addition of intrathecal narcotics (fentanyl 10–25 µg, sufentanil 5–20 µg or intrathecal morphine 0.25 mg).

Epidural anesthesia

Epidural anesthesia can provide as effective operative anesthesia as spinal anesthesia, but can be titrated to a desired sensory level, with less potential for the rapid development of systemic hypotension. The benefit of an indwelling epidural catheter includes the ability to provide prolonged surgical anesthesia (if needed) and also prolonged postoperative analgesia.

Surgical epidural anesthesia in pregnancy is provided with 2% lidocaine, 0.5% bupivacaine, 3% 2-chloroprocaine, or 0.5% ropivacaine.[48] Reports of fatal maternal cardiac arrhythmias with 0.75% bupivacaine occurred in the 1980s; therefore use of epidural bupivacaine in obstetric populations is limited to 0.5% solutions. An excellent review of epidural local anesthetic dosing safety issues exists.[49] Epinephrine in 1:200 000 to 1:400 000 concentrations is often added to epidural local anesthetics to enhance analgesia, motor blockade, or prolong duration. Clinical studies

have been done in obstetrics that indicate this practice is safe if maternal hypotension is avoided.[50]

Epidural narcotics (fentanyl 50–100 µg, sufentanil 10–20 µg, or preservative-free morphine 3–5 mg) provide intraoperative alleviation of visceral pain sensation and their effect extends into the postoperative period as well. Epidural catheters can be left in place for several days for postoperative pain control utilizing bolus dosing of epidural narcotics or continuous infusion techniques.

Peripheral regional anesthesia techniques

Brachial plexus blockade (axillary, interscalene approaches) can provide excellent anesthesia for isolated upper extremity injuries, with the benefit of minimal fetal effects if intravascular injection and local anesthetic toxicity are avoided.[51] Intravenous regional anesthetic techniques (Bier block) can be used for isolated forearm injuries, if tourniquet malfunction is avoided. This technique is less practical for lower extremity operations because of the requirement for large doses of local anesthetics with an added risk of venous stasis and thrombophebitis in pregnancy.[52] However, an ankle block can be utilized for distal foot surgery. Peribulbar or retrobulbar ophthalmologic blockade may be valuable in eye injuries. Local infiltration techniques for the management of traumatic lacerations are well described in a review[53] and each of these techniques is described more fully in corresponding chapters of this text.

Perioperative pain management

Intrathecal narcotics are possibly the ideal analgesic for the acute trauma patient with a lower extremity injury. There is a lower incidence of hypotension with intrathecal narcotic administration than with local anesthetics. Additionally, there is less systemic absorption of intrathecal narcotics than with parenteral use (dependent to some extent on lipid solubility of the narcotic). The onset of analgesia is quick with lipophilic narcotics, such as fentanyl or sufentanil, but the duration of action is short. The hydrophilic narcotic morphine has a delayed onset, but its action can last 6 to 18 hours. Intrathecal administration of combinations of short duration narcotics and morphine are described that combine the benefits and side effects of both.[54] If a combined spinal epidural technique is performed, the epidural catheter could be used later for an operative procedure or further pain control.

Multiple rib fractures or crush injuries of the chest can be managed by placing thoracic epidural catheters. A dilute local anesthetic (with or without narcotic) can be infused to manage pain under these circumstances. These techniques help to avoid artificial ventilation, enable earlier ventilator weaning, and maximize the need for pulmonary toilet, thus minimizing infectious sequelae.[55] Intercostal nerves blocks and intrapleural catheters have also been used for these patients and after thoracotomy procedures. Both techniques are less efficacious if the integrity of the chest wall is interrupted, and are associated with higher local anesthetic absorption levels, as well as a higher incidence of inadvertent pneumothorax.[56]

Postoperative regional techniques

Postoperative epidural narcotic regimens are described after abdominal procedures through lumbar epidural catheters, as well as after upper abdominal and chest operations through thoracic catheters.[57] Combinations of dilute local anesthetics and narcotics administered continuously via these catheters may minimize the need for supplemental narcotics. Table 17.5 lists some suggested initial epidural-dosing regimens that may require adaptation to suit the demands of the situation. These regimens are conservative and have been adjusted for the altered anesthetic responses in pregnancy. Proper monitoring regimens and education of postoperative nursing personnel enhance the efficacy and safety of these techniques.[58]

Common side effects of the epidural narcotics include pruritus, nausea and vomiting, and uri-

Table 17.5 Suggested initial epidural narcotic and combined local anesthetic with narcotic dosing regimens

Drug	Solution	Bolus[a] dose	Basal[c] infusion	Rescue[b] dose
Morphine	0.1 mg/mL 0.01%	3–5 mg[c]	0.5–0.8 mg/h[c]	0.2–0.3 mg q 10–15 min
Fentanyl	10 µg/mL 0.001%	100 µg	50–100 µg/h	10–15 µg q 10–15 min
Sufentanil	1 µg/mL 0.0001%	10 µg	5–10 µg/h	5–7 µg q 10–15 min
Hydro-morphone	0.05 mg/mL 0.005%	0.8–1.5 mg[c]	0.15–0.3 mg/h	0.14–0.3 mg q 10–15 min
Morphine Bupivacaine	0.005% 0.0625%	0.125%* Bupivacaine	4–8 mL/h	1–2 mL q 10–15 min
Fentanyl Bupivacaine	0.0005% 0.0625%	0.125%* Bupivacaine	4–8 mL/h	1–2 mL q 10–15 min
Sufentanil Bupivacaine	0.00005% 0.0625%	0.125%* Bupivacaine	4–8 mL/h	1–2 mL q 10–15 min
Morphine Ropivacaine	0.005% 0.05–0.1%	0.1–0.2%* Ropivacaine	6–8 mL/h	1–2 mL q 10–15 min
Fentanyl Ropivacaine	0.0005% 0.05–0.1%	0.1–0.2%* Ropivacaine	6–8 mL/h	1–2 mL q 10–15 min
Sufentanil Ropivacaine	0.00005% 0.05–0.1%	0.1–0.2%* Ropivacaine	6–8 mL/h	1–2 mL q 10–15 min

*Initial volume of local anesthetic will vary from 4–6 mL for thoracic catheters to 6–10 mL for lumbar catheters; and appropriate test and sequential 4–5 mL aliquots dosing.
[a]The bolus dose recommended assumes that lipophilic narcotics (fentanyl and sufentanil) are used; the epidural catheter tip is located is near dermatome that lies in the middle of all dermatomes innervating the entire injury site; and the narcotics are diluted in 5 mL preservative-free normal saline.
[b]Rescue regimens may require larger volumes with prolonged use.
[c]Lower doses for thoracic catheters; higher doses for lumbar catheters.
Adapted from DeLeon-Caseola,[57] doses modified owing to pregnant physiology.

nary retention. Respiratory depression is very rare but more common with concomitant administration of sedative agents or excessive narcotic administration.[59]

SPECIAL CONSIDERATIONS IN REGIONAL ANESTHESIA

Ropivacaine

Ropivacaine is a new, long-acting local anesthetic that became available for general clinical use in the USA in early 1997, and offers some advantages over bupivicaine in the pregnant population. Animal and human studies indicate a lower potential for toxicity and animal studies predict a higher success rate with resuscitation from inadvertent intravascular injections.[60,61] Additional advantages of ropivacaine include better motor-sensory separation at lower concentrations as seen in Figure 17.3.[62] Also improved frequency-dependent block potential,[63] and faster clearance from the bloodstream are beneficial properties (Table 17.6).[64,65] These properties of ropivacaine make it an ideal agent for infusions for postoperative pain control in injured pregnant patients. Continuous ropivacaine infusions for postoperative pain control are now in general use.[66]

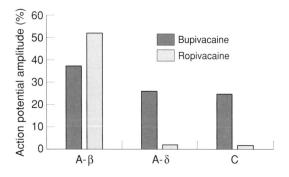

Fig. 17.3 Differential sensitivity of A-δ and C fibers to ropivacaine and/or bupivacaine. Ropivacaine = 25 μM = Bupivacaine 50 μM with 8 minutes bathtime. Note that the A-δ and C fibers are much more sensitive to ropivacaine than to bupivacaine. Motor fibers (A-β) appear to be more sensitive to bupivacaine. Based on Rosenberg.[62]

Table 17.6 Pharmacokinetics of ropivacaine in comparison to bupivacaine following IV infusion. (0.67 mL/min of 50 mg ropivacaine)

	Ropivacaine	Bupivacaine
Disposition half-life (h)	1.9*	3.5
Volume of distribution (L)	59	73
Clearance (L/min)	0.82*	0.58
Protein binding (%)	94	95

*significantly different from the corresponding value with bupivacaine.
Based on data from McClure.[64]

SUMMARY

In providing regional anesthesia to the pregnant trauma patient, the important physiologic and anatomical changes that occur with pregnancy must be taken into account. The possibility of unique conditions occurring in pregnancy such as placental abruption, premature rupture of membranes, isoimmunization, embolic phenomenon (thrombotic and amniotic), preeclampsia/eclampsia, and uterine trauma must be remembered. The involvement of obstetric, intensivist, and neonatal specialists should be obtained as early as feasible. Fetal monitoring with continuous heart rate tracings, tocodynometry, and ultrasound (as clinically indicated) also should be obtained, and performed by qualified individuals.

Regional anesthesia may not be feasible in certain circumstances such as uncorrected hypovolemia, maternal coagulopathy, vertebral and head trauma, overwhelming maternal sepsis, or infection at the site of the intended procedure. If regional anesthesia is feasible however, it is the preferred technique because of maternal and fetal considerations. The aforementioned regional techniques are acceptable practice. Prehydration and prevention of maternal hypotension are mandatory, so as to preserve uteroplacental perfusion (with use of left lateral uterine displacement devices after mid-second trimester gestations). If hypotension occurs, it should be treated first with intravenous isotonic volume administration, prior to the use of vasopressor agents that potentially vasoconstrict uterine blood vessels. Epidural catheters are valuable in providing perioperative analgesia, with minimal systemic passage of drug to the fetus. Ropivacaine is a promising, new, local anesthetic with potentially less maternal toxicity and decreased motor blocking properties.

REFERENCES

1. Lane PL. Traumatic fetal deaths. J Emerg Med 1989; 7: 433.

2. Sachs BP, Brown DAJ, Driscoll SG, et al. Maternal mortality in Massachusetts: trends and prevention. N Engl J Med 1987; 316: 667.

3. Sherer DM, Schenker JG. Accidental injury during pregnancy. Obstet Gynecol Surv 1989; 44: 33.

4. Esposito TJ, Gens DR, Smith LG, Scorpio R. Trauma during pregnancy: a review of 79 cases. Arch Surg 1991; 126: 1073–1079.

5. Smith CV, Phelan JP. Trauma in pregnancy. In: Clark S, et al, eds. Critical care obstetrics. 2nd ed. Boston: Blackwell Scientific; 1991: 601.

6. Esposito TJ. Trauma during pregnancy. Emerg Med Clin North Am 1994; 12: 167.

7. Crosby W. Traumatic injuries during pregnancy. Clin Obstet Gynecol 1983; 26: 902.

8. Rode H, Millar AJW, Cywes S, et al. Thermal injury in pregnancy–the neglected tragedy. S Afr Med J 1990; 77: 346.

9. George ER, Vanderkwook T, Schalten DJ. Factors influencing pregnancy outcome after trauma. Am Surg 1992; 58(9): 594–598.

10. Trauma in women. In: Advanced Trauma Life Support. 6th ed. Chicago: American College of Surgeons 1997; 11: 377–387.

11. Kissinger DP, Rozycki GS, Morris JA. Trauma in pregnancy–predicting pregnancy outcome. Arch Surg 1991; 126: 1079.

12. Conklin KA. Physiologic changes of pregnancy. In: Chestnut DH, ed. Obstetric Anesthesia; Principles and practice. St Louis: Mosby; 1994; 2: 1–41.

13. Marx GF, Bassel GM. Physiologic considerations of the mother. In: Marx GF, Bassel GM, eds. Obstetric analgesia and anesthesia. New York: Elsevier; 1980: 21–54.

14. Special resuscitation situations: cardiac arrest associated with pregnancy. In: Cummings RO, ed. American Heart Association: Advanced Cardiac life support. Dallas, Texas: American Heart Association; 1997; 10: 10.

15. Katz VL, Dotters DJ, Droegemueller W. Perimortem cesarean delivery. Obstet Gynecol 1986; 68: 571–576.

16. Cooper SD, Beunumof JL, Reisner LS. The difficult airway; risk, prophylaxis, and management. In: Chestnut DH, ed. Obstetric anesthesia: Principles and practice. St Louis: Mosby; 1994; 572.

17. Pearlman MD, Tintinalli JE, Lorenz RP. A prospective controlled study of outcome after trauma during pregnancy. Am J Obstet Gynecol 1990; 162: 1502.

18. Higgins SD, Garite TJ. Late abruptio placentae in trauma patients: implications for monitoring. Obstet Gynecol 1984; 63(suppl): 10.

19. Trauma During Pregnancy. Washington, DC: American College of Obstetricians and Gynecologists; 1991: 161.

20. Gilstrap LC, Cotton DB, Phelan ST, et al. Obstetric complications. In: Hauth JC, Merenstein GB, eds. Guidelines for perinatal care. 4th ed. Washington, DC: American College of Obstetricians and Gynecologists; 1997; 6: 127–146.

21. Conklin KA. Maternal adaptations during gestation, labor, and the puerperium. Seminars in Anesthesia 1991; 10: 221.

22. Albright G. Cardiac arrest following regional anesthesia with etidocaine and bupivacaine. Anesthesiology 1979; 51: 285–287.

23. Santos AC, Arthur GE, Finster M. Comparative systemic toxicity of ropivacaine and bupivacaine in non-pregnant and pregnant ewes. Anesthesiology 1995; 82: 734–740.

24. Rothmell JP, Viscomi CM, Ashburn MA. Management of nonobstetrical pain during pregnancy and lactation. Anesth Analg 1997; 85(5): 1074–1087.

25. Friedman JM, Little BB, Brent RL, Cordero JF, Hanson JW, Shepard TH. Potential human teratogenicity of frequently prescribed drugs. Obstet Gynecol 1990; 75: 594–599.

26. Amaro H, Fried LE, Cabral H, Zuckerman B. Violence during pregnancy and substance use. Am J Public Health 1990; 80: 575.

27. Kain ZW. Cocaine abusing parturients undergoing cesarean section; a cohort study. Anesthesiology 1996; 85: 1028.

28. Hannah RS, Moore KL. Effects of fasting and insulin on skeletal development in rats. Teratology 1971; 4: 135.

29. Abramson JH, Singh AR, Mbambo V. Antenatal stress and the baby's development. Arch Dis Child 1961; 36: 42.

30. Abboud TK, Sarkis F, Blikian A, Varakian L, Earl S, Henriksen E. Lack of adverse neonatal neurobehavioral effects of lidocaine. Anesth Analg 1983; 62: 473.

31. Safra MJ, Oakley GP. Association between cleft lip with or without cleft palate and prenatal exposure to diazepam. Lancet 1975; 2: 478.

32. Beeley L. Adverse effects of drugs in later pregnancy. Clin Obstet Gynecol 1981; 8: 275.

33. Sloane D, Siskind V, Heinonen OP, Monson RR, Kaufman DW, Shapiro S. Antenatal exposure to the phenothiazines in relation to congenital mal-

formations, perinatal mortality rate, birth weight, and intelligence quotient score. Am J Obstet Gynecol 1977; 128: 486.

34. Stimmel B, Goldberg J, Reisman A, Murphy RJ, Teets K. Fetal outcome in narcotic-dependent women: the importance of the type of maternal narcotic used. Am J Drug Alcohol Abuse 1982; 9: 383.

35. Ramanathan S, Porges RM. Anesthetic care of the injured pregnant patient. In: Capan LM, Miller SM, Turndorf H, eds. Trauma anesthesia and intensive care. Philadelphia: JB Lippincott; 1991; 19: 599–625.

36. Bergland F, Flodh H, Lundborg P. Drug use during pregnancy and breast-feeding: a classification system for drug information. Acta Obstet Gynecol Scand 1984; 5: 126.

37. Crosby WM, Haycock CE, Carbal SS. An emergency care protocol for trauma in pregnancy. In: Crosby WM, Haycock CE, Carbal SS, eds. Emergency Medicine Reports 1987; 8: 73.

38. Hunt TM, Semple MJ. Blood transfusion. In: Churchill-Davidson HC, ed. A practice of anaesthesia. Chicago: Year Book Medical Publishers; 1984; 587.

39. Baker B. Trauma. In: Chestnut D, ed. Obstetrical anesthesia: Principles and practice St Louis: Mosby; 1994; 53: 996–1005.

40. Hawkins L, Koonin LM, Palener SK, Gibbs C. Anesthesia-related deaths during obstetric delivery in the United States 1979–1990. Anesthesiology 1997; 86(2): 277–283.

41. Morgan M. Anaesthetic contribution to maternal mortality. Br J Anaesth 1987; 59: 842–855.

42. Hirose M, Hara Y, Hosokawa T, Tanaka Y. The effect of postoperative analgesia with continuous epidural bupivacaine after cesarean section on the amount of breast feeding and infant weight gain. Anesth Analg 1996; 82: 1166–1169.

43. Wilhelm S, Standl T, Esch JS. Comparison of continuous spinal with combined spinal epidural anesthesia using plain bupivacaine 0.5% in trauma patients. Anesth Analg 1997; 85: 69–74.

44. Rigler ML, Lambert DH, Krejac TC. Cauda-equina syndrome after continuous spinal anesthesia. Anesth Analg 1991; 72: 275–281.

45. Drasner K. Lidocaine spinal anesthesia; a vanishing therapeutic index? Anesthesiology 1997; 87(3): 469–471.

46. Rout CC. A reevaluation of the role of crystalloid and colloid preload in the prevention of hypotension associated with spinal anesthesia for elective cesarean section. Br J Anaesth 1993; 79: 262–269.

47. Ramanathan S, Grant GJ. Vasopressor therapy for hypotension due to epidural anesthesia for cesarean section. Acta Anaesthesiol Scand 1988; 32: 559.

48. Alahunta S, Rosanen J, Jouppilla P. The effects of epidural ropivacaine and bupivacaine for cesarean section on uteroplacental and fetal circulation. Anesthesiology 1995; 83: 23–32.

49. Mulroy MF, Norris MA, Spenser SL. Safety steps for epidural injection of local anesthetics: review of the literature and recommendations. Anesth Analg 1997; 85: 1346–1356.

50. Joupilla R, Jouppilla P, Kuilka J. Placental blood flow during cesarean section under lumbar extradural analgesia Br J Anaesth 1978; 50: 275.

51. Bridenbaugh DL. The upper extremity: somatic blockade. In: Cousins MJ, Bridenbaugh PO, eds. Neural bloackade: in clinical anesthesia and management of pain. 2nd ed. Philadelphia: JB Lippincott; 1997; 10: 405.

52. Henderson CL, Warringer CB, McElwen JA, Merrick PM. A North American survey of intravenous regional anesthesia. Anesth Analg 1997; 85: 858–863.

53. Singer AJ, Hallander JE, Quinn JV. Evaluation and management of traumatic lacerations. N Engl J Med 1997; 337(16): 1142–1149.

54. Leighton BL, DeSimone CA, Norris MA. Intrathecal narcotics revisited; the combination of fentanyl and morphine intrathecally provides rapid onset of profound, prolonged analgesia. Anesth Analg 1989; 69: 122–125.

55. Dittman M, Ferst A, Wolf G. Epidural analgesia for the treatment of multiple rib fractures. Eur J Intens Care Med 1975; 1: 71.

56. Symreng T, Gomez MN, Rossi N. Intrapleural bupivacaine–technical considerations and intraoperative use. J Cardiothorac Anesth 1989; 3: 139.

57. DeLeon-Caseola OA, Lema MJ. Postoperative epidural opioid analgesia: what are the choices? Anesth Analg 1996; 83: 867–875.

58. Ready LB, Loper KA, Nessley M, Wild L. Postoperative epidural morphine is safe in the surgical ward. Anesthesiology 1991; 75: 452–456.

59. Cousins M, Mather L. Intrathecal and epidural administration of opioids. Anesthesiology 1984; 61: 276–310.

60. Nancarrow C, Rutten AJ, Runciman WG. Myocardial and cerebral drug concentrations and the mechanisms of death after fatal intravenous doses of lidocaine, bupivacaine, and ropivacaine in sheep. Anesth Analg 1989; 69: 276–283.

61. Scott DB, Lee A, Fagan D. Acute toxicity of ropivacaine compared with that of bupivacaine. Anesth Analg 1989; 69: 563–569.

62. Rosenberg PH, Heinonen E. Differential sensitivity of A and C nerve fibers to long-acting amide local anaesthetics. Br J Anaesth 1983; 55: 163–166.

63. Wildsmith JAW, Brown DT, Paul D, Johnson S. Structure-activity relationships in differential nerve

block at high and low frequency stimulation. Br J Anaesth 1989; 63: 444–452.

64. McClure JH. Ropivacaine. Br J Anaesth 1997; 76(2): 300–307.

65. Datta S, Camann W, Bader A. Clinical effects and maternal and fetal plasma concentrations of epidural ropivacaine versus bupivacaine for cesarean section. Anesthesiology 1995; 82: 1346–1353.

66. Scott DA, Emanuelson BM, Mooney PH. Pharmacokinetics and efficacy of long-term epidural ropivacaine infusion for postoperative analgesia. Anesth Analg 1997; 85: 1322–1330.

18

Burn patient

Lauren J DeLoach and Judith L Stiff

Introduction	**Management of burn pain**
	Pharmacologic management of burn pain
The pain experience in burn patients	Non-pharmacologic management of burn pain
Pain mechanisms	**Summary**
Pain mechanisms specific to burns	
Types of burns and pain	
Stages of burn and pain	

INTRODUCTION

Each year, an estimated 1.5 million Americans require medical attention for burn injuries. Of this number, approximately 52 000 are hospitalized for treatment of moderate-to-severe burns and 5500 die of their injury.[1]

The healing from moderate-to-severe burn injuries is a process that occurs over many months and during that time patients experience variable amounts of pain, not only from the injury itself but also from therapeutic procedures. Therefore, it is impossible to have any standardized pain protocols. Even the pain management protocols used as starting points vary from burn center to burn center.[2]

THE PAIN EXPERIENCE IN BURN PATIENTS

The pain experience consists of more than the simple sensation and can be divided into several aspects. For example, the McGill Pain Questionnaire uses word descriptions of pain and divides responses into sensory, affective and evaluative components.[3] The affective aspect rates pain using words describing categories such as fear and punishment. The evaluative words are for intensity range from 'mild' to 'excruciating'. This type of pain rating indicates that in addition to the actual sensory part of pain, the affective aspects may need adjunctive therapy. In a study of 42 patients, it was found that when overall pain scores increased, both within the McGill scheme and with other measurement scales, the affective and evaluative components also increased.[4]

In addition to these aspects, burn patients also experience varying degrees of purely psychological stress because of their anticipation of further medical procedures, loss of mobility, social worries (financial, family, future work prospects), and worry about disfigurement. Thus, they suffer from disturbances such as anxiety, depression and post-traumatic stress disorder which add to the affective component of their pain experience. Any pain management strategy for burn patients should thus include both pharmacologic and psychological interventions. Appropriate pain management strategies can reduce pain, improve patient well-being, and reduce the length of hospitalization.

PAIN MECHANISMS

While the precise mechanisms for pain associated specifically with burn injuries have not been completely elucidated, general pain-generating mechanisms that apply to burn injuries include nociception, primary and secondary hyperalgesias, and neuropathies. Anatomically, the presence of nociceptors that respond to tissue-damaging stimuli is well-established (see Ch. 3). Stimulation of cutaneous nociceptors, A and C fibers, is transmitted to the dorsal area of the spinal cord. Glycine and γ-aminobutyric acid (GABA), two amino acids, inhibit synaptic transmission and are important mediators of pain. Pain impulses are then transmitted to the brain via various ascending pathways including the spinothalamic tract and spinoreticular tract. A division of the spinothalamic tract, the paleospinothalamic tract, is thought to be associated with the autonomic and unpleasant emotional perceptions of pain. The spinoreticular tract probably produces arousal associated with pain perception and motivational-affective responses to pain.[5] There are also descending pathways from the brain to the spinal cord that inhibit pain. The periaqueductal gray area of the midbrain has high concentrations of opioid receptors and endogenous opioids and may mediate inhibition of pain impulses in the spinal cord. Environmental factors such as pain and stress may produce increases in the pain threshold while anxiety, depression, and emotional distress may decrease the pain threshold.[5]

Pain mechanisms specific to burns

Beyond the general pain mechanisms, repeated tissue injury and inflammation from repeated burn wound debridement may lead to sensitization of pain receptors causing hyperalgesia. Hyperalgesia is a decrease in the pain threshold and an increase in pain in response to a suprathreshold stimulus. The amines, 5-hydroxytryptamine and histamine, and the peptide bradykinin are endogenous chemical sensitizers. In addition, prostaglandins may potentiate the action of bradykinin to cause pain. It has been shown that hyperalgesia occurs after thermal injury; pain impulses are carried via A and C nociceptive fibers, and A fibers probably code for hyperalgesia.[6]

Mechanisms for pain occurring after the acute burn injury are poorly understood. Patients continue to have variable amounts of pain. As the burn injury heals, neural tissue is reorganized. Chronic pain syndromes such as dysesthesias, causalgias, and phantom pain, although rare, may develop.[7,8]

Types of burns and pain

The depth and extent of the burn injury are important determinants of the resultant pain, both from the injury itself and secondary to the required therapy. Burn types have traditionally been described as first, second, third, and fourth degree, however a more description classification based on the depth of the burn is preferred (Table 18.1).

First degree, or superficial, burns affect only the epidermis. They are painful, but since they require no procedures and heal rapidly, minimal pain management is necessary.

Second degree burns are partial thickness burns, but the basal layer of the dermis is unaffected. They affect variable amounts of dermis causing variable amounts of pain. Superficial partial thickness burns form blisters, and can be quite painful. Healing occurs in 14 to 17 days. Deep partial thickness burns are associated with dermal destruction and skin grafting is often required. These burns may heal spontaneously in 3 to 4 weeks or may progress to a full thickness burn and cause hypertrophic scar formation.

Table 18.1   Burn depth classification

Type	Example	Appearance	Pain	Procedures
1st degree	Sunburn	Dry, red	Painful, can be hyperesthetic topical analgesia helpful	Not needed, healing in 4 to 6 days
Superficial 2nd degree	Flash burn, spill scald	Red, blisters	Painful, can be hyperesthetic	Debridement, may heal spontaneously in 3 to 4 wks
Deep 2nd degree	Brief flame burn, brief immersion scald	Dark red to pale yellow, no exudate	Painful, can be hyperesthetic	Debridements, skin grafts
3rd degree	Immersion scalds, flame burns	White or charred, dry, thrombosed vessels	Anesthetic	Debridements, skin grafts
4th degree	Electrical, prolonged flame burn	Charred, dry	Anesthetic	Debridements, skin grafts, muscle flaps, amputation

Donor sites have the pain characteristics of 1st or superficial 2nd degree burns.
Donor sites and superficial 2nd degree burns often 'convert' to deep 2nd degree or 3rd degree injury.

Third degree burns are full thickness burns. They are not painful initially as the nerve fiber-containing dermis is completely destroyed. However, at the edges of third degree burns there may be areas of first and second degree injury causing pain. Although ingrowth of epithelium from the margins of the wound may occur, skin grafting is required for any large third degree burn. As the burn heals, neural function and pain sensation return.

Fourth degree burns result in the total destruction of skin and involve adjacent structures such as fat, fascia, muscle, and sometimes bone. The pain is quite unpredictable. Healing requires skin grafting and often regional flaps to cover the wounds. Electrical injury frequently results in fourth degree injury. Electrical injury or any fourth degree burn of an extremity may require amputation and is the cause of chronic pain syndromes.

The extent of the various types of burns is quantified in terms of percent of total body surface (TBSA). Although it would seem that the greater the extent of the burn, the greater the pain, this is not necessarily so. No correlation between pain scores and burn size has been found in several studies.[4] This may be due to the distribution of first, second, and third degree burns in the patients. However, in a study of 42 children, aged 7 to 17, a correlation was found between the amount of third degree size and pain scores during dressing changes.[9] If, however, psychological factors, particularly the anxiety scale, are also considered, burn size did correlate with pain scores in 103 patients.[10]

Stages of burn and pain

The *early phase* of recovery for a moderate to severe burn consists of resuscitation, much like a non-thermal trauma patient. Patients may be critically ill, requiring intubation and massive fluid resuscitation. Physiologic stressors such as anoxia, electrolyte imbalances, infection, and edema occur at this time. The onset of pain may be immediate or may be delayed by as much as 2 days. Some early debridement is often necessary to remove char and clothing. At the point where pain or procedures start, pain management also starts. Psychological disturbances such as delirium, anxiety, sleep disturbances, and confusion may also begin at this time, and appropriate therapy should be considered.

The *intermediate phase* consists of acute rehabilitation and begins within 48 hours after the injury. The burn patient commonly undergoes procedures such as surgical excision and skin grafting, dressing changes, wound debridement, splinting, and physical therapy. The patient may experience considerable pain at rest and pain associated with treatment procedures. Psychologically, patients begin to focus on the ramifications of their injuries. The most common psychological problems experienced are depression and post-traumatic stress disorder. Nightmares, anxiety, hostility, and dependence also occur.

The *long-term phase* of rehabilitation begins at the time of discharge from the hospital. Patients may still experience pain during physical therapy. Also, compression garments may cause discomfort and there often is pruritus. Physically, the burn scar matures and the patient must cope with the limitations imposed by the injury. The most common psychological problems during this phase are anxiety and depression which diminish in intensity after 1 year.[11]

MANAGEMENT OF BURN PAIN

The management of burn pain varies immensely among patients because of differences in the extent of the burn injury, differences in pain thresholds among patients, and psychological factors. Even within the time of treatment of a single patient, the management changes because of procedures, healing, and changing response to the pain experience. Thus, the management must be frequently reviewed and modified.

Pharmacologic management of burn pain

In the management of burn pain, it is necessary to consider the various effects of the burn injury on the pharmacology of the drugs to be used. In the acute, resuscitative phase, blood flow to the organs and tissues is decreased.[12,13] Drugs given by the enteral, subcutaneous, or intramuscular route of administration will have delayed absorption with decreased peak concentrations and possibly decreased bioavailability. In these patients, the intravenous route of administration is preferred.[14]

In the intermediate, rehabilitation phase, blood flow to tissues and organs is increased and the patient becomes somewhat hypermetabolic. However, few clinical studies have been done to specifically evaluate the variation in the pharmacology of pain management drugs that this might cause. There also are additional factors present during the treatment of burn victims that may alter drug action such as sepsis, malnutrition, parenteral nutrition, as well as hepatic, renal, cardiac, and pulmonary disease. Careful attention must be given to individual patients and their potential drug interactions and toxicities.

Burn patients experience pain at rest and pain associated with treatment procedures. Pain at rest, or 'background pain' is usually managed with opioids. Although opioids are most commonly given on an as needed (prn) basis, patients may benefit from a regular medication schedule during phases associated with intense pain. Procedural pain occurs during dressing changes, wound debridement, and physical therapy and has a greater intensity than background pain. For procedural pain, the analgesic regimen should be directed at obtaining therapeutic drug levels prior to initiating the procedure. Ideally, the agents used should have a fast onset, high potency, and short duration of action to minimize post-procedure sedation and respiratory depression.

Pain is often undertreated in burn patients for several reasons.[2,15,16] Patients are underdosed because of the fear of drug side effects, especially respiratory depression, the fear of addiction to opioids, and the lack of routine evaluations of pain.[2] Iatrogenic addiction was not documented in a survey of 93 burn centers in the USA.[2] Careful selection and appropriate dosing of analgesics, and monitoring of the patient may reduce the occurrence of respiratory depression. Finally, evaluation of pain should be multidisciplinary as patients are in daily contact with the physician, nursing and physical therapy staff.

Because psychological disturbances may influence pain intensity, anxiolytics and anti-depressants also have a role in pain-management strategies. Additionally, psychological interventions involving cognitive and behaviour modifications may have an important role in reducing pain.

Opioids

Opioids are the main component of pain-management therapy in the burn patient. Patients receiving opioids and other drugs that cause cardiorespiratory depression via the intravenous route of administration should have vital signs monitored closely, with resuscitative equipment immediately available. Reversal agents such as naloxone for opioids (as well as flumezanil for benzodiazepines) should also be available. Opioids, as well as other drugs may also be administered orally, intramuscularly, nasally, and transdermally. However, intramuscular injections are painful, the onset of action is delayed, and absorption may be erratic. Difficulty in achieving an adequate dose may lead to more than one injection which not only increases the risk for respiratory depression, but also may increase anxiety. Thus, intramuscular routes of administration should be avoided. Therapeutic drug levels are more quickly obtained with intravenous administration and titration to desired effect for treatment procedures. Table 18.2 lists commonly-used opioids.

Morphine. There is some evidence for altered pharmacology of morphine in burn patients. In the acute phase of burn injury, or when a burn patient has not received opioids for several hours, there is evidence for increased potency.[17,18] In children with burns, the distribution and elimination half-life of morphine was found to be shortened.[19] However, in another study, the distribution and elimination half-life of morphine in burn patients was not significantly different compared to non-burn groups.[20] In a study which examined the analgesic efficacy of oral sustained-release morphine (morphine sulfate – MS Contin) versus the continuous infusion of morphine in 10 patients, the analgesic qualities of morphine sulfate were comparable to those of the continuous intravenous morphine infusion.[21] Advantages of morphine sulfate include oral administration and long duration of action with a 12-hour dosing schedule. Morphine sulfate is commonly used in chronic pain patients and may be an efficacious drug in burn patients.[22] However, burn patients may develop tolerance during prolonged use. Other oral, semi-synthetic and synthetic opioid agents are also useful.

Patient-controlled analgesia (see Ch. 11). Patient-controlled analgesia (PCA) enables patients to deliver a specific amount of opioid at a specific time interval via an infusion pump. There is a wide variation in patient drug requirements so the PCA settings must be individualized. PCA allows patients

Table 18.2 Commonly-used opioids

Drug	Route of administration	Equivalent dosage (mg)	Onset (min)	Peak effect (min)	Duration (h)
Morphine	IV	10	3–5	10–20	3–4
	IM	10	15–60	30–60	3–4
	Oral soln	30	30	45	3–4
	Oral tabs	30	30	45	3–4
	Oral sustained-release tabs	30	30	60–120	12–14
Fentanyl	IV	0.1	1–5	3–5	0.5–1.5
	Buccal (adults)	5 microg/kg	10–20	30	1–1.5
	Buccal (peds)	10–15 microg/kg	10–20	30	1–1.5
Sufentanil	IV	0.01	1–3	3–5	0.5–1
Alfentanil	IV	0.75	1–3	1.5–2	0.2–0.3
Meperidine	IV	100	5–7	10–20	2–4
	IM	100	15–60	30–60	2–3
	PO	200	15–60	60–120	2–3
Codeine	PO	200	15–30	60	4–6
Oxycodone	PO	30	15–30	60	4–6
Hydromorphone	PO	7.5	15–30	60	2–3
Methadone	PO	20	15–30	30–60	3–4

to self-medicate and is associated with a high degree of patient satisfaction. Total drug use is less than when opioids are administered by a physician or nurse.[23] PCA has been studied in burn patients and found to be effective.[24,25] Although morphine is useful for both background and procedural pain, side effects such as urinary retention and decreased gastrointestinal motility may occur. Shorter-acting opioids are useful for procedural pain, but accumulation may occur with repeated dosing so the patient should be closely monitored.

Fentanyl. Fentanyl may be given via the oral, nasal, and transdermal routes of administration. The pharmacokinetic profile of transbuccal fentanyl is similar to its profile following intravenous administration, therefore patients should be similarly monitored.[26] Transbuccal fentanyl has not been studied in burn patients, however anecdotal reports indicate its usefulness in both pediatric and adult patients. The fentanyl analogs, alfentanil and sufentanil, have shorter half-lives than fentanyl and may be useful for brief procedures. They have not been studied in burn patients.

Partial agonists/mixed agonists–antagonists. Partial agonists and mixed agonists–antagonists, such as butorphenol and nalbuphine, have the advantage of having a ceiling effect on side effects such as respiratory depression and gastrointestinal dysmotility. However a ceiling effect also exists for analgesia, therefore limiting the usefulness of these agents in burn patients. Certainly they can be considered for a burn patient experiencing lesser amounts of pain. Butorphanol may also be administered intranasally but there is a ceiling effect on its analgesic properties.

Benzodiazepines

Anxiety commonly occurs in patients with burn injuries and is often intensified during dressing changes and wound care. Benzodiazepines can be used to reduce anxiety and may be given concomitantly with opioids to aid in the management of both background and procedure pain. However, benzodiazepines are believed to potentiate the effects of opioids, both the analgesic effects and the potential for respiratory depression.[27] Pharmacokinetic studies of *diazepam* and *lorazepam* in burn patients demonstrate that diazepam had a shorter hypnotic effect than lorazepam owing to its high lipid solubility and rapid tissue uptake.[14] The elimination half-life of diazepam was prolonged, thus repeated doses may result in prolonged sedation.

Midazolam has a more rapid onset than diazepam and lorazepam, a shorter elimination half-life and a low incidence of phlebitis and

Table 18.3   Commonly-used benzodiazepines

Drug	Route of administration	Dosage (mg)	Onset (min)	Peak effect (min)	Duration (min)
Diazepam	IV	1–5	1–5	10	15–60
	IV	5–10	15–30	30–60	180–240
	PO	10–20	20–30	30–60	180–240
Midazolam	IV	1–2.5	1–3	15	120–240
	IM	2.5–5.0	15	30–60	60–120
Lorazepam	IV	0.5–2.0	15–20	60–90	12–24 h
	IM, PO	2–4	60–120	60–120	12–24 h

IM, intramuscular; IV, intravenous; PO, by mouth.

would be appropriate for patients undergoing procedures. Intravenous midazolam (0.08 mg/kg) and fentanyl (4–8 microg/kg) were given together over 5 to 10 minutes to 256 patients with burns prior to dressing changes.[28] A restrospective review showed that 'superior' pain relief was described by patients and staff, patients were more responsive to physical therapy post-dressing change, and respiratory depression did not occur. The pharmacokinetics of midazolam in burn patients have not been studied. Commonly-used benzodiazepines are listed in Table 18.3.

Ketamine

Ketamine is a potent analgesic agent that does not produce respiratory depression when given to burn patients in subanesthetic doses (0.5–1.0 mg/kg).[29] Ketamine is commonly used in pediatric patients undergoing burn dressing changes and wound debridement and has proven to be a safe and effective analgesic.[30,31] Tolerance develops and patients may experience unpleasant emergence reactions. These reactions are more common in adults and the incidence can be decreased by pre-treatment with a benzodiazepine. Other side effects include increased oral secretions, tachycardia, and systemic and pulmonary hypertension. Medical personnel unfamiliar with ketamine need to be advised that eye movements and vocalizing under ketamine do not indicate patient awareness.

Nonsteroidal anti-inflammatory drugs

Nonsteroidal anti-inflammatory drugs (NSAIDs) are useful in managing mild-to-moderate pain. NSAIDs have an additive effect when given as adjuncts to opioids[32,33] and may be useful when the

opioid dose must be decreased because of adverse opioid side effects. NSAIDs may be given orally and intravenously. The pharmacokinetics of oral ibuprofen after burn injury was examined in 10 patients.[34] The half-life varied from 1.4 to 5.1 hours, with the reported half-life of ibuprofen suspension being 1.8 to 2 hours. Enteral administration resulted in levels below the targeted 10–20 microg/mL for the traditional 6-hour dosing interval. Ibuprofen may attenuate the post-burn hypermetabolic response.[35] Adverse effects of NSAIDs include gastrointestinal bleeding, prolonged bleeding times, and impaired renal function. There is one case report of a 71-year-old woman with a 12% TBSA burn who experienced transient renal insufficiency after receiving diclofenac 50 mg tid for 8 days.[36] Thus, NSAIDs should probably be used cautiously in patients with burn injuries.

Inhalational agents

Nitrous oxide is an inhalation agent that may be used for wound debridement and dressing changes and provides satisfactory analgesia in a 50% concentration with 50% oxygen.[37] Nitrous oxide has a rapid onset and short duration of action.

In a report on 24 patients who received 50% nitrous oxide and 50% oxygen along with morphine, 0.25 mg/kg prior to debridement, patients were randomly divided into two groups to receive either nitrous oxide/oxygen or compressed air.[38] Patients were also allowed to use nitrous oxide/oxygen for non-study debridement periods. 20 patients withdrew from the study because they felt they were getting inconsistent pain relief on study days.

Side effects associated with nitrous oxide include nausea, giddiness, increased verbalizations, dream-like states, and non-specific tremors. Changes in liver function have not been reported. A case of progressive myelopathy has been reported in a 23-year-old male who received 40 000 L of nitrous oxide on an as-needed basis over a 3-month period.[39] He developed bilateral foot drop, bilateral hand weakness, and his symptoms progressed to leg weakness, diarrhea, and impotence. 6 months after discharge, all symptoms except for the leg weakness resolved. However, such side effects are uncommon with short-term administration. Environmental contamination is of concern as scavenging is not available with portable nitrous oxide delivery systems.

Methoxyflurane and enflurane are fluorinated inhalational agents demonstrated to provide satisfactory analgesia for procedures in burn patients, but their usefulness is limited by the risk of nephrotoxicity.

Other adjuvants

It has been observed that anti-depressant drugs, particularly tricyclics, can be useful in patients with certain kinds of chronic neuropathic pain.[40] The mechanism appears not to be the anti-depressant action and smaller doses are used. Although this approach has not been studied in burn patients, there may be a role for tricyclics, since part of burn pain may be neuropathic as a result of reorganization of nerve tissue.

Regional analgesia

Regional anesthetic techniques have a limited role in burn patients. Critically-ill burn patients may be hypotensive and septic and the injuries may be widespread, precluding the use of regional techniques.

When regional anesthesia is not contraindicated, excellent analgesia may be obtained for both background and procedural pain. Local anesthetics administered through an epidural catheter cannot only provide anesthesia for operative procedures but also for analgesia for dressing changes and wound debridement. A disadvantage is that long-term administration of local anesthetics results in tachyphylaxis. Epidurally- and intrathecally-administered opioids may provide excellent analgesia for 12 to 24 hours following a single injection.[41] Upper and lower extremity regional blocks may be used for operative proce-

dures and an indwelling catheter may be used to provide postoperative analgesia.

Non-pharmacologic management of burn pain

It has long been recognized that psychological factors play a large role in an individual's perception of pain. When patients continue to report severe pain despite receiving sufficient quantities of opioids and/or anxiolytics, incorporating non-pharmacologic pain control techniques into burn patient management is useful. Consideration should be given to incorporating these techniques as soon as the patient is sufficiently alert to participate.

In a study examining the efficacy of morphine for relief of pain and anxiety at rest and with hydrotherapy, patients who received no morphine or morphine derivatives were found to have lower levels of pain and anxiety than the patients who received morphine. It is hypothesized that morphine administration increased attention to the pain experience, and that patients relied on morphine for pain relief while excluding other coping mechanisms such as distraction techniques. Additionally, the expectation of the patient and staff is that morphine administration will relieve pain. If pain relief does not occur, anxiety and pain may increase. Though not specifically studied, it is possible that coping techniques aided patients in the 'no morphine' group and contributed to the lower pain scores.[42]

Cognitive interventions

Cognitive interventions attempt to influence the way a patient perceives a painful sensation and consist of reappraisal and distraction techniques. Reappraisal techniques teach patients to reinterpret the meaning of painful sensations, for example, choosing to perceive that pain during wound debridement is not harming or injuring the patient, but instead is allowing healing to occur; or imagining that the affected area is numb. Distraction techniques encourage patients to focus on something other than the pain. This can be a place or a pleasantly remembered experience, or can be done by listening to music, watching a video or concentrating on the surroundings, for example counting ceiling tiles. To achieve this most patients need some help and training to determine on what specifically they will focus.

The evidence on the usefulness of cognitive therapies is not clear, perhaps because in such a study investigators cannot be sure that control subjects are not using cognitive therapies of their own invention.

Preparatory information technique

Preparatory information technique attempts to alter a patient's appraisal of a painful procedure, to make it more benign and less anxiety-producing. It involves describing the procedure and the expected sensations to the patient, and it has been shown to reduce pain and anxiety.[43,44] This approach works well with some, but not all patients.

Behavioral techniques

Behavioral techniques include relaxation, hypnotherapy, and behavior reinforcement approaches. Hypnosis may facilitate procedural pain control.[45] Hypnotherapy has been studied in burn patients and while some patients do obtain pain relief, the evidence is largely anecdotal.[45,46] There have been small studies comparing hypnosis with no hypnosis. One study showed a reduction in pain medication usage in the hypnosis group. This was more pronounced in children aged 7 to 18.[47] Another study showed a decrease in Visual Analog Scale measurements for pain during debridement compared to the previous debridement after hypnosis, but no decrease in the controls.[48] For hypnosis to be successful, a therapist is needed and adequate time must be provided for the intervention.

Relaxation and biofeedback techniques have been studied in pediatric patients with severe burns and it has been concluded that anxiety and pain are reduced as compared to the control group.[49]

Obviously, there are many situations where these non-pharmacologic approaches will not help: very young children, semi-conscious or confused patients, and patients resistant to suggestion. Some burn centers now use parent participation during painful procedures in pediatric burn patients.[50,51] Although no study has shown a measurable advantage, caretakers and parents who participate seem to feel it to be a useful strategy. It should not be undertaken without consent and preparation of the parent.

For any of these techniques to be utilized to their full potential, a clinical psychologist–therapist is necessary. However, health care providers need not have special training to suggest and/or enhance a patient's own strategy. It is easy in a brief conversation to come upon an image attractive to a patient and then continue to reinforce it, or to find a video that an adolescent patient likes and use it during procedures. Some patients will accept suggestion readily and benefit. These therapies may well be enhanced by appropriate pharmacological agents (see also Ch. 15).

SUMMARY

The management of pain in the burn patient requires an understanding that there is no 'standard' burn pain. Therefore, pain management strategies must accommodate acute pain, pain associated with therapeutic procedures, and pain that may occur after healing is complete. Psychological factors may alter and worsen the pain experience in burn patients, thus psychological interventions may be useful adjuncts.

More research is necessary in describing burn pain mechanisms, evaluating pain, and treating pain in the burn patient. Ongoing research in developing opioids with better side effects profiles and efficacious non-opioid analgesics will also lead to better pain management.

REFERENCES

1. Brigham PA, McLoughlin E. Burn incidence and medical care use in the United States: estimates, trends, and data sources. J Burn Care Rehabil 1996; 17: 95–107.
2. Perry S, Heidrich G. Management of pain during debridement: a survey of U.S. burn units. Pain 1982; 13(3): 267–280.
3. Melzack R. The McGill Pain Questionnaire: major properties and scoring methods. Pain 1975; 1(3): 277–299.
4. Choiniere M, Melzak R, Rondeau J, et al. The pain of burns: characteristics and correlates. J Trauma 1989; 29(11): 1531–1539.
5. Willis WD. The orgin and destination of pathways involved in pain transmission. In: Melzak R, Wall PD, eds. Textbook of pain. New York: Churchill Livingstone; 1984: 88–97.
6. Meyer RA, Campbell JN. Myelinated nociceptive afferents account for the hyperalgesia that follows a burn to the hand. Science 1981; 213: 1527–1529.

7. Aldrete JA, Ghaly R. Delayed sympathetically maintained pain caused by electrical burn at the current's entry and exit sites. J Pain Symptom Manage 1994; Nov9(8): 541–543.

8. Isakov E, Boduragin N. Reflex sympathetic dystrophy of both patellae following burns. Burns 1995; 21(8): 616–618.

9. Atchison NE, Osgood PF, Carr DB, et al. Pain during burn dressing change in children: relationship to burn area, depth and analgesic regimes Pain 1991; 47(1): 41–45.

10. Doctor JN, Patterson DR, Summer G, et al. Psychological factors that influence pain reports during hospital stay for patients recovering from severe burn. (Abstract) J Burn Care Rehabil 1997; 18 Part 3: S82.

11. Roberts ML, Pruitt BA. Nursing care and psychological considerations. In: Artz CP, Moncrief JA, Pruitt BA, eds. Burns: A team approach. Philadelphia: WB Saunders; 1979: 371–392.

12. Moncrief JA. Burns. N Engl J Med 1973; 288(9): 444–454.

13. Wilmore DW, Goodwin CW, Aulick LH, et al. Effect of injury and infection on visceral metabolism and circulation. Ann Surg 1980; 192(4): 491–504.

14. Martyn J. Clinical pharmacology and drug therapy in the burned patient. Anesthesiology 1986; 65(1): 67–75.

15. Perry S, Heidrich G, Ramos E. Assessment of pain in burned patients. J Burn Care Rehabil 1981; 2: 322–326.

16. Heidrich G, Perry S, Armand R. Nursing staff attitudes about burn pain. J Burn Care Rehabil 1981; 2: 259–261.

17. Furman WR, Munster AM, Cone EJ. Morphine pharmacokinetics during anesthesia and surgery in patients with burns. J Burn Care Rehabil 1990; 11(5): 139–141.

18. Silbert BS, Lipkowski AW. Enhanced potency of receptor-selective opioids after acute burn injury. Anesth Analg 1991; 73(4): 427–433.

19. Perry S, Inturrisi CE. Analgesia and morphine disposition in burn patients. J Burn Care Rehabil 1983; 4: 276–279.

20. Osgood PF, Szyfelbein SK. Management of burn pain in children. Pediatr Clin North Am 1989; 36(4): 1001–1003.

21. Alexander L, Wolman R, Blache C, et al. Use of morphine sulfate (MS Contin) in patients with burns: a pilot study. J Burn Care Rehabil 1992; 13: 581–583.

22. Herman RA, Veng-Pederson P, Miotto J, et al. Pharmacokinetics of morphine sulfate in patients with burns. J Burn Care Rehabil 1994; 15(2): 95–103.

23. White PF. Use of patient-controlled analgesia for the management of acute pain. JAMA 1988; 259(2): 243–247.

24. Kinsella J, Glavin R, Reid WH, et al. Patient-controlled analgesia for burn patients: a preliminary report. Burns Includ Therm Inj 1988; 14(6): 500–503.

25. Choniere M, Grenier R, Paquette C. Patient-controlled analgesia: a double-blind study in burn patients. Anaesthesia 1992; 47(6): 467–472.

26. Streisand JB, Varuel JR, Stanski DR, et al. Absorption and bioavailability of oral transmucosal fentanyl citrate. Anesthesiology. 1991; 75(2): 223–239.

27. Bailey PL, Pace NL, Ashburn MA, et al. Frequent hypoxemia and apnea after sedation with midazolam and fentanyl. Anesthesiology 1990; 73(5): 826–830.

28. Kyff JV, Prasad JK. Use of intravenous fentanyl and midazolam for dressing changes in burned patients. Presented at the Twenty-first Annual Meeting of the American Burn Association, New Orleans, Louisiana. March 29–April 1, 1989.

29. Slogoff S, Allen GW, Wessels JV, et al. Clinical experience with subanesthetic ketamine. Anesth Analg 1974; 53(3): 354–358.

30. Sage M, Laird SM. Ketamine anaesthesia for burns surgery. Postgrad Med J 1972; 48(357): 156–161.

31. Groeneveld A, Inkson T. Ketamine. A solution to procedural pain in burned children. Can Nurse 1 1992; 88(8): 28–31.

32. Beaver WT. Aspirin and acetominiphen as constituents of analgesic combinations. Arch Intern Med 1981; 141: 293–300.

33. Sushine A. Analgesic efficacy of two ibuprofen–codeine combinations for the treatment of postepisiotomy and postoperative pain. Clin Pharmacol Ther 1987; 42: 374–380.

34. Cone JB, Wallace BH, Olsen KM, et al. The pharmacokinetics of ibuprofen after burn injury. J Burn Care Rehabil 1993; 14(6): 666–669.

35. Wallace BH, Caldwell FT Jr, Cone JB. Ibuprofen lowers body temperature and metabolic rate of humans with burn injury. J Trauma 1992; 32: 154–157.

36. Jonsson CE, Ericsson F. Impairment of renal function after treatment of a burn patient with diclofenac, a non-steroidal anti-inflammatory drug. Burns 1995; 21(6): 471–473.

37. Baskett PJ. Analgesia for the dressing of burns in children: a method using neuroleptanalgesia and entonox. Postgrad Med J 1972; 48(557): 138–142.

38. Filkin SA, Cosgrav P, Marvin JA, et al. Self-administered anesthesia: a method of pain control. J Burn Care Rehabil 1981; 2: 33–34.

39. Hayden PJ, Hartemink RJ, Nicholson GA.

Myeloneuropathy due to nitrous oxide. Burns Includ Therm Inj 1983; 9(4): 267–270.

40. Egbunike IG, Chaffee BJ. Antidepressants in the management of chronic pain syndromes. Pharmacotherapy 1990; 10: 262–270.

41. Cousins MJ, Mather LE. Intrathecal and epidural administration of opioids. Anesthesiology 1984; 61(3): 276–310.

42. Foertsch CE, O'Hara MW, Kealey GP, et al. A quasi-experimental, dual-center study of morphine efficacy in patients with burns. J Burn Care Rehabil 1995; 16: 118–126.

43. Moss BF, Everett JJ, et al. Psychologic support and pain management the burn patient. In: Richard RL, Staley MJ, eds. Burn care and rehabilitation: Principles and practice. Philadelphia: FA Davis; 1994: 475–498.

44. Everett JJ, Patterson DR. Cognitive and behavioral treatments for burn pain. Pain Clin 1990; 3: 133–145.

45. Margolis CG, DeClement FA. Hypnosis in the treatment of burns. Burns 1980; 5: 253.

46. Patterson DR, Questad KA, de Lateur BJ. Hypnotherapy as an adjunct to narcotic analgesia for the treatment of pain for burn debridement. Am J Clin Hypn. 1989; 31(3): 156–163.

47. Wakeman JR, Kaplan JZ. An experimental study of hypnosis in painful burns. Am J Clin Hypn 1978; 21: 3–12.

48. Patterson DR, Everett JJ, Burns GL, et al. Hypnosis for the treatment of burn pain. J Consult Clin Psychol 1992; 60(5): 713–717.

49. Knudson-Cooper MS. Relaxation and biofeedback training in the treatment of severely burned children. J Burn Care Rehabil 1981; 2102: 109.

50. Doctor ME. Parent participation during painful wound care procedures. J Burn Care Rehabil 1994; 15(3): 288–292.

51. George A, Hancock J. Reducing pediatric burn pain with parent participation. J Burn Care Rehabil 1993; 14(1): 104–107.

Trauma patient with thoracic and abdominal injuries

Raymond S Sinatra and Sean J Ennevor

Introduction

Anatomy and physiology

Thoracic and upper abdominal trauma

Nociceptive responses associated with thoracic
   and upper abdominal trauma
   Peripheral sensitization
   Central facilitation
   Sympathoadrenal activation
   Neuroendocrine responses
   Deep venous thrombosis

Phases of thoracic trauma
   Emergent phase
   Acute phase
   Rehabilitative phase
   Chronic phase

Parenteral analgesic techniques
   Traditional on-demand administration
   Intravenous patient-controlled analgesia

Neuroaxial analgesia
   Technical considerations

Intermittent dosing
Continuous epidural infusions
Patient-controlled epidural analgesia
Contraindications and adverse effects

Neural blockade for acute pain management
   Infiltration
   Intercostal nerves blockade
   Interpleural analgesia
   Paravertebral block
   Central neural blockade

Oral analgesics

Other techniques

Clinical evaluations

Recommendations for optimal pain management
   following thoracic trauma

Pain control and diagnostic interference

Conclusion

INTRODUCTION

Of the various forms of violent and accidental trauma, injuries to the thorax and upper abdomen are associated with significant morbidity, long-term disability, and some of the highest mortality.[1,2,3,4,5] The causes of thoracoabdominal or torso injury include penetrating etiologies such as knives, missiles, and other foreign bodies, and blunt trauma including deceleration injuries, crush injuries, and direct blows. Regardless of the traumatic cause, the resultant organ and musculoskeletal damage may be extensive and associated with severe, often debilitating, pain.[2,6,7]

Blunt and penetrating chest trauma is associated with a spectrum of injuries including pneumothorax, hemothorax, myocardial and pulmonary contusions, and rib, scapular, and clavicular fractures.[1,2] Serious injuries occurring with lower incidence include rupture of the thoracic aorta, and bronchial, tracheal, esophageal, and diaphragmatic tears. Injuries to the brachial plexus, recurrent laryngeal nerve may also occur (Table 19.1).[1,2]

Upper abdominal injuries include laceration and blunt compressive injuries to the liver and spleen which present with upper quadrant pain, intra-abdominal internal hemorrhage, and shock. Injuries to stomach, duodenum and pancreas are less likely to result in hemorrhagic shock but are nevertheless associated with significant morbidity.[1,8] Abdominal trauma is investigated radiographically, or by peritoneal lavage, and may require extensive laparotomy to control hemorrhage, resect devitalized tissues, and to drain digestive fluids.

Poorly controlled pain following thoracoabdominal trauma can evoke a number of pathophysiologic responses which can adversely affect patient outcome and duration of hospital stay. The presenting symptomatology is influenced by the extent of the injury and the physical status of the patient. Patients may present with severe musculoskeletal dysfunction, hemorrhagic shock, alterations in pulmonary mechanics, and life-threatening cardiovascular instability.[8]

Thirty to forty years ago, patients presenting with thoracic trauma were managed with external traction and stabilization. Avery et al[9] pioneered the use of mechanical hyperventilation to decrease morbidity and mortality following serious injury to the thorax. Nevertheless, studies performed in the 1970s in patients with flail chest[3] demonstrated an 87% incidence of pulmonary infection, and a mortality rate of 30%. Improved ventilators that allowed intermittent mandatory ventilation (IMV) with positive end-expiratory pressure (PEEP) provided additional clinical benefits; however, the morbidity and mortality rate in patients with flail chest remained high, until Trinkle et al[5] developed the concept of spontaneous ventilation and aggressive treatment of pulmonary injuries. A significant component of their management included optimization of analgesia using a combination of intravenous morphine and intercostal nerves blocks. In recent years the importance of optimal pain control in restoring pulmonary mechanics and increasing ambulation in an effort to minimize atelectasis and pneumonia has become widely recognized.[7,10,11] Thus, anesthesiologists and other acute pain specialists are now commonly consulted to provide pain control and minimize pathophysiologic responses in posttraumatic settings which include rib fractures, flail chest, and pulmonary injury (see Ch. 14).[7,10,12,13]

ANATOMY AND PHYSIOLOGY

Prior to choosing the modality of pain control a thorough understanding of the musculoskeletal and the neural innervation of thorax and upper abdomen is needed.

The thorax is an osteocartilaginous frame providing protection to the principal organs of respiration and circulation. The thoracic cavity is formed by the sternum and 12 pairs of ribs, attached to thoracic vertebra. True ribs articulate directly with the sternum via costal cartilage, while the lower five pairs, false ribs, do not. The last two sets of ribs, 11 and 12, terminate in cartilaginous tips embedded in the abdominal wall.[14]

The most inferior portion of the thoracic cavity is formed by the diaphragm. This structure is a dome-shaped, muscular-fibrous septum that moves in accordance with respiration, enlarging or contracting the thoracic cavity as needed.[8] Through the cavity pass structures that are potential targets for injury including the esophagus, inferior vena cava, and the abdominal aorta. The thoracic cage and diaphragm function as a unit to promote ventilation, and cough, as well as altering cardiopulmonary physiology.[1,8,15] Thoracic expan-

Table 19.1 Incidence of thoracic injuries found in closed thoracic trauma*

Injury type	Incidence (%)
Fractured ribs Myocardial contusion Pulmonary contusion	> 50
Hemopneumothorax Flail segment Thoracic wall contusion	10–50
Fractured thoracic spine Ruptured thoracic aorta Ruptured diaphragm Pulmonary laceration Fractured sternum	< 10
Ruptured trachea or main bronchus Ruptured innominate artery Ruptured pulmonary artery or vein Hemopericardium Ruptured esophagus Disrupted aorta or tricuspid valve	Rare

*Data summarized from references[1-3].

sion decreases intrathoracic pressure and air flow resistance, allowing air to enter the pulmonary tree.[15] Respiratory excursions are greatest in the sternally attached ribs. Vertebralchondral ribs not only increase the size of the thorax, but also allow for an increase in upper abdominal space. This is essential, since upper abdominal viscera are displaced by diaphragmatic excursion.

Diaphragmatic excursion is responsible for almost all tidal volume during quiet respiration.[15,16] Deep inspiration is characterized by more active contraction of the scalene and intercostal musculature, and diaphragm. Quiet expiration is predominantly the result of elastic recoil of the lungs and the thoracic wall, while forceful expiration requires contraction of the abdominal muscles. This raises intra-abdominal pressure moving the diaphragm up and drawing the lower ribs downward and medially.[16]

Sensory, motor, and sympathetic innervation of the thorax evolves from the 12 pairs of thoracic ventral rami. Innervation of the thoracic wall is provided predominantly by the third to sixth intercostal nerves, while the next five innervate the thorax as well as the upper abdominal wall. Intercostal nerves one and two supply the axilla and upper arm. Each intercostal nerve, at the level of two to six, gives rise to a collateral, and a lateral cutaneous branch (Fig. 19.1). Lateral cutaneous branches of nerves three to six, pierce the intercostals obliquely, and innervate the region between the anterior axillary line and midclavicular line.

The intercostal space is of critical importance, since it provides access to ventral neural rami for clinical intervention. Bony landmarks of the space are defined by the angle of the rib, which is the most superficial part of the rib, and the sub-

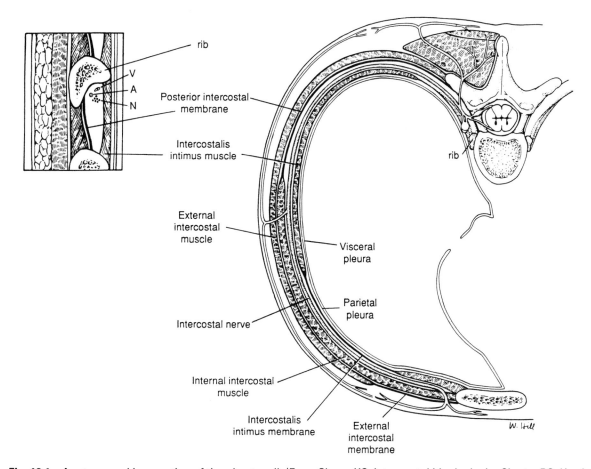

Fig. 19.1 Anatomy and innervation of the chest wall. (From Chung KS. Intercostal blockade. In: Sinatra RS, Hord AH, Ginsberg B, Preble LM, eds. Acute pain mechanisms and management. St Louis: Mosby-Yearbook; 1992: p 358, Fig. 32.1, with permission.)

costal groove, which is the inferior notched aspect of the rib that extends 15 cm beyond the spinous process. Triangular in appearance, the intercostal space is largely filled with fat, through which run the intercostal vein, artery, and nerve, from cephalad to caudad. The space is specifically defined by the subcostal groove, the posterior intercostal membrane, and by the intercostalis intimus. An external intercostal muscle lies posterior to the triangular space and the space is further protected by the relatively impervious intercostal membrane. It is this membrane that prevents the spread of local anesthetic outward after infiltration into the intercostal space. In contrast, the intercostalis intimus is permeable, and allows for the diffusion of compounds into adjacent intercostal spaces, and the subpleural space[17,18] (Fig. 19.2).

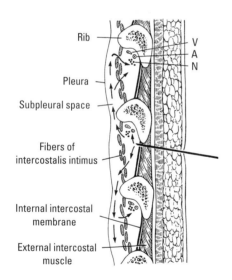

Fig. 19.2   Anatomy of the intercostal space. Notice the thin, non-continuous, structure of the intercostalis intimus and the thick, aponeurotic, internal, intercostal membrane; the former is permeable to local anesthetic solutions. Local anesthetic continuously infused at one interspace can spread to adjacent spaces, blocking 3–5 intercostal nerves. Extent of spread is volume dependent. (From Chung KS. Intercostal blockade In: Sinatra RS, Hord AH, Ginsberg B, Preble LM, eds. Acute pain mechanisms and management. St Louis: Mosby-Yearbook; 1992: 359, Fig. 32.2, with permission.)

THORACIC AND UPPER ABDOMINAL TRAUMA

The anterolateral portion of the thorax is more prone to injury, than the more heavily muscled posterior portion.

Lung contusion is common following blunt trauma to the thorax, but also results from the blast effect of penetrating trauma and high velocity missiles.[1,2] Contusion and associated interstitial edema or hemorrhage may significantly decrease lung compliance, and create a functional shunt that limits pulmonary venous oxygenation. If the traumatic event compromises the integrity of the chest wall or the visceral pleura, a communication between the atmosphere and the pleura may occur. This communication provides a conduit of air that serves to disrupt the balance between the outward expansion and inward recoil of the chest wall. Lung parenchyma eventually collapses causing a pneumothorax, and if the air leak accumulates with each negative inspiratory effort, a tension pneumothorax may occur.[1,2,3] Hemorrhage following disruption of the pleura or chest wall may result in a hemothorax. Hemothorax can accommodate approximately one-third of a patient's blood volume leading to severe hypotension. Compression of the underlying lung results in altered compliance and derangement of the tissues responsible for elastic recoil.[15] If hemothorax is large enough, compression of the contralateral lung can occur by displacement of mediastinal structures.

Compressive trauma to the thorax frequently results in rib fracture at its weakest structural point, which is just in front of the angle of the rib.[1,2] Direct impact may fracture a rib anywhere, and as a result the broken jagged ends may be directed inward and damage thoracic or upper abdominal organs. Periosteal injury is further aggravated during continued respiratory movement of the thorax. Injury may also occur at the costovertebral, sternocostal, interchondral, costochondral, or sternal joints, and can invoke dramatic pain responses, secondary to rich innervation of these structures. Sternal fractures are less common since the ribs provide effective suspension and shock absorption.

Flail chest is the abnormal movement of the chest wall following fracture of two or more ribs in two places on the same side. During inspiration the floating segment moves paradoxically inward upon the lung, preventing adequate expansion, and the reverse occurs during spontaneous exhalation.[1,2,12,13,15] Alterations in chest wall motion reduce lung compliance and require an increased work of breathing if effectual respiration is to be achieved. Splinting, secondary to pain, exaggerates this process by decreasing respiratory effort and furthers this process of unopposed elastic lung recoil. Perfusion is maintained to this unventilated portion of lung, assuming no pulmonary vasculature damage from the trauma. A shunt then develops leading to hypoxia, and severe respiratory distress.[1,15]

Penetrating trauma to the torso between the nipple line to below the costal margin may injure either thoracic or upper abdominal organs or the diaphragm itself, since the diaphragm and associated thoracoabdominal contents move over 15 cm between full inspiration and exhalation.[8]

Blunt, high force trauma may result in diaphragmatic rupture. Since the liver functions as a stabilizing mass, the majority of ruptures occur on the left side. Extensive diaphragmatic disruption results in significant thoracic dysfunction and ineffectual respiration.[19] Small or large tears allow for abdominal viscera to enter the thorax with resultant pulmonic compression. Small tears may entrap and strangulate the stomach, small bowel, spleen, omentum, liver, and kidney.[8,20,21] Inhibition of diaphragmatic function is a major factor responsible for respiratory dysfunction and morbidity following acute thoracoabdominal injury. The precise mechanism underlying diaphragmatic dysfunction is unknown; however, afferent nociception from the diaphragm, chest wall, and upper abdominal viscera result in reflex inhibition of phrenic nerve motor drive.[19,22–24]

Pain associated with thoracic and upper abdominal trauma as well as procedural intervention is effort-dependent (dynamic) reflecting pleuritic and diaphragmatic injury as well as reflex spasm of the chest wall (secondary hyperalgesia).[8,25] As was previously mentioned, severe postsurgical pain and diaphragmatic irritation that follow thoracotomy and extensive upper abdominal exploration may compromise pulmonary function to a greater extent than the presenting injury. Thoracic and upper abdominal injuries result in significant deterioration of pulmonary function, especially in the presence of hyperalgesia and splinting.

Acute alterations in pulmonary function were first described by Beecher[26] who examined pulmonary responses to upper abdominal surgery. Acute alterations included an increase in respiratory rate and diminution in tidal volume (TV), vital capacity (VC), functional residual capacity (FRC), and forced expiratory volume (FEV_1) (Fig. 19.3).[26,27,28] Reductions in FEV_1 and FRC are most pronounced during the first 24 hours following injury. The magnitude of change is directly related to the degree of pain and site of trauma. In this regard, the percentage reduction in TV, VC, and FEV_1 is highest after upper thoracic injury and upper abdominal exploration and lowest in patients recovering from extra-abdominal, non-thoracic procedures.[26,28] Poorly controlled dynamic pain is associated with shallow inspirations, an inability to cough effectively and clear secretions.[1,4,8,28,29] Atelectasis, progressive airway closure, and ventilation-perfusion mismatch are common post-traumatic events that lead to clinically significant hypoxemia and hypocapnia.[1,8,27] As the patient becomes fatigued, acute respiratory failure with hypercarbia and respiratory acidosis mandate intubation and mechanical ventilation.

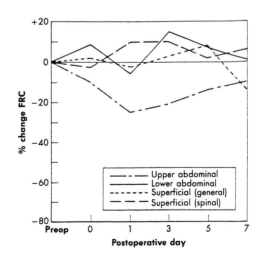

Fig. 19.3 Changes in functional residual capacity (FRC) relative to preoperative values in patients recovering from different surgical procedures. Significant decreases were observed after upper abdominal surgery. (From Ali J. Am J Surg 1974; 376–382, reprinted with permission.)

Despite such support, adult respiratory distress syndrome and pneumonia are frequent complications that lead to prolonged hospitalization and patient mortality.[1–3,6]

NOCICEPTIVE RESPONSES ASSOCIATED WITH THORACIC AND UPPER ABDOMINAL TRAUMA

Pain perception or nociception reflects activation of nociceptors following thermal, mechanical or chemical injury, eventual afferent transmission to the spinal cord dorsal horn, and relay to supraspinal centers for processing and reaction.[30] Pain perception from the thorax can be divided into two major components. The first is a sensory discriminative component, which describes the location and quality of the stimulus, and is transmitted via myelinated A-δ fibers, (see Ch. 3 for further discussion of neural innervation etc.). The second, termed the affective–motivational component is more slowly conducted via peripheral unmyelinated C fibers and is responsible for the suffering and emotional components of pain.[25,30]

Although splinting and other pain-related behaviors serve to limit further tissue injury and promote wound healing, subsequent alterations in physiology and emotional responses are less desirable in post-traumatic settings[25] (Table 19.2). The

Table 19.2 The acute injury response: potential benefits versus disadvantages following severe trauma

Beneficial effects	Adverse effects
1. Maintenance of blood pressure, maintenance of cerebral perfusion	1. Hypertension, hemorrhage, stroke
2. Maintenance of cardiac output	2. Tachycardia, arrhythmias, cardiac ischemia, congestive heart failure
3. Maintenance of intravascular volume	3. Hypercoagulable state, increased risk of infection and deep venous thrombosis
4. Enhanced hemostasis	4. Hyperglycemia, negative nitrogen balance
5. Substrate mobilization, enhanced energy production	5. Hypervolemia, hypernatremia hypokalemia
6. Immobilization, minimizing further tissue injury	6. Reduction in respiratory volumes or flow rates, hypoxia, pneumonia
7. Learned avoidance behavior	7. Anxiety, fear, demoralization, prolonged convalescence

following physiologic responses may increase pain intensity and associated morbidity following acute injury in thoracic trauma.

Peripheral sensitization

Following the injury, a local neurohumoral reflex is established whereby bradykinin, prostaglandin, and substance P sensitize nociceptors immediately adjacent to the site of tissue damage resulting in a heightened inflammatory response, neurogenic edema, and hyperalgesia.[25,31,32] Continued sensitization secondary to compression, pleural inflammation, infection, and hematoma may lead to a progressive worsening of acute pain, development of persistent pain syndromes, and impaired rehabilitation.[25,32,33] Nociceptor sensitization may also elicit reflex motor and sympathetic responses that result in severe muscle spasm myofascial pain, vasoconstriction, and sympathetically maintained pain (Fig. 19.4). The goal of providing optimal pain management is to break this cycle.[33–36]

Central facilitation

Central facilitation describes an enhancement of synaptic transmission and nociceptive processing within the dorsal horn that accentuate hyperalgesia. Central facilitation is initiated by the action of substance P and excitatory amino acids such as aspartate and glutamate upon N-methyl-D-aspartate (NMDA) receptors.[36] The initial phase, termed 'wind-up', is characterized by an immediate increase in dorsal horn wide dynamic range (WDR) firing rate. This is followed by a second phase, termed 'long-term potentiation', in which WDR neurons exhibit enhanced and prolonged sensitivity to noxious stimulation.[35,36] Clinical manifestations associated with central facilitation include secondary hyperalgesia, the elaboration of ipsilateral and contralateral flexion reflexes (splinting), and alterations in regional sympathetic tone.[25,31,32] As a result, pain is perceived in dermatomes above and below the site of injury. This situation is worsened by continuous, yet essential, respiratory movements and forceful secretion-clearing actions of the chest wall and upper abdomen.

Sympathoadrenal activation

In addition to effects on pulmonary function, poorly controlled pain, is associated with anxiety,

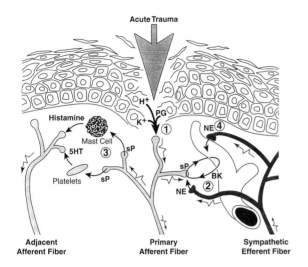

Fig. 19.4   Peripheral responses to acute injury: (1) Following tissue injury, potassium, serotonin, and histamine released from damaged cells, and bradykinin released from damaged vessels activate the terminal endings of sensory afferent fibers (nociceptors). Bradykinin (BK) initiates prostaglandin (PG) release at nociceptive endings. Prostaglandin has been implicated in nociceptor sensitization, further increases in vascular permeability, and primary hyperalgesia. (2) Orthodromic transmission in sensitized afferents results in the release of substance P (sP) in and around the site of injury. Substance P is responsible for further release of BK. (3) Substance P also stimulates histamine release from mast cells, and 5HT from platelets which, in turn, activate additional nociceptors and exacerbate the inflammatory response. (4) Reflexes mediated by sympathetic efferents may sensitize nociceptors directly via secretion of noradrenaline (NA), indirectly via further release of BK and PG, or by localized vasoconstriction. (Modified from Fields HL, Basbaum AI. Endogenous pain control mechanisms. In: Wall PD, Melzack R, (eds. Textbook of pain. New York: Churchill Livingstone; 1989: 206–217, with permission.)

important causal factor for cardiac morbidity and stroke, particularly in patients with poorly compensated coronary and cerebral artery disease.[35,37–39] Reductions in circulation have been associated with impaired wound healing, enhanced sensitization of nociceptors, increased muscle spasm, and visceral–somatic ischemia and acidosis.[25,35] These negative effects are further compounded following thoracic trauma, particularly in settings of myocardial or great vessel injury.

Neuroendocrine responses

Severe pain following acute thoracoabdominal injury can activate neuroendocrine responses and alter hypothalamic–adrenal function.[32,40,41] This 'stress response' to injury is characterized by elevations in plasma cortisol, glucagon, and epinephrine levels resulting in glycogenolysis, hyperglycemia, and a negative nitrogen balance.[32,42–44] While providing the injured organism with short-term benefits of enhanced energy production, prolonged tissue catabolism may adversely affect post-traumatic outcome.[41,42] Metabolic responses to trauma have been well described, and include an initial phase in which the metabolic rate is depressed.[41–43] In 24 to 48 hours post-injury, a catabolic phase exists with increased metabolic activity leading to mobilization of glycogen stores, carbohydrates, proteins, and fats.

Energy expenditure is known to be increased in trauma, starvation states, severe infections, or burns. Increased sympathetic tone is a major determinant of increased energy expenditure, which fuels elevations in cardiac output, and blood pressure.[38,42,44] Catecholamine outflow, and its sometimes deleterious effects, can be mediated, via effective pain control.[32,39,42] especially when cardiovascular and pulmonary systems have stabilized.

Deep venous thrombosis

The likelihood for deep venous thrombosis increases in settings where severe effort-dependent pain limits ambulation, and decreases venous return.[25,35,45] It has also been demonstrated that catecholamines, angiotensin, and factors associated with severe acute pain, increase platelet adhesiveness, leading to a hypercoagulable state.[45] This combination of venous stasis and hypercoagulabil-

sleeplessness, and release of stress hormones and catecholamines that can have deleterious effects upon patient outcome. The magnitude and duration of this response is directly related to the extent of the injury.[32,37,38] Pathophysiologic changes associated with increased sympathetic tone include tachycardia, hypertension, and altered circulation. Cardiovascular instability is an

ity increases risk of clot formation and deep venous thrombosis. The pathophysiologic response to acute pain is presented in Figure 19.5.

PHASES OF THORACIC TRAUMA

In an effort to minimize post-traumatic morbidity and mortality, patients presenting with serious thoracic injuries require optimal pain control at each phase of their recovery. Modalities for the pain control are varied in complexity and overall efficacy is dependent upon the severity of the injury and the organ system involved, be it musculoskeletal, skin, or visceral. When possible, the severity of pain prior to and following therapy should be assessed with a standardized method of analysis including visual analog and verbal descriptor scales.[46,47]

Pain management is determined not only by the presenting injury, but often by the necessary medical procedural interventions.[47] For instance,

not only does the noxious periosteal and ligamentous pain of a rib fracture need to be addressed, but also the iatrogenic pain associated with chest tube insertion or thoracotomy.[1,15] At this point, optimal pain control can prevent splinting, and help re-establish baseline pulmonary function. The same premise is evident in following upper abdominal injuries; for instance, patients suffering blunt abdominal trauma may require an extensive exploratory laparotomy for diagnosis and treatment of acute abdomen.

The pain specialist can assist in the recovery from the traumatic injury (see Ch. 14) as well as a painful procedural interventions, which further compromise respiratory effort. Optimal pain control also the physiotherapy (including chest wall percussion, deep breathing, incentive spirometry, and range of motion exercises) needed to maintain adequate ventilation and prevent atelectasis or pneumonia.[1,48]

The initial traumatic event can be subdivided

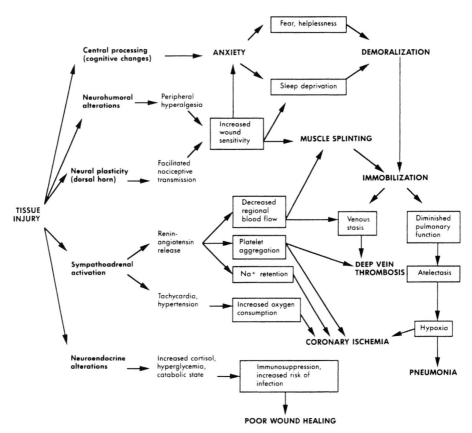

Fig. 19.5   An outline of pathophysiological responses associated with surgical trauma and their impact upon key target organs. (From Sinatra RS. The pathophysiology of acute pain. In: Sinatra RS, Hord AH, Ginsberg B, Preble LM, eds. Acute pain mechanisms and management. St Louis: Mosby-Yearbook; 1992: 54, with permission.)

into phases, which can be utilized in formulating a plan for pain intervention. The *emergent phase* which focuses on stabilizing vital signs and stabilization of pulmonary function; the *acute phase* where optimization of analgesia is the critical key to continued stabilization of pulmonary function; the *rehabilitative phase* where effective pain control improves exercise tolerance; and finally, the *chronic phase* where patients return to baseline function.

Emergent phase

The emergent phase starts with first contact with the patient and includes stabilization of the patient's airway, breathing, and circulation. Advanced trauma life support protocols (ATLS) are typically followed and control the patient's respiratory and cardiovascular system. Patients presenting with thoracic trauma may also suffer head injuries leaving them unconscious. The response to pain in the unconscious patient is that of hypertension, tachycardia, diaphoresis, and pupillary dilatation.[47] Paradoxically, a vagal response to pain may result in bradycardia, as well as hypotension.

The benefit of acute pain at this early interval is that it limits movement and further damage to injured anatomy.[1,8,25,47] Sympathetic response to injury may support blood pressure and cardiac output in patients who have lost large volumes of blood. This initial benefit may become a significant detriment if myocardial oxygen consumption (secondary to increased heart rate contractility), and afterload outstrips ventilation and vascular supply.[32,37–39]

Treatment of pain is initiated in the emergency room, operating room, or intensive care unit (ICU), provided the patient's ventilatory and cardiovascular status can appropriately be maintained. Care must be taken to treat pain, and not agitation. Nevertheless, judicious use of short-duration sedatives which reduce conscious perception may provide benefits particularly in tachypneic and highly anxious patients.[49]

Acute phase

Aggressive pain management provides greatest clinical benefits during the acute phase. Therapy is based upon the patient's injuries and clinical presentation. Many clinical situations may preclude one modality versus another (Table 19.3). For instance, patient spinal fractures may contraindicate intrathecal/epidural placement, while continuous chest tube suctioning reduces the

Table 19.3 Methods of controlling pain following thoracoabdominal trauma at various phases of recovery

Phase	Primary therapy	Adjunctive therapy
Emergent phase[1]	1. IV morphine (1–2 mg q10–30 min) 2. IV fentanyl (12.5–50 microg q10–30 min)	1. Ketamine 5–25 mg PRN 2. Diazepam 1–2 mg PRN 3. Midazolam 0.5–1 mg PRN
Acute phase[1]	1. Continuous epidural analgesia[2] (bupivacaine, fentanyl, hydromorphone) 2. IV-PCA[3] (morphine, hydromorphone, fentanyl) 3. Intercostal blockade 4. Interpleural infusions 5. Paravertebral block	1. NSAIDs 2. Anxiolytics
Rehabilitative phase	1. IV-PCA 2. Switch to oral opioid analgesics (morphine, oxycodone) 3. Transdermal fentanyl	1. NSAIDs 2. Transdermal clonidine 3. Tricyclic anti-depressants
Chronic phase	1. Oral opioids (PRN) 2. NSAIDs 3. Local anesthetic injections 4. Corticosteroids injections	1. Tricyclic anti-depressants 2. Anti-convulsants (Gabapentin)

[1]Administer analgesics to treat pain not agitation.
[2]Clear cervical spine for fractures, assess coagulation status.
[3]Not for use in agitated or confused patients.
IV-PCA, intravenous patient-controlled analgesia; NSAIDs, Nonsteroidal anti-inflammatory drugs.

effectiveness of interpleural analgesia. The ultimate goal in aggressively treating pain is to help limit cardiopulmonary morbidity and mortality. Other important goals include reducing the need for intubation and ventilatory support, the duration of ICU stay, and overall hospitalization costs.

Rehabilitative phase

The transfer of the patient from the ICU to the ward usually signals the initiation of the rehabilitative phase. Patients may continue to be affected by alterations in pulmonary or cardiovascular mechanics depending upon the mechanism of injury and remain susceptible to pneumonia, myocardial dysfunction, and deep venous thrombosis.[1,47]

Continuation of nerve blocks, epidural, or intravenous analgesia may proceed on wards where nurses have been trained to manage such therapy, or new techniques initiated as the patient's clinical status allows. For example, the patient may now have regained consciousness, possess a spinal fracture now deemed to be stable, or no longer be coagulopathic. In settings where epidural analgesia is to be maintained for periods longer than 5 days, a catheter placed 7–10 cm subcutaneously is recommended to reduce risks of epidural infection. A number of analgesic adjuncts may be employed to augment opioid-mediated analgesia[35,44] including nonsteroidal anti-inflammatory agents (NSAIDs), transdermal clonidine, tramadol, and nightly doses of tricyclic anti-depressant drugs.

Chronic phase

Thoracic trauma patients may be troubled by chronic skeletal, visceral, or neuralgic type pain. Costochondral injuries often take months to years to heal, or may never heal. Injections of corticosteroids and local anesthetics at the affected costochondral joints may provide symptomatic relief, permit physical therapy, and speed healing.[1,45] Neuropathic pain secondary to intercostal nerve neuromas, or myofascial pain syndromes created by the initial injury or the procedural trauma, also require prolonged intervals until resolution of symptoms.

Patients may require a chronic pain consultation and treatment with a series of intercostal steroid/local anesthetic blocks and oral-administered modulators of neuropathic pain including tricyclic anti-depressants and anti-convulsants. Aggressive pain management during the chronic phase can be crucial, so that the neuropathic pain syndromes such as reflex sympathetic dystrophy or causalgia may be avoided.

PARENTERAL ANALGESIC TECHNIQUES

Traditional on-demand administration

Intramuscular (IM) and intravenous (IV) analgesic regimens are commonly employed during the emergent and rehabilitative phases of thoracic injury. While most physicians are comfortable with the ease and simplicity of on-demand (PRN) administration schedules, pain control is often delayed, and effectiveness is generally suboptimal.[52–54]

These deficiencies are poorly tolerated by patients suffering severe dynamic pain. The length of time patients wait for analgesia is dependent upon the nursing workload at the time of the request.[52] When the level of pain is deemed significant to warrant treatment, the nurse must requisition the medication, prepare an injection, and administer the dose. The drug must then be absorbed from the IM or subcutaneous (SC) site of administration, and activate central nervous system (CNS) receptor sites. These steps delay the onset of effective relief and worsen pain-induced anxiety, helplessness, and sleep deprivation[55] (Fig. 19.6).

A second problem associated with PRN dosing is its inability to maintain therapeutic plasma concentrations. Doses are rarely adjusted for pharmacokinetic/pharmacodynamic variables including inter-individual differences in pain perception, age, weight, and body surface.[55,56] Despite these deficiencies, PRN doses of IV and IM opioids administered by trained critical care professionals remain the analgesic technique of choice during the acute phase of recovery from thoracic trauma.

Administration of opioids as intravenous boluses eliminates absorption variabilities associated with IM or SC dosing and shortens the delay to peak analgesic effect; however, the high dose frequency is labor-intensive.

Continuous intravenous infusions are less labor-intensive and overcome other shortcomings observed with intermittent IM- or IV-dosing regimens.[16] Intravenous infusions of morphine (1–5 mg/h) or fentanyl (50–200 microg/h) are particularly useful in patients who remain intubated

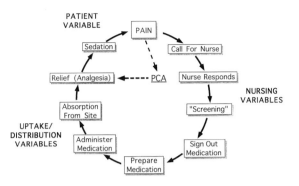

Fig. 19.6 The traditional acute pain cycle as managed with intramuscular or intravenous 'PRN' doses of opioid analgesics. Patient-controlled analgesia avoids nursing pain dispensing as well as the uptake and distribution variables, thereby eliminating the cycle. (From Preble LM, Guveyan J, Sinatra RS. Patient characteristics influencing postoperative pain management. In: Sinatra RS, Hord AH, Ginsberg B, Preble LM, eds. Acute pain mechanisms and management. St Louis: Mosby-Yearbook; 1992: 144, with permission.)

as they provide effective pain control and a level of sedation that facilitates mechanical ventilation. Drawbacks associated with continuous opioid infusions include tolerance development requiring an increased infusion rate, and a progressive increase in plasma levels of drug which may lead to excessive sedation and respiratory depression. In this regard, depression of the cough reflex and progressive depression of respiratory rate remain the most feared complications associated with parenterally administered opioids and are the principal cause of intentional under-medication of pain. Careful patient monitoring including continuous oxygen saturation monitoring during the acute and emergent phases can prevent these complications.

Morphine remains the standard opioid analgesic for control of thoracic injuries as it effectively blocks musculoskeletal and visceral pain. Onset of analgesia is appreciated within 5 minutes after IV and 15 minutes following IM and SC administration while duration ranges from 2 to 4 hours depending upon dose and site of administration. Administration of morphine may release histamine and has been associated with hypotension and biliary colic.

Hydromorphone and meperidine provide effec-

tive alternatives in patients intolerant of morphine. Doses of meperidine exceeding 1 g/day may result in seizures secondary to accumulation of its excitatory metabolite, normeperidine. The parenteral potency of meperidine is one-tenth that of morphine with a duration of effect that is only two-thirds as long. Hydromorphone is three to six times as potent as morphine with an equivalent duration of effect.

Fentanyl and alfentanil have been advocated for use in patients with marked hemodynamic instability as parenteral administration has minimal effects on the cardiovascular system.

Other parenteral agents employed during acute and emergent phases include sedative hypnotic agents such as midazolam, diazepam and lorazepam, and the disassociative analgesic, ketamine.[49]

Mixed agonist–antagonist and partial agonist opioids, including nalbuphine and butorphanol, have been prescribed for control of acute thoracic trauma as they possess a ceiling effect for respiratory depression. Unfortunately, these agents also possess an analgesic ceiling and generally provide poor pain control during the emergent phase following injury.

Parenteral forms of NSAIDs have become available (ketorolac, diclofenac) and offer analgesic potentiation of opioid-based therapy or regional blockade.[50] NSAIDs reduce pain intensity by reducing prostaglandin synthesis at the peripheral site of injury as well as by effects on pain processing in the CNS.[57] These agents are particularly useful in managing post-traumatic musculoskeletal pain and pleuritic irritation and are not associated with excessive sedation or respiratory depression. Major side effects, including increased risk of hemorrhage, gastric ulceration, and renal toxicity limit their usefulness during the acute and emergent phases following injury.

Intravenous patient-controlled analgesia

Patient-controlled analgesia (PCA) allows patients to titrate small doses of pain medication in amounts proportional to a perceived pain stimulus (also see Ch. 11).[55,58,59] Such therapy avoids cycles of excessive sedation and ineffective pain control observed with either on-demand or 'by the clock' IM dosing, and limits variabilities related to inappropriate screening, delays in administration, and drug absorption[55,59] (see Fig. 19.6). PCA delivery compensates for the fact that pain intensity associated with thoracic injuries is rarely constant, and is intensified by movement and physical therapy, coughing, and incentive spirometry.

Since opioid dose and dosing interval are titrated by the patient, optimal analgesic concentration is more likely to be maintained while interindividual variations in pharmacokinetics and pain perception are more easily accommodated.[55,59,60] An opioid 'loading' dose, which provides baseline plasma levels of analgesic, is administered prior to initiating PCA. The patient-activated bolus dose initiates a lockout interval ranging from 5 to 10 minutes, during which time a second bolus cannot be delivered. Morphine remains the most widely administered PCA analgesic for controlling thoracic musculoskeletal pain.[58,59] Other suitable agents include rapid-acting, intermediate-duration opioids including hydromorphone, meperidine, and oxymorphone.[55,59]

A continuous (basal) opioid infusion may be added to supplement patient-controlled delivery. This form of administration may improve pain control and sleep patterns. It is generally offered to intubated patients, patients recovering from extremely painful injuries, and individuals presenting with some degree of opioid tolerance. Patients receiving basal opioid infusions should be carefully observed since continuous (non-patient controlled) delivery may increase the risks of adverse effects.[59]

IV-PCA is commonly employed during the emergent phase following thoracic trauma in awake–alert patients. Such therapy may be offered to selected alert–oriented, intubated patients where it offers acceptable pain relief and increased satisfaction, but may not reduce the stress response to acute injury.[40] A number of adjunctive agents and interventions including NSAIDs, clonidine, and intercostal nerves block may be employed to provide multimodal analgesia, thereby improving the effectiveness of IV-PCA while reducing dose-dependent side effects.[50] IV-PCA dosing guidelines are presented in Table 19.4.

NEUROAXIAL ANALGESIA

Technical considerations

Epidural administration of opioids, local anesthetics, and opioid–local anesthetic combinations offers a level of pain control and improved pulmonary performance following thoracoabdominal injury that is unsurpassed by alternative analgesic techniques.[61–65] Whenever possible the epidural catheter should be placed at the level of the neuraxis immediately adjacent to the site of injury, particularly when lipophilic opioids or local anesthetics are administered.[65,66]

The high thoracic approach is employed for upper thoracic and clavicular fractures and requires epidural catheter placement at an interspace between T1 and T4.[16] The epidural space is entered with the patient in the sitting position. Placement is facilitated by employing a 40° angle of insertion, an off-midline approach, and a saline loss of resistance technique. Dilute solutions of local anesthetic and segmentally acting opioids such as fentanyl or sufentanil are utilized for analgesia. Midthoracic approaches utilizing interspaces between T5 and T9 are most commonly employed for control of pain following thoracic and upper abdominal trauma. Because of the steep overhang of the thoracic spines, a paramedian approach with 50° angle of needle insertion is generally required to ensure placement (Fig. 19.7a).

Table 19.4 Dosing guidelines for IV-patient-controlled analgesia

Opioid	Concentration	Loading dose	Incremental bolus dose	Lockout interval	Basal infusion (Rate)	Comments
Morphine	1 mg/mL	3–10 mg	0.5–1.5 mg	6–8 min	0.5–1.5 mg/h surgical pain	Major abdominal/orthopedic
Meperidine	10 mg/mL	25–50 mg	5–15 mg	6–8 min	not recommended	Useful for visceral pain, limit dose to 600 mg/24 h
Hydromorphone	0.2 mg/mL	0.5–1 mg	0.1–0.3 mg	6–8 min	0.1–0.3 mg/h	Rapid onset, fewer side effects than morphine or meperidine
Fentanyl	20 microg/mL	30–100 microg	10–20 microg	5–6 min	10–20 microg/h	Rapid onset, short duration of effect, requires basal infusion

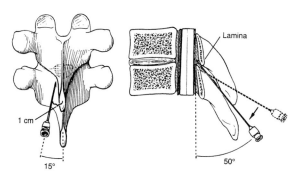

Fig. 19.7a   Needle placement for thoracic epidural analgesia; (1) midline approach may be difficult in the mid-thoracic region (T6–T8); (2) paramedian approach. Notice the steep orientation of the spinous processes and recommended angle of needle insertion. (From Wagner F. Thoracic epidural anesthesia. In: Hoerster W, Kreushcher H, Niesel HC, Zenz M, eds. Regional anesthesia. 2nd ed. St Louis: Mosby-Yearbook; 1990: 167, Fig. 137, with permission.)

One exception is the T6 interspace (directly in line with the lower tip of each scapula) which is usually well defined and permits midline insertion.

A variety of opioid analgesics including fentanyl, hydromorphone, and morphine alone or in combination with bupivacaine may be administered as bolus doses or continuous infusion.

Low thoracic and upper lumbar approach utilizes interspaces between T10 and L2 for control of pain following upper abdominal and lower thoracic trauma. A 20–30° angle of needle insertion and 'loss-of-resistance' technique is employed. Morphine and hydromorphone are commonly administered at this site as they provide a greater rostral spread of analgesia than the more segmental effects of highly lipophilic opioids such as fentanyl (also see Ch. 12).[66]

Intermittent dosing

Preservative free morphine in doses ranging from 5–8 mg can be administered via lumbar catheters for control of pain following upper abdominal surgery. Hydrophilic morphine molecules are retained in cerebrospinal fluid (CSF) and spread rostrally to higher levels of the spinal cord, resulting in a widespread non-segmental band of analgesia. Onset of analgesia with epidural morphine is appreciated within 30 to 60 minutes, peak effect

at 90 to 120 minutes, and duration ranges from 8 to 16 hours.[66–68]

Thoracic administration of morphine offers more efficient relief of pain originating at higher dermatomal segments. Patients treated with thoracic epidural (T6–7) morphine required significantly less drug than others with lumbar catheters (L2–3) although no intragroup differences in post-thoracotomy pain scores or pulmonary function were detected. In this regard only 3–5 mg morphine provide highly effective analgesia for patients recovering from thoracotomy or acute thoracic trauma.[7,67,68]

Intermittent doses of epidural hydromorphone (0.5–1.5 mg) offer advantages over morphine including a more rapid onset of analgesia and a reduced incidence of adverse effects.[69,70] In patients recovering from thoracotomy, reduction in pain intensity is noted within 15 minutes following administration, peak effect occurs at 30 minutes while duration of effect ranges from 4 to 8 hours.[70] Bolus doses of highly lipophilic opioids (fentanyl 50–100 microg) provide rapid pain relief of limited duration, but may be combined with morphine in an effort to minimize delays in analgesic onset.[67]

Intrathecal bolus doses of morphine provide prolonged analgesia in settings where epidural catheters are contraindicated or technically difficult to place.[71] Morphine dosage ranges from 0.5 mg to over 2 mg in patients who are expected to remain intubated for 24 hours. A major disadvantage of intrathecal morphine is the limited duration of analgesia such therapy provides. Benefits include excellent pain control during the immediate post-traumatic period and a reduction in subsequent overall IV-PCA or IM narcotic dose requirements. One important role for single dose therapy is to provide a pain-free period while weaning a patient off ventilator support.

Continuous epidural infusions

Continuous epidural infusions allow opioid analgesics to be titrated to patient comfort and rapidly terminated if problems should occur. The high CSF concentrations associated with intermittent epidural boluses are avoided and risk of rostral spread/delayed respiratory depression are reduced.[67,72] Other benefits include decreased time spent administering agents and assessing effect, and a reduced risk of contamination and medication errors. Epidural infusions also provide greater therapeutic versatility since shorter-acting opioids and dilute local anesthetic solutions may be continuously administered.[72–74]

In patients recovering from thoracotomy, continuous epidural morphine (0.5 mg/h) infusions provide superior analgesia than intermittent boluses of morphine or bupivacaine.[66,72] Patients receiving continuous infusion experienced less pruritus and oversedation than individuals treated with intermittent doses of morphine and less urinary retention and hypotension than individuals receiving bupivacaine. Epidural infusions of hydromorphone (0.5%) also provide safe and highly effective pain control with less pruritus and oversedation than morphine.[75,76] Continuous epidural infusions of fentanyl have been advocated for pain control following thoracic and upper abdominal injury.[77–79] Administration via thoracic catheters improves epidural specificity, analgesic effectiveness, and reduces total dose requirements.[78–81] Dosing guidelines for intermittent opioid bolus doses and continuous epidural infusions are presented in Table 19.5.

Patient-controlled epidural analgesia

Patient-controlled epidural analgesia PCEA offers improved pain relief with lower opioid dose requirements than IV-PCA, while providing increased control and higher patient satisfaction than either single doses or continuous infusions of epidural opioids (also see Ch. 14).[82]

The technique involves thoracic placement of an epidural catheter, administration of an analgesic loading dose (opioids, local anesthetic, or both), and initiation of patient-activated epidural boluses alone, or in combination with a continuous epidural infusion.

With PCEA, total morphine dose and plasma concentrations required to provide analgesia were significantly less than amounts observed with IV-PCA.[82] Lipophilic opioids including fentanyl, sufentanil, and hydromorphone have also been advocated for control of pain following thoracic injury as they offer greater analgesic titratability and fewer side effects than morphine.

The major advantage of PCEA for patients

Table 19.5 Dosing guidelines for epidural opioid analgesia

Opioid	Site of administration	Intermittent bolus technique*	Continuous infusion technique*	Adjunctive therapy
Morphine	Lumbar catheters for incisions below T8; thoracic catheters for upper abdominal and thoracic surgery	Administer 3–8 mg bolus in 10 mL preservative-free saline every 8–24 h as clinically indicated	2–4 mg bolus followed by infusion (50 microg/mL) at 8–12 mL/h (lumbar catheters), 4–8 mL/h (thoracic catheters)	IV ketorolac 15–30 mg q6 h, epidural bupivacaine (0.1–0.03%)
Hydromorphone	Lumbar catheters for incisions below T8; thoracic catheters for upper abdominal and thoracic surgery	0.5–1.5 mg bolus in 10 mL saline every 5–10 h	0.5–1.5 mg bolus followed by infusion (10 microg/mL) at 8–15 mL/h (lumbar catheters), 4–8 mL/h (thoracic catheters)	IV ketorolac 15–30 mg q6 h, epidural bupivacaine (0.1–0.03%)
Fentanyl	Lumbar catheters for incisions below T12; thoracic catheters for almost everything else	50–100 microg bolus every 2–3 h	50–100 microg bolus followed by infusion (5 microg/mL) at 8–15 mL/h (lumbar catheters), 4–8 mL/h (thoracic catheters)	Ketorolac 15–30 mg q6 h, epidural bupivacaine (0.05–0.1% or less)

*Dependent on age, physical status, height, etc.

Table 19.6 Patient-controlled epidural analgesia dosing guidelines

Opioid	Concentration*	Loading dose**	PCEA dose*	Lockout (min)	Continuous rate*	4-h limit
Morphine	50 microg/mL	2–4 mg	2–4 mL	10–15	6–8 mL/h	40–70 mL
Hydromorphone	10 microg/mL	500–1500 microg	2–4 mL	6–10	6–8 mL/h	40–70 mL
Fentanyl	5 microg/mL	75–100 microg	2–4 mL	6	6–10 mL/h	40–70 mL

*Concentration of infusate solution.

**From preservative-free vial diluted in 10–15 mL sterile saline, loading and PCEA doses are dependent upon site of epidural catheter placement, site and extent of acute trauma, patient physical status.

recovering from thoracoabdominal injuries is the fact that pain control is more selective, opioid exposure is minimized and the incidence of dose-dependent side effects is reduced. In this regard a relatively low baseline infusion rate generally covers pain at rest, while patient-activated bolus doses allow rapid control of brief increases in pain stimulus that follow chest physical therapy, and movement out of bed. Dosing guidelines for PCEA are presented in Table 19.6. A decision tree for managing an epidural infusion is depicted in Fig. 19.7b.

Contraindications and adverse effects

Consideration of epidural analgesia requires assessment of coagulation status, cervical radiographs (to rule out vertebral fractures/instability), and neurological examination. We avoid placement of epidural catheters in patients with con-

sumptive or drug-induced coagulopathy unless the underlying cause is corrected. Other contraindications are infection at the insertion site, septicemia, and coagulopathy.

Cervical spine instability

Cervical spine imaging and clearance are highly desired, but difficult to perform during the acute and early phases of recovery. We will place epidural catheters in patients with uncleared cervical spine films provided they wear a cervical collar, and when a note from the trauma specialist states that the benefits of therapy outweigh associated risks.

Respiratory depression

Respiratory depression is the most feared complication associated with neuroaxial opioids.[67,83,84]

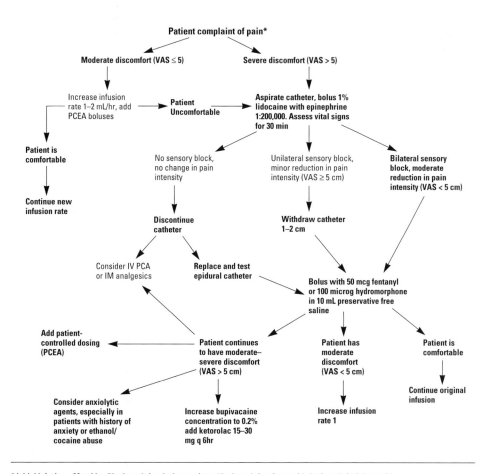

* Initial infusion – Morphine 50 microg/mL or hydromorphone 10 microg/mL or fentanyl 3–5 microg/mL plain or with-bupivacaine 0.05–0.1%; PCEA, patient-controlled epidural analgesia; VAS, visual analog scale score; IV PCA, intravenous patient-controlled analgesia; IM- intramuscular

Fig. 19.7b Decision tree for managing an epidural infusion.

Respiratory depression following administration of epidural or intrathecal morphine occurs at two different intervals.[67,84] An *early phase* observed soon after administration reflects rapid systemic absorption and is of similar magnitude as that noted following parenteral dosing. A *late phase*, more insidious depression occurring after 8 to 12 hours, has been related to rostral flow of CSF and delivery of morphine molecules to the brainstem respiratory centers.[67,84] Mild depression of CO_2 responsiveness is common following administration of 3–5 mg of morphine; however the incidence of clinically significant respiratory compromise has been found to range between 0.1 and 0.4%.[84]

Single epidural or intrathecal boluses of more lipophilic opioids including fentanyl and hydromorphone are not associated with delayed respiratory depression, but 'early onset' depression, usually occurring within 30 minutes of administration, has been observed.[70,85]

The speed with which epidural opioid-induced respiratory depression develops is not fast, but slowly progressive, and is generally preceded by nausea, vomiting, and increased sedation.[67,69,83] Vigilant nursing observation, and documentation of inadequate respiratory effort, slow respiratory rate, or unusual somnolence represents the best form of monitoring. Patients with optimal levels of spinal opioid analgesia will almost always maintain an elevated PCO_2. Unless deemed clinically inappropriate, we set our 'target' at 42–44 mmHg.

Increasing respiratory depression is promptly treated with naloxone (40–80 microg IV) followed by a naloxone infusion (300–400 microg/L of crystalloid every 8 hours). Prophylactic IV infusions of naloxone (400–800 microg/L, at 50–125 mL/h have been advocated to reduce the risk of opioid-induced respiratory depression in elderly or debilitated patients.[1,86,87] In our experience this rate of infusion maintains optimal $PaCO_2$ and level of consciousness while maintaining effective analgesia.

Intoxication

A final concern is related to the fact that thoracoabdominal trauma may be associated with intoxication.[1,2] Patients presenting with a history of ethanol abuse often appear anxious, highly irritable, and dissatisfied with epidural analgesia despite the fact that they are experiencing highly effective pain control. In this setting, anxiolytic therapy and ethanol withdrawal prophylaxis may dramatically improve patient cooperation and satisfaction.

NEURAL BLOCKADE FOR ACUTE PAIN MANAGEMENT

Infiltration

Peripheral neural blockade minimizes exposure to opioids and is ideally suited for patients sensitive to opioid-induced ileus and bowel obstruction. Other indications include avoidance of opioid-induced ventilatory depression, particularly in patients with underlying pulmonary disease.

Peripheral neural blockade is accomplished by a variety of techniques including intercostal blockade, intermittent or continuous, interpleural catheters, or oral medications. Infiltration techniques employ injections of local anesthetic at the site of surgery and offer several hours of post-traumatic analgesia. Injection into wound blockade is useful for chest tube placement and closure of epidermal and subcutaneous injuries. The technique employs an undiluted local anesthetic, such as 0.25–0.5% bupivacaine, infiltrated into skin, subcutaneous tissues, and fascia.[88] More effective and prolonged anesthesia/analgesia may be provided by direct neural blockade or by continuous infusions of local anesthetic into the intercostal, epidural, paravertebral, and interpleural spaces.

In these settings bupivacaine has become the local anesthetic of choice for a number of reasons: (1) dilute solutions provide selective (C fiber) nociceptive blockade while sparing motor fibers;[74,89] (2) tachyphylaxis, or reduction in clinical efficacy with continued administration, develops more slowly with bupivacaine than with other local anesthetics. Bupivacaine dose requirements remain fairly constant during short courses (24 to 36 hours) of therapy,[16,89] thereafter escalation in dose requirements, complaints of inadequate analgesia, and risk of toxicity make it difficult to continue pain management with this agent alone.

Intercostal nerves blockade

Blockade of intercostal nerves T5–T11 offers segmental analgesia, reduces opioid dose requirements, and is particularly useful following traumatic thoracic injury and thoracotomy.[18,90] Intercostal nerves may be blocked either at the angle of the rib or posteriorly at the mid-scapular

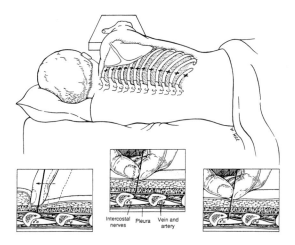

Fig. 19.8 Posterior intercostal nerves block Patient positioning, sites of needle insertion, and retracting finger method of 'walking off' rib to enter the intercostal space. (From Chung KS. Intercostal blockade. In: Sinatra RS, Hord AH, Ginsberg B, Preble LM, eds. Acute pain mechanisms and management. St Louis: Mosby-Yearbook; 1992: 360, Fig. 32.3, with permission.)

line (Fig. 19.8). A 2 inch, blunt-tipped 25 gauge needle is inserted at the lower rib margin and walked off the rib until it pops through the external fascial sheath. Following a negative aspiration of air or blood, 5–6 mL of 0.5% bupivacaine is administered per nerve (see Ch. 14).

In general, nerves at the site of fracture and one to two segments above and below are blocked. To avoid local anesthetic toxicity, no more than six nerves should be blocked per session. The duration of nerve block ranges from 6 to 12 hours during which time the patient benefits from improved pain control and pulmonary function, as well as reductions in opioid dose requirements.[18,90]

Supplemental analgesia is generally required and may be provided by restricted dose IV-PCA morphine or intermittent doses of IV ketorolac (15 mg q6 h/48 h max). In addition to risks of pneumothorax and lung perforation, a major drawback of the technique is the high local anesthetic dose requirement. In this regard therapeutic doses of bupivacaine may be associated with plasma levels which approach toxicity.[18]

Continuous intercostal blockade provided by infusions of bupivacaine (0.125–0.25%) administered via an 19 gauge epidural-type catheter offers effective pain relief for patients recovering from rib fracture, and mini-thoracotomy. At high rates of infusion (8–12 mL/h), the local anesthetic solution spreads to intercostal and paravertebral spaces above and below the site of administration providing multisegmental blockade[18,91,92] (see Fig. 19.2). The technique is relatively easy to perform as well as being more efficient, less labor-intensive, and potentially safer than multiple intercostal blocks.

Continuous intercostal blockade can be used when epidural placement is contraindicated (coagulopathy, neuroaxial injury). In contrast to epidural blockade, continuous intercostal analgesia does not block sensory/motor, sympathetic, and sacral parasympathetic nerves and is not associated with cardiovascular instability, urinary retention, and lower extremity weakness. Patients with multiple rib fractures and concomitant head injuries have presumed contraindications for intravenous opioids or thoracic epidural analgesia. Neurologic assessment can be difficult when intravenous opioids are administered, and a dural puncture or spinal injury during the placement of a thoracic epidural could result in significant morbidity. Graziotti[91] reported that intercostal catheterization and continuous blockade was beneficial in patients with head injuries and multiple rib fractures.

A recent variation of the technique termed 'patient-controlled intercostal analgesia', adds self-administration of bolus doses to supplement the continuous intercostal infusion. This combination allows patients to titrate additional medication in response to an increase in pain stimulus, and allows a reduction in the basal infusion rate.[93]

Interpleural analgesia

Interpleural analgesia provides a therapeutic option in managing pain localized to the thorax and upper abdomen.

The technique is for patients who would be at more than the usual risk for opioid-induced respiratory depression.[17,94-98] Interpleural dosing requires insertion of 17 gauge Tuohy epidural needle at the anterior axillary line and placement of a 19 gauge, open-tip, epidural catheter (Fig. 19.9). A distinct click is noted following penetration of the parietal pleura and is associated with a loss of resistance noted in a saline-filled syringe.[17,96,97] The catheter is carefully advanced 3–5 cm (toward the shoulder) and taped in place. 2 mL increments of bupivacaine 0.5% are injected every 2 to 3 minutes (also see Ch. 14).[17]

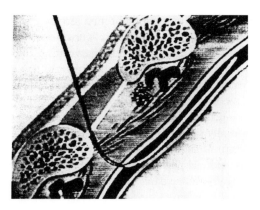

Fig. 19.9 Computed tomogram of a properly inserted interpleural catheter. The catheter penetrates skin, external and internal intercostal muscles and fascia, and parietal pleura and is advanced 6–8 cm in the space between visceral and parietal pleural surfaces. Placement over the superior edge of the rib minimizes trauma to the intercostal neurovascular bundle. (From Rocco A, Reiestad F, Gudman J, et al. Interpleural administration of local anesthetics for pain relief in patients with multiple rib fractures – Preliminary report. Reg Anaesth 1987; 12: 10–13, with permission.)

The mechanism of action of interpleural analgesia includes back diffusion of local anesthetics through the parietal pleura producing multiple intercostal blocks.[16,17,94,97] Additional effects include direct blockade of pleural nerve endings and paravertebral and/or epidural effect resulting from the accumulation of local anesthetic in the posterior thoracic cage. In general, pain relief is noted within 5 to 10 minutes following administration of 15–30 mL of 0.5% bupivacaine. The interval between intermittent doses varies between 4 to 8 hours and is associated with high plasma bupivacaine levels immediately following rebolus.

Continuous interpleural infusions of bupivacaine 0.25% (at a rate of 8–10 mL/h), are less labor-intensive and offer reduced dose requirements and greater analgesic uniformity than intermittent dosing.[99] Rocco et al[98] noted that interpleural infusions of 0.25% bupivacaine (5–10 mL/h) did not provide complete pain relief, in patients presenting with multiple rib fractures, while 0.5% bupivacaine at similar rates of infusion resulted in subjective pain relief and unilateral analgesia to pinprick. In a double-blind, placebo-controlled study, Schneider et al[100] questioned the effectiveness of interpleural analgesia in controlling pain following thoracotomy. They found no significant difference in pain relief, supplemental opioid requirements, and pulmonary function/morbidity between patients receiving interpleural bupivacaine or placebo solution.

Interpleural analgesia like other forms of regional analgesia may be associated with 'windows' or regions of less effective analgesia, particularly during cough and chest physical therapy. Patients complaining of inadequate analgesia may benefit from concomitant administration of IV-PCA opioids, and ketorolac. An alternative method of improving pain relief may be gained by adding fentanyl (1–2 microg/mL) to the interpleural bupivacaine infusion.[93]

Placement of interpleural and intercostal catheters are frequently associated with clinically insignificant side effects such as small hematoma, non-leaking lung puncture, or small pneumothoraces. The risk for serious complications such as tension pneumothorax is low but exists irrespective of technique, needle, or syringe used.[16,17,97] We avoid placement of interpleural catheters in patients receiving PEEP ventilation, and individuals with pleural fibrosis, pleural adhesions, pleuritis, pleural effusion, and infection at proposed sites of insertion. Because of local anesthetic volume and concentration constraints, the technique is restricted for use in patients with unilateral thoracic injuries.[95]

Paravertebral block

The thoracic paravertebral space contains the proximal portions of the intercostal nerves and the rami communicantes of the sympathetic nervous system. Injection of local anesthetic (20–30 mL bupivacaine 0.5–0.25%) into this space provides up to 12 hours of unilateral somatic analgesia with some degree of sympathetic blockade.[16,101] Complications associated with paravertebral block include epidural or intrathecal injection with risk of severe hypotension and respiratory insufficiency, and pneumothorax.[16] Continuous paravertebral blockade requires insertion of a 19 gauge catheter and infusion of dilute solutions of bupivacaine. The space is entered by advancing a standard epidural needle off-midline and walking off the transverse process. As the needle penetrates the costotransverse ligament a distinct loss of resistance is noted[101] (Fig. 19.10).

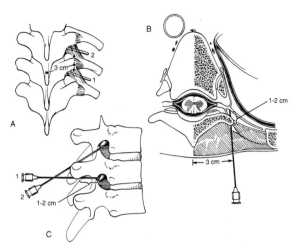

Fig. 19.10 Thoracic paravertebral nerve block. Care must be taken to avoid inappropriate needle placement. (1) The presence of pleura and lung necessitates that needles are not directed laterally. (2) Ribs may be mistaken for transverse processes, advancing a needle beyond them (ribs) will risk pneumothorax.(3) Because the thoracic vertebrae are smaller than those in the lumbar region and nerve root sheaths may extend beyond the intervertebral foramen, care must be taken to avoid unintentional intrathecal or epidural injection. (From Kopacz DJ Regional anesthesia of the trunk. In: Brown DL, ed. Regional anesthesia and analgesia. Philadelphia: WB Saunders; 1996: 309, Fig. 18.11, with permission.)

In a case report[101] a 59-year-old presenting with head injury and subdural hematoma as well as fractures of ribs 1–9 required optimization of pain control to improve pulmonary function while avoiding opioids and NSAIDs that might increase sedation or worsen his neurological status. A diagnostic paravertebral block at the levels of the fourth and seventh thoracic vertebrae provided satisfactory analgesia, and marked improvement in SpO_2. A catheter was then inserted and 10 mL bupivacaine 0.5% was administered every 6 hours for the next 48 hours resulting in resolution of pulmonary distress while permitting continuous neurological assessment.

Central neural blockade

Epidural infusion of local anesthetics or central neural blockade offers highly effective segmental analgesia for patients recovering from traumatic thoracoabdominal injury.[102] The technique avoids exposing patients who are at risk for opioid-induced respiratory depression to this class of analgesic.

Central neural blockade is associated with clinically significant sensory/motor and sympathetic blockade particularly when relatively large amounts of local anesthetic are administered at lumbar interspaces. In this regard, hypotension and impaired micturition occur more frequently with epidural local anesthetics than with opioid analgesics.[16,67,72] To ensure patient safety a balance between optimal pain relief and unacceptable side effects must be reached. This is accomplished by placing the epidural catheters at segments immediately adjacent to the injury (i.e. T3–6 for thoracotomy incision), and infusing dilute solutions of 0.1–0.125% bupivacaine continuously at rates of 5–8 mL/h.

ORAL ANALGESICS

The oral administration of analgesics offers the simplest, safest, least invasive, and least labor-intensive method of controlling pain. Alterations in gastrointestinal function and perfusion that follow traumatic injury markedly reduce the reliability and effectiveness of such therapy particularly during the acute and emergent phases of recovery.[57] However, the oral route of administration offers clinical usefulness during the rehabilitation phase in patients who were initially treated with parenteral or neuroaxial analgesics.

Useful agents include morphine elixir, and hydromorphone and oxycodone tablets for patients who continue to suffer moderate-to-severe pain. Acetaminophen plus codeine and tramadol (50–100 mg) may be prescribed in patients with mild-to-moderate pain, and as supplements to patients treated with regional neural blockade. Sustained-release opioid preparations including morphine sulfate (MS-Contin) and oxycodone (Oxycontin) offer less frequent administration intervals (decreased labor-intensiveness) and greater analgesic uniformity. These preparations are ideally suited for patients suffering discomfort during rehabilitation and chronic pain.

Tramadol is a centrally-acting analgesic that blunts noxious perception via weak interactions at opioid and α-adrenergic receptors. Doses of 50–100 mg provide analgesia comparable to meperidine with a lower incidence of respiratory depression.[103] Combinations of tramadol and NSAIDs may provide more effective pain control. Tramadol offers an analgesic alternative in patients at risk for opioid-induced ileus, and individuals with gastric ulceration or treated with anticoagulants for whom aspirin and NSAIDs may be contraindicated. At present, only an oral dose form of tramadol is available, thus it would only be of use in the rehabilitative and chronic phases of recovery.

Oral transmucosal fentanyl citrate (OTFC) is a lozenge-shaped preparation attached to a plastic stick that provides rapid onset, yet short-lived duration of intense analgesia. The OTFC system offers effective analgesic supplementation during dressing changes and physical therapy. Oral opioid preparations are commonly associated with ileus and constipation. Such therapy should always be supplemented with stool softeners, bulk laxatives, and occasional enemas.

OTHER TECHNIQUES

Oral transmucosal and delivery systems have been introduced for acute pain management.

Transdermal fentanyl is supplied in 25–100 microg/h patches which provide effective and prolonged analgesia. Although disadvantages, including a 6 to 8-hour latency to analgesic onset and progressive narcosis, limit their overall usefulness in acute settings, the preparation may be employed to wean patients off parenteral opioids and for use in patients intolerant of oral opioids.

The use of transcutaneous electric nerve stimulation (TENS) represents a conservative method of reducing periosteal pain and skeletal muscle spasm associated with thoracic injury.[104] The stimulating electrodes may be placed on either side of the fractured rib(s) or adjacent to the site of thoracotomy or upper abdominal incision. Frequencies of 40–70 Hz provide useful pain relief following acute thoracic injury and are well accepted by patients.[105,106] While unable to relieve the most intense aspects of acute pain, TENS provides useful non-pharmacological analgesic supplementation and important reductions in IM, IV-PCA, and epidural opioid dose requirements. TENS may be combined with intercostal block and/or IV ketorolac to offer a more effective analgesic, that has a minimal risk of sedation and respiratory depression.[93]

Temporary destruction of intercostal nerves using cryoneurolysis has been recommended for control of post-thoracotomy pain.[1,16,104,107] The technique is performed with a frozen cryoprobe during surgical exposure. The intercostal nerve is lifted by a hook and contacted by the cryoprobe cooled to $-20°C$, for 20 to 30 seconds. The region of thorax innervated by the nerve is rendered pain-free for up to 2 months until axonal regeneration restores neural function. In general, two nerves above and below the thoracotomy incision must be frozen to obtain effective pain control.[16] Cryoanalgesia by itself may not provide complete pain relief following acute thoracic injury, but decreases in opioid dose requirements and improvements in negative inspiratory force and force vital capacity (FVC) represent important clinical benefits.[104,107]

CLINICAL EVALUATIONS

A variety of pain management modalities have been evaluated for the treatment of thoracoabdominal trauma. In general, the more invasive techniques including epidural and continuous intercostal infusions offer greatest clinical benefit in patients with moderate-to-severe pulmonary dysfunction secondary to rib fractures, flail chest, and lung contusion. Advantages are also observed in elderly high-risk populations, particularly individuals with baseline cardiovascular and pulmonary disease.[32,37–39]

Thoracotomy is associated with among the highest intensity of post-surgical discomfort resulting from incisions of skin, intercostal muscles and parietal pleura, periosteal and ligamentous injury, and pleuritic irritation secondary to chest tubes. Patients recovering from extensive upper abdominal procedures also experience severe pain as well as diaphragmatic irritation and dysfunction. These forms of surgical injury have allowed the benefits of differing analgesic techniques to be evaluated in a more controlled setting than that following traumatic injury.

The advantages of epidural analgesia in patients recovering from thoracic surgery were first recognized by Crawford et al in the early 1950s.[102] Investigations which followed found that patients treated with epidural morphine or morphine–local anesthetic combinations experienced more effective pain control following thoracotomy and upper abdominal surgery, with less sedation, and lower opioid dose requirements than individuals treated with parenteral analgesics.[61,62,68,70,72,75,81] Patients also benefited from improvements in pulmonary flow rates (including FVC, FEV_1, and peak expiratory flow rate), and improved arterial oxygenation.[61,68,70] In patients recovering from upper abdominal surgery, the combination of epidural morphine and dilute bupivacaine resulted in superior pain control and more rapid return of gastrointestinal function than morphine alone, and was associated with less hypotension than more concentrated solutions of bupivacaine alone.[62]

Comparisons of analgesic modalities pitting epidural morphine versus intercostal nerves block (ICNB), interpleural analgesia or intramuscular narcotics have also been performed.[7,64,108–110] Grosmanova et al[108] reported that pulmonary complications following thoracotomy (specifically, atelectasis, hypoxemia, hypercarbia, or hypocarbia) could be minimized regardless of the analgesic technique. In their experience, boluses of IV morphine were equivalent as epidural morphine, provided that effective analgesia was maintained. Richardson et al[7] reported that patients recovering from thoracotomy and treated with either lumbar epidural morphine or extrapleural ICNBs experienced equivalent analgesia and improvements in pulmonary mechanics as compared with parenteral opioid analgesics.

In another study,[110] the safety, analgesic efficacy, and pulmonary benefits of ICNB, interpleural analgesia, and thoracic epidural blockade were evaluated in 40 patients recovering from thoracotomy. Patients in the thoracic epidural group experienced the most effective pain control, lowest requirement for supplemental opioids, and had the lowest plasma levels of epinephrine. This finding was confirmed by Salomaki et al[65] who noted that patients treated with thoracic epidural infusions of fentanyl experienced highly effective pain control as well as inhibition of hormonal and metabolic stress responses. High-risk patients treated with epidural analgesia for recovery following extensive surgical procedures have a lower incidence of infectious complications and pneumonia.[111] These benefits may be related to the fact that patients receiving epidural analgesia had a decreased duration of endotracheal intubation, and a reduced ICU stay with less need for invasive monitoring.

The finding that immune competence is better maintained in patients treated with epidural analgesia may provide an additional factor.

Less information is available at present regarding the benefits of epidural local anesthetics and opioids in the patient with upper abdominal and thoracic trauma. Several uncontrolled evaluations have found that patients treated with epidural analgesia benefit from fewer pulmonary complications, shortened duration of mechanical ventilation and ICU stay, and reduced morbidity/mortality than individuals treated with parenteral narcotics.[6,10–12,112] Excellent control of pain following blunt chest injuries has been observed with epidural doses of bupivacaine, and opioid analgesics including morphine, fentanyl, and hydromorphone.[10–13,93]

In a prospective randomized trial, Luchette et al[13] evaluated the clinical benefits of epidural versus interpleural analgesia in patients presenting with blunt chest wall trauma. Thoracic epidural infusions of bupivacaine (0.125% at 8–10 mL/h) significantly reduced pain at rest and motion, and decreased the need for supplemental narcotic analgesics, compared with interpleural analgesia (20 mL bupivacaine 0.5% every 8 h) (Fig. 19.11). Patients in the epidural group benefited from improved pulmonary function including increased negative inspiratory pressure and TV; however, mild hypotension was a common clinical complication.

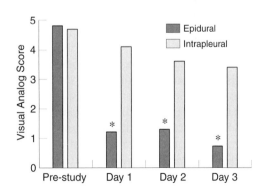

Fig. 19.11 Pain with movement or coughing in patients recovering from thoracic trauma; *significantly less epidural versus interpleural, $P < 0.05$. (From Luchette FR, Radafshan SM, Kaiser R, Flynn W. Prospective evaluation of epidural versus interpleural catheters for analgesia in chest wall trauma. J Trauma 1994; 36: 865–869, Fig. 2.)

Cicala et al[113] compared two different epidural analgesic techniques (bupivacaine 0.5% administered via thoracic catheters and morphine given via lumbar catheters) for pain relief in patients recovering from thoracic trauma. Subjective pain scores decreased in both treatment groups (when compared with pre-epidural treatment with parenteral narcotics).

However, patients treated with bupivacaine benefited from significant improvements in pulmonary function including increased VC and FEV, when compared with individuals receiving morphine. Two of seven patients in the bupivacaine group experienced hypotension. It is unclear why the authors chose not to administer morphine via thoracic catheters where its onset to peak effect is more rapid and its analgesic efficacy is greater.[66,67] This study nevertheless underscores the observation that factors other than pain intensity may be responsible for deterioration in pulmonary function, and that local anesthetic blockade of afferent reflexes may be required to reduce intercostal muscle spasm, and to restore phrenic nerve activity and diaphragmatic contractility. In this regard, epidural opioids by themselves do not improve diaphragmatic dysfunction following upper abdominal surgery despite providing effective pain control.[24] In contrast, thoracic administration of 0.5% bupivacaine (8–12 mL) abolishes phrenic nerve inhibition, improves diaphragmatic tone, and increases TV and VC.[19,23] As observed in patients recovering from thoracotomy and upper abdominal surgery[62] the epidural combination of opioid and dilute bupivacaine may offer the best treatment option for pain control following traumatic injury as it provides additive analgesic and respiratory benefits with a lower risk of hypotension and excessive sedation.

Intravenous morphine has been compared with epidural morphine in trauma patients with flail chest stratified for age, number of ribs fractured, and type of thoracic injury.[112] Patients treated with epidural morphine benefited from improvements in respiratory parameters, such as TV, ICU time, duration of mechanical ventilation, and incidence of tracheostomy. The authors indicated that optimal pain control, in particular a decrease in dynamic pain, was responsible for the improvement in outcome in these patients.

The concept of varying modalities of pain control was studied by Iwama et al[95] who evaluated 12 chest trauma patients treated with interpleural analgesia (since epidural blockade was difficult to induce). All patients had multiple rib fractures, hemopneumothorax, or pulmonary contusion, and thus had thoracostomy tubes in place at time of evaluation. After interpleural analgesia was begun these patients had significant pain relief from their chest sites.

Intercostal and paravertebral catheterization appears particularly useful in patients with multiple rib fractures and head injury. Such therapy is safer than epidural catheterization which requires manipulation of the neuroaxis and may result in dural puncture, and is preferable to large doses of parenteral opioids which can alter mental status.[91,101]

RECOMMENDATIONS FOR OPTIMAL PAIN MANAGEMENT FOLLOWING THORACIC TRAUMA

Patients presenting to Yale New Haven hospital with acute thoracic trauma are aggressively managed by the Acute Pain Service. For the acute phase of thoracoabdominal trauma the patient is given small intravenous doses of fentanyl or morphine titrated to effect. During the emergent phase, optimal pain control is provided with thoracic epidural, continuous regional blockade, or IV-PCA. We remain convinced that thoracic epidural analgesia provides highest analgesic efficacy with an acceptable degree of safety. Benefits, including effective control of dynamic musculoskeletal as well as static incisional pain and high efficacy in terms of low opioid dose requirement, outweigh technical or logistic difficulties and therapy-associated adverse effects.

Epidural morphine and hydromorphone are utilized for pain control following blunt chest trauma and in patients recovering from upper abdominal exploration and thoracotomy. In agreement with previous reports,[44,74,89,115] we have found that the addition of dilute concentrations of bupivacaine improves control of dynamic pain, without increasing the incidence of orthostatic hypotension or interfering with safe-assisted ambulation. This multimodal analgesic combination offers rapid control of pain-associated thoracic and diaphragmatic injury, more effectively blunts the autonomic stress response, and provides greater improvement in pulmonary function than epidural opioids alone.[61,75,93,114]

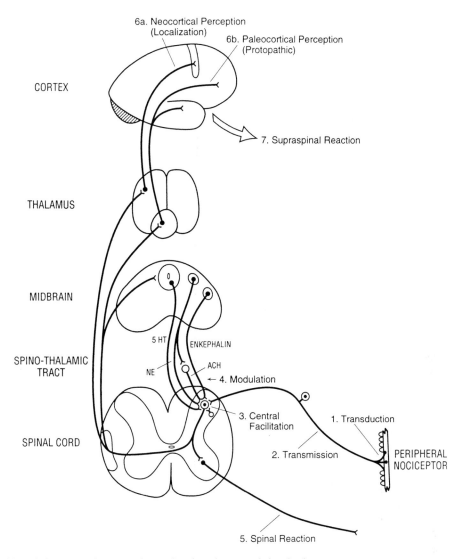

Fig. 19.12 Multimodal approach to treating pain after thoracoabdominal trauma.

1. **Transduction**—refers to the activation of peripheral nociceptors. Transduction is inhibited by NSAID, antihistaminics, and topical local anesthetics
2. **Transmission**—propagation of action potentials from peripheral nociceptive endings to second order cells in dorsal horn. Nociceptive impulses ascend via the spinothalamic tract to reach supraspinal targets. Transmission is blocked by local anesthetics (peripheral/central neural blockade)
3. **Central facilitation**—activation of N-methyl-D-aspartic acid NMDA receptors is associated with increased sensitivity and firing frequency of dorsal horn neurons. Central facilitation is inhibited by NMDA antagonists such as ketamine.
4. **Modulation**—mediated by descending enkephalinergic, adrenergic and cholinergic nerve fibers, which either inhibit release of nociceptive transmitters from primary afferents or blunts responses of second order cells. Modulation is enhanced by neuroaxial administration of opioids, clonidine, and neostigmine
5. **Spinal reaction**—increased motor and sympathetic outflow results in hypertension, tachycardia, adrenal activation, muscle spasm/splinting. Spinal reactions are suppressed by benzodiazepines, β-adrenergic antagonists, and metaclopramide
6. **Supraspinal perception**—includes the neocortical epicritic component which is responsible for pain localization and the paleocortical protopathic component, responsible for severe discomfort, and suffering aspects of pain. Protopathic perception is blunted by opioid analgesics
7. **Supraspinal reaction**—describes neocortical- and paleocortical-limbic responses including fear, anxiety, depression and other pain-related behaviours, and pituitary–hypothalamic responses including release of stress hormones, neuropeptides, and activation of the sympathetic axis. Supraspinal reactions are blunted by regional blockade, adrenergic agonists, and anxiolytics. Consider administration of substrate (glucose, branched chain amino acids) and glucocorticoids to ablate the catabolic responses.

Epidural infusions are administered via lumbar or thoracic catheters and supplemented with dilute concentrations of bupivacaine (see Table 19.12). Bupivacaine is omitted from the epidural infusate in hypovolemic patients at risk for hypotension. Continuous infusions of fentanyl are also administered via thoracic catheters and supplemented with dilute concentrations of bupivacaine.[74,81] PCEA is initiated in alert-oriented patients who have received a loading dose of 0.5–1.0 mg hydromorphone with 0.25% bupivacaine 5–7 mL. A basal infusion of hydromorphone (10 microg–20 microg/mL) at a rate of 5–7 mL/h is started in the SICU. When the patient is extubated, PCA doses of 1–2 mL with a 6-to-8-minute lockout are added. 24 hours following epidural placement the continuous rate is decreased by 50% while the PCA bolus dose is increased as required. Intravenous ketorolac (15 mg q6 h) is used to supplement PCEA hydromorphone unless medical or surgical contraindications exist (also see Fig. 19.7b).

In reviewing records of patients recovering from thoracic trauma and/or thoracotomy and treated with PCEA hydromorphone with 0.03% bupivacaine, more than 90% reported good-to-excellent analgesia.[93] Side effects, especially pruritus, nausea, and sedation were significantly less common than those previously observed with epidural morphine.

In situations where thoracic epidural placement is contraindicated secondary to location of the patient's injuries, incisions, etc., continuous intercostal and interpleural techniques offer useful alternatives. IV-PCA morphine augmented with NSAIDs and other pain modulators represent a less desirable option, that nevertheless provides greater uniformity of pain control than traditional administration of parenteral analgesics. A multimodal approach that provides additive analgesic benefits following thoracoabdominal trauma is presented in Figure 19.12.

PAIN CONTROL AND DIAGNOSTIC INTERFERENCE

Early intervention and multimodal pain control not only limit suffering and associated responses, but often prevent or greatly limit the need for intubation and ventilator support. One question that has been raised is whether such therapy obscures clinical diagnosis. There has been little research performed to answer this question, but case reports have documented asymptomatic worsening of clinical status in patients receiving dense local anesthetic blockade. In this regard, Pond et al[116] reported a case of delayed traumatic splenic rupture that went undetected in a patient receiving interpleural blockade with 1.5% lidocaine and 0.5% bupivacaine. Although the patient manifested signs of hypovolemia, pain of the expanding subcapsular hematoma did not become evident until after interpleural analgesia was discontinued. We avoid concentrated local anesthetics for epidural and peripheral regional analgesia and instead rely upon continuous dilute infusions supplemented with hydromorphone or fentanyl. Such therapy does not obscure progression of clinical signs following trauma or surgery. We have been able to detect wound dehiscence, abscess formation, and hemothorax by changes in the quality or intensity of pain. In patients with head injuries complicating thoracoabdominal trauma, we follow guidelines which employ regional blockade or epidural analgesia while avoiding large doses of parenteral opioids.

CONCLUSION

Poorly controlled pain following thoracic and upper abdominal injury incites several pathophysiologic responses that increase post-traumatic morbidity. By appreciating the severity and character of the pain stimulus, optimal control may be provided at each phase of the recovery process. Analgesic regimens including opioid infusions, IV- and epidural-PCA, and continuous regional blockade not only provide effective pain relief and high patient satisfaction, but also lead to improved pulmonary function, decreased ICU stay, and shortened hospitalization. Large scale investigations are needed to compare analgesic efficacy and outcome benefits versus cost and inherent risks associated with each form of therapy.

REFERENCES

1. Cicala RS. Pain management. In: Grande CM, ed. Textbook of trauma anesthesia and critical care. St Louis: Mosby–Yearbook; 1993: 958–970.
2. Newman RJ, Jones IS. A prospective study of 413 consecutive car occupants with chest injuries. J Trauma 1984; 24: 129–135.

3. Relihan M, Litwin MS. Morbidity and mortality associated with flail chest injury: a review 85 cases. J Trauma 1973; 13: 663–669.

4. Stanik-Hutt JR. Strategies for pain management in traumatic thoracic injuries. Crit Care Nurs Clin of NA 1993; 5: 713–722.

5. Trinkle KJ, Richardson DJ, Franz JL, et al. Management of flail chest without mechanical ventilation. Ann Thorac Surg 1975; 19: 355–363.

6. Wisner DH. A stepwise regression analysis of factors affecting morbidity and mortality after thoracic trauma: Effect of epidural analgesia. J Trauma 1990; 30: 799–804.

7. Richardson J, Sabanathan S, Eng J, et al. Continuous intercostal nerve block versus epidural morphine for postthoracotomy analgesia. Ann Thorac Surg 1993; 55(2): 377–380.

8. Ali J. Torso trauma. In: Hall JB, Schmidt GA, Wood LD, eds. Principles of critical care. New York: McGraw-Hill; 1992: 736–755.

9. Avery EE, Morch ET, Benson DW. Critically crushed chests (a new method of treatment with continuous mechanical hyperventilation to produce alkalotic apnea and internal pneumatic stabilization. J Thorac Surg 1956; 323: 291–298.

10. Dittman M, Keller R, Wolff G. A rationale for epidural analgesia in the treatment of multiple rib fractures. Intensive Care Med 1982; 4: 89–92.

11. Dittman M, Ferstl A, Wolff G. Epidural analgesia for the treatment of multiple rib fractures. Eur J Intensive Care Med 1975; 1(2): 71–75.

12. Johnston JR, McCaughey W. Epidural morphine: A method of management of multiple rib fractures. Anaesthesia 1980; 35: 155–157.

13. Luchette FR, Radafshan SM, Kaiser R, Flynn W. Prospective evaluation of epidural versus interpleural catheters for analgesia in chest wall trauma. J Trauma 1994; 36: 865–869.

14. Hahn MB. Intercostal nerve. In: Hahn MB, McQuillan PM, Sheplock GJ, eds. Regional anesthesia, an atlas of anatomy and technique. St Louis: Mosby; 1996: 241–246.

15. Moulton AL, Greenburg AG. The pulmonary system. In: O'Leary JP, ed. The physiologic basis of surgery. Philadelphia: Williams & Wilkins; 1993: 512–524.

16. Banoub M, Nugent M. Thoracic anesthesia. In: Rogers MC, Tinker JH, Covino BJ, Longnecker D, eds. Principles and practice of anesthesiology. St Louis: Mosby-Yearbook; 1992: 1719–1926.

17. Abraham ZA. Interpleural analgesia. In: Sinatra RS, Hord AH, Ginsberg B, Preble LM, eds. Acute pain mechanisms and management. St Louis: Mosby-Yearbook 1992: 326–339.

18. Chung KS. Intercostal blockade. In: Sinatra RS, Hord AH, Ginsberg B, Preble LM, eds. Acute pain mechanisms and management. St Louis: Mosby-Yearbook; 1992: 357–363.

19. Polaner DM, Kimball WR, Fratacci MD. Thoracic epidural anesthesia increases diaphragmatic shortening after thoracotomy in the awake lamb. Anesthesiology 1993; 79: 808–816.

20. Shulman A, van Gelderen F. Bowel herniation through the torn diaphragm: Intestinal herniation. Abd Imaging 1996; 21: 400–403.

21. Sutter JP, Carlisle RB, Stephenson SE. Traumatic diaphragmatic hernia. Ann Thorac Surg 1967; 3: 136–150.

22. Dureuil B, Viires N, Cantineau J. Diaphragmatic function after upper abdominal surgery. J Appl Physiol 67: 1986; 1775–1780.

23. Mankikian B, Cantineau JP, Bertrand M, et al. Improvement of diaphragmatic function after abdominal surgery. Anesthesiology 1988; 68: 379–386.

24. Simmoneau G, Vivien A, Sartene R. Diaphram dysfunction induced by upper abdominal surgery: Role of postoperative pain. Am Rev Respir Dis 1983; 128: 899–893.

25. Cousins MJ. Acute pain and the injury response: immediate and prolonged effects. Reg Anesth 1989; 14: 162–176.

26. Beecher HK. The measured effect of laparotomy on the respiration. J Clin Invest 1933; 12: 639–650.

27. Marshall BE, Longnecker DE, Fairley HB. Anesthesia for thoracic procedures. Boston: Blackwell Scientific; 1988: 1–90.

28. Ali J, Weisel RD, Layug AB, et al. Consequences of postoperative alterations in respiratory mechanics. Am J Surg 1974; 128: 376–382.

29. Reeder MK, Goldman MD, Loh L, et al. Postoperative hypoxaemia after major abdominal vascular surgery. Br J Anaesth 1992; 68: 23–26.

30. Bonica JJ. Definitions and taxonomy of pain. In: Bonica, JJ ed. Management of pain. Philadelphia: Lea & Febiger; 1990: 18–94.

31. LaMotte RH, Thalhammer JG, Robinson CJ. Peripheral neural correlates of magnitude of cutaneous pain and hyperalgesia. J Neurophysiol 1983; 50: 1–26.

32. Kehlet H. Modification of responses to surgery by neural blockade: Clinical implications. In: Cousins MJ, Bridenbaugh PO, eds. Neural blockade in clinical anesthesia and management of pain. Philadelphia: JB Lippincott; 1987: 145–190.

33. Crile GW, Lower WE. Anoci-association. Philadelphia: WB Saunders; 1914: 223–225.

34. Armitage EN. Postoperative pain prevention or relief. Br J Anaesth 1989; 63: 136–137.

35. Brown DL, Carpenter RL. Perioperative analgesia: a review of risks and benefits. J Cardiothorac Anesth 1990; 4: 368–383.

36. Woolf CJ, Chong MS. Preemptive analgesia-treating postoperative pain by preventing the establishment of central sensitization. Anesth Analg 1993; 77: 362–379.
37. Beattie WS, Buckley DN, Forrest JB. Epidural morphine reduces the risk of postoperative myocardial ischemia in patients with cardiac risk factors. Can J Anaesth 1993; 40: 523–541.
38. Breslow MJ. Neuroendocrine responses to surgery. In: Breslow MJ, Miller CF, Rogers MC, eds. Perioperative management. St Louis: Mosby–Yearbook; 1990.
39. Breslow MJ, Jordan DA, Christopherson R, et al. Epidural morphine decreases postoperative hypertension by attenuating sympathetic nervous system hyperactivity. JAMA 1989; 261: 3577–3581.
40. Moller IW, Dinesen K, Sondergard S, et al. Effect of patient controlled analgesia on plasma catecholamine, cortisol and glucose concentrations after cholecystectomy. Br J Anaesth 1988; 61: 160–164.
41. Udelsman RL, Holbrook NJ. Endocrine and molecular responses to surgical stress. Curr Probl Surg 1994; 31(8): 655–720.
42. Brandt MR, Fernandes A, Mondhorst R, et al. Epidural analgesia improves postoperative nitrogen balance. Br Med J 1978; 1: 1106–1112.
43. Cuthbertson DP. Post-shock metabolic response. Lancet 1942; 1: 433.
44. Dahl JB, Rosenberg J, Dirkes WE, et al. Prevention of postoperative pain by balanced analgesia. Br J Anaesth 1990; 64: 518–520.
45. Modig J, Borg T, Bagge L, Saldeen T. Role of extradural and general anesthesia in fibrinolysis and coagulation after total hip replacement. Br J Anaesth 1983; 55: 625–631.
46. McIlvaine WB, Knox RF, Fennessey PV, et al. Continuous infusion of bupivacaine via interpleural catheter for analgesia after thoracotomy in children. Anesthesiology 1988; 69: 261–264.
47. Stevens DS, Dunn WT. Acute pain management for the trauma patient. In: Sinatra RS, Hord AH, Ginsberg B, Preble LM, eds. Acute pain mechanisms and management. St Louis: Mosby–Yearbook; 1992: 412–421.
48. Ciesla N. Postural drainage, positioning and breathing exercises. In: Mackenzie CF, ed. Chest physiotherapy in the intensive care unit. 2nd ed. Baltimore: Williams & Wilkins; 1989: 321–344.
49. Ward CM, Diamond AW. An appraisal of ketamine in the dressing of burns. Postgrad Med 1976; 52: 222–225.
50. Sevarino FB, Sinatra RS, Paige D, et al. The efficacy of intramuscular ketorolac in combination with intravenous PCA morphine for postoperative pain relief. J Clin Anesth 1992; 4: 285–288.
51. Landerscaper J, Coghill TH, Lindesmith LA. Long term disability after flail chest injury. J Trauma 1984; 24: 410–414.
52. Cohen FL. Postsurgical pain relief: Patients' status and nurses' medication choices. Pain 1980; 9: 265–274.
53. Collins JG. Historical overview of pain management: from undermedication to state of the art. In: Sinatra RS, Hord AH, Ginsberg B, Preble LM, eds. Acute pain mechanisms and management. St Louis: Mosby–Yearbook; 1992: 1–8.
54. Cronin M, Redfern PA. Psychometry and postoperative complaints of pain in surgical patients. Br J Anaesth 1973; 45: 879–882.
55. Perry S, Heidrich G. Management of pain during debridement: a survey of U.S. burn units. Pain 1982; 13: 267–271.
56. Ferrante FM, Covino BG. Patient-controlled analgesia: a historical perspective. In: Ferrante FM, Ostheimer GW, Covino BG, eds. Patient-controlled analgesia. Boston: Blackwell Scientific; 1990.
57. Dow AC, Baskett PJ. Anesthesia and analgesia in the field. In: Grande CM, ed. Textbook of trauma anesthesia and critical care. St Louis: Mosby–Yearbook; 1993.
58. Harrison DM, Sinatra R, Morgese L. Epidural narcotic and patient controlled analgesia for post-cesarean section pain relief. Anesthesiology 1988; 68: 454–457.
59. White PW. Use of patient-controlled analgesia for management of acute pain. JAMA 1988; 259: 243–247.
60. Egbert AE, Parks LH, Short LM, Burnett ML. Randomized trial of postoperative patient-controlled analgesia vs intramuscular narcotics in frail elderly men. Arch Int Med 1990; 150: 1897–1903.
61. Jayr C, Thomas H, Rey A, et al. Postoperative pulmonary complications: Epidural analgesia versus parenteral opioids. Anesthesiology 1993; 78: 666–676.
62. Liu S, Carpenter RL, Mackey DC, Thirlby RC et al. Effects of perioperative analgesic technique on rate of recovery after colon surgery. Anesthesiology 1995; 83: 757–765.
63. Rawal N, Sjostrand UH, Christofferson E. Comparisons of intramuscular and epidural morphine for postoperative analgesia in the grossly obese: influence on postoperative ambulation and pulmonary function. Anesth Analg 1984; 63: 584–592.
64. Rawal N, Sjostrand UH, Dahlstrom B, et al. Epidural morphine for postoperative pain relief: a comparative study with intramuscular narcotic and intercostal block. Anesth Analg 1982; 61: 93–98.
65. Salomaki TE, Leppaluoto J, Laitinen JO, et al.

Epidural versus intravenous fentanyl for reducing hormonal, metabolic, and physiologic responses after thoracotomy. Anesthesiology 1993; 79: 672–679.

66. Grant GJ, Zakowski M, Ramanathan S, et al. Thoracic versus lumbar administration of epidural morphine for postoperative analgesia after thoracotomy. Reg Anesth 1993; 18(6): 351–355.

67. Cousins MJ, Mather LE. Intrathecal and epidural administration of opioids. Anesthesiology 1984; 61: 276–310.

68. Shulman M, Sandler AN, Bradley JW, et al. Post-thoracotomy pain and pulmonary function following epidural and systemic morphine. Anesthesiology 1984; 61: 569–575.

69. Bromage PR, Camporesi EM, Chestnut D. Epidural narcotics for postoperative analgesia. Anesth Analg 1980; 59: 473–480.

70. Shulman MS, Wakerlin G, Yamaguchi L, Brodsky JB. Experience with epidural hydromorphone for post-thoracotomy pain relief. Anesth Analg 1987; 66: 1331–1335.

71. Gwirtz KH. Single-dose opioids in the management of acute postoperative pain. In: Sinatra RS, Hord AH, Ginsberg B, Preble LM, eds. Acute pain mechanisms and management. St Louis: Mosby–Yearbook; 1992.

72. El-Baz NMI, Faber LP, Jensik RJ. Continuous epidural infusion of morphine for treatment of pain after thoracic surgery: a new technique. Anesth Analg 1984; 63: 757–764.

73. Akerman B, Arwenstrom E, Post C. Local anesthetic potentiates spinal morphine antinociception. Anesth Analg 1988; 67: 943–947.

74. Badner NH, Bhandari R, Komar WE. Bupivacaine 0.125% improves continuous postoperative epidural fentanyl analgesia after abdominal or thoracic surgery. Can J Anesth 1994; 41: 387–392.

75. Geurts AM, Jessen HJG, Megans JH, et al. Continuous high thoracic epidural administration of morphine with bupivacaine after thoracotomy. Reg Anesth 1995; 20(1): 27–32.

76. Brodsky JB, Chaplan SR, Brose WG, Mark JBD. Continuous epidural hydromorphone for post-thoracotomy pain relief. Ann Thorac Surg 1990; 50: 888–893.

77. Chaplan SR, Duncan SR, Brodsky JB, Brose WG. Morphine and hydromorphone epidural analgesia: A prospective, randomized comparison. Anesthesiology 1992; 77: 1090–1094.

78. Welchew EA, Thorton JA. Continuous thoracic epidural fentanyl. Anesthesia 1982; 37: 309–316.

79. Salomaki TE, Laitinen JO, Nuutinen LS. A randomized double-blind comparison of epidural versus intravenous fentanyl infusion for analgesia after thoracotomy. Anesthesiology 1991; 75: 790–795.

80. Sawchuck CW. Thoracic versus lumbar epidural fentanyl for postthoracotomy pain. Ann Thorac Surg 1993; 55: 1472–1478.

81. Guinard JP, Mavrocordatos P, Cuttat JF, Carpenter R. A randomized comparison of intravenous versus lumbar and thoracic epidural fentanyl for analgesia after thoracotomy. Anesthesiology 1992; 77: 1108–1115.

82. Wamsley PNH. Patient-controlled epidural analgesia. In: Sinatra RS, Hord AH, Ginsberg B, Preble LM, eds. Acute pain mechanisms and management. St Louis: Mosby–Yearbook; 1992.

83. Bromage PR, Camporesi EM, Durant PAC, et al. Non-respiratory side effects of epidural morphine. Anesth Analg 1982; 61: 490–495.

84. Etches RC, Sandler A, Daley MD. Respiratory depression and spinal opioids. Can J Anaesth 1989; 36: 165–179.

85. Horan CT, Beeby DG, Brodsky JB, Oberhelman MD. Segmental effect of lumbar epidural hydromorphone: A case report. Anesthesiology 1985; 62: 84–85.

86. Johnson A. Influence of intrathecal morphine and naloxone intervention on postoperative ventilatory regulation in elderly patients. Acta Anaesthesiol Scand 1992; 36: 436–444.

87. Rawal N, Schott U, Dahlstrom B, et al. Influence of naloxone infusion on analgesia and respiratory depression following epidural morphine. Anesthesiology 1986; 64: 194–201.

88. Thomas DFM, Lambert WG, Lloyd-Williams K. The direct perfusion of surgical wounds with local anesthetic solutions: an approach to postoperative pain. Ann R Coll Surg Engl 1983; 65: 226.

89. De Leon-Casasola OA, Parker B, Lema MJ, et al. Postoperative epidural-bupivacaine-morphine therapy: Experience with 4,227 surgical cancer patients. Anesthesiology 1994; 81: 368–375.

90. Crawford RD, Thompson GE. Intercostal block. In: Cousins MJ, Phillips GD, eds. Acute pain management. New York: Churchill Livingstone; 1986.

91. Graziotti PJ, Smith GB. Multiple rib fractures and head injury–an indication for intercostal catheterization and infusion of local anesthetics. Anaesthesia 1988; 43: 964–968.

92. Murphy DF. Continuous intercostal nerve blockade for pain relief following cholecystectomy. Br J Anaesth 1983; 55: 521–525.

93. Sinatra RS. Unpublished observations, 1994–1996. Yale University Acute Pain Service.

94. Carabine UA, Gilliland H, Johnstone JR, McGuigan J. Pain relief for thoracotomy: Comparison of morphine requirements using interpleural bupivacaine. Reg Anesth 1995; 20(5): 412–417.

95. Iwama H, Kawamae K, Katsumi, et al. [Interpleural regional analgesia in pain manage-

ment after chest trauma.] Japanese Journal of Anesthesia 1993; 42(5): 669–676.

96. Kambam JR, Handte RE, Parris WC, et al. Interpleural anesthesia for post-thoracotomy pain relief. Reg Anesth 1987; 12: 106–107.

97. Reiestad F, Stromskag KE. Interpleural catheter in management of postoperative pain. Reg Anesth 1986; 11: 89–90.

98. Rocco A, Reiestad F, Gudman J, et al. Interpleural administration of local anesthetics for pain relief in patient with multiple rib fractures. Reg Anesth 1987; 12: 10–14.

99. Laurito CE, Kirz LI, VadeBoncouer TR, et al. Continuous infusion of interpleural bupivacaine maintains effective analgesia after cholecystectomy. Anesth Analg 1991; 72: 516–521.

100. Schneider RF, Villamena PC, Harvey J, et al. Lack of efficacy of interpleural bupivacaine for postoperative analgesia following thoracotomy. Chest 1993; 103: 414–419.

101. Williamson S, Kumar CM. Paravertebral block in head injured patient with chest trauma. Anesthesia 1997; 52: 284–285.

102. Crawford OB, Ottosen P, Buckingham WW. Peridural anesthesia in thoracic surgery, a review of 677 cases. Anesthesiology 1951; 12: 73–78.

103. Lehmann KA. Tramadol for the management of acute pain. Drugs 1994; 47:(Suppl 1) 19–32.

104. Rooney SM, Jain S, McCormack P, et al. A comparison of pulmonary function tests for postthoracotomy pain using cryoanalgesia and transcutaneous nerve stimulation. Ann Thorac Surg 1986; 41: 204–209.

105. Brown RE. Transcutaneous electrical nerve stimulation for acute and postoperative pain. In: Sinatra RS, Hord AH, Ginsberg B, Preble LM, eds. Acute pain mechanisms and management. St Louis: Mosby–Yearbook; 1992.

106. Warfield CA, Stein JM, Frank HA. The effect of transcutaneous electrical nerve stimulation after

thoracotomy. Ann Thorac Surg 1985; 39: 462–469.

107. Roxburgh JC, Markland CG, Ross BA, et al. Role of cryoanalgesia in the control of pain after thoracotomy. Thorax 1987; 42: 292–299.

108. Grosmanova T, Koutna J, Sceinarova A. Analgesia after intercostal thoracotomy. Acta Universitatis Palackianae Olomucensis Facultatis Medicae 1993; 136: 53–55.

109. Perttunen K, Nilsson E, Heinonen J, et al. Extradural, paravertebral, and intercostal nerve blocks for post-thoracotomy pain. Brit J Anaesth 1995; 75: 541–547.

110. Bachmann-Mennenga, Biscoping J, Kuhn DF, et al. Intercostal nerve block, interpleural analgesia, thoracic epidural block or systemic opioid application for pain relief after thoracotomy. Eur J Cardiothorac Surg 1993; 7: 12–18.

111. Yeager MP, Glass DG, Neff RK. Epidural anesthesia and analgesia in high-risk surgical patients. Anesthesiology 1987; 66: 729–736.

112. Ullman DA, Fortune JB, Greenhouse BB, et al. The treatment of patients with multiple rib fractures using continuous thoracic epidural narcotic infusion. Reg Anesth 1989; 14: 43–47.

113. Cicala RS, Voeller GR, Fox T. Epidural analgesia in thoracic trauma: effects of lumbar morphine and thoracic bupivacaine on pulmonary function. Crit Care Med 1990; 18: 229–234.

114. Kehlet H, Dahl JB. The value of 'multimodal' or 'balanced analgesia' in postoperative pain treatment. Anesth Analg 1993; 77: 1048–1056.

115. Terjani GA, Rattan AK, McDonald JS. Role of spinal opioid receptors in the antinociceptive interactions between intrathecal morphine and bupivacaine. Anesth Analg 1992; 74: 726–734.

116. Pond WW, Somerville GM, Thong SH, et al. Pain of delayed traumatic splenic rupture masked by interpleural lidocaine. Anesthesiology 1989; 70: 154.

20

Trauma patient with neurologic injuries

Irene P Osborn, Haroon F Choudhri and George Sandor

Introduction

Initial evaluation and resuscitation
  Considerations in head injury
  Airway management
  Control of intracranial pressure
  Neurodiagnostic evaluation: anesthesia/critical
    care support function
  Intracranial pressure monitoring

Perioperative considerations
  Anesthetic preparation

Intraoperative concerns
Postoperative period

Sedation objectives
  Sedation/analgesia in the mechanically-ventilated
    patient
  Propofol and head injury
  Muscle relaxants in the intensive care unit
  Miscellaneous agents

Conclusion

INTRODUCTION

The anesthesiologist plays an important role in the resuscitation and management of trauma patients. Priorities include securing and maintaining an airway, monitoring of the patient throughout diagnostic evaluation, and control of pain. When concurrent neurologic injuries are diagnosed or suspected, the management becomes more challenging. The goals for pain management in patients with neurotrauma may include sedation for control of intracranial pressure as well as for tolerance of an endotracheal tube. Relief of pain in these patients is a puzzling dilemma because neurologic assessment usually depends on their ability to perceive and respond to painful stimuli. Yet, pain is common in these critically-ill patients and has often been undertreated for fear of masking recognition of surgical pathology and of depressing ventilation. Most importantly, the management of pain and/or sedation should not profoundly interfere with the ability to evaluate the patient's neurologic status. There are a number of valuable techniques, anesthetic agents, and monitoring parameters to benefit these patients.

This discussion will highlight important considerations for pain management of trauma patients with neurologic injuries.

INITIAL EVALUATION AND RESUSCITATION

Considerations in head injury

To minimize mortality and morbidity, severely head-injured patients require effective management from hospital admission through intensive care unit (ICU) discharge. One powerful determinant of outcome is 'secondary brain injury'. This is characterized by ischemic neurologic damage associated with post-injury hypotension, hypoxemia, and intracranial hypertension (Fig. 20.1). Potential mechanisms contributing to secondary ischemia include cerebral vasoconstriction and impaired autoregulation of cerebral blood flow (CBF).[1] Previously, head injury management emphasized the reduction of intracranial pressure (ICP) as the primary goal. Current management principles are based on diminishing elevated ICP and improving cerebral perfusion by maintaining adequate blood pressure.[2] Cerebral perfusion

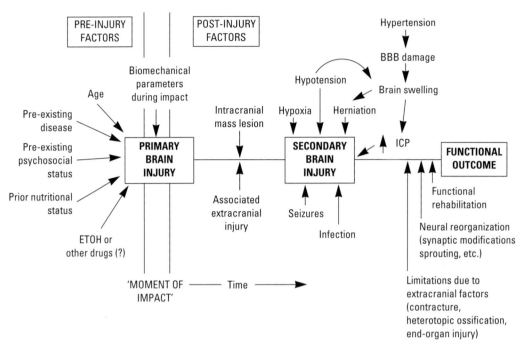

Fig. 20.1   Schematic representation of factors and events that influence outcome after head injury. ETOH, alcohol; BBB, blood–brain barrier; ICP, intracranial pressure. (From Volmer DG, Dacey TG. Prediction and assessment of outcome following closed head injury. In: Pitts LH, Wagner FC Jr, eds. Craniospinal trauma. New York: Thieme Medical; 1990.)

pressure (CPP) is classically defined as mean arterial pressure (MAP) minus ICP. The lower limit of CPP acceptable in adults is 50 mmHg. Many investigators now recommend maintaining CPP greater than 70 mmHg in head-injured patients to minimize cerebral ischemia and prevent the cascade of effects from inadequate perfusion.[3] Either a decrease in MAP or an elevation in ICP will deleteriously alter the effective perfusion pressure.

Typically head-injured patients without other major systemic injuries demonstrate a hyperdynamic circulatory response which produces hypertension, tachycardia, and increased cardiac output. Consequently, the patient with multiple trauma including head injury may be vulnerable to the effects of hypotension as a result of blood loss. Cerebral autoregulation is impaired in patients after traumatic brain injury.[4] Further decreases in marginally adequate CBF could produce cerebral ischemia.

Airway management

One of the first decisions which must be made is whether or not to intubate a patient with trau-matic injury to the head. There is little debate that the patient who has severe head injury (Glasgow Coma Scale (GCS) score = 8 or less) (Table 20.1) or who is unable to breathe should have an airway secured. Effective and timely management of the airway is essential for resuscitation and recovery. Secondary neurologic damage from raised ICP can be minimized by preventing hypoxemia, hypercarbia, and acidosis.[2] In addition, patients may present in various states of consciousness which can change rapidly. Endotracheal intubation should be performed expeditiously if not done previously in the field.[5] Tracheostomy or cricothyrotomy is indicated in patients with significant facial or cervical injury, and/or when oral or nasal intubation attempts are frustrated by abnormal anatomy or bleeding.

In approximately 10% of head-injured patients there is a concomitant injury to the cervical spine.[6] Cervical spine injury should be suspected when the patient reports neck pain and/or is flaccid, has diaphragmatic breathing, hypotension, and bradycardia. Techniques to minimize head movement should be employed during the intubation of these patients. Once the airway is secured, patients are

Table 20.1 Glasgow Coma Scale

	Score
Eye opening	
Spontaneous	4
To speech	3
To pain	2
None	1
Best verbal response	
Oriented	5
Confused	4
Inappropriate	3
Incomprehensible	2
None	1
Best motor response	
Obeys commands	6
Localizes pain	5
Withdraws from pain	4
Flexes to pain	3
Extends to pain	2
None	1

likely to need ventilatory assistance and this should be maintained throughout the diagnostic evaluation sequence. The presence of an endotracheal tube is generally quite stimulating; patients should not be allowed to thrash about excessively as this increases ICP as well as blood pressure and heart rate. The patient who does not require airway control may benefit from the use of small doses of narcotic (Table 20.2) in order to relieve pain, facilitate line placement, and allow position-

Table 20.2 Agents for analgesia and sedation of intubated patients

	Advantages	Disadvantages
Opioids		
Morphine sulfate 0.05–0.15 mg/kg	Analgesia Sedation Reversible	Respiratory depression Hypotension
Fentanyl 1–2 microg/kg	Analgesia Sedation Reversible	Short duration Respiratory depression Hypotension
Benzodiazepines		
Midazolam 0.01–0.04 mg/kg	Anxiolysis Amnesia Reversible	Respiratory depression Hypotension Opioid interaction
Diazepam 0.1–0.3 mg/kg	Similar effect Long duration Anti-convulsive	Not as profound
Lorazepam 2–4 mg		Long duration

ing for radiologic studies. This may be better than prophylactic intubation, yet requires careful monitoring of the patient. Ideal is a patient who becomes cooperative and is able to 'show two fingers' (follows complex commands). Titration of morphine sulfate with oxygen supplementation and pulse oximetry often achieves this purpose. Midazolam, in increments of 0.5 mg (0.015 mg/kg), may also be used. Both agents are reversible in the event of oversedation.

Control of intracranial pressure

When elevated profoundly, ICP alters perfusion of cortical and subcortical structures. Sedation, pain control, and neuromuscular blockade can be utilized as part of the global treatment of increased ICP.[7] The management of intracranial hypertension involves aggressive surgical intervention if warranted. A ventriculostomy may be performed in the emergency department if necessary to prevent further neurologic deterioration caused by herniation. Prior to this, a number of maneuvers may be employed to reduce suspected ICP (Table 20.3). These include elevating the patient's head, use of diuretics to decrease brain bulk, institution of moderate hyperventilation and sedatives to prevent straining, coughing, or seizures.[8] Significant hemodynamic alterations can occur as ICP rises and approaches the levels of diastolic blood pressure. Hemodynamic manifestations probably reflect brainstem compression or distortion secondary to elevated ICP but are not the direct result of intracranial hypertension.

The triad of hypertension, bradycardia, and respiratory irregularities was first reported by Cushing in 1901, which he believed to be the sequelae of medullary ischemia.[9] The Cushing triad, as it is called, is rare and has most commonly been reported in association with

Table 20.3 Management of acute intracranial hypertension

- Head elevation 30° (if tolerated)
- Mild hyperventilation
- Mannitol
- CSF withdrawal
- Intravenous sedation/relaxants
- Barbiturates
- Early surgical intervention

infratentorial mass lesions.[7] Patients with intracranial pathology deteriorate in the following order:

1. consciousness declines
2. there is a sustained increase in ICP
3. pupillary dilation occurs
4. hypertension is noted
5. bradycardia ensues.

The best monitor of neurologic function is the neurologic exam. Deterioration will be detected later in a patient who is intubated and has an ICP monitor than one who can be examined. There is no need to place an ICP monitor in a patient who can follow complex commands since this patient is receiving adequate CBF and oxygenation. If a patient suspected of having an intracranial mass lesion or non-operative pathology must be intubated and/or sedated, then ICP monitoring may be indicated since this will provide an earlier sign of neurologic deterioration. These patients may receive analgesia and sedation as deemed appropriate. For all other patients, including those appearing to be intoxicated, it is important to determine that no intracranial pathology exists. These patients should not receive sedation or narcotics. If the computed tomography (CT) scan is negative for intracranial pathology (hematoma, excessive swelling) and the patient is neurologically intact, then the patient can be treated like any other trauma patient requiring analgesia and/or sedation.

Neurodiagnostic evaluation: anesthesia/critical care support function

Most head-injured patients are sent directly for CT scan after evaluation and stabilization in the emergency department. The condition of the patient (GCS score) will determine whether he or she will be intubated, somnolent, or awake and oriented. The intubated patient should be transported with oxygen and ventilation controlled or assisted as needed. These patients should be monitored via pulse oximetry and/or electrocardiogram (ECG) and non-invasive blood pressure.[10] Oxygen sources, suction units, and monitoring equipment should be available in the diagnostic suite. During the scanning procedure a mechanical ventilator is sufficient to maintain respiratory support for the comatose, sedated, or pharamacologically-paralyzed patient. Alternatively, an anesthesia machine with functioning ventilator is also useful. The patient should continue to be monitored via pulse oximetry.

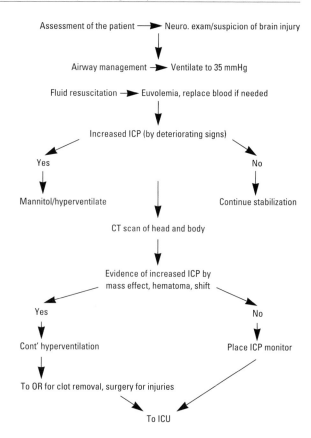

Fig. 20.2 Algorithm for management of the trauma patient with neurologic injuries.

Patients who received non-depolarizing relaxants for intubation or transport may begin to cough or struggle when the effects have subsided. Unless the patient is now fully awake and extubation is planned, excessive straining should not be allowed as it may seriously increase ICP. The agitated or unruly patient presents a diagnostic and treatment challenge. The patient who is semi-conscious yet requires airway control may benefit from a number of pharmacologic choices (See Table 20.2). After the head and body CT evaluation, the patient may move directly to surgery or may require more diagnostic/therapeutic intervention for other injuries or will be transported to the ICU (Fig. 20.2).

Intracranial pressure monitoring

The intraventricular catheter (or ventriculostomy) was introduced by Lundberg in 1960 and has remained the gold standard for ICP monitoring.

Over the years, newer monitoring modalities have been developed, and ICP can be recorded from an epidural, subdural, subarachnoid, ventricular, or intraparenchymal location (Fig. 20.3). Monitoring devices in use include catheters, bolts, screws, and fiberoptic cables.

In addition to recording ICP, an intraventricular catheter has the added therapeutic advantage of cerebrospinal fluid (CSF) drainage and can be used simultaneously to treat intracranial hypertension. Placement of an intraventricular catheter requires more skill than other monitoring devices, has a higher incidence of infection, and has a greater potential to cause injury during placement. It is presumed that once the monitor is in position the ICP recorded is reflective of pressure in the supra- and infratentorial compartments in the absence of obstruction.

An ICP monitor does not replace the neurologic exam but can guide treatment when the patient is comatose and intracranial hypertension is suspected. A monitor is generally placed by the neurosurgeon with local anesthetic infiltration in the obtunded or intubated adult.

PERIOPERATIVE CONSIDERATIONS

Anesthetic preparation

The primary anesthetic objectives are to continue the initial resuscitation and maintenance of the patient's existing vital organ function and to avoid secondary brain injury. This may be caused by inadequate CBF secondary to arterial hypotension, elevated ICP, excessive hyperventilation, and/or hypoxemia. By this time, intra-arterial monitoring should be established to continually assess MAP. The craniotomy procedure is characterized by periods of anticipated, intense stimulation which may occur with head pinning, skin incision, muscle flap elevation, and closure of the scalp. Once the dura is opened, there is little requirement for analgesia, as minimal or no pain is perceived. In order to minimize intraoperative hemodynamic changes, local anesthetic infiltration should be administered at the anticipated pin sites as well as in the area of the planned incision.[10,11]

Scalp block

A more effective means of providing supplemental analgesia during and after craniotomy is to perform a 'scalp block' (Fig. 20.4). This technique

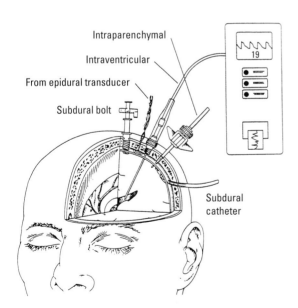

Fig. 20.3 Methods of intracranial pressure (ICP) measurement. Locations used to monitor ICP include intraventricular, subarachnoid, epidural, subdural, and intraparenchymal. (From Schell RM, Cole DJ. Neurophysiologic monitors. In: Lichtor JL, ed. Preoperative preparation and intraoperative monitoring. New York: Churchill Livingstone; 1997.)

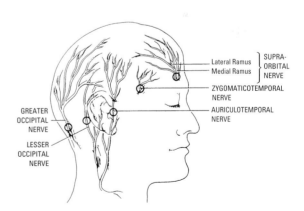

Fig. 20.4 Cutaneous nerves providing sensory innervation to the scalp. Open circles show the points at which nerves can be blocked most easily by local anesthetic injections. (From Girvin J. Neurosurgical considerations and general methods for craniotomy under local anesthesia. In: Varkey GP, ed. Anesthetic considerations for craniotomy in awake patients. Int Anesthesiol Clin 1986; 24.)

was first advocated by Harvey Cushing and developed by Penfield.[12] It is commonly used for awake craniotomy procedures and provides for extensive and effective analgesia. This block may be performed while the patient is asleep as the landmarks are easily palpated.

It is recommended that bupivacaine 0.5% be used with epinephrine at a concentration of 1:200,000. Local anesthesia is administered bilaterally to anesthetize the supraorbital nerves, zygomaticolotemporal nerves, auricilotemporal nerves, and greater and lesser occipital nerves.[13] A volume of 2–5 mL of solution is administered with careful aspiration at each site for a total of 18–20 mL. While the onset time is 15 to 20 minutes, this block provides analgesia for at least 8.5 hours.

The benefits of performing supplemental regional anesthesia for craniotomy are:

1. minimal hemodynamic response to skull pinning and skin incision
2. decreased requirement for opioids intraoperatively
3. potential for more rapid awakening/recovery from anesthesia
4. postoperative analgesia and potential for improved hemodynamic stability.[14] (Fig. 20.5).

Intraoperative concerns

Patients for emergent craniotomy are best managed with a technique that does not compromise intracranial dynamics and allows maintenance of adequate perfusion pressure. Intraoperative management is thoroughly discussed in other references.[15,16] Generally, once the hematoma is evacuated or swelling decreased, patients may be prepared for PACU or ICU admission unless other surgical procedures are to be subsequently performed.

Most patients are not expected to be extubated if they were obtunded prior to the procedure; however, young patients, following evacuation of epidural hematomas, may recover consciousness quite rapidly. If stable and following commands, they may be extubated and carefully monitored postoperatively.

Patients with head injury not requiring craniotomy may undergo surgery for treatment of other injuries. These patients are best managed with the consideration of potential development of intracranial hypertension. An ICP monitor, if placed, is useful during the procedure to evaluate changes that may occur with positioning, noxious stimuli, and hemodynamic fluctuations. The use of a 'steep' Trendelenberg position should be avoided and normocapnia should be maintained unless increases in ICP are noted or suspected. One must be aware that prior mannitol administration may aggravate intraoperative hypovolemia.

Postoperative period

Postoperatively, attempts to maintain ICP at controlled levels are undertaken as the patient emerges from anesthesia. The decision will likely have been made regarding when the patient should emerge. This is often a joint decision among caretakers based upon the patient's condition preoperatively, the intraoperative course and findings, the duration of surgery, and subsequent diagnostic plans.

Before emergence the patient should:

1. be normothermic
2. be hemodynamically stable
3. have effective analgesic agents or nerve blocks.

The patient who is to undergo additional radiologic studies should have them at this time. Once the patient emerges (i.e. follows commands) further criteria should be met before extubation.

SEDATION OBJECTIVES

Many patients will not rapidly return to consciousness and will be maintained on mechanical

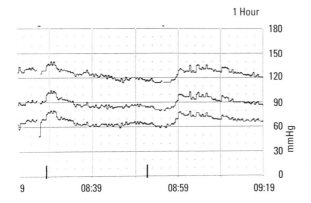

Fig. 20.5 Blood pressure trends when scalp block has been administered for craniotomy. Application of pins followed by incision in patient with combined technique.

ventilation for some time. Care of the patient with intracranial pathology requires a working knowledge of how much pain control and sedation may be given without masking important aspects of the neurologic exam. Some procedures involving the posterior fossa will have an increased risk of bulbar palsy, and the patient should not be extubated until an adequate gag reflex has returned. If a patient is neurologically intact, and has a GCS score of 15, he or she is unlikely to harbor any clinically significant intracranial pathology.

Neurosurgical patients, especially postcraniotomy patients, are usually monitored in critical care environments that allow close observation of responses to analgesic regimens. However, conventional therapy of prescribing intermittent doses of analgesics in response to patient demands is often ineffective and is recognized as suboptimal management. Codeine has been used by neurosurgeons for many years without effective relief. Pain associated with craniotomy is primarily derived from trauma to the scalp and muscle but also represents the discomfort of a pneumocephalus which likely exists. Some degree of pain is relieved by providing a 'scalp block' before or after surgery, particularly for incisions in the suboccipital region. The awake, extubated patient complaining of headache may best benefit from the use of acetaminophen or nonsteroidal anti-inflammatory agents.

Sedation/analgesia in the mechanically-ventilated patient

Critically-ill patients who require mechanical ventilation often have high levels of anxiety and discomfort. Most victims of severe head injury will be sedated and ventilated while there is still a risk of raised ICP. Patient discomfort in the ICU takes on many forms; foremost among these are dyspnea and pain. Dyspnea may result from impaired gas exchange or the need for suctioning. Multiple causes of pain include surgical incision sites, chest tubes, arterial or venous punctures, or ischemia to the limbs. Pain, whether continual, intermittent, or episodic, elicits a fear response, which exacerbates the patient's underlying anxiety.[17]

Pain and nociceptive stimuli such as endotracheal tube mobilization and chest physiotherapy may induce increases in ICP in patients with low cerebral compliance and induce a secondary decrease in cerebral perfusion pressure. In the past, deep sedation in which the patient was completely detached from the environment was considered the ideal. Neuromuscular relaxants were used liberally and the effects contributed to prolonged immobility, decubitus ulcers, pulmonary congestion, and occasional aspiration of feeding material.[18] The preferred level of sedation is one in which the patient is asleep but easily roused and able to cooperate with care. Benzodiazepines, opiates, and muscle relaxants are usually administered to provide good conditions for mechanical ventilation by avoiding fighting against the ventilator and concomitant intracranial hypertension.

Benzodiazepines

These are the agents most commonly used in the ICU to relieve anxiety, restore normal sleep, provide amnesia, and relax skeletal muscles. They are often used concomitantly with opiates or neuroleptics, creating a synergy that allows for lower doses of each agent. These agents appear to bind with benzodiazepine receptor sites in the CNS where they potentate or mimic γ-aminobutyric acid, the inhibitory neurotransmitter. All produce some degree of respiratory depression and can potentially cause hypotension. The most commonly administered benzodiazepines in the ICU are diazepam, lorazepam, and midazolam.

Diazepam is a long-acting sedative that has become less frequently used in the ICU because of its prolonged duration and undesirable side effects. It has a rapid onset, provides relief of anxiety, and is often effective for the acute cessation of seizures. For mild-to-moderate agitation, diazepam is given slowly in a 2–5 mg dose. For moderate-to-severe agitation, a 5–10 mg dose may be used. Its elimination half-life is 24 to 72 hours and its active metabolite can produce more prolonged effect. Diazepam injection intravenously may produce phlebitis because of propylene glycol in its solution.

Lorazepam (Ativan) is an intermediate-acting sedative with a slower onset than diazepam. Because it does not have an active metabolite, its sedating effects are removed as it is metabolized by the liver. A 1–2 mg dose is administered for mild-to-moderate agitation. This may be followed by regularly scheduled intravenous boluses or by a continuous infusion of 1–2 mg/h. Like diazepam, it precipitates easily which makes infusions difficult.

Midazolam is a short-acting benzodiazepine with good sedating and amnesic properties. A water-soluble preparation, midazolam does not irritate peripheral veins, nor does it precipitate in solutions or intravenous lines. It has a rapid onset, and when used for fewer than 3 to 5 days, has an elimination half-life of 2 to 4 hours. However, after long-term use, midazolam's elimination half-life may extend from 5 to 26 hours as the drug is sequestered in poorly perfused tissue. Midazolam is more potent than diazepam and tends to produce an exaggerated response in combination with opioids, causing hypotension and respiratory depression. There is no consensus on the dose which might guarantee amnesia; however, when administered for sedation prior to a noxious stimulus, it is very effective.

The specific antagonist, flumazenil, may be used to reverse or modify the hemodynamic and sedative effects of the benzodiazepines. It must be administered by repeated bolus injections or continuous infusion because of its short duration of action.[19]

Analgesics

Opiates are the mainstay of pain control in critical care. Their efficacy has been well-established, and their side effects are known and in most cases controlled by adjusting the dose and rate of administration or by taking countermeasures such as intravenous fluids for transient hypotension. Opiates bind to several known receptor sites in the brain and spinal cord. Past concerns about inducing addiction have proved unfounded. The persistence of apparent undertreatment of pain argues strongly for the use of pain assessment scales and accurate measuring techniques (Table 20.4). Opiates decrease gastric motility, and may lead to constipation and a potential small bowel ilius.[18]

Morphine sulfate is a pure opiate agonist that binds to receptor sites in the central and peripheral nervous system. It blocks the transmission and perception of pain. Because it is not lipophilic, morphine has a slower onset than agents such as fentanyl. Once a therapeutic blood level is established, it provides relief for 2 to 4 hours. Morphine's actions can affect the cardiac, pulmonary, gastrointestinal and neurohumoral systems. It is known to stimulate histamine release, causing peripheral vasodilatation and hypotension.[19] Morphine produces some degree

Table 20.4 The Ramsay Scale for assessment of sedation

Level	Clinical description
I	Anxious and agitated
II	Cooperative, oriented, tranquil
III	Responds to verbal commands
IV	Asleep with brink response to light stimulation
V	Asleep without response to stimulation
VI	No response

of sedation and euphoria in many patients, but given alone can also cause confusion and delirium in some elderly patients. With good pain relief, the patient is able to relax, allowing for easier chest excursion, improving thoracic compliance. The patient is able to cooperate with suctioning and chest physiotherapy.

Fentanyl is an opiate agonist that is rapidly becoming popular in the ICU because of its rapid onset. A highly lipophilic drug, fentanyl readily crosses the blood–brain barrier and binds to receptor sites in the brain and spinal cord. Like morphine, it can cause hypotension and decreased respiratory rate. Constipation, nausea, and decreased gastric emptying may occur. Despite its rapid onset, fentanyl has a longer elimination half-life than morphine. This effect is more likely to occur in patients who have received infusions for more than 3 to 5 days or who have hepatic or renal failure.[19] This may lead to oversedation or to resedation after the medication is discontinued. Careful titration and monitoring with a sedation scale, along with attention to factors that extend the drug's efficacy, will prevent excessive accumulation in the body.

Propofol

Propofol, an alkyl-phenol, is now used extensively as an induction agent, for maintenance of anesthesia and for sedation of adult, ventilated patients in the ICU. Many studies have indicated a lack of accumulation after incremental administration. When propofol is administered as a continuous infusion for anesthesia lasting over 2 hours, it gives rapid, clear-headed recovery. Propofol is rapidly metabolized in both hepatic and extrahepatic sites, and studies indicate no significant hepatic effects when it is used for up to 120 hours.[20] Benzodiazepines had been the frequent choice of sedative agent in the ICU before propofol was available. Both sedatives produce acceptable cardiovascular stability, but recovery takes longer with midazolam and the sedative level is less easily controlled.

Propofol has been utilized for sedation in most recent years with generally good results. The patient does not receive a loading dose, as is common with other agents. Some anesthesiologists administer a small test dose to detect if there is an allergic reaction. Because it can be irritating to the vein, the infusion is initiated slowly and gradually increased as the patient becomes somnolent. Intravenous lidocaine 1% may be given to prevent or relieve this discomfort.

The most common side effect is hypotension from peripheral vasodilatation, which is more likely in elderly, debilitated patients or in patients with excessive opiate blood levels. The most serious unwanted side effect reported in the literature is bacteremia. There have been documented cases of sepsis owing to contamination of the propofol

solute. Some hospital protocols require that the intravenous solution containing propofol and the tubing be changed every 12 hours to prevent contamination.[21] Propofol infusions may be titrated to achieve virtually any level of consciousness. The infusion may be increased in anticipation of noxious stimuli such as suctioning (Fig. 20.6) or may be decreased to a level that allows the patient to undergo a neurologic exam. It has been known to provoke sexual dreams in some patients, and therefore, family members and caregivers should be aware of this phenomenon.[22]

Propofol and head injury

Propofol has been used widely in neuroanesthesia despite initial warnings about the potential for hypotension and decreased perfusion pressure. Its advantages for intracranial procedures outweigh even the concerns over its cost (Table 20.5). Most reliably, it has been used for sedation of neurosurgical patients for radiologic procedures with rapid recovery. This has led to its current use for neurosurgical patients in the ICU. Neurologic patients in the ICU require the same considerations as other patients; sedation should provide adequate comfort, reduce stress, and facilitate ventilation (Table 20.6). In addition, the use of drugs allowing rapid recovery rates following cessation of sedation is beneficial, allowing early neurologic assessment.[23] Drugs reducing ICP and the cerebral metabolic rate for oxygen may provide a degree of cerebral protection. A number of recent studies have demonstrated the efficacy of propofol sedation in adult patients following head injury. An infusion of propofol at 30–50 microg/kg/min is effective in maintaining sedation in head-injured patients without reducing CPP.[24] When given in increments, it can also reduce the effects on ICP of stressful interventions, such as tracheal suction.

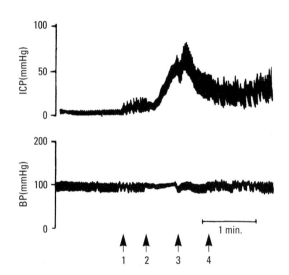

Fig. 20.6 Intracranial hypertension resulting from carbon dioxide retention during endotracheal suctioning. $Paco_2$ during controlled ventilation immediately prior to suctioning was 21 torr. Arrows indicate: 1, manual hyperventilation; 2, apnea followed by endotracheal suctioning; 3, return to mechanical ventilation; 4, manual ventilation reinstated. (From Shapiro H. Intracranial hypertension: Therapeutic and anesthetic considerations. Anesthesiology 1975; 43: 460.)

Table 20.5 Propofol and its effects on the central nervous system

---

- Decreased cerebral blood flow (inc. resistance)
- Decreased intracranial pressure
- Decreased $CMRo_2$
- No change in cerebral autoregulation

Adapted from Farling P, Johnson JR, Coppel DL. Propofol infusion for sedation of patients with head injury in intensive care. A preliminary report. Anaesthesia 1989; 44: 222.

Table 20.6   Propofol infusion – ICU clinical trials

ICU patient type	Sedation dose microg/kg/min
Post-CABG	0.1–100
Postsurgical	6–82
Neurological/head trauma	8.3–87
Medical ICU	3.1–131
ARDS/respiratory failure	10–142

ARDS, adult respiratory distress syndrome; CABG, coronary artery bypass graft. From Lund N, Papadakos PJ. Barbiturates, neuroleptics, and propofol for sedation. In Sedation of the critically ill patient. Critical Care Clinics 11:827, 1995; p. 880.

The policy for use of propofol by given healthcare institutions depends also on the availability of suitably trained personnel.[25]

Muscle relaxants in the intensive care unit

There has been a dramatic reduction in the use of muscle relaxants in the ICU because of certain conditions: modern, synchronized intermittent mandatory ventilators have become available, newer sedatives have been introduced, and problems with the use of relaxants have been realized.[26] Immobility leads to an increased incidence of infection and pressure sores as well as deep venous thrombosis and pulmonary emboli. The risks of paralyzing patients without sedating them adequately have been highlighted as well as dramatically reported by patients.[27,28] It is essential that the caregivers provide sufficient anesthesia to all degrees of stimulation and that all staff appreciate that relaxants do not provide sedation or analgesia, nor do they prevent seizures.

Relaxants are useful at certain times, particularly in the early stages of recovery when patients are on high doses of analgesics for pain, and ventilatory support is critical to treat or prevent adult respiratory distress syndrome.[21] Relaxants are most useful for short procedures such as endotracheal intubation or bronchoscopy, where movement (or struggling) will impair or prolong the procedure. The ideal muscle relaxant for use in the ICU is one that is pharmacokinetically suitable for infusion without having an unexpected prolonged action (Table 20.7). Patients receiving muscle-relaxant infusions should be monitored with a nerve stimulator.[22]

Table 20.7   Qualities of the ideal muscle relaxant in the ICU

- Pharmacologically suitable for infusion
- Should not rely on renal or hepatic function for elimination
- Should be free from side effects
- Should be inexpensive

Miscellaneous agents

Haloperidol is the drug of choice for delirium in the ICU. It has no analgesic or sedating properties, but because it relieves confusion it may help the patient achieve a calm state when confusion is frightening. Haloperidol acts by blocking surges of dopamine from several regions of the brain, including the limbic system. By suppressing the effects of this neurotransmitter, haloperidol relieves restlessness, tremors, and uncontrolled muscle movements, as well as disorientation. Intravenous administration of 2–10 mg improves symptoms in 10–15 minutes. After 30 minutes, the dose can be doubled until the patient improves.[20]

CONCLUSION

Achieving and maintaining adequate levels of analgesia and sedation in critically-ill patients is a fundamental part of modern anesthetic care. Awareness of the physiology and pathology of neurologic injury is essential in the management and for the potential recovery of these patients. Understanding of the clinical pharmacology of commonly-used sedative agents enables clinicians to choose the best dose of these drugs for the desired clinical effect while minimizing the risk of excessive sedation and cardiopulmonary depression. The role of monitoring in the course of recovery is important, whether it is invasive and numerical or the ability to 'show two fingers'. The ultimate goal of patient recovery requires dedication, knowledge, and vigilance.

REFERENCES

1. Chestnut RM, Marshall LF, Klauber MR, et al. The role of secondary brain injury in determining outcome from severe head injury. J Trauma 1993; 34: 216.

2. American Association of Neurological Surgeons. Guidelines for the management of severe head injury. New York: Brain Trauma Foundation; 1995.

3. Rosner MJ, Daughton S. Cerebral perfusion pressure management in head injury. J Trauma 1990; 30: 933.

4. Reilly PL, Lewis SB. Progress in head injury management. J Clin Neurosci 1997; 4:9. Muizelaar JP, Marmarou A, Ward JD, et al. Adverse effects of prolonged hyperventilation in patients with severe head injury: a randomized clinical trial. J Neurosurg 1991; 75: 931.

5. Redan JA, Livingston DH, et al. The value of intubating and paralyzing patients with suspected head injury in the emergency department. J Trauma 1991; 31: 371.

6. Hastings RH, Marks JD. Airway management of trauma patients with potential cervical spine injuries. Anesth Analg 1991; 73: 471.

7. Sulek CA. Intracranial pressure. In: Cucchiara, Black, Michenfelder, eds. Clinical neuroanesthesia. New York: Churchill Livingstone; 1998: 82.

8. Feldman Z, Kanter MJ, Robertson CS, et al. Effect of head elevation on intracranial pressure, cerebral perfusion pressure, and cerebral blood flow in head injured patients. J Neurosurg 1992; 76: 207.

9. Cushing H. Concerning a definite regulatory mechanism of the vaso-motor centre which controls blood pressure during cerebral compression. Bull Johns Hopkins Hospital 1901; 12: 290.

10. Doblar DD, Lim YC, Baykan, et al. Preventing the hypertensive response to skull pin insertion: A comparison of four methods. J Neurosurg Anesthesiol 1994; 6: 314(A).

11. Pinosky ML, Fishman RL, Reeves ST, et al. The effect of skull block on the hemodynamic response to craniotomy. Anesth Analg 1996; 83: 1256.

12. Penfield W. Combined regional and general anesthesia for craniotomy and cortical exploration, neurologic considerations. Proceedings of the International Anesthesia Research Society, Quebec, October 26, 1953.

13. Archer In: Girvin JP, ed. Considerations for craniotomy in the awake state. Int Anesthesiology Clinics 1986; 24(3), 89.

14. Osborn IO, Ferson DZ, Tran DQ, et al. Combined regional and general anesthesia for craniotomy. J Neurosurg Anesthesiol 1994; 6: A329.

15. Prough DS. Perioperative management of head trauma. IARS Review Course Lectures 1998; p. 91.

16. Avellino AM, Lam AM, Winn HR. Management of acute head injury. In: Albin MS, ed. Textbook of neuroanesthesia with neurosurgical and neuroscience perspectives. New York: McGraw-Hill; 1997: 1137.

17. Burns AM, Shelly MP, Park GR. The use of sedative agents in critically ill patients. Drugs 1992; 43: 507.

18. Watson D. Sedation in the mechanically ventilated patient. In: Watson D, ed. Conscious sedation/analgesia. St Louis: Mosby; 1998: 160.

19. Aitkenhead AR. Analgesia and sedation in intensive care. Br J Anaesth 1989; 63: 196.

20. Chiolero RL. Sedatives and antagonists in the management of severely head injured patients. Acta Neurochir (Wein) 1992; Suppl 55: 43.

21. Wheeler A. Sedation, analgesia and paralysis in the intensive care unit. Chest 1993; 104: 566.

22. Shapiro B, Greenbaum D, Schein R, et al. Practice parameters for intravenous analgesia and sedation of adult patients in the intensive care unit: An executive summary. Crit Care Med 1995; 21: 1596.

22. Chan KH, Dearden WM, Miller JD, et al. Multimodality monitoring as a guide to treatment of intracranial hypertension after severe brain injury. Neurosurgery 1993; 32: 547.

23. Shapiro HM. Intracranial hypertension: therapeutic and anesthetic considerations. Anesthesiology 1975; 43: 460.

24. Farling P, Johnson JR, Coppel DL. Propofol infusion for sedation of patients with head injury in intensive care. Anaesthesia 1989; 44: 222.

25. Buckley PM. Propofol in patients needing long-term sedation in intensive care: as assessment of the development of tolerance. A pilot study. Intensive Care Med 1997; 23: 969.

26. Lund N, Papadakos PJ. Barbiturates, neuroleptics, and propofol for sedation. In Sedation of the critically ill patient. Crit Care Clin 1995; 11: 875.

27. Barr J, Donner A. Optimal dosing strategies for sedatives and analgesics in the intensive care unit. In Sedation of the critically ill patient Crit Care Clin 1995; 11: 827.

28. Paralysed with fear. (Editorial) Lancet 1981; 427.

21

Trauma patient with orthopedic injuries

Ralph L Bernstein, Andrew D Rosenberg and David B Albert

Advantages of regional anesthesia in the trauma victim

Analgesic modalities available for pain relief in orthopedic trauma
Oral analgesics
Intramuscular analgesia
Intravenous analgesia
Nonsteroidal anti-inflammatory drugs
Infiltration of local anesthetics
Intravenous regional anesthesia
Peripheral nerve blocks
Subarachnoid analgesia
Epidural analgesia
Pain management in patients with injuries of the spine

Peripheral nerve blocks
The nerve stimulator and insulated needles

Superficial skin stimulation

Perioperative pain management for injuries to the extremities

Interscalene brachial plexus block
The shoulder region
Technique for interscalene brachial plexus block

Infraclavicular brachial plexus block
Technique for infraclavicular brachial plexus block

Axillary brachial plexus block
Continuous infusion technique

Use of individual nerve blocks

The patient with a fractured hip
Management of a patient with a fractured hip and severe respiratory insufficiency
Anesthetic management
Assess intravascular volume
Management of a patient with a fractured hip and chronic obstructive pulmonary disease and aortic stenosis
Technique for lumbar plexus block
A fractured hip repaired under individual nerve blocks
Technique for femoral nerve block
Technique for block of the lateral femoral cutaneous nerve of the thigh
Technique for block of the obturator nerve
Postoperative pain control in patients with fracture of the hip
Lower extremity trauma

Femoral and sciatic nerve blocks
Technique for sciatic nerve block using anterior approach
Management of trauma to the lower extremity using femoral and sciatic nerve blocks
Technique for sciatic nerve block using posterior approach

Fractures of the pelvis

Conclusion

Pain management of orthopedic injuries in the multiple trauma patient is a challenge since the type of injury impacts on the choices and techniques of pain management. While some trauma patients suffer only an isolated orthopedic injury, frequently the orthopedic injury is only one component of multiple trauma. The entire patient must be carefully evaluated prior to treating orthopedic pain since neurologic, cardiac, pulmonary, and hemodynamic abnormalities may be present.[1,2] For example, pain management of the orthopedic injury is not the first priority of the patient who is hemodynamically unstable, intubated, with a flail chest and a femur fracture. Patients with orthopedic injuries who appear obtunded may be suffering from associated head injuries or from the effects of fat embolism.[1,2] Hypoxemia from pneumothorax, hemothorax, or lung contusion can be exacerbated by pain medication.

Appropriate use of pain medications through carefully chosen routes such as intravenous, epidural, spinal, or regional blockade can relieve pain, improve respiratory function, decrease the stress response, and improve the rehabilitation process. While concern exists that pain medication not be administered too early resulting in some untoward effect, pain management does not have to wait until the patient reaches the post-anesthesia care unit. Once a patient is stable, a pain management plan can be initiated that can be utilized pre-, intra- and postoperatively. This chapter will review the current concepts of perioperative pain management and regional anesthesia for patients with orthopedic injuries utilizing case reports to aid in understanding the best route for administration based on the injury present and the status of the patient.

ADVANTAGES OF REGIONAL ANESTHESIA IN THE TRAUMA VICTIM

While many do not consider regional anesthesia an alternative when caring for acute trauma patients, and frequently this view is correct, there are circumstances in which this modality is not only effective but beneficial[3–6] (Table 21.1). The patient in whom regional anesthesia is to be employed must be cooperative, and be able to maintain an adequate airway. Spinal or epidural anesthesia, when administered to a hemodynami-

Table 21.1   Benefits of regional anesthesia

Provide prolonged pain relief
Supplement or replace general anesthesia
Decrease incidence of deep vein thrombosis (spinal epidural)
Reduce sympathetic tone
Improve blood supply
Decrease stress response
Improve local and systemic hemodynamics

cally stable patient, can reduce sympathetic tone, improve perfusion, and decrease blood loss and deep vein thrombosis.[3,4] Long-acting neuraxial narcotics administered at the time of surgery provide excellent postoperative pain relief. Alternatively, an epidural catheter can remain in place and provide prolonged pain relief via infusion or intermittent injection (see Ch. 12). Proper dosage adjustment can provide sensory blockade while allowing motor function to remain intact.

If an epidural catheter is placed for the surgical procedure and postoperative pain relief it must be borne in mind that systemic anticoagulation may be administered to prevent deep vein thrombosis. Therefore, it is essential that proper procedures be followed in removing the catheter (see Ch. 12).

Peripheral nerve blocks can provide prolonged pain relief in the postoperative period. This may be especially useful after reimplantation of digits or a free muscle flap.[7–11] When performing peripheral nerve blocks for pain management consider the extent of the injuries present. For example, when the patient develops a hemidiaphragmatic paralysis after an interscalene block will respiratory status be compromised? Will a Horner's syndrome confound neurologic examination? Complications of regional anesthesia that also must be considered include pneumothorax, intravascular injection, and seizures.

Another concern is that a patient with injuries to an extremity may develop a compartment syndrome. Physicians must be alert for this complication, especially when pain, which is a major sign of a compartment syndrome, is blocked by the administration of local anesthetics and opioids.[1,5,12–14]

Remember that there are some risks related to the use of neuraxial regional anesthesia including hypotension in the patient who has not been properly stabilized or who has continued bleeding (Table 21.2).[3,4]

Table 21.2   Risks of regional anesthesia

Hypotension
Intravascular injection
Systemic hemodynamic changes in patient unable to
    compensate because of concurrent injuries
Pneumothorax
Masking compartment syndrome
Hemidiaphragmatic paralysis (interscalene block)
Horner's syndrome (interscalene)

ANALGESIC MODALITIES AVAILABLE FOR PAIN RELIEF IN ORTHOPEDIC TRAUMA

When it is deemed appropriate to administer pain medication to a patient suffering from orthopedic trauma, type, route of administration, rate of absorption, and interval dosing must be taken into account.

Oral analgesics

Oral analgesics should be avoided in the immediate post-injury period. There is a possibility of vomiting and aspiration as well as decreased gastrointestinal (GI) activity with lack of predictable absorption at this time. The oral route is very useful in the postoperative period after the GI system is functioning adequately.

Intramuscular analgesia

Intramuscular (IM) medications are not optimal in the immediate post-injury period since poor perfusion of peripheral tissues will not allow the drug to be absorbed when administered. After adequate perfusion is established, large amounts of narcotics may be absorbed leading to overdose.

Intravenous analgesia

The intravenous (IV) route provides a reliable method of making certain that uptake and distribution of the administered medication are effective. IV morphine is very useful. Doses should be titrated until effect is achieved, thereby avoiding overdosing. The patient must be monitored for respiratory depression and hypotension. Patient-controlled analgesia (PCA) is very effective in the postoperative period. It is important that the patient understands the concept behind PCA including the lockout interval and that no one else pushes the PCA button (see Ch. 11).

Nonsteroidal anti-inflammatory drugs

Nonsteroidal anti-inflammatory drugs (NSAIDs) are now available in injectable form. Medications such as ketoralac provide significant pain relief without respiratory depression and are frequently used as adjuvants to narcotics. However, the antiplatelet effect of NSAIDs must be considered in the preoperative period since bleeding may occur. Postoperative indications are changing since some physicians believe these agents retard bone healing and thus should not be administered to patients with fractures or those who undergo procedures involving the use of bone grafts since pseudarthroses may result.

A new class of medications Cox 2 inhibitors may come to play an important role in perioperative pain relief since they are purported to not inhibit platelet function.

Infiltration of local anesthetics

After careful sterile preparation local anesthetics can be injected into the hematoma of a fracture, such as that of the wrist, to provide analgesia for closed reduction. However, if there is an open fracture it is not recommended that local anesthetic agents be infiltrated into the area since infection may be spread.

Intravenous regional anesthesia

IV regional anesthesia is a safe and effective technique for anesthesia of an extremity. Advantages of regional anesthesia are that the technique is easy to perform, onset is rapid, and anesthesia and muscle relaxation can be obtained. Disadvantages include possible toxic effects of local anesthetics upon release of the tourniquet, no postoperative analgesia, and the possibility of increased swelling. If exsanguination of the extremity by means of an Esmarch bandage is not feasible because of pain, gravity drainage is useful. Our practice at the Hospital for Joint Diseases Orthopaedic Institute (HJDOI) is to use 0.5% xylocaine preservative-free, epinephrine-free.[12] Others add various medications to IV regional anesthesia. McGlone et al added 2 mg of atracurium to IV regional blocks to improve ease of reduction and quality of analgesia.[15] Remember that since atracurium is not metabolized in an ischemic limb it will circulate centrally when the tourniquet is released. As a result, some patients have difficulty with vision after tourniquet release.[15] Therefore, McGlone recommends atracurium only for larger more muscular patients where reduction is difficult.[15]

Case study

A 20-year-old male involved in a motor vehicle accident resulting in a T4 fracture with paraplegia, a scapular fracture, a brachial plexopathy, and a forearm fracture was scheduled for repair of the forearm fracture. The patient had undergone anterior and posterior spine stabilization with a residual pleural effusion after removal of a chest tube placed during surgery. An arterial blood gas revealed a PaO_2 of 57 mmHg and a $PaCO_2$ of 57 mmHg. The patient was not intubated. The pulmonary status made general anesthesia a poor choice and the brachial plexopathy on the side of the forearm fracture contraindicated a brachial plexus block. Administering a general anesthetic might have made him respiratory-dependent for some time. Lidocaine 0.5% preservative-free, epinephrine-free was administered via an intravenous regional technique and the patient tolerated the procedure well. The patient had no episodes of respiratory insufficiency in the immediate postoperative period.[6]

Peripheral nerve blocks

This is an effective method of providing analgesia to injuries of the extremities. Peripheral nerve blocks, such as a femoral nerve block, can be used in the field for relief of pain secondary to trauma (see Ch. 6). An interscalene block of the brachial plexus for shoulder injuries, an infraclavicular block of the brachial plexus for injuries of the upper extremity below the shoulder, and an axillary brachial plexus block for injuries below the elbow are useful to provide excellent surgical conditions and pain relief. Femoral, lateral femoral cutaneous, and sciatic nerve blocks will provide analgesia for injuries of the hip, thigh, knee, and ankle. In addition, indwelling catheter techniques with long-acting local anesthetics, such as bupivacaine or ropivacaine, can provide prolonged analgesia. This topic was covered in detail in Chapter 13.

Subarachnoid analgesia

Combined with the local anesthetic used for spinal anesthesia, a single dose of preservative-free morphine (0.3–0.4 mg) can provide analgesia for as long as 24 hours.

Epidural analgesia

This modality can be very effective in providing postoperative pain relief for pelvic fractures and lower extremity surgery. Intermittent bolus doses or infusions can be employed (see Ch. 12).

Pain management in patients with injuries of the spine

Following evaluation and stabilization of injury to the spine, pain relief can be obtained by the judicious use of IV narcotics. The ability to perform neurological evaluation must not be hindered by the effects of pain management. Also, somnolence or sedation from narcotics must not mask changes that may be occurring as a result of unrecognized neurologic injury. If injury to the spine affects respiratory function, narcotics should be avoided. Patient-controlled analgesia is very effective following spinal stabilization (see Ch. 11).

PERIPHERAL NERVE BLOCKS

The nerve stimulator and insulated needles

At HJDOI peripheral nerve blocks are performed with the aid of a nerve stimulator and insulated needle.[12] This technique places an insulated needle in very close proximity to the nerves to be anesthetized without seeking a paresthesia. By obtaining a maximal twitch response at the lowest milliamperage (mA) in the nerve distribution of the area requiring anesthesia, it is believed that the tip of the insulated needle will be on the same side of a fascial sheath as the nerves. It is important that the nerve stimulator has a digital readout in a low current range (0.1 or 0.2 mA) since twitch responses obtained at this level indicate close proximity to the nerve. An insulated needle isolates the current to the tip of the needle ensuring that the local anesthesia is administered where the twitch is obtained (Fig. 21.1).

Obtaining a twitch response at the lowest mA possible improves success rate. This is explained

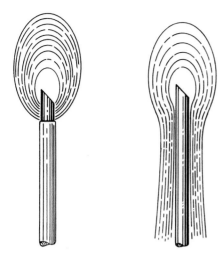

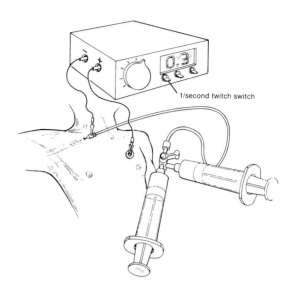

1/second twitch switch

Fig. 21.1 Electric current is concentrated at tip of insulated needle but is diffuse in uninsulated needle. From Bernstein and Rosenberg, with permission.[12]

Fig. 21.2 Nerve stimulator set-up. Block needle is attached to negative electrode of nerve stimulator; ground to positive terminal. Injection is performed where maximal twitches are obtained at lowest amperage. From Bernstein and Rosenberg, with permission.[12]

by understanding Coloumb's law, the inverse square law, which states that the current necessary to stimulate a nerve decreases by the inverse square as you approach the nerve: the closer to the nerve, the less current is required to stimulate the nerve.[16] Conversely, if the needle is at a far distance from a nerve, the nerve can be stimulated but it will require much higher currents to achieve the response. It thus becomes obvious that if a nerve is stimulated with a very low current (0.1–0.2 mA), the needle must be in very close proximity to the nerve. Just as obvious is the concept that if a twitch response is obtained at a higher current such as 0.5–1.5 mA, the observer cannot be certain that the needle is right next to the nerve, or in fact, if the needle and applied current may be stimulating the nerve across a fascial sheath.

The negative lead of the nerve stimulator is placed on a metal connector on the insulated needle and the positive lead is attached to an electrocardiogram (ECG) electrode (the ground electrode) placed on the opposite side of the body from that being blocked (Fig. 21.2).

The process of obtaining the appropriate twitch response can be divided into two stages, the *search mode* and the *fine tune mode*. During the search mode, a twitch response is sought in the muscle groups of the nerves to be blocked. The insulated needle is advanced using an initial current of 1.0–1.5 mA and a twitch response is sought. Once a twitch is obtained, the fine tune mode is used. The nerve stimulator is 'dialed-down' while still

observing for a twitch response using as an end-point the best twitch response at the lowest mA possible. If the twitch response is lost, the needle may need to be advanced, withdrawn, or the angle changed until a twitch is again obtained. If twitches are lost, the twitch monitor mA can be dialed back up to the 1.0–1.5 mA range while twitches are again sought. Once twitches are obtained and maximized, the nerve stimulator can be dialed back down and the needle manipulated until a twitch response is obtained in the 0.1–0.3 mA range. The end-point varies for different blocks: 0.1–0.2 mA for axillary; 0.1–0.3 mA for interscalene; 0.1–0.4 mA for infraclavicular; and 0.1–0.2 mA for femoral nerve block. Once this is achieved, stabilize the needle, aspirate to insure that the needle tip is not intravascular, and inject 2 mL of local anesthetic. It is noted that with only 2 mL of local anesthetic the twitch response is abolished. If the twitch response is not lost after 2 mL of local anesthetic is injected, withdraw the needle slightly, reconfirm a good twitch response at 0.2 mA, aspirate to make certain the needle is not intravascular, and reinject 2 mL. If the twitch response becomes abolished, the remainder of the local anesthetic is administered with intermittent aspiration.

SUPERFICIAL SKIN STIMULATION

Use of the nerve stimulator and an insulated needle is a 'blind procedure' since the tip of the needle is not visualized when obtaining a twitch response. Because of this, there is a 'search process' that occurs when trying to initially obtain a twitch response. At times the 'search process' is uncomfortable for the patient and unsatisfactory for the anesthesiologist.

The process of locating nerves such as those in the brachial plexus or the femoral nerve can be facilitated by stimulating the skin over the area where the nerves are thought to be located and obtaining a response in the nerve distribution to be blocked. By locating the nerves prior to sticking the patient with a needle, the patient is more comfortable and the physician appears more facile. The site now becomes the entry point of the needle or the location toward which the needle is advanced when performing an unpadavacular block. Superficial skin stimulation has been very helpful especially in obese patients where anatomy is difficult to delineate. In a number of circumstances when the operator has been advancing and withdrawing an insulated needle numerous times without a successful twitch response, location of the brachial plexus by superficial skin stimulation has facilitated achieving a successful block.

Technique for use of the nerve stimulator for superficial skin stimulation

- Open the inside of an ECG pad and remove the metallic inside component.
- Connect the ECG metal component to the 'alligator' clip of the negative lead of the nerve stimulator.
- Place a ground ECG pad on the patient and attach the positive lead to this ECG pad.
- With the current set at about 5 mA, palpate the area in the axilla where the axillary artery is pulsating or where you believe the brachial plexus is located (Fig. 21.3).
- Press the ECG metallic component into the skin over that area while searching for a twitch response.
- Maximize the location of the twitch response and mark this with a skin-marking pen.
- Use this site as the entry point for performing an axillary block or the direction that you will be

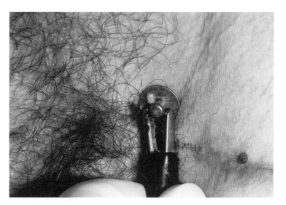

Fig. 21.3   Superficial skin stimulation being utilized to help locate the bracheal plexus in the axilla (see text).

aiming toward when performing an infraclavicular block.

PERIOPERATIVE PAIN MANAGEMENT FOR INJURIES TO THE EXTREMITIES

Advantages of regional anesthesia for upper extremity surgery include excellent surgical operating conditions, prolonged postoperative pain relief, improved blood flow to extremities after reimplantation, and capability of placing patients in continuous passive motion (CPM) machines shortly after surgery.[1,4–6,12]

Pain relief can be obtained by repeating nerve blocks via a catheter utilizing intermittent injections or infusion techniques. For upper extremity injuries, block of the brachial plexus by interscalene, infraclavicular, and axillary techniques can be utilized (see Ch. 13). The block should be chosen based on the location of surgery[1] (Table 21.3). An axillary block will occasionally spare the thumb, and an interscalene block may miss areas supplied by the ulnar nerve. The musculocutaneous nerve may be spared with axillary blocks, since it exits from the brachial plexus and enters the substance of the coracobrachialis muscle above the level where an axillary block is performed.

While a prolonged block can be obtained with proper choice of local anesthetic agent, e.g. bupivacaine or ropivacaine, catheters can provide prolonged relief via infusion or intermittent injection (Ch. 13). Successful use of catheter techniques have been described. In 1979, Rosenblatt utilized

Table 21.3 Block of choice[1]

Injury	Interscalene	Infraclavicular	Axillary
Shoulder dislocation	✓		
Rotator cuff	✓		
Fracture of the proximal humerus	✓		
Biceps rupture	✓		
Triceps tendon rupture	✓		
Humeral shaft	✓		
Distal humerus	✓	✓	
Olecranon	✓	✓	✓
Forearm fasciotomy		✓	
Elbow dislocation		✓	
Open reduction internal fixation radius		✓	
Boxer's fracture (5th metacarpal)		✓	✓
Thumb	✓	✓	
Reimplantation		Continuous	Continuous

a continuous infusion of bupivacaine to provide postoperative pain relief after a traumatic hand injury was repaired in a 15-year-old boy.[9] Matsuda, Selander, and Berger have all described successful use of continuous brachial plexus catheters.[8,10,11] Bupivacaine in concentrations of 0.125–0.25% at rates of 7–10 mL/h appears to be safe and effective[17] (see Ch. 13).

INTERSCALENE BRACHIAL PLEXUS BLOCK

The shoulder region

Anesthesia for surgery of the shoulder for fractures, rotator cuff repair, and arthroscopy can be performed using an interscalene brachial plexus block.[12] Since performance of an interscalene block requires some movement of the neck, cervical spine injury must first be ruled out. As mentioned previously, an interscalene block causes a Horner's syndrome on the ipsilateral side which may confuse neurologic examination of the patient.[12] This may be construed as a sign of intracranial pathology. Hemidiaphragmatic paralysis will also occur on the side of the block.[18]

Following shoulder surgery it may be necessary to place patients in a CPM machine to prevent a frozen shoulder. These machines move the shoulder through a continuous range of motion. Pain management for CPM can be obtained by daily nerve blocks with long-acting local anesthetic agents or via continuous infusion techniques.

Case studies

A 76-year-old female with a history of coronary artery and valvular heart disease as well as chronic obstructive pulmonary disease presented for repair of a humeral head fracture. An interscalene block was performed. The patient tolerated the surgery without problem.

A 25-year-old male underwent rotator cuff repair under general anesthesia. The patient had severe pain postoperatively and was given an interscalene block of 40 mL ropivacaine 0.2% with epinephrine with excellent relief.

Technique for interscalene brachial plexus block (Fig. 21.4)

- The patient is placed on the OR table in the supine position or may be placed in the sitting position for shoulder surgery.[1,5,6,12,19]
- A ground electrode is attached to an ECG pad on the opposite side of the body.
- The head is turned to the opposite side from that being blocked.
- The neck area is prepped, and sterile gloves are worn.
- The posterior border of the sternocleidomastoid muscle is palpated at the level of the cricoid cartilage.

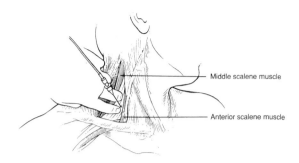

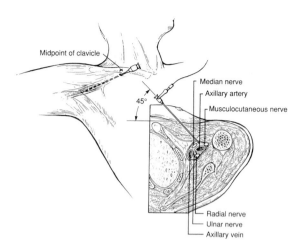

Fig. 21.4 Interscalene brachial plexus block. Needle is inserted between anterior and middle scalene muscles. Needle is directed caudad, mesiad, and posterior. From Bernstein and Rosenberg, with permission.[12]

- The index and middle fingers are slipped off the posterior border of the sternocleidomastoid muscle and into the groove between the anterior and middle scalene muscles and then slightly separated.
- A skin wheal is raised.
- An insulated needle is attached to the negative lead of the nerve stimulator. With the nerve stimulator set at 1.0–1.5 mA, the needle is passed into the neck in a backward and downward direction to avoid an intravascular or intrathecal injection.
- As the needle is advanced, observe for twitches of muscles below the shoulder, or any response in the arm or hand.
- Once twitches are obtained, adjust the stimulation to achieve maximal twitches at the lowest current (0.2–0.3 mA). This may require moving the needle in or out and adjusting mA levels.
- If twitches are obtained that stimulate the diaphragm, the needle is too anterior – it is on the anterior scalene muscle.
- If twitches are obtained that stimulate the back of the shoulder, the needle is too posterior.
- Once maximal twitch is obtained at lowest mA, stabilize the needle and aspirate to make certain that the needle tip is not intravascular or intrathecal.
- Inject 2 mL of local anesthetic which should abolish the twitch.
- Inject remainder of 40 mL of local anesthetic with intermittent aspiration.
- Infiltrate 5 mL of local anesthetic along the mid-point of the posterior border of the sternocleidomastoid muscle in order to block the superficial cervical plexus.

Fig. 21.5 Infraclavicular brachial plexus block. Operator stands on side opposite one to be blocked. Needle is inserted 1 inch below mid-point of the clavicle at a 45° angle and directed toward pulsations of axillary artery. From Bernstein and Rosenberg, with permission.[12]

INFRACLAVICULAR BRACHIAL PLEXUS BLOCK

Block of the brachial plexus by the infraclavicular approach will anesthetize all the nerves of the brachial plexus including the musculocutaneous nerve. This block provides anesthesia for surgery on the arm below the shoulder. A nerve stimulator is used to perform the block[1,5,6,12,20] (Fig. 21.5).

Technique for infraclavicular brachial plexus block

- The patient is placed on the OR table in the supine position.
- The head is turned away from the side to be blocked. The mid-point of the clavicle is identified and a point 2.5 cm below the mid-point is marked.
- The axillary artery is palpated as high in the axilla as possible and marked.
- The brachial plexus can be located in the axilla by superficial skin stimulation.
- A line can be drawn from the skin wheal toward the pulsations of the axillary artery which will give an indication of the direction for the needle.
- A skin wheal is raised 2.5 cm below the mid-point of the clavicle. A tiny hole is made with an

18 gauge needle in the center of the skin wheal if a blunt needle is to be used for the block.

- Through the skin wheal an insulated needle is passed at a 45° angle toward the pulsations of the axillary artery in the axilla with the nerve stimulator set at 1.0–1.5 mA. Some practitioners insert the needle 1–2″ lateral to described point of insertion but still at a 45° angle.
- Muscle twitches in the distribution of the musculocutaneous nerve are ignored (biceps twitch) since the nerve may be stimulated after it has exited from the brachial plexus. The musculocutaneous nerve may also be stimulated at a low mA across a fascial plane since it is the most superficial nerve in the brachial plexus at the level where an infraclavicular nerve block is performed.
- When the maximum twitch in the muscle of the forearm or hand is achieved at the lowest current possible (0.2–3 mA), 2 mL of local anesthetic is injected after aspiration which should abolish the twitch.
- 40 mL of local anesthetic are then injected with intermittent aspiration.

For continuous block, a catheter passed through a needle or a catheter over a needle may be used (see Ch. 13).

The catheter is inserted and secured to the skin and an antibacterial dressing is applied. Successful pain relief has been achieved utilizing both intermittent bolus injections of local anesthetic or a continuous infusion.

AXILLARY BRACHIAL PLEXUS BLOCK

This block is useful for surgery in the hand.[1,12,19] When performing a brachial plexus block at the axillary level it must be remembered that the musculocutaneous nerve has already exited from the brachial plexus and therefore the musculocutaneous nerve must be blocked by a separate injection in the coracobrachialis muscle. Continuous infusion techniques are very successful. Chapter 13 outlines this technique.

Continuous infusion technique

The infusion rate can start at 5–7 mL per hour using 0.125% bupivacaine. The rate and concentration can be adjusted as needed by evaluating the patient's response.[17] The dose and rate of administration can affect sensory, sympathetic, and motor function. If motor function is to be maintained, it may be necessary to decrease the concentration of the local anesthetic.

Infection prophylaxis for continuous catheter technique

When using a continuous infusion, attention to sterility should be observed to avoid infection at the catheter site. Povidine ointment should be placed at the site and a transparent occlusive dressing applied. The time and date should be noted at the catheter site.

USE OF INDIVIDUAL NERVE BLOCKS

Frequently, victims of major trauma suffer from isolated injuries to an extremity which requires immediate attention. However, the patient may not be able to undergo general anesthesia, or, because of hemodynamic instability, may not be able to tolerate spinal or epidural anesthesia. The use of nerve blocks in such instances is of great value and can aid in early stabilization of fractures and debridement of open wounds without any effects on hemodynamic stability.

The reduction of fractures early in the management of the victim suffering from major trauma can aid in stabilizing the patient, decrease the chances of infection, decrease the chances of fat and pulmonary emboli, and will definitely decrease pain.[21–23]

THE PATIENT WITH A FRACTURED HIP

Patients who suffer from fractures of the hip should have the fracture repaired as soon as possible. However it is imperative that physiologic stabilization be carried out to bring the patient into the best possible condition prior to embarking on formal surgical repair.

The amount of bleeding associated with a fractured hip is determined by the site of the fracture. In patients with subcapital fractures there is usually a small amount of bleeding since the fracture is within the capsule. Intertrochanteric fractures will probably have more bleeding. Blood and fluids should be administered as necessary to achieve hemodynamic stability. Associated medical problems should be evaluated and treated in order to bring the patient into the best possible condition. Upon admission these patients are usually placed in traction to stabilize the fracture which usually decreases the amount of pain. Pain relief may be obtained in these patients while they are awaiting surgery by a femoral and lateral femoral cutaneous nerve block.

Management of a patient with a fractured hip and severe respiratory insufficiency

Case study

An 85-year-old female presented for repair of a fractured hip. On arrival to the OR her O_2 saturation was noted to be 70% and an arterial blood gas test revealed a PaO_2 of 37 mmHg. The patient was evaluated for a pulmonary embolism. She complained of severe pain in her hip. To provide pain relief, spinal morphine 0.5 mg was administered which was very successful. A pulmonary embolism was ruled out and the patient underwent surgery under spinal anesthesia.

A 51-year-old female sustained a fractured hip after falling. She had a history of chronic obstructive pulmonary disease with an increased anterior–posterior chest diameter, scattered rhonchi, occasional wheezing, and decreased breath sounds. An arterial blood gas test revealed a PaO_2 of 50 mmHg with an oxygen saturation of 88%.[1,5,6,12]

Anesthetic management

In many patients regional anesthesia is chosen in order to avoid the possibility of the need for prolonged ventilatory care. A spinal anesthetic using 3 mL of isobaric bupivacaine 0.5% with 0.3 mg of epinephrine, and 0.3–0.4 mg of preservative-free morphine is an appropriate dose. This technique is useful since the spread of the spinal anesthetic is usually well controlled and does not interfere with respiration. The use of intrathecal morphine provides pain relief without the use of parenteral narcotics. It is clear that a patient with a PaO_2 of 37 mmHg, even if it is of long-term duration, would do well to avoid the respiratory depressant effects of systemic opioids. Respiratory depression, pruritus, and urinary retention are side effects that must be considered after administering epidural or intrathecal narcotics (see Ch. 12).

Assess intravascular volume

Prior to administering spinal anesthesia to a patient with a fractured hip, intravascular volume status and hematocrit level must be assessed and if there is any deficiency it should be reconstituted with blood and crystalloid as indicated. If there should be a drop in blood pressure following administration of the spinal anesthetic, judicious use of fluids plus vasopressors are recommended. The infusion of large volumes of fluid to treat a drop in blood pressure from systemic vasodilatation may lead to postoperative pulmonary edema as the spinal anesthetic recedes. If there is any question concerning volume status and there is a fear of congestive heart failure, a pulmonary artery catheter may be inserted to guide treatment.

Management of a patient with a fractured hip and chronic obstructive pulmonary disease and aortic stenosis

Case study

An 80-year-old patient was scheduled for repair of a non-displaced subcapital fracture of the hip. She suffered from chronic obstructive pulmonary disease and had moderate-to-severe aortic stenosis. A regional anesthetic technique was considered preferable in order to avoid general anesthesia with endotracheal intubation. However, because of the moderate-to-severe aortic stenosis, the side effects of spinal anesthesia: sympathetic blockade, vasodilatation, and afterload reduction made that an unacceptable choice. Therefore it was elected to perform a lumbar plexus block[1,5,6] (Fig. 21.6).

Technique for lumbar plexus block

- The patient is placed on the OR table with the fracture site up.[5,12,24,25] A line is drawn along the lumbar spinous processes

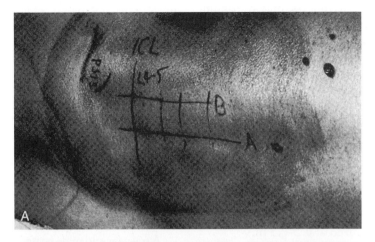

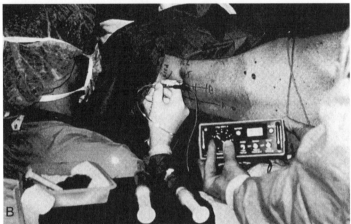

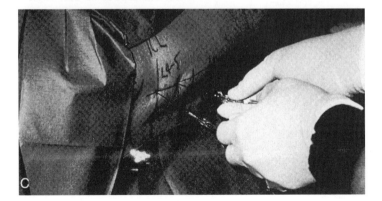

Fig. 21.6 Lumbar plexus block. (A) Anatomy marked out. PSIS, posterior superior iliac spine; ICL, intercristal line; A, line along spinous process; B, line parallel to line A through PSIS. (B) Block with nerve stimulator. (C) Close-up of lumbar plexus block. From Rosenberg and Bernstein, with permission.[5]

- A line parallel to this line is drawn passing through the posterior–superior iliac spine.
- Lines drawn at the L4–5 and L3–4 interspaces intersect the line from the posterior–superior iliac spine (Fig. 21.7).
- At the point of intersection of these two lines, skin wheals are raised.
- Through these wheals insulated needles are passed until the transverse processes are encountered. The needles are then directed off the transverse processes caudally and into the psoas compartment.
- Twitches in the area supplied by the nerves from the lumbar plexus are sought.
- Twitches are maximized at 0.2–0.3 mA
- 10 mL of lidocaine 1.5% with epinephrine 1:200 000 are injected at each site where the maximum twitch is achieved at the lowest current.[5]

Using this method anesthesia is achieved with the patient in the position needed for the surgery with the fracture site uppermost. Afterload reduction, which may have resulted from the spinal

anesthetic, is avoided.[5] The lumbar plexus block was employed by Chayen et al to provide anesthesia and analgesia for 100 patients undergoing surgery including repair of hip fracture, femoral plating, amputation, and removal of femoral nails.[24] The results were reported as excellent.[24] Chapter 13 has a detailed discussion comparing two different approaches to the lumbar plexus.

A fractured hip repaired under individual nerve blocks

Case study

A 63-year-old male sustained a non-displaced subcapital fracture of his hip which was scheduled to be repaired with Knowles pins. The patient had a history of mitral stenosis and atrial fibrillation. Echocardiography revealed an ejection fraction of 40% and left ventricular dysfunction. A pulmonary artery catheter revealed a pulmonary artery pressure of 75/35 mmHg. His systemic blood pressure was 140/40 mmHg.[1,5,6] *Femoral, lateral femoral cutaneous, and obturator nerve blocks were performed.*

In this operation a small incision is made on the lateral aspect of the thigh and pins are inserted through the neck of the femur across the fracture and into the head of the femur. This fracture was non-displaced and required no reduction.

To provide adequate analgesia for the procedure, femoral, lateral femoral cutaneous, and obturator nerve blocks were performed using lidocaine 2% and bupivacaine 0.5%. Epinephrine was not used since tachycardia may have been detrimental to this patient and may have interfered with left ventricular filling. The femoral and obturator nerve blocks were performed with the use of a nerve stimulator. Remember, to keep the stimulating current low to avoid violent, muscle twitches and pain at the fracture site.[1,5]

The patient was sedated with midazolam and fentanyl. Anesthesia was provided using peripheral nerve blocks so that there was no chance for any hemodynamic changes secondary to the anesthesia. The techniques used in this patient provided complete anesthesia for the surgical procedure as well as postoperative pain relief because of the long action of the bupivacaine. The

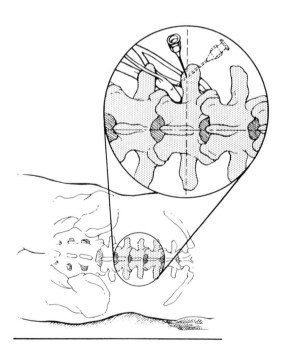

Fig. 21.7 Lumbar plexus block. Patient is placed in lateral position. Needle is inserted until transverse process is encountered and redirected deeper while observing for twitches. From Bernstein and Rosenberg, with permission.[12]

pain control provided by the nerve blocks is beneficial since it decreases the stress response with the
attendant tachycardia in this patient.

Technique for femoral nerve block

- After the area is prepped, the femoral artery is
  palpated[12] (Fig. 21.8).
- A skin wheal is raised just lateral to pulsations of
  the femoral artery at approximately 2.5 cm
  below the inguinal ligament (Fig. 21.8).
- Insert an insulated needle through the wheal do
  not use a pencil-point type insulated needle for
  a femoral nerve block. You may have the tip of
  the needle on one side of the fascia with the
  femoral nerve and the injection port on the
  other side of the fascia.
- The negative lead is attached to the needle and
  the ground lead to an ECG pad on the patient.
- Set the mA at 0.5 mA.
- Remember that since the femoral nerve is
  located approximately 1 cm below the skin, the
  needle need not be inserted too deeply.
- Once twitches are obtained, decrease the mA to
  obtain twitch at 0.1–0.2 mA.
- Aspirate and inject the local anesthetic.[12]

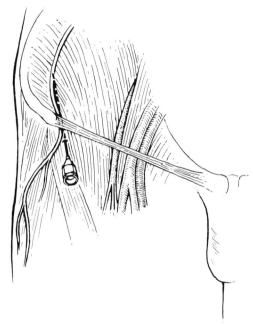

Fig. 21.9   Lateral femoral cutaneous nerve block.
Needle is inserted 1 inch medial and 1 inch inferior to
anterior superior iliac spine. Anesthetic solution is
infiltrated in a fan-wise direction. From Bernstein and
Rosenberg, with permission.[12]

Technique for block of the lateral femoral cutaneous nerve of the thigh

- This nerve supplies sensory innervation from the
  lateral aspect of the thigh to the knee (Fig. 21.9).
- The patient is placed on the OR table in the
  supine position.[12]
- The area of the thigh medial and inferior to the
  anterior superior iliac spine (ASIS) is prepped.
- A skin wheal is raised 2.5 cm medial and 2.5 cm
  inferior to the ASIS (Fig. 21.9).
- Through this wheal a 22 gauge needle is passed
  and 5–7 mL of 1.5% lidocaine with epinephrine
  1:200 000 is injected in a fan-wise manner
  superiorly and laterally toward the iliac crest.[12]

Technique for block of the obturator nerve

The obturator nerve supplies the skin on the
anteromedial aspect of the thigh down to the knee
and provides a nerve to the hip joint.

- The patient is placed on the OR table in the
  supine position.[12]
- The pubic tubercle is identified.

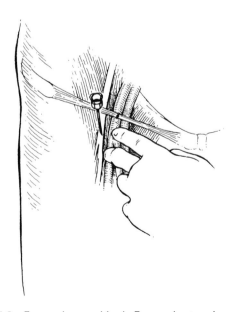

Fig. 21.8   Femoral nerve block. Femoral artery is
palpated below inguinal ligament. Needle is inserted
perpendicular to skin lateral to femoral artery. Twitch
monitor is used. From Bernstein and Rosenberg, with
permission.[12]

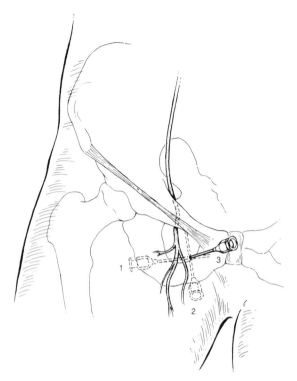

Fig. 21.10 Obturator nerve block. Needle is inserted 1–2 cm below and 1–2 cm lateral to the pubic tubercle. (1) Medial direction – identity ramus of pubis. (2) 45° cephalad – superior portion of canal. (3) Lateral and inferior – into canal. From Bernstein and Rosenberg, with permission.[12]

- The skin wheal is raised 2.5 cm lateral and 2.5 cm inferior to the pubic tubercle (Fig. 21.10).
- Through this wheal an insulated needle is passed and attached to a nerve stimulator.
- Manipulate needle as described in Figure 21.10.
- Twitches at 0.1–0.2 mA are sought on the medial aspect of the thigh.
- 5 mL of 1.5% lidocaine with epinephrine 1:200 000 injected.[12]

Postoperative pain control in patients with fracture of the hip

If a continuous epidural catheter is placed for the surgery, intermittent or continuous administration of local anesthetics and narcotics can be used (see Ch. 12). If a spinal anesthetic is used for the operative procedure, 0.3 mg of preservative-free morphine can be placed with the local anesthetic. This will provide pain relief for approximately 24 hours. The patient must be observed for and treated for respiratory depression, pruritus, and

urinary retention. Femoral and lateral femoral cutaneous nerve blocks can be repeated at approximately 12-hour intervals for 1 to 2 days postoperatively to provide pain relief.

Lower extremity trauma

For other traumatic injuries of the lower extremity, femoral, lateral femoral cutaneous, and sciatic nerve blocks are also useful. Femoral and lateral femoral cutaneous nerve blocks have already been described. For anesthesia of the posterior aspect of the thigh and below the knee, block of the sciatic nerve is necessary. In instances where the patient must remain in the supine position, block of the sciatic nerve by the anterior approach is useful.

FEMORAL AND SCIATIC NERVE BLOCKS

Case study

A young male sustained a fracture of the femur as a result of a motor vehicle accident. He was placed in traction at another hospital but as no surgical repair was carried out, the patient developed respiratory distress and a PaO_2 of 60 mmHg on room air. He was transferred to our institution where chest X-ray revealed acute respiratory distress syndrome. A diagnosis of fat embolism was made. Despite his acute situation, it was felt that surgery should be performed. In the OR holding room a femoral nerve block was performed in order to provide analgesia. Because of the hypoxemia secondary to fat embolism it was elected not to administer general anesthesia. Regional anesthesia was administered via femoral and sciatic nerve blocks. Since the patient could not lift his leg, a sciatic nerve block was performed via the anterior approach.[26]

The femoral fracture was reduced and intramedullary rods were inserted through a small incision at the knee. On the first postoperative day, the hypoxemia disappeared and the chest X-ray cleared. The residual effect of the femoral and sciatic nerve blocks provided analgesia for the first 24 hours following the procedure. The patient was allowed out of bed on the first postoperative day at which time his pain was controlled with parenteral analgesics.[26]

WARNING When carrying out a femoral nerve block for patients who have pain secondary to a fracture of the femur, do not start with the nerve stimulator on a high mA since the contraction of the muscles may cause severe pain. Start with a low mA to avoid violent muscle contraction when beginning the stimulation.

Technique for sciatic nerve block: using anterior approach

- The patient is placed on the OR table in the supine position.[6,26,27]
- The anterior–superior iliac spine and the pubic tubercle are palpated.
- A line is drawn between them (Fig. 21.11).
- Another line parallel to this line is drawn passing through the greater trochanter.
- The first line is divided into three equal parts.
- A perpendicular is dropped from the point between the medial and middle third of the first line to the line parallel to that passing through the greater trochanter. Where these two lines intersect, a skin wheal is raised.
- Through this wheal an insulated needle is passed while using a nerve stimulator. Twitches in the area supplied by the sciatic nerve are sought (calf, ankle). The sciatic nerve lies just posterior to the femur at the level of the lesser trochanter. If the lesser trochanter is encountered, the needle may have to be moved slightly medially and advanced posteriorly. After a twitch is obtained

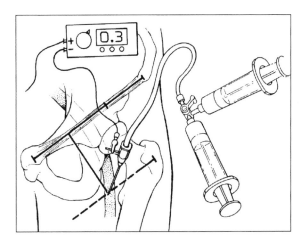

Fig. 21.11 Sciatic nerve block: anterior approach. From Rosenberg, Bernstein, Marshall and Albert, with permission.[26]

at 0.4 mA and aspiration is negative, 30 mL of 2% xylocaine with epinephrine 1:200 000 is injected after intermittent aspiration.[6,26,27] Alternatively a longer acting local anesthetic can be utilized.

Posterior approach to sciatic nerve

Case study

A 19-year-old male with a history of asthma sustained an injury to his neck and right knee as a result of a motorcycle accident. Although there was a temporary loss of consciousness, a CT scan of the head was negative. Neck pain led to further imaging studies which revealed a nondisplaced fracture of the odontoid necessitating placement of a halo. The patient was scheduled for arthroscopy of the knee for evacuation of a hematoma. Since the halo vest extended to the lumbar area, spinal anesthesia was not possible. General anesthesia was complicated by the presence of the halo and would have required an awake fiberoptic intubation which may have induced an asthmatic attack. It was elected to utilize peripheral nerve blocks of the femoral, sciatic, and lateral femoral cutaneous nerves to provide anesthesia for the surgical procedure. A femoral nerve block was performed by injection of chloroprocaine 2%, 10 mL 2.5 cm below the inguinal ligament immediately adjacent to the pulsations of the femoral artery. This was accomplished utilizing a nerve stimulator. A sciatic nerve block was then performed with the patient supine, and the hip and knee flexed at 90°.[1,5,6]

Technique for sciatic nerve block using posterior approach

The patient is placed in the supine position with the hip and knee flexed at 90°.[27] The surface anatomy is identified (Fig. 21.12).

- The ischial tuberosity and the greater trochanter are palpated.
- A line is drawn between the ischial tuberosity and the greater trochanter, and the area is prepped.

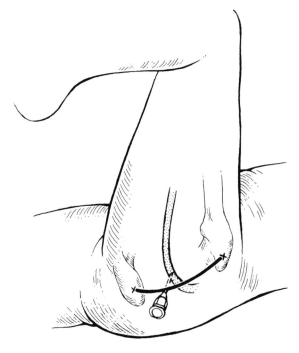

Fig. 21.12 Supine approach sciatic nerve block. Needle is inserted between ischial tuberosity and greater trochanter and advanced. Needle is kept parallel to table. From Bernstein and Rosenberg, with permission.[12]

- A skin wheal is raised slightly medial to the midpoint of this line.
- An insulated needle is passed perpendicular to the skin and parallel to the OR table with the current in the 1.5–2.0 mA range.
- As the needle is advanced, twitches are noted in the gluteal muscles. These result from direct muscle stimulation, not from stimulation of the sciatic nerve and should be ignored.
- The needle is then advanced until twitches are noted in the calf or ankle, indicating stimulation of the sciatic nerve.
- A maximal twitch response is obtained at the lowest mA (0.1–0.4 mA).
- 20–30 of local anesthetic are injected after intermittent aspiration.[12,27]

A lateral femoral cutaneous nerve block was performed by infiltrating local anesthesia agent in a fanwise direction from a point 1 inch medial and 1 inch inferior to the anterior superior iliac spine.

These three blocks, sciatic, femoral, and lateral femoral cutaneous, provided anesthesia for the surgical procedure.

In this patient the nerve block techniques used in the management of the trauma were tailor-made since the patient suffered from a head injury, a cervical spine injury, and asthma.

FRACTURES OF THE PELVIS

Pelvic fractures can be associated with massive blood loss and significant mortality.[29–31] An organized approach to care of these patients includes careful evaluation, fluid resuscitation, consideration for angiogram and embolization, and surgery if necessary.[29] To stabilize fractures of the pelvis and to decrease bleeding external fixators may be applied in the ER.[2,5] Imaging studies delineate the type of fracture so that proper planning for surgery can be carried out. In fact, fracture type is associated with different degrees of blood loss.[31] Bleeding occurs from laceration of the extensive arterial anastamoses that are present in the pelvis. In addition, venous drainage flows into a valveless system and this also increases blood loss. Brotman has described the importance of the extensive anastamoses in exacerbating blood loss (Fig. 21.13).[30] Pelvic fractures are associated with massive bleeding which results in development of retroperitoneal hematomas. The retroperitoneal hematoma that develops tamponades the arterial and venous bleeding sites and surgery may be contraindicated because it could cause these tamponaded vessels to bleed. Therefore angiography and embolization have become popular methods for managing these patients.[32] After proper blood and fluid resuscitation and evaluation patients may be brought to the OR for repair.[2,29,30] These procedures, however, are associated with large blood loss, hemodynamic instability, and long operations.

IV-PCA or an epidural infusion is useful to control postoperative pain. Epidural analgesia is an excellent modality after pelvic fracture repair (see Ch. 12). This is the case even though the procedure is performed under general anesthesia. Three sources of pain are present after pelvic surgery and all are controlled with an epidural infusion: surgical pain, pain from transportation to the radiology department for radiation therapy which is used to prevent heterotopic bone formation, and pain occurring as a result of the patient being placed in a CPM machine.

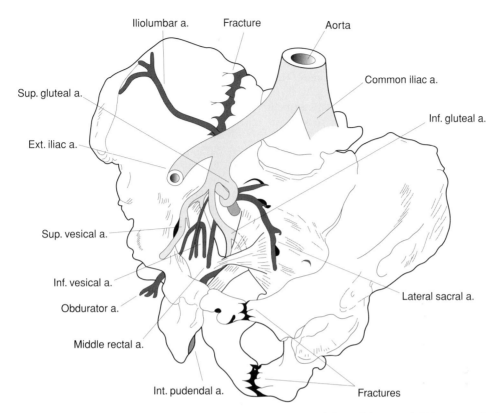

Fig. 21.13   Closely intertwined anatomical relationship of the bony pelvis and the arterial blood supply. From Brotman, et al, with permission.[30]

CONCLUSION

The patient with orthopedic trauma provides the anesthesiologist with the unique opportunity to provide pain relief to the extremity that is injured without necessarily requiring systemic medication. However, it is important that the orthopedic injury be understood in the context of the patient's other injuries. Regional blocks, spinal anesthesia, and epidural infusions can produce significant pain relief, improve the rehabilitation process, and increase patient satisfaction.

REFERENCES

1. Rosenberg AD, Bernstein RL, Grande CM, eds. Trauma anesthesia and critical care for orthopedic injuries. Problems in anesthesia. Philadelphia: JP Lippincott; 1994; 8(3).

2. Rosenberg AD, Bernstein RL. Perioperative anesthetic management of orthopedic trauma. In: Grande C, ed. Textbook of trauma anesthesia and critical care. St Louis: Mosby; 1992.

3. Dow AC. Regional anesthesia. In: Grande C, ed. Textbook of trauma anesthesia and critical care. St Louis: Mosby; 1993.

4. Desai SM, Bernhard WB, McAlary B. Regional anesthesia: management considerations in the trauma patient. Crit Care Clin 1990; 6.

5. Rosenberg AD, Bernstein RL. Regional anesthesia and trauma. In: Gotta AW, ed. Trauma. Anesthesia Clinics of North America 1996; 14(1): 101–123.

6. Rosenberg AD, Bernstein RL. Anesthesia for major orthopedic trauma. In: Smith C, Grande CM, eds. Anesthesia Clinics of North America 1999.

7. Ang ET, Lassale B, Goldfarb G. Continuous axillary brachial plexus block–a clinical and anatomical study. Anesth Analg 1984; 63: 680–684.

8. Selander D. Catheter technique in axillary plexus block presentation of a new method. Acta Anaesthesiol Scand 1977; 21: 324–329.

9. Rosenblatt R, Pepitone-Rockwell F, McKillop MJ. Continuous axillary analgesia for traumatic hand injury. Anesthesiology 1979; 51: 565–566.

10. Matsuda M, Kato N, Hosoi M. Continuous brachial plexus block for reimplantation in the upper extremity. The Hand 1982; 14: 129–134.

11. Berger A, Tizian C, Zenz M. Continuous plexus blockade for improved circulation in microvascular surgery. Ann Plast Surg 1985; 14: 17.

12. Bernstein RL, Rosenberg AD. Manual of orthopedic anesthesia and related pain syndromes. New York: Churchill Livingstone; 1993.

13. Strecker WB, Wood MB, Bieber EJ. Compartment syndrome masked by epidural anesthesia for postoperative pain. J Bone Joint Surg Am 1986; 68A: 1447–1448.

14. Bourne RB, Rorabeck CH. Compartment syndromes of the lower leg. Clin Orthop 1989; 240: 97.

15. McGlone R, Heyes F, Harris P. The use of a muscle relaxant to supplement local anesthetics for Bier's blocks. Arch Emerg Med 1988; 5: 79–85.

16. Pither C. Nerve stimulation. In: Raj PP, ed. Clinical practice of regional anesthesia. New York: Churchill Livingstone; 1991: 161–169.

17. Concepcion M. Continuous brachial plexus catheter techniques. In: Ferrante FM, VadeBoncover TR, eds. Postoperative pain management.

18. Urmey WF, Talts KH, Sharrock NE. One hundred percent incidence of hemidiaphragmatic paralysis associated with interscalene brachial plexus anesthesia or diagnosed by ultrasonograph. Anesth Analg 1991; 72: 498.

19. Winnie AP. Plexus anesthesia: Perivascular techniques of brachial plexus block. Philadelphia: WB Saunders; 1983.

20. Raj PP, Montgomery SJ, Nettles D, et al. Infraclavicular brachial plexus block. A new approach. Anesth Analg 1973; 52: 897.

21. Johnson KD, Cadambi A, Seibert GB. Incidence of adult respiratory distress syndrome in patients with multiple musculoskeletal injuries: effect of early operative stabilization of fractures. J Trauma 1985; 25: 375.

22. LaDuca JN, Bone LL, Seibel RW, et al. Primary open reduction and internal fixation of open fractures. J Trauma 1980; 20: 580.

23. Seibel R, LaDuca J, Hassett JM, et al. Blunt multiple trauma (ISS 36), femur traction, and the pulmonary failure–septic shock state. Ann Surg 1985; 202: 283.

24. Chayen B, Nathan H, Chayen B. The psoas compartment block. Anesthesiology 1976; 45: 95.

25. Winnie AP, Ramanurthy S, Durrani Z, et al. Plexus blocks for lower extremity surgery. Anesth Rev 1974; 1: 11.

26. Rosenberg AD, Bernstein RL, Marshall MH, Albert, DB. Anterior approach to the sciatic nerve–a radiographic correlation. Am J Anesthesiol 1997; 24: 166–167.

27. Beck GP. Anterior approach to sciatic nerve block. Anesthesiology 1963; 24: 222.

28. Raj PP, Parks RI, Eatson TD, et al. New single position spine approach to sciatic–femoral nerve block. Anesth Analg 1975; 54: 489.

29. Mucha P, Welch TJ. Hemorrhage in major pelvic fractures. Surg Clin North Am 1988; 68: 757.

30. Brotman S, Soderstrom CA, Oster-Granite M, et al. Management of severe bleeding in fractures of the pelvis. Surg Gynecol Obstet 1981; 153: 823.

31. Cryer HM, Mitler FB, Evers BM, et al. Pelvic fracture classification. Correlation with hemorrhage. J Trauma 1988; 28: 973.

32. Panetta T, Scalfani JJ, Goldstein AS, et al. Percutaneous transcatheter embolization for massive bleeding from pelvic fractures. J Trauma 1985; 25: 1021.

22

Chronic pain after trauma: complex regional pain syndrome and phantom limb pain syndrome

Pedro Alejandro Mendez-Tellez and Mark J Lema

COMPLEX REGIONAL PAIN SYNDROME: REFLEX SYMPATHETIC DYSTROPHY AND CAUSALGIA

Introduction

Taxonomy and classification of complex regional pain syndrome: reflex sympathetic dystrophy and causalgia
Complex regional pain syndrome
Sympathetically-maintained and sympathetically-independent pain

Pathogenesis of complex regional pain syndrome
Peripheral processes
Central processes

Clinical features and natural course of complex regional pain syndrome
First stage: the acute 'hyperemic' phase
Second stage: the dystrophic 'ischemic' phase
Third stage: the 'atrophic' phase

Diagnosis of complex regional pain syndrome
Clinical diagnosis
Ancillary tests
Diagnostic sympathetic block

Management of complex regional pain syndrome
Sympathetic block

PHANTOM LIMB PAIN SYNDROME

Introduction

History

Definitions

Clinical characteristics
Telescoping

Pathogenesis and pathophysiology
Peripheral
Spinal
Central (supraspinal)

Treatment
Surgical intervention
Epidural blockade
Spinal analgesia
Regional anesthesia
Intravenous infusion
Oral pharmacologic strategies
Transcutaneous electrical nerve stimulation
Other methods

Summary

COMPLEX REGIONAL PAIN SYNDROME: REFLEX SYMPATHETIC DYSTROPHY AND CAUSALGIA

INTRODUCTION

Reflex sympathetic dystrophy (RSD), causalgia, and phantom limb pain produce chronic noxious sensations known as neuropathic pains. The term neuropathic pain is applied to any acute or chronic condition in which the sustaining mechanism for the pain is inferred to involve aberrant somatosensory processes in the peripheral or central nervous system.[1]

Evans introduced the term of RSD in 1943.[3] Since then, RSD has acquired many synonyms (Table 22.1). Earlier classifications of RSD divided it into major and minor RSD on the basis of the presence or absence of actual neural injury and/or neurological deficit.[4] Major RSD was characterized by the presence of constant, spontaneous, severe, and burning pain, usually following either partial or complete peripheral nerve trunk injury, and often associated with hyperalgesia, hyperesthesia, and hyperpathia, along with vasomotor and sudomotor disturbances, and trophic changes. In addition to causalgia and phantom limb pain, central pain, thalamic syndrome, cerebral lesions, brainstem lesions, and spinal cord lesions can produce these symptoms. Similarly, vasomotor, sudomotor, and trophic changes characterize minor RSD, but they were not associated with overt damage to the nerve trunks.

The term RSD has been used to describe

a complex group of disorders that may develop as a consequence of trauma usually affecting limbs, with or without an obvious nerve lesion. RSD may also develop after visceral diseases, central nervous system lesions, or, without any antecedent event. Its symptoms consist of pain and related sensory abnormalities, abnormal blood flow, decreased or increased sweating, altered motor function, and changes in the structure of both superficial and deep tissues such as muscle and bone ('trophic changes'). It is not necessary that all components be present to diagnose RSD.

Thus, the term reflex sympathetic dystrophy is used in a descriptive sense and does not imply specific underlying mechanisms.[2]

Several precipitating factors and diseases also are associated with RSD (Table 22.2). Trauma secondary to accidental injury is probably the most common cause of RSD, but there is usually no correlation between the severity of injury and the severity of the resultant syndrome. The classic lesion that predisposes to the development of causalgia is a low- or high-velocity missile injury that stretches, but does not transect, a peripheral nerve. RSD occurs more commonly in whites; women seem to be more predisposed than men; ratios 2.9:1 frequently are observed, and it seems

Table 22.1 Synonyms used to describe complex regional pain syndromes I and II

Acute peripheral trophoneurosis
Algoneurodystrophy
Causalgia
Chronic traumatic edema
Neurovascular post-traumatic painful syndrome
Post-traumatic chronic edema
Post-traumatic pain syndrome
Post-traumatic osteoporosis
Post-traumatic sympathetic dystrophy
Reflex neurovascular dystrophy
Reflex neurovascular sympathetic dystrophy
Shoulder–hand syndrome
Spreading neuralgia
Sudeck's atrophy
Sympathalgia
Traumatic angiospasm
Traumatic vasospasm
Thermalgia

Table 22.2 Predisposing factors associated with reflex sympathetic dystrophy

- **Peripheral and post-traumatic**
  Soft tissue injuries (fracture, dislocation, sprain), immobilization or disuse, arthritis, infection, venous and arterial thrombosis, surgery, tumors, aortic aneurysm, myelography, arthroscopy, spinal anesthesia, paravertebral alcohol injection, Herpes zoster, brachial plexopathy, radiculopathy, or nerve plexus or trunk injury, vasculitis, myocardial infarction, Weber–Christian disease, polymyalgia rheumatica and pulmonary fibrosis
- **Central**
  Brain tumor, severe head injury, cerebral infarction, subarachnoid hemorrhage, cervical cord injury, subacute combined degeneration, syringomyelia, poliomyelitis and amyotrophic lateral sclerosis
- **Other** idiopathic, familial

unlikely in patients younger than 16 years of age.[5] The percentage of patients with RSD after an injury or accident varies widely from region to region and may have cultural implications. Reports show an incidence rate ranging from 0.05 to 15% of all trauma cases.[5]

Although injury to bone or soft tissue in an extremity appears to be the most common predisposing factor for RSD, there have been no systematic epidemiological studies of this phenomenon. RSD can also occur in the head and trunk.[1] It is not clear why, after similar injuries, some patients develop RSD and others do not. Several predisposing factors have been considered:

1. Genetic predisposition: Mailis & Wade[6] observed in a pilot study, that in 15 Caucasian women, certain HLA profiles seemed to be predisposed to develop refractory RSD. A twofold increase of A3, B7, and DR2 (15) MHC antigens was observed in the study population compared to control frequencies. 80 (five of six) of DR2 (15)-positive patients proved to be resistant to treatment.[6] Likewise, familial presentation suggests a genetic predisposition[7].
2. Disuse of an extremity might contribute to the onset or persistence of RSD.
3. Psychological factors: there is some evidence that suggests RSD is a psychogenic condition. It is likely that anxiety, stress, and chemical dependence increase nociception in RSD.

TAXONOMY AND CLASSIFICATION OF COMPLEX REGIONAL PAIN SYNDROME: REFLEX SYMPATHETIC DYSTROPHY AND CAUSALGIA

Complex regional pain syndrome

Recently, the International Association of the Study of Pain (IASP) introduced a new terminology for the chronic pain syndromes formerly recognized as RSD and causalgia. The term RSD implied a reflex (which has never been demonstrated), a linkage of the sympathetic nervous system (which was not always present), and the presence of dystrophy (which has also been inconsistently present). Since RSD was no longer a useful term to describe this clinical entity, it was, then, recommended that it and causalgia be called Complex Regional Pain Syndrome (CRPS).[8]

The new CRPS terminology describes a variety of painful conditions following injury that appear regionally, having a distal predominance of abnormal findings exceeding in both magnitude and duration the expected course of the inciting event. These findings often result in significant impairment of motor function and show variable progression over time.[8] CRPS, therefore, should be suspected if regional pain and sensory changes following a trauma exceed, in magnitude, duration, or both, the anticipated healing period. CRPS is further classified into types I and II (Table 22.3).

Table 22.3 Criteria for complex regional pain syndrome

CRPS I (Reflex Sympathetic Dystrophy)
- Type I is a syndrome that develops after an initiating noxious event
- Spontaneous pain or allodynia/hyperalgesia occurs, is not limited to the territory of a single peripheral nerve, and is disproportionate to the inciting event
- There is or there has been evidence of edema, skin blood flow abnormality, or abnormal sudomotor activity in the region of the pain since the inciting event
- This diagnosis is excluded by the existence of conditions that otherwise would account for the degree of pain and dysfunction

CRPS II (Causalgia)
- Type II is a syndrome that develops after a nerve injury
- Spontaneous pain or allodynia/hyperalgesia occurs and is not necessarily limited to the territory of the injured nerve
- There is or has been evidence of edema, skin blood flow abnormality, or abnormal sudomotor activity in the region of the pain since the inciting event
- The diagnosis is excluded by the existence of conditions that otherwise would account for the degree of pain and dysfunction

From: Stanton-Hicks M. Complex regional pain syndrome: a new name for reflex sympathetic dystrophy and causalgia. Current Review of Pain 1996; 1: 34–40.

Complex regional pain syndrome I

The first sub-group of disorders, CRPS I, describes the phenomena previously known as RSD. CRPS I (RSD) is a syndrome that develops after an initiating noxious event, and is characterized by continuous or spontaneous pain, allodynia, and/or hyperalgesia, which are disproportionate to the inciting event. There is evidence at some time, not necessarily at the time of diagnosis, of edema and abnormal vasomotor and sudomotor activities. This definition does not imply that the sympathetic nervous system was the source of the changes in skin blood flow, edema, or the sudomotor activity.[9]

Complex regional pain syndrome II

The second sub-group of painful conditions is CRPS II, previously known as causalgia. CRPS II also implies the presence of continuing pain, allodynia, and/or hyperalgesia after a nerve injury that is not necessarily limited to the distribution or territory of the injured nerve. As in CRPS I, there is evidence at some time of edema as well as vasomotor and sudomotor disturbances in the region of the injured nerve.[9]

Finally, the diagnosis of CRPS I or II is excluded by the presence of any condition that would otherwise account for the degree of pain and dysfunction.

Sympathetically maintained and sympathetically independent pain

In certain patients with CRPS, the pain depends on sympathetic activity in the affected areas. In 1986, Roberts[10] introduced the term sympathetically maintained pain (SMP) to describe that aspect of pain which is sustained, at least in part, by sympathetic efferent activity, and that is relieved by blockade of the efferent sympathetic nervous system. In contrast, sympathetically independent pain (SIP) refers to the aspect of pain, which is unresponsive to sympathetic blockade.[11] Therefore, CRPS may or may not have components of SMP. Clinically, a patient with CRPS may present with SMP or SIP, or part of the chronic pain syndrome may be SMP and part of it may be SIP. Patients with CRPS may or may not improve with sympathetic block. Thus, unequivocal response to sympathetic blockade establishes the diagnosis of SMP. It is important to understand that the SMP/SIP terminology is an operational definition, which categorizes a chronic pain according to the response to sympathetic blockade. These distinctions are important from a clinical perspective because treatment is accordingly influenced.

PATHOGENESIS OF COMPLEX REGIONAL PAIN SYNDROME

Despite the numerous theories that have been proposed to explain the mechanism giving rise to CRPS, no single pathophysiologic hypothesis explains the origin of CRPS adequately. Most hypotheses revolve around the notion of an abnormal reverberatory circuit at some level in the nervous system that contributes to a cycle of afferent sensory input and efferent sympathetic hyperactivity. Early explanations of this disorder included the suggestion that the sympathetic nerve fibers themselves transmitted pain impulses to the central nervous system. Mitchell et al[12] suggested that the pain and dystrophic changes were caused by alterations in peripheral blood flow resulting from sympathetic hyperactivity. Another hypothesis suggested that metabolic alterations in the extremity itself would activate the autonomic nervous system, producing the characteristic symptoms. It was postulated that excitation of the efferent fibers released a substance in the peripheral end organs that caused vasodilatation and subsequent sensitization of afferent neuronal pathways.[5] The involvement of the sympathetic nervous system in the pathophysiology of CRPS has been assumed for many decades on the basis of several clinical observations. These include the therapeutic response to sympathetic blockade, the worsening of causalgia following stimulation of the ipsilateral sympathetic chain, and the flare in pain that may be produced by subcutaneous injection of epinephrine in the affected area.[1] However, it is now recognized that the syndrome may not be mediated by sympathetic activity (e.g. SIP). Thus, RSD/causalgia has been ascribed to both peripheral and central processes (Table 22.4).

Peripheral processes

The peripheral mechanisms of RSD involve the following:

1. Ephaptic 'electrical' activity originated in damaged nociceptors[13]
2. Ephaptic 'chemical' irritation
3. 'Backfiring' by injured polymodal C fibers (ABC phenomenon or indirect coupling)[14]
4. Hypersensitization as a result of injury to the primary afferent nociceptors (Cannon's phenomenon) can cause aggravation of the pain.[15]

Table 22.4   Pathogenesis of complex regional pain syndrome

Peripheral mechanisms
- Doupe and Barnes' 'cross-talk' or 'artificial synapse' (ephaptic transmission) theory (ephaptic electrical discharge)
- Ephaptic substance P and norepinephrine secretion
- ABC Phenomenon ('Angry backfiring C fibers' theory)
- Hypersensitization (Cannon's phenomenon)

Central mechanisms
- Livingston's 'reverberatory circuit' theory
- Melzack & Casey's 'gate-control' theory
- Roberts' 'wide dynamic range (WDR) neurons sensitization' theory
- Turbulence of Sutherland

The 'Cross-talk' or 'artificial synapse' (ephaptic transmission) theory was proposed in 1944 by Doupe.[13] As a result of a trauma such as a crush injury, there is destruction of the biophysical insulation of nerves resulting in 'shunting' or 'short circuiting' of impulses, thus creating an artificial synapse or so-called ephapse between primary afferent nociceptors and efferent sympathetic impulses. Thus, direct cross-stimulation and cycle formation may cause exacerbation of pain during increased sympathetic activity.[5]

Indirect coupling is thought to occur when nociceptive visceral afferent neurons are sensitized by certain algogenic substances (such as substance P, prostaglandins, bradykinin, serotonin, and lactic acid) released peripherally. A release of such substances may cause vasodilatation and/or sensitization of afferent neural pathways,[5] resulting in hyperalgesia and allodynia owing to polymodal hyperpathia.[16]

Also ephaptic 'chemical' irritation may occur when, after local trauma, damaged nerves have increased sensitivity to the catecholamines released by sympathetic terminals (chemical coupling). The number of α-adrenergic receptors on regenerating nerve fibers (neuroma) increases, and ectopic activity produced by these nociceptive sensory fibers fluctuates with levels of circulating catecholamines. This mechanism may be mediated by α-adrenergic receptors on damaged peripheral nerves in humans, specifically contributing to the development of SMP.[1]

Central processes

The most compelling evidence that central mechanisms are fundamental in RSD/causalgia development is that complete isolation of the painful part from the central nervous system by neurectomy or rhizotomy does not reliably eradicate the pain.[1] Other relevant observations include the occurrence of classic RSD/causalgia following damage of the central nervous system or viscera, the immediate appearance of the pain after injury in many patients before the neuroma can develop, and the development of spreading pain and bilateral symptoms in many patients.[1] A variety of central mechanisms may be involved in the pathogenesis of CRPS.

First, the 'wide dynamic range (WDR) neurons sensitization' theory as proposed by Roberts[10] suggested that activation of peripheral unmyelinated C polymodal (CPM) nociceptors by minor trauma can sensitize these WDR neurons located in the dorsal horn of the spinal cord. A possible chronologic development of sympathetic dystrophy is as follows: cutaneous trauma initially generates afferent traffic in the CPM nociceptors that travels through the dorsal root ganglion into the spinal cord where it activates and sensitizes the WDR whose axons subsequently send nociceptive information to higher centers. These sensitized WDR neurons can respond to activity in the larger A mechanoreceptors activated by light touch. This mechanism produces the condition of allodynia. The same sensitized WDR neurons are hypothesized to transmit, not only painful information to higher centers, but also to initiate the sympathetic efferent activity that may further affect the sensory receptors further and induce a circuitous reverberating pain pathway. Roberts[10] suggested that SMP is a result of tonic activity in mechanoreceptor afferents and that this activity is induced by sympathetic efferent stimulation of these sensory receptors.

Second, Livingston's 'reverberatory circuit' theory[4,17] proposed that three factors were required for sympathetic dystrophy. First, a nerve injury, be it partial severance of a nerve, or an injury to smaller nerve endings or in close proximity thereto, occurs that serves as a focus of chronic irritation from which an abnormally increased number of afferent impulses arise that constantly bombard the spinal cord and are probably interpreted as pain. Second, as a result of increased afferent neuronal traffic, there is an upset in the normal activity of the internuncial pool of the gray matter of the cord. Third, because of the increased activity in the internuncial pool there is an increased activity of the anterior and lateral horn cells, which in turn produces increased motor activity to the affected segment. As the intensity of the process is increased, more and more neuron systems become involved, and the process becomes self-sustaining.

Third, Melzack et al's[4,5,18–20] 'gate-control' or 'central biasing' theory states that the perception of pain depends on two factors: the balance between large and small fiber input; and the modulating functions of the higher centers in the brain (the 'central biasing' mechanism). Under normal circumstances, the central biasing mechanism exerts a tonic inhibitory influence on neuronal synaptic transmission at all levels of the somatic protection system. When the amount of input to the reticular formation is decreased, inhibitory influence from the reticular formation also decreases. A decrease in the inhibitory influence from the biasing mechanism of the reticular formation, therefore, could produce self-sustaining activity at all neural levels, and it can be triggered repeatedly by noxious impulses from the site of injury. Pain occurs when the output of the self-sustaining neuron pools reaches a critical level. Because this activity can recruit adjacent neurons, and because it occurs at several levels, trigger zones can spread to distant areas.[4,5]

CLINICAL FEATURES AND NATURAL COURSE OF COMPLEX REGIONAL PAIN SYNDROME

As previously described, CRPS I and II are characterized by spontaneous and touch-evoked pain, with or without associated hyperalgesia, as well as vasomotor and sudomotor disturbances, and trophic changes of the skin and its appendages. Clinically, CRPS I (RSD) progresses through three stages[4,21,22] (Table 22.5). which will now be discussed.

First stage: the acute 'hyperemic' phase

Earlier signs and symptoms of CRPS I may appear at the time of injury or, more often, they may be delayed for several weeks. During the first stage,

Table 22.5 Complex regional pain syndrome I – clinical stages

First stage: the acute 'hyperemic' phase
- Burning or aching spontaneous pain, hyperpathia, and/or allodynia
- Increased skin blood flow and temperature, with rubor, soft edema, decreased sweating, and increased hair and nail growth

Second stage: the dystrophic 'ischemic' phase
- Hyperpathia, allodynia, and burning pain are more pronounced than in the first stage
- Decreased skin blood flow (cold, cyanotic, and sweaty skin)
- Decreased hair and nail growth
- Brawny edema
- Muscle atrophy, decreased range of motion of the joints, and early osteoporosis

Third stage: the 'atrophic' phase
- Hyperpathia, allodynia, and burning pain become less prominent
- Normalization of skin blood flow and temperature (less sweating and less difference in hair and nail growth)
- Marked trophic structural changes in the form of tight, thin skin, and subcutaneous tissues
- Pronounced muscle atrophy, osteoporosis, pericapsular fibrosis, and ankylosis leading to a marked limitation of function of the affected extremity

signs of sympathetic denervation or underactivity are present. The disturbances in vasomotor and sudomotor activities cause increases in blood flow, vasodilatation, hyperemia, hyperthermia, and anhydrosis of the affected extremity. The patient complains of spontaneous aching and/or burning pain in the extremity, restricted to a vascular, neural, or radicular territory. The pain may be constant and out of proportion to the severity of the antecedent injury. Hyperesthesia or hypesthesia may be present, as well as hyperpathia or allodynia. As a result, the patient protects the extremity from motion and physical contact resulting in disuse atrophy. The skin is warm and dry, with localized edema, dependent rubor, and increased growth of hair and nails. Treatment at this stage appears to be most effective.

Second stage: the dystrophic 'ischemic' phase

If untreated, the acute 'hyperemic' stage may progress to a second 'dystrophic' stage, usually within 2 to 3 months, during which signs of sympathetic overactivity will become quite promi-nent. Throughout this vasoconstrictive phase, spontaneous pain is prominent and may spread to the entire extremity; hyperpathia and/or allodynia is also more pronounced. The skin becomes cold and cyanotic, and frequently mottled. There is increased sweating. Edema becomes brawny and indurated. The cutaneous appendages of the extremity become scant and brittle. Hair growth decreases and the nails become cracked and ridged, with heavy grooves. Muscle wasting occurs, and joint capsules and ligaments become less flexible. Limited joint range of motion and pain leads to joint stiffening and contractures. Radiographically, patchy demineralization develops.[4,23] If this stage is not adequately treated, it progresses to the final atrophic stage, usually within 6 to 12 months of the precipitating event.

Third stage: the 'atrophic' phase

During the 'atrophic' phase, symptoms of diffuse sympathetic dystrophy appear in the subsequent months to years. During this stage, the pain that originally was distal in location spreads proximally and becomes less prominent; hyperpathia or allo-dynia is also less prominent. Irreversible trophic changes in the skin and subcutaneous tissues occur with loss of connective tissues. The skin is cool, thin, shiny and either cyanotic or pale because of decreased blood flow. Similarly, sweat-ing may be increased or decreased. Severe muscle wasting and bone demineralization also pro-gresses. Pericapsular fibrosis, ankylosis of joints, and contractures lead to marked limitation of function and resorption of the affected extremity. In addition, central nervous system involvement may be shown by bilateral limb involvement.[5] During the third stage, generalized systemic responses to chronic illness include malnutrition, disturbances of the diurnal rhythms, and emo-tional fixation on the pain problem.[5] The intractable pain eventually may cause mental deterioration, chronic invalidism, drug addiction, and possible suicide.[5]

DIAGNOSIS OF COMPLEX REGIONAL PAIN SYNDROME

To date, there are no validated diagnostic criteria for CRPS. Clinically, a patient with CRPS may present with SMP or SIP. Unfortunately, the clin-ical presentation of CRPS alone does not allow one to conclude whether the sympathetic system is involved in the generation or perpetuation of the CRPS. Thus, the diagnosis of CRPS should be based primarily on the medical history, clinical findings, ancillary tests, and a high index of suspi-cion (Table 22.6). Since some patients with CRPS may improve with sympathetic block, an important aspect during the diagnostic stage is to establish whether the pain is SMP. Pain relief with sympathetic nerve block confirms that the pain syndrome is also SMP.

Table 22.6   Diagnosis of complex regional pain syndrome

1. **Clinical diagnosis**
2. **Ancillary tests**
• Skin temperature measurements
Infrared thermography
Contact thermography
• Skin blood flow measurements
Digital plethysmography
Transcutaneous oxygen monitoring
• Sweating measurements
Q-SART sweat response test
• Skin conductance response
• Radiographic bone density
• Bone scan
3. **Diagnostic sympathetic block**
• Local anesthetic sympathetic ganglion blockade
• Intravenous phentolamine infusion
• Intravenous guanethidine blockade

Clinical diagnosis

A careful interview may reveal a traumatic precipi-tating event, which is always true in causalgia, but not so in all cases of RSD. A clinical description of the pain is very helpful. In the earlier stages it is described as aching and/or burning in nature and restricted to a vascular, neural, or radicular areas. It may radiate proximally or distally from the site of injury during the second stage. Hyperpathia, allodynia, hyperesthesia, or hypoesthesia may accompany the pain in the initial atrophic phase, but becomes less prominent in late stages. Other findings include skin, hair, and nail growth changes; in the early stages the skin is cold, cyan-otic, and sweaty owing to sympathetic overactivity accompanied by local spongy edema, later the edema spreads and becomes brawny. Initially, hair and nail growth is increased, but then it decreases during the second stage; the nails become cracked, grooved, and ridged. Any additional precipitating, aggravating, or mitigating factor should be fully described.

Ancillary tests

It is necessary to make a number of objective measurements during the evaluation of RSD in order to define baseline values. These measurements can then be used to monitor the progression or resolution of the condition and to guide therapy.

Skin temperature measurements

Early in the course of this syndrome, signs of sympathetic denervation or underactivity are present; there may be increased cutaneous blood flow, vasodilatation, hyperemia, hyperthermia, and anhydrosis of the affected extremity. Later, however, skin blood flow and temperature may be reduced.[24] Skin temperature provides a crude estimation of the severity of the disorder. It is most accurately measured by infrared methods, using telethermometry or thermography, liquid crystallography or by direct measurement with a surface thermometer.[24] Consistent differences between the affected and normal limb may indicate the presence of sympathetic involvement.[24]

Infrared thermography is one of the most sensitive tests in the diagnosis of RSD. Infrared thermography identifies subtle temperature gradients in different parts of the skin. Infrared thermography is capable of recording instantaneous skin temperature with greater than $0.1°C$ accuracy over an area as small as a few square millimeters. Although there have been numerous studies of this technique, its diagnostic role is still controversial. Virtually any physical or emotional stimulus can alter peripheral skin blood flow. The interpretation may be further complicated when the putative stages of the condition are considered, i.e. initial high skin temperature, then low, and finally reversion to normal temperature. It is therefore conceivable for skin temperature to be normal in RSD.[24]

Contact thermography is a precise technique that compares the affected and unaffected extremities.

The extremity is either sprayed with heat-sensitive crystals or is placed against a plate containing similar crystals which change color in response to different temperatures. Thus, a permanent photographic record of the skin temperature color pattern may be made and can be used to document the cutaneous manifestation of the disorder and the presence or absence of improvement after therapy.[5]

Skin blood flow measurements

Peripheral blood flow can be assessed by several methods including venous occlusion plethysmography, laser Doppler, and xenon clearance techniques.[24]

Digital plethysmography and oscillometry permit the clinician to record a magnification of the peripheral pulse waves. It is useful to document the paucity of peripheral perfusion under conditions of sympathetic dystrophy and indicate early improvement in flow after an effective sympathetic block is administered. However, there are few data on the effects of RSD on blood flow or the responses to therapeutic interventions[24] to warrant it as a valid diagnostic or therapeutic test.

Transcutaneous oxygen monitoring may reveal decreased peripheral perfusion as a result of RSD. Thus, Sonneveld et al[25] reported that sympathetic hyperactivity resulted in reduced peripheral perfusion that could be detected by comparing transcutaneous oxygen content signals with the contralateral unaffected extremity. They also found that effective treatment to correct the sympathetic hyperactivity produces gradual return of transcutaneous oxygen content in the affected extremity to levels seen in the contralateral extremity.[5]

Sweating measurements

Q-SART sweat response test. The Q-SART (Quantitative sudomotor axon reflex test) measures sweat production.[24] A Perspex capsule is placed on the skin, and the increase in humidity of air blown through the capsule is measured. The mass of water/unit area/time may be calculated. Acetylcholine is then iontophoresed into the skin, and the resulting sweat output is measured. It is believed that the stimulated sweat output is higher and prolonged when sympathetic hyperactivity is present. It can therefore be used to assess both presynaptic and postsynaptic activity of the sympathetic sudomotor system.[24]

Skin conductance response

Skin conductance response (SCR) is used in some laboratories based on the fact that disturbance of sympathetic dysfunction causes an altered SCR. This is useful in assessment of effectiveness of sympathectomy postoperatively. It is not a sensitive test in the early stages of the illness.[15]

Radiographic bone density

Earliest radiographic changes of sympathetic dysfunction and disuse include patchy epiphysial demineralization of the short bones of hands and feet.[24] Subperiosteal bone resorption, cortical striation, and tunneling may occur as well. Soft tissue swelling or atrophy may also be apparent.[24] These changes are not diagnostic of RSD and may occur in any condition producing disuse of one limb.[24]

Bone scan

Bone scan is helpful in the dystrophic and atrophic stages but rarely in the hyperemic stage. Three-phase technetium bone scanning may reveal reduction in flow during the early phase but it shows increased periarticular uptake during the late phase[24], and asymmetry of technetium uptake in the bones of the extremity involved with RSD. This test is nonspecific, and many other conditions such as arthritis, infection, malignancy, and gout can show similar changes.[15]

Diagnostic sympathetic block

Even though the diagnosis of CRPS is a clinical one, determining if a component of the pain is mediated or maintained by the sympathetic nervous system is very important when deciding on a specific therapeutic approach. SMP is ameliorated or eliminated by blockade of the appropriate sympathetic efferent innervation. Therefore, different tests are indicated to assess whether the patient has SMP or SIP. These tests include local anesthetic sympathetic blocks, and phentolamine and guanethidine infusions.

Local anesthetic sympathetic ganglion blockade

Diagnostic ganglion sympathetic block with local anesthetics is frequently done to confirm the clinical impression of a SMP syndrome. Sympathetic blockade is able to abolish sympathetic efferent activity to the limb, with a resulting increase in blood flow and a decrease in sweating. It is argued that pain relief, in such circumstances, by blockade of sympathetic efferent activity is the sine qua non of RSD. However, the results of local anesthetic sympathetic blocks need to be interpreted with caution, particularly if there is a condition of combined sympathetic and somatic pain.[24] It is important to know whether the sympathetic block is complete, especially in those patients who do not experience significant pain relief.[26] The efficacy of sympathetic blockade can objectively be assessed evaluating the effects of sympathetic sudomotor and vasoconstriction function, measuring changes in skin blood flow, skin temperature, and skin resistance.[26] Stellate ganglion blockade and lumbar sympathetic blockade can provide 'pure' sympathetic denervation for upper and lower extremities respectively, but neither block necessarily provides unequivocal results. In patients who have pain relief from local anesthetic sympathetic blockade it is important to do a careful sensory examination, since local anesthetic can directly spread to nearby nerve roots, resulting in a somatic nerve block, that may have significant effects on the patient's pain. Depending on the total dose of local anesthetic used, pain relief may also be due to systemic uptake of the local anesthetic.[26]

Intravenous phentolamine infusion

An alternative test to block sympathetic activity and to evaluate for SMP has been introduced using intravenous phentolamine infusion.[26] The rationale for this test is that excitation of nociceptive sensory neurons through norepinephrine released from postganglionic axons is prevented by blockade of α-adrenergic receptors. If pain is reduced during the phentolamine infusion, the sympathetic nervous system is likely to be involved in the generation of pain.[26] Phentolamine is a nonspecific α-adrenergic blocker, with a short serum half-life (17 minutes) when infused via a peripheral vein. The efficacy of phentolamine in blocking adrenoreceptor function is dose-dependent.[26] Since phentolamine decreases peripheral vascular resistance, patients are preloaded with 300–500 mL of isotonic saline solution, followed then, by the administration of phentolamine 1 mg/kg over 10 minutes. Reflex tachycardia can be controlled by the administration of a beta-blocker prior to the phentolamine infusion.[26] Major advantages to the IV phentolamine administration are minimal risk or discomfort for the patient, lack of invasive neural injections, ease of obtaining repetitive pain assessments, and a placebo control.[26] Several investigators[27,28] have demonstrated a high correlation between a positive phentolamine infusion response and pain relief achieved by regional intravenous guanethidine,[27] and local anesthetic sympathetic blockade.[28]

Regional intravenous guanethidine blockade

Several investigators have used regional intravenous blockade with guanethidine for the diagnosis of SMP.[29] Patients who have prolonged relief lasting 2 weeks to 6 months are classified as having SMP. Patients, who have no relief or minor pain relief lasting less than 5 days, are classified as having SIP.[30] Guanethidine is, however, not available for this use in the USA. For this reason, some investigators have used regional bretylium,[31] and ketanserin,[32] an S_2 serotoninergic antagonist, as alternatives to regional intravenous guanethidine blockade.

In summary, Raja[33] recommends that a local anesthetic sympathetic ganglion block be used as an initial screening test. The blockade should be considered adequate if cutaneous temperature approaches core temperature. If, in the presence of an appropriate sympathetic blockade, the patient experiences less than 30% pain relief, the patient is diagnosed as having predominantly SIP. If, on the other hand, the patient achieves greater than 30% relief of pain and/or hyperalgesia without any clinical evidence of somatic blockade, he or she should be then subjected to a placebo-controlled phentolamine test on a separate occasion. A patient who achieves significant pain relief with both the local anesthetic and the phentolamine sympathetic blocks would be considered to have a clinically important component of SMP.[33]

MANAGEMENT OF COMPLEX REGIONAL PAIN SYNDROME

Multiple therapeutic modalities have been recommended for the management of CRPS (Table 22.7). Some of these therapeutic interventions are aimed at blocking the sympathetic hyperactivity (SMP), while other treatments attempt to reduce the sympathetically-independent component of CRPS (SIP). These therapeutic interventions include conservative measures such as physical therapy, massage, early ambulation, and several psychologic approaches such as thermal biofeedback and behavioral techniques. Other therapeutic modalities include acupuncture, transcutaneous electrical nerve stimulation (TENS), sympathetic ganglion blocks, intrathecal or epidural infusion of local anesthetics with and without opioids; systemic intravenous administration of phentolamine; intravenous regional administration of bretylium, reserpine, or guanethidine; and several surgical approaches. Several pharmacological agents have also been used; nonsteroidal anti-inflammatory drugs (NSAIDs), systemic steroids, β-adrenergic and calcium channel blocking agents among others. Despite their number none of these therapies has proven consistently effective.

Table 22.7   Management of complex regional pain syndrome

Conservative therapies
- Early diagnosis, physical therapy and mobilization
- Psychological approaches
- Trigger point injections, TENS

Sympatholysis
- Percutaneous techniques
- Intravenous techniques
- Oral therapy
- Topical therapy
- Surgical approaches

Adjuvant pharmacotherapy
- Anti-depressants
- Anti-convulsants/ Antiarrhythmics
- Opioids (systemic, pumps)
- NSAIDs
- Calcitonin
- Nitrates
- Corticosteroids
- Neurostimulatory techniques

Sympathetic block

As discussed earlier, determining the component of the CRPS that is mediated or maintained by the sympathetic nervous system (SMP) is very important when deciding a specific treatment. During the assessment stage, any 'diagnostic block' is directed specifically to block the sympathetic nervous system, and to avoid any added sensory or motor block. Once the diagnosis of SMP is made, the mainstay treatment is sympatholysis. Most patients will undergo a trial period during which several sympathetic blocks are performed before the technique is considered a failure. Sympathetic blockade can be achieved by several means, either by pharmacologic or interventional techniques (Table 22.8). Extended sympathetic blockade may lead to long-term, or even permanent resolution of the SMP. When deciding on a sympatholytic technique, one must take into consideration its safety as well as its efficacy. To date, however, there have been very few studies evaluating the effectiveness, or the unwanted effects of the techniques.

Table 22.8 Techniques for therapeutic sympathetic block

---

1. **Percutaneous techniques**
- Sympathetic ganglion blocks
- Peripheral nerve blocks
- Epidural administration of local anesthetics
- Sympathetic neurolytic (sympathetic chain) block (phenol, alcohol)
- Percutaneous radio-frequency sympathectomy

2. **Intravenous techniques**
- Systemic (phentolamine)
- Regional (phentolamine, guanethidine, bretylium, reserpine)

3. **Oral therapy**
- Prazosin, terazosin or doxasozin
- Phenoxybenzamine
- Topical therapy
- Clonidine

4. **Surgical approach**

Percutaneous sympatholytic techniques

Sympathetic ganglion blocks are routinely done with local anesthetic or with neurolytic drugs such as alcohol or phenol, when long-term sympathectomy is warranted. Injections into the appropriate sympathetic ganglion can be diagnostic, as well as therapeutic. The choice of block is tailored to the patient's physical status, the severity and duration of the syndrome, and the ease of access to medical care. Cervicothoracic (stellate) ganglion block is indicated for SMP of the upper extremity, above T8. Likewise, brachial plexus block can provide sympathectomy to the upper extremity. Thoracic ganglion block provides sympathectomy of the chest wall and parietal pleura. Interpleural local anesthetics can block sympathetic nerves to the thorax, head, and neck. This technique is a reasonable alternative for patients who are not candidates for other regional sympathetic procedure.[34] Celiac plexus block interrupts afferent input from the abdominal viscera. Hypogastric plexus block denervates the pelvic viscera. For SMP of the lower extremity, lumbar (L2–L4) sympathetic block is indicated.[34]

A stellate ganglion block is usually administered using either lidocaine or bupivacaine, with the patient in a semi-Fowler, inclined position, and the neck hyperextended. The usual point of needle insertion is at the lateral border of the trachea and medial border of the sternocleidomastoid muscle, i.e., the angle between these two structures and 1 cm below Chassaignac's tubercle. This point lies anterior to the transverse process of C7. The carotid sheath and sternocleidomastoid muscle is retracted laterally, and the needle is directed at right angles to the skin in all directions. The needle is then advanced until bone is contacted; and then withdrawn 0.5 cm and aspiration is carried out to rule out intravascular or subarachnoid location.[43] 10–20 mL of local anesthetic is then injected. Complications of stellate ganglion block include Horner's syndrome, pneumothorax, bradycardia, vertebral artery injection, brachial plexus block, inability to cough, and epidural or subdural injection.

Lumbar sympathetic blockade is administered preferably with the patient in the prone position. The one-needle or 'lateral technique'[5,43] and the three-needle or 'paramedian technique' using a paravertebral approach with needles inserted at approximately L2, L3, and L4 have been described.[42] With the three-needle technique, each needle is inserted at an angle of 10° to the parasagittal plane and advanced so as to contact the transverse process of the lumbar vertebra. At this point, the needle is re-directed slightly to pass caudad to the edge of the transverse process and is advanced an additional 1¾–2 inches until it slides past the vertebral body lying on its anterolateral aspect.[42,43] With the 'lateral technique',[44] a single needle is inserted at the level of L2 or L3, 8–10 cm from the midline. With this technique, the transverse process is not contacted. The needle is inserted at an angle of approximately 35° to the parasagittal plane, directed to contact the vertebral body and then slightly re-directed to slide off and remain placed at its anterolateral position. Initially, 3–5 mL of lidocaine 1% is injected to exclude subarachnoid or epidural injection. Subsequently, an additional 15–18 mL of bupivacaine 0.25% with 1:200 000 epinephrine then is injected. Fluoroscopy or cross-table X-rays are useful to document the needle position. Frequently, within 1 or 2 minutes after injection, the skin temperature on the blocked side increases. Lumbar sympathetic block may be repeated as required. Generally, the response to sympathetic block continues from a few hours to many days.[5]

Percutaneous neurolytic blockade, using either phenol or up to 100% alcohol, may provide long-term relief of SMP. However, its use has been discouraged because of its target inaccuracy and more importantly because phenol or alcohol leaves new scars and new sources of pain.[37] Computed tomography scan-guided neurolytic block may lessen the risk of damage to adjacent structures.

Epidural sympathetic blocks. Continuous sympathetic blockade of the lower extremity can be accomplished by lumbar epidural administration of local anesthetics with or without opioids, and by clonidine.[35] Epidural blockade will produce continuous sympatholysis, good analgesia, and only partial somatic block. Lumbar epidural block may be of less diagnostic benefit than sympathetic block techniques. However, continuous epidural blockade allows intensive physical therapy.

Peripheral nerve blocks can provide a degree of sympathetic block, as there are sympathetic fibers that travel for variable distances with the somatic nerves. The nerve supply can be blocked for 6 to 24 hours. During this period of sensory, motor, and sympathetic blockade, the patient may undergo intensive physical therapy. Continuous techniques, such as axillary,[36] interscalene, and sciatic nerve catheter infusions, have also been reported.[24] In general, the more distally the block is done, the lower the likelihood of providing significant sympatholysis.[34]

Radiofrequency percutaneous sympatholysis. Despite demonstration of its safety,[38,39] radiofrequency percutaneous upper thoracic sympathectomy has gained only a limited popularity. The sympathectomy technique has evolved over a 15-year period and is currently in its third phase.[40] The phase III technique relies on neuroleptoanalgesia with superficial local anesthesia only and does not require general anesthesia, intubation, or lung collapse. Two 18 gauge radiofrequency TIC needle electrodes (Radionics, Burlington, MA) are used. A series of lesions are rostrocaudally made at each of the ganglion sites selected in an attempt to destroy the entire fusiform ganglion. Lesion sites are targeted by C-arm fluoroscopy and electrical stimulation. Lesion effectiveness is monitored by bilateral finger plethysmography and hand skin temperature measurement. With the phase III technique, the sympathetic activity in 96% of operated limbs after 2 years and in 91% of operated limbs after 3 years continues to be completely or largely interrupted.[40] When necessary, a subsequent operation can easily be repeated should the symptoms recur.

Intravenous sympatholytic techniques

Systemic intravenous phentolamine administration. The therapeutic administration of intravenous phentolamine to block adrenergic receptors to treat SMP has several advantages over other techniques. It does not require repeated invasive procedures, it causes minimal discomfort and risk for the patient, it provides adrenergic block throughout the body, and it is safe.[41] Several investigators have reported good long-term success.[61,62] Others, on the other hand, question the concept of SMP, based on the response to phentolamine. Verdugo & Ochoa[63,64] administered placebo-controlled phentolamine sympathetic blocks to 14 patients with painful polyneuropathies to test for the presence of SMP. Six received IV infusion of saline for 30 minutes, followed by phentolamine (35 mg). In eight patients, the saline phase was followed by double-blind infusion of phentolamine or phenylephrine (500 microg), a second saline phase, and then the other active drug. Five patients reported significant diminution of pain

(>50%), all in response to placebo. Neither phentolamine nor phenylephrine provided relief, although all patients had signs of physiologic abnormalities reputed to be determinants or predictors of SMP. They concluded that their results complemented previous studies demonstrating the non-existence of SMP among RSD patients and further question the concept of SMP.

Intravenous regional sympathetic block (Bier's block). Intravenous regional blockade (IVRB) can cause sympatholysis by depletion of adrenergic transmitters from sympathetic nerve endings. Sympatholysis is accomplished by the intravenous administration of reserpine, guanethidine, bretylium, or phentolamine. Bier's block avoids side effects such as pneumothorax, intradural and extradural injections, Horner's syndrome, anhydrosis, and death from injection into the vertebral artery.[37] Its effect also may last longer than the sympathetic ganglion block. Regional block should be promptly followed by joint manipulation and physical therapy.[37] A regional intravenous sympathetic blockade should be considered for those patients with suspected SMP who are unable or unwilling to undergo neural blockade.

Reserpine produces sympathetic block by reducing storage vessel reuptake of cathecolamines, thereby slowly depleting norepinephrine stores in sympathetic nerve endings.[5] Reserpine (1–2 mg) is diluted in 40 mL of lidocaine 0.25% and then injected into an exsanguinated extremity. The tourniquet will remain inflated for 30 to 45 minutes to allow the drug to bind to the tissues. Side effects include burning pain on the injection site, postural hypotension lasting 12 to 24 hours, and facial flushing persisting for 24 hours postblock.[5] Morros & Cedo[45] reported their results after treating 165 patients with RSD. Altogether 540 IVRB with reserpine were performed. Results obtained were excellent in 57 (34%) patients, good in 77 (45%), fair in 29 (17%) and nil in 7 (4%). Benzon et al[47] also reported the successful treatment of RSD using IVRB with reserpine. Chuinard et al[49] reported the efficacy of reserpine in relieving the pain of reflex sympathetic dystrophy in 25 patients – 21 with upper extremity and 4 with lower extremity involvement. After the extremity was exsanguinated and the cuff was inflated, 1 mg of reserpine diluted to 50 mL with normal saline was injected intravenously into the

upper extremity. In the lower extremity, 2 mg of reserpine diluted to 100 mL was injected. The tourniquet was removed after 15 minutes. Injection of the drug relieved the acute signs and symptoms in the upper extremity in 12 of 17 patients. Four patients with quiescent reflex sympathetic dystrophy of upper extremities had prophylactic injection at the time of reconstructive surgery; they had no flare of symptoms. Relief was obtained in the four cases of lower extremity dystrophy. No patient had significant side effects. Duncan et al[50] treated 20 patients with RSD involving the upper extremity with associated joint stiffness by manipulation under Bier's blocks composed of lidocaine, methylprednisolone, and reserpine or guanethidine. Range of motion in the affected joints (primarily the hand and wrist) improved from a pre-block mean of 46 to 81% of normal following the blocks. Patients also reported an 80% mean improvement in their pain. Therefore, the treatment of advanced RSD using joint manipulation under sympatholytic Bier's blocks appears to be a safe and effective method of treatment.

In an attempt to improve the results and lessen the side effects during intravenous regional reserpine blocks, Hannington-Kiff[29] introduced the technique of intravenous regional sympathetic block with parenteral guanethidine. Guanethidine appears to bind to sympathetic nervous tissue, thus displacing norepinephrine from presynaptic vesicles and preventing its reuptake. Guanethidine has a biphasic action, initially releasing norepinephrine and then interfering with its reuptake and inhibiting further release.[4] The half-life of guanethidine is quite prolonged. A single injection of guanethidine has a 50% excretion rate of 2 to 3 days through the kidneys. The intravenous regional block is performed similarly to a local anesthetic Bier block. An IV catheter is placed distally in the affected limb. A tourniquet is applied proximally in the affected limb, and the extremity is exsanguinated, either by elevating it or with an Esmarch bandage. Following exsanguination, the tourniquet is inflated 50–100 mmHg above the systolic pressure. 20 mg of guanethidine is diluted in 30 mL of 0.9% saline[4] or 40 or 50 mL of 0.25% lidocaine.[5] The tourniquet should remain inflated for at least 20 minutes to allow the guanethidine to 'fix' to the tissues. The tourniquet is then deflated but left in place in the extremity for 5 minutes in case reinflation is needed.[4] Early tourniquet deflation may cause transient hypertension, because of guanethidine's initial inducement of norepinephrine release from post-ganglionic neuronal storage sites. Other side effects include orthostatic hypotension, vertigo, nausea, vomiting, somnolence, and apnea.[4,5] Complete sympathetic blockade and excellent pain relief can be achieved for 3 to 4 days and as long as up to 6 months.[29] Guanethidine is most effective in patients who have hyperesthesia as the prominent symptom.[29] The effectiveness of guanethidine IVRB is controversial. Randomized trials have used guanethidine, but none showed significant analgesic effect to relieve pain caused by RSD. Bonelli et al[59] compared guanethidine IVRB and stellate ganglion block in a randomized trial. 19 patients, randomly allocated to two groups of therapy and exhibiting severe reflex sympathetic dystrophy, were enrolled. The intravenous guanethidine group showed a persistent and significant increase of the skin temperature and of the plethysmographic traces in the blocked side 24 hours and 48 hours after blockade in comparison with the patients treated with stellate ganglion block. Concerning the therapeutic effects, an intravenous guanethidine block carried out every 4 days up to a total of four blocks was comparable with a stellate ganglion block every day up to a total of eight blocks. The results of this study show that regional sympathetic block with guanethidine was a good therapeutic tool in the treatment of reflex dystrophies, especially on account of its negligible risks and contraindications.[59]

Gschwind et al[57] performed a prospective, randomized, double-blind study in 71 patients undergoing fasciectomy for Duputyren's disease. Guanethidine IVRB was performed perioperatively with the intention of protecting their patients from postoperative dystrophy. Perioperative guanethidine did not prevent postoperative RSD. Ramamurthy and Hoffman[58] in a double-blind, randomized, multicenter study, enrolled 60 patients to receive four intravenous regional blocks at 4-day intervals with either guanethidine or placebo in 0.5% lidocaine. Each patient was randomized to receive either one, two, or four blocks with guanethidine. At 4 days after the initial block, the group treated with placebo experienced a greater decrease in pain scores than those treated with guanethidine, although this difference was not statistically significant. On long-term follow-up there was no difference in pain scores between groups receiving one, two, or four guanethidine blocks. Overall, only 35% of patients experienced clinically significant relief on long-term follow-up even though all were treated early in the evolution of RSD.

Blanchard et al,[46] compared the effectiveness of IVRB using guanethidine, reserpine, and normal saline, in a double-blind, randomized study. 21 patients with RSD of an upper or lower extremity were enrolled and received IVRB with one of the three medications. There was significant pain relief in all three groups at 30 minutes. There were no significant differences among the three groups in the degree of pain relief, the number of patients obtaining pain relief in the 30 minutes after the block, or the number of patients reporting more than 50% pain relief for more than 24 hours. The saline group's high rate of pain relief could be partially due to a mechanism of tourniquet-induced analgesia. Similarly, Rocco et al[48] compared the efficacy of IVRB with guanethidine and reserpine in a controlled, randomized, double-blind cross-over study. 12 patients, 10 of whom had previous stellate or lumbar sympathetic blocks, were entered into this double-blind, cross-over study. Each patient successively received 20 mg guanethidine in 50 mL 0.5% lidocaine, 1.25 mg reserpine in 50 mL 0.5% lidocaine, and 50 mL 0.5% lidocaine with a 1-week interval between medications. Changes in pain intensity for the first 3 days did not differ significantly among guanethidine, reserpine, and control groups. Pain relief from 2 to 14 months was achieved in two patients receiving reserpine, one receiving guanethidine, and none receiving lidocaine. None of the patients experienced permanent relief. No difference was found between reserpine and guanethidine.

Another agent used is bretylium.[51–56] Bretylium produces sympatholysis by being taken up and concentrated in adrenergic nerve terminals. With initial uptake of bretylium there is some displacement and release of norepinephrine as in the case of guanethidine. Bretylium, however, releases much less norepinephrine compared with guanethidine. Bretylium 100–200 mg diluted in 30 mL of 0.9% saline is used. The sympatholysis produced is short-lived. Therefore, the bretylium IVRB should be repeated on a daily basis.[4] Only one randomized study[52] has been reported. Hord et al[52] enrolled patients with RSD, who had received transient pain relief from sympathetic ganglion blocks and had abnormal isolated cold stress tests. Each patient received two control treatments (0.5% lidocaine) and two treatments with 0.5% lidocaine and bretylium 1.5 mg/kg in a randomized, double-blind fashion. Bretylium and lidocaine provided more than 30% pain relief for a mean of 20.0 (+/– 17.5) days, whereas lidocaine alone provided relief for only 2.7 (+/– 3.7) days (Mann–Whitney U-test, $P < 0.001$). The investigators concluded that the combination of bretylium and lidocaine was significantly more effective than lidocaine alone when an intravenous block is used to treat RSD.

Surgical management

Surgical intervention is usually reserved for patients who have failed to achieve long-lasting pain relief from conservative sympatholysis. These procedures, which include neurectomy, rhizotomy, cordotomy, mesencephalic tractotomy, and thalamotomy, are designed to isolate the painful part from the central nervous system. Except for sympathectomy in selected cases, surgical approaches are usually ineffective and not currently recommended in the management of SMP.[1] Surgical sympathectomy can be considered when the diagnosis has been clearly established and other options for sympatholysis provide only transient pain relief.[26] An open sympathectomy offers a substantial advantage over neurolytic injections because it is performed under direct vision, minimizing the potential damage to non-targeted tissue. The short-term results tend to be very good, but, unfortunately, there appears to be a high recidivism rate, with recurrence of some symptoms 3 to 6 months after the procedure. Failures of surgical sympathectomy may reflect inadequacy of diagnosis and lack of adequate sympathetic denervation.[33] Surgical failures can also occur because of collateral reinnervation of post-ganglionic sympathetic efferent fibers.[65] Likewise, differences in timing of the procedure, skills of the surgeon, extent of sympathectomy, and length of follow-up care account for differences in reported success rates.[33]

Pharmacologic sympathectomy (Table 22.9)

α_1-**blockers.** Both phenoxybenzamine and prazosin have been reported to be effective for the treatment of SMP. Phenoxybenzamine (dibenzyline) is a potent α_1-receptor blocker. Usually the

Table 22.9 Sympathetic blocking agents

1. **Adrenergic receptor blockers**
- Phenoxybenzamine
- Phentolamine
- Terazocin
- Prazosin
- Doxazosin
- Propanolol
2. **Calcium channel blockers**
- Nifedipine
- Diltiazem
- Verapamil
- Nicardipine
3. **Central α-$_2$ agonist**
- Clonidine

dosage starts at 10 mg at bedtime with very gradual increase to no more than 10 mg tid. Secondary side effects (dizziness and hypotension) preclude adequate dosing in many patients.[66] Prazosin (Minipress), another α_1-blocker, given at 2 mg/day by mouth twice daily, has resulted in good relief in causalgia. The side effects consist of postural hypotension, tachycardia, poor ejaculation, myosis, and nasal congestion.[67] Terazocin (Hytrin) is a very well-tolerated α_1-blocker and can be an excellent substitute if the patient cannot tolerate the former α_1-blockers.[37]

Calcium channel blockers such as nifedipine (Procardia), relax smooth muscles, increases peripheral blood flow, and counteract the effects of norepinephrine on arterial and venous smooth muscle.[22] Such blockers also suppress abnormal calcium conductance at areas of nerve degeneration in ephaptic scars.[22,37] Nifedipine, given 10–30 mg three times a day, resulted in complete relief of pain in 7 out of 13 patients.[68]

Central α_2-agonists. Clonidine (Catapress) stimulates the presynaptic-receptors in the brainstem thus decreasing sympathetic outflow. Clonidine is quite a helpful treatment in doses as much as 0.1–0.2 mg up to three times a day. However, it has its own side effects in the form of postural hypotension, insomnia, and depression.[37] Topical clonidine can also be used to provide more extended pain relief.[69,70]

β-**adrenergic blocking agents.** Propanolol in relatively high doses has been suggested for patients this RSD.[71,72] This form of treatment decreases the β-adrenergic response and thus helps the central origin types of RSD such as migraine and other forms of atypical face pain of central pain.[37] Its use has not proved useful in the treatment of SMP. A double-blind, cross-over trial was not effective in patients with causalgia.[73]

Neurostimulatory techniques

Invasive neurostimulatory procedures. These include acupuncture, percutaneous electrical nerve stimulation, dorsal column stimulation, and deep brain stimulation. Dorsal column stimulation has been used with some success in a small number of patients with causalgic pain (see Ch. 23).[74]

Transcutaneous electrical nerve stimulation (TENS) is reported to be effective for a variety of acute post-surgical and chronic painful conditions. The mechanisms underlying the analgesic effects of TENS are not established. TENS may activate endogenous segmental pain modulating systems through selective stimulation of large diameter myelinated (A-β) fibers. These systems presumably inhibit the central transmission of nociceptive input through slower, unmyelinated C fibers. Although only a few patients attain long-term analgesia from TENS, the safety of this approach supports a trial in any patient with RSD/causalgia who fails to respond promptly to sympathetic blockade combined with adjunctive psychiatric and pharmacologic approaches.

PHANTOM LIMB PAIN SYNDROME

INTRODUCTION

Phantom limb sensation is a common occurrence in patients who have undergone an amputation, brachial plexus avulsion, or spinal cord injury.[75] It is the persistent awareness of the lost body part and it may be vague or vivid. Phantom sensations cover almost the entire spectrum of feelings that normal body parts offer, including pain.[75] Herein lies the problem, because the pain is sometimes so great that it is debilitating.

From 1981 to 1987 it was estimated that 230 000 surgical amputations occured each year and approximately 6.0/1000 injuries resulted in an amputation, including major and minor extremities.[76] This estimate means that about 1.3 million traumatic amputations occur per year.[76] About 72% of amputations lead to phantom limb pain 1 week after amputation and 60% of amputees have phantom pain 6 months later. The same finding of 60% occurs 7 years later.[77,78] As Melzack points out, only 10–12% of phantom limb pain sufferers ever obtain pain relief.[79] There are at least 68 published treatments and more are published each year.[80] These statistics lead one to believe that the problem of phantom pain has not been resolved.

HISTORY

Phantom limb sensation, first associated with amputations during wartime (Fig. 22.1), can also occur after the loss of other organs such as the tongue, breast, teeth, penis, bladder, and nerve avulsion.[81–89] Ambroise Pare (1510–1590), a French military surgeon, first described phantom limb pain.[90] The American neurologist, Silar Weir Mitchell (1829–1914), first published his article on phantom limbs anonymously in the Atlantic Monthly, a non-scientific journal in order to test for his contemporaries' reactions to the concept without risking his eminent reputation.[75] Charles Bell (1774–1842) also described and coined the

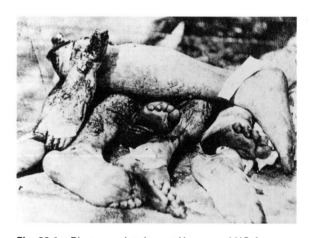

Fig. 22.1 Photograph taken at Harewood US Army Hospital 1865 entitled 'A Morning's Work' gives an impression of the volume of amputations performed daily during the US Civil War. (Photograph courtesy Stanley B. Burns, The Burns Archive.)

phrase 'phantom limbs' in his monograph entitled *The Nervous System of the Human Body* in 1830 before Mitchell's article.[91,92]

DEFINITIONS

Since the original accounts of phantom limb phenomena, four clinical entities have been described. *Phantom limb sensation* is the sensory perception of a missing limb that does not include pain[93] and occurs in virtually all amputees.[94–96] It usually dissipates during the first year after amputation.[81] In contrast, *phantom limb pain* is a noxious sensory phenomenon of the missing limb/organ.[94,96–98] *Stump pain*, distinct from phantom pain, is the painful sensory phenomenon perceived in the region of amputation that may be localized to one small area or occur diffusely throughout the amputated region. Some form of pain occurs in all patients after surgery but usually subsides within a few weeks. However, up to 50% of the patients can experience chronic painful conditions so severe they become incapacitated.[99] *Super-added* phantom sensation is the sensation of an object like a ring or wristwatch[100,101] attached to the phantom limb. Two remarkable examples are the sensation of holding a cane handle when the hand was accidentally amputated[101] or blood felt in the boot of an amputee soldier.[102] As will be discussed, it becomes very important to distinguish between these clinical entities, especially between phantom pain and stump pain, because the treatment modalities for each are quite different.[103] We will focus on phantom pain in this review.

CLINICAL CHARACTERISTICS

Three clinical characteristics of the phantom phenomenon have been described by Jensen & Rasmussen.[93] First, *kinesthetic sensations* involve posture, length, and volume. Second, *kinetic sensations* consist of willed, spontaneous, and associated movements. Third, *exteroceptive* or *cutaneous sensations* consist of touch, temperature, pressure, and pruritus.[93] Virtually all normal limb sensations might be experienced, including, for example, the sensation of having one's foot fall asleep. Phantom sensation occurs most commonly in distal limbs that are more richly innervated[104] and often diminishes with time. It is also true that after 1 year, the phantom sensation is not apt to change much.[93] The quality of phantom pain is variable

but two types generally predominate. One type is a burning or throbbing pain while the other presents as an abnormal ischemic discomfort of the phantom limb ranging in intensity from mild to excruciating.[96]

Telescoping

Gueniot (1861) first used the phrase 'heterotopie subjective' to describe a phenomenon experienced by limb amputees, also known as regressive deformation or 'telescoping'.[80,105,106] Telescoping is the process in which the phantom limb shrinks and the digits of the phantom hand or foot become attached to the stump (Fig. 22.2). This process occurs gradually with an incidence of 25–75% and is completed within the first year after amputation. Telescoping is more likely to occur in the arm rather than the leg[107] and is more commonly seen in the painless phantom limb. In contrast, super-added phantom pain may prevent or retard telescoping. The physiologic explanation of telescoping is unknown.[103]

36% of these patients after 2 to 6 years reported the telescoping of the phantom hands so that they accommodated the bifurcated shape of the stump,[108–116] i.e. some fingers fused or disappeared, as well as shortened to coincide with the length of the stump.[108,116]

It is interesting that complete spinal cord transection or complete brachial plexus avulsion does not result in telescoping of the phantom limb.[117–120] Katz hypothesizes that telescoping probably does not occur if somatosensory input from the periphery does not reach the central nervous system or dorsal root ganglion.[108]

Another interesting correlation is that phantom limb pain usually does not coincide with telescoping. The amputated limb of phantom limb pain sufferers is generally of normal length or temporarily longer during bouts of pain.[93,121,122] Further studies are needed to explain this phenomenon. If it is true that somatosensory reorganization is actually the cause of telescoping, then perhaps the facilitation of these processes by stump retraining can possibly reduce phantom pain in amputees.[108]

PATHOGENESIS AND PATHOPHYSIOLOGY

The pathophysiology of phantom pain remains elusive,but three hypotheses have been proposed: peripheral, spinal, and central (supraspinal) medi-

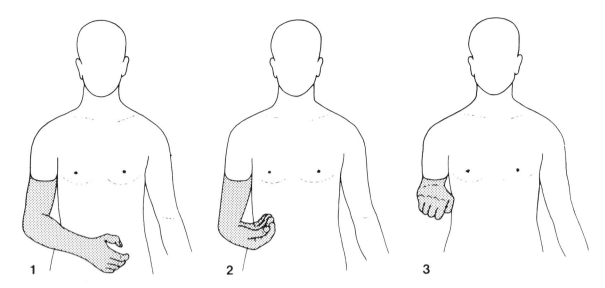

Fig. 22.2 A 34-year-old man who was injured when he drove his moped into a lamp-post in September 1980. There was a right-sided humerus fracture and a total paralysis of the entire upper extremity. The paralyzed arm felt localized in the position in which it was at the time of the accident: as if the patient held the handlebars of the moped. (1) After a few weeks the patient had pains in the hand and fingers and the distal third of the forearm. The pains were squeezing and of increasing intensity during the following 3 months. Simultaneously the phantom began shrinking and 6 months after the injury the hand felt as if it were localized distally to the elbow joint. (2) Amputation was performed in May 1981, but it had no effect on the pains. The shrinking continued, and from December 1981, the hand felt as if placed directly on the amputation stump and clenched more tightly. (3) Electrocoagulation in the cervical medulla (Lissauer) in May 1982 had no effect on the phantom pain.

ation.[103] It is possible that all three mechanisms together explain phantom limb pain.

Peripheral

Although peripheral nerves are involved in the generation of phantom pain, this requisite does not explain the phenomenon entirely. Neuromas from regenerating axons might contribute to the overall phantom limb sensation. Peripheral mechanisms are implicated in modulation of phantom sensation by stump manipulation, alteration in stump blood flow, and after local stump anesthesia.[96,97,103,123,124] Nystrom & Hagbarth studied two patients with phantom limb pain after traumatic limb amputations with increased mechanosensitive neuromas in their stumps.[125,126] Spontaneous or ectopic activity arising proximal to the neuroma was also found in some of the unmyelinated efferents innervating the neuromas in these patients.[125] Although it is suggested that these peripheral stimuli contribute to the phantom pain, Nystrom & Hagbarth have proposed that additional central

factors must also be involved because phantom limb pain itself is not altered by conduction blockade of peripheral neurons although electrical stimulation of the stump exaggerates the phantom limb experience.[125]

Katz has shown that changes in the sympathetic nervous system may be related to phantom limb sensation (Fig. 22.3);[108,127] skin conductance and surface skin temperature are lower at the stump than the contralateral limb in patients with phantom limb sensation only, and in those with phantom limb pain but not in those without phantom limb sensation.[108,127] Stump skin conductance is shown to correlate with the intensity of phantom limb paresthesias.[108,127]

The mechanism drawn up to explain these paresthesias, the 'sympathetic–efferent/somatic–afferent mechanism,'[108,128] consists of a cycle where input from the cortex excites sympathetic neurons in the spinal cord that excite post-ganglionic noradrenergic cutaneous vasoconstrictor and cholinergic sudomotor fibers in the stump resulting in increased release of acetylcholine

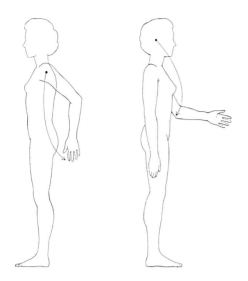

Fig. 22.3   Referred sensations in a painful phantom arm were reported by a woman receiving electrical stimuli at two different places (dots). Stimulation at the stump gave the sensation of electric shocks that jumped from finger to finger. Stimulation on the right ear made the phantom elbow feel warm and caused a pulsing sensation that traveled down the phantom wrist and thumb. The observations were made by Joel Katz, now at the University of Toronto, and the author.

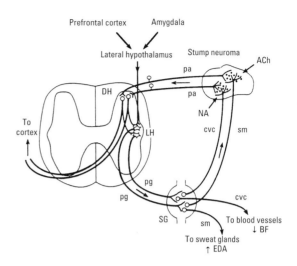

Fig. 22.4   The 'sympathetic-efferent/somatic-afferent mechanism' (see text at foot of p. 386 onwards).

(ACh).[10,108,126,129] The result is increased electrodermal activity and decreased blood flow occurring at the stump. ACh and NA activate primary afferents which stimulate the pre-ganglionic sympathetic neurons and result in the perception of phantom limb sensations. Pain might result if certain changes occur in the dorsal horn cells or abnormal activation by nociceptors of primary afferents occurs after injury[10,108,126,129] (Fig. 22.4).

It has been shown that stress and anxiety can cause increased reflex bursting activity in cutaneous sudomotor and vasomotor sympathetic fibers,[108,130,131] while distraction, attention diversion, and intense concentration can reduce this sympathetic activity.[108,113,132] The same can be said for phantom limb pain.[108,133–135] Stress and anxiety exacerbate phantom limb sensations and pain [108,136] but in some patients progressive relaxation and electromyogram biofeedback techniques applied to the stump and forehead can help reduce the phantom pain for up to 3 years.[108,134,137] Hence, there might be some central modulation of the 'sympathetic–efferent/somatic–afferent' mechanism.[108]

Spinal

Loss of afferent nerves through spinal cord lesions or root avulsions[88] elicits disinhibition of dorsal horn neurons,[138] allowing transmission of phantom pain (Fig. 22.5). Recent reports show that the onset of spinal anesthesia in amputees can cause the appearance or re-appearance of phantom limb pain and thus supports this theory. Melzack has reported that anesthetic blockade of the spinal cord decreases somatic input to the cortex thereby reducing the level of inhibition and permitting pain recognition.[139] Prevoznik et al contended that the last impulses received by the proprioceptive fibers before blockade became 'locked in' the memory.[140] Accordingly, patients who experienced phantom sensations during spinal anesthesia had their limbs in unusual positions before administration of the sensory and motor block, for example, a flexed leg. Phantom sensations did not occur if the patient was in a neutral supine position with legs extended. Prevoznik et al differentiated between a natural phantom limb that can be moved at will, and a proprioceptive phantom limb that remains fixed in the position it was in before initiation of spinal anesthesia. However, either phantom limb may be distressing to the patient and require therapeutic intervention.

Davis describes the mechanism which leads to plasticity in the dorsal horn neurons which then result in the creation of pain without stimulus. Pain messages are carried by fast A-δ neurons via

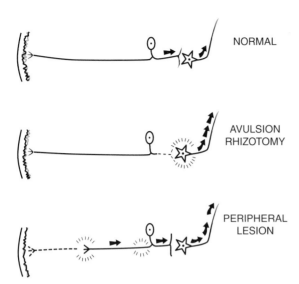

Fig. 22.5 The mechanism which leads to plasticity in the dorsal horn neurons which then result in the creation of pain without stimulus (see text below).

excitatory amino acids (EAAs), like aspartate and glutamate, which activate the NMDA receptors on wide dynamic range (WDR) neurons and slow unmyelinated fibers that release neurokinins like substance P.[141-146] (Fig. 22.5). Substance P is important because of its ability to depolarize secondary nociceptive neurons in the dorsal horn and possibly to increase the sensitivity of WDR neurons to EAAs.[147-149]

Nerve avulsion or noxious stimulation can cause the development of hyperirritable foci in the dorsal columns. Hyperactivity of cells in lamina V was found in rat spinal cords following the cutting of dorsal roots innervating that section of spinal cord.[105,126] This phenomenon has been shown to begin about 6 hours after cutting the dorsal roots and usually subsides after 3 months (Fig. 22.5). Lamina V is known to contain many nociceptive cell synapses.[105,126] Under such conditions EAAs and neurokinins are released. Secondary nociceptive neurons in the dorsal horn are depolarized by the **sustained** release of EAAs, leading to the removal of the Mg^{2+} blocking the NMDA receptor channel. This could result in more depolarization by EAAs and substance P or other neurokinins.[141,150-153]

Eventually, 'wind-up' or temporal summation of the membrane potential occurs, leading to long-term depolarization and toxicity from increased Ca^{2+} uptake. This could lead to inacti-

vation or death of interneurons which are required for inhibition and result in increased pain. Ca^{2+} is also a second messenger in the secondary neuron where it can cause the activation of certain DNA transcriptional regulators. The result could be the accumulation of products that spontaneously depolarize the secondary nociceptive neurons and lead to increased pain transmission as proposed by Davis.[141,154-160]

Central (Supraspinal)

Melzack contends that sensation of phantom pain is authentic because it is produced by the same brain processes that operate when the body is intact. He further proposes that the brain creates the nature of the experience tempered by the inputs from the body that are not essential. These experiences or inputs of the body set up a neuromatrix that is unique to each individual. Consequently, Melzack constructs the concept of a unique self, created by the experiences of both the body and the innate neuromatrix, which exists as a neural engram in the thalamus producing a three-dimensional image of the body[161] (Fig. 22.6).

He has proposed a central (supraspinal) origin consisting of a *neuromatrix*, or a network of neurons, loops between cortex and thalamus as well as cortical and limbic system that is subsequently modified by life experiences[79] (Fig. 22.7). These interconnections have been supported by a report of phantom pain disappearance after focal brain infarction in the posterior internal capsule, confirmed by CT scan, presumably disrupting thalamocortical sensory fibers. This patient ultimately recovered cutaneous sensation without the reappearance of phantom pain.[162]

The neuromatrix imparts a pattern, or a *neurosignature*, on all sensory inputs or experiences of the body that create a unique neural motif. This pattern is created by cyclical processing and synthesis of nerve impulses through the neuromatrix creating a characteristic pattern. A specialized part of the neuromatrix, or *neuromodule*, is necessary for processing information coming from major sensory events like injury or temperature change, etc., creating a subsignature within a neurosignature. Sensory inputs modulating the neurosignature are converted to an ever-changing awareness by the *sentient neural hub*. If the neurosignature is to produce a movement by activating a neuromatrix, two pathways then occur. One goes to the

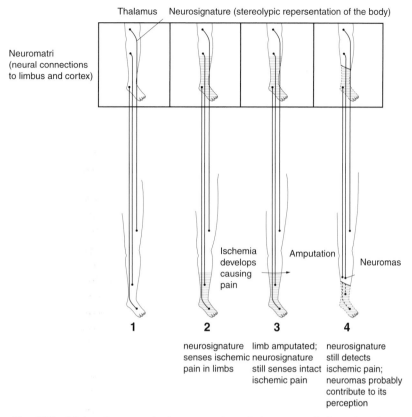

Thalamus   Neurosignature (stereolypic repersentation of the body)

Neuromatri
(neural connections
to limbus and cortex)

Ischemia
develops
causing
pain

Amputation

Neuromas

1   **2**   **3**   **4**

neurosignature limb amputated; neurosignature
senses ischemic neurosignature still detects
pain in limbs   still senses intact ischemic pain;
                 ischemic pain   neuromas probably
                                  contribute to its
                                  perception

Fig. 22.6 Melzack contends that sensation of phantom pain is authentic because it is produced by the same brain processes that operate when the body is intact (see text p. 388).

sentient neural hub to create the sensation or experience of movement, while the other runs through an action neuromatrix that actually turns on the spinal cord neurons that signal the muscles for movement.[79]

Further evidence is presented by paraplegics who have higher level complete spinal breaks, and yet, they experience all normal bodily sensations in the absence of inputs. Melzack also states that without inhibitory inputs, increased firing of spinal cells above the break can trigger the neuromatrix. The overactive action neuromatrix interacts with the sentient neural hub in an abnormal fashion, producing a hot, burning, cramping pain. Without limbs, the frequency and intensity of the messages grow stronger, trying to move the non-existent limb and possibly result in shooting pain[79] (Fig. 22.8).

Removal of the somatosensory areas of the cortex or thalamus does **not** relieve phantom limb pain. It is impossible to destroy the neuromatrix since it interconnects throughout the brain.

However, it is possible to inject lidocaine to the lateral hypothalamus (as performed in rats) resulting in decreased pain in formalin tests.[163] Conversely, no effect was observed when adjacent hypothalamic structures were injected with lidocaine.[163] Lidocaine injected into the cingulum also decreases pain in the formalin test and decreases self-mutilation or autotomy after peripheral nerve lesions.[164,165] The frequency of autotomy in rats is an indicator for how much pain is experienced after nerve damage.[79,166–168]

A corollary for the central origin of phantom limb pain proposes that the ensuing pain is actually a 'memory' of pain in the limb before amputation. Katz & Melzack[100] reported that these somatosensory memories are so vivid that in the mind of amputees, they do not believe the operation had occurred. Approximately 56% of the patients in their study reported that the phantom limb pain resembles pre-amputation pain in quality and location, differing only in intensity. Consequently, Katz & Melzack hypothesized a

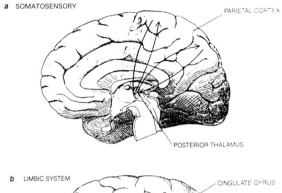

a SOMATOSENSORY

PARIETAL CORTEX

POSTERIOR THALAMUS

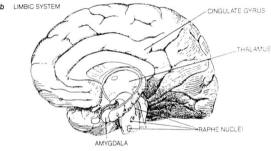

b   LIMBIC SYSTEM

CINGULATE GYRUS

THALAMUS

RAPHE NUCLEI

AMYGDALA

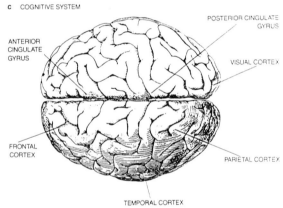

c   COGNITIVE SYSTEM

POSTERIOR CINGULATE GYRUS

ANTERIOR CINGULATE GYRUS

VISUAL CORTEX

FRONTAL CORTEX

PARIETAL CORTEX

TEMPORAL CORTEX

Fig. 22.7   Source of phantom limbs is thought by the author to involve activity in three of the brain's neural circuits. One of them (a) is the somatosensory receiving areas and the adjacent parietal cortex, which process information related to the body. The second area (b) is the limbic system, which is concerned with emotion and motivation. The third (c) encompasses the widespread cortical networks involved in cognitive activities, among them the memory of past experience and the evaluation of sensory inputs in relation to the self.

physical basis for this somatosensory memory (i.e. the engram), established in the brain before amputation.[100,123,139,169,170] Conversely, Wall et al reported that only 12.5% of the patients in their study experienced the same pain before amputation. These studies differed only in what necessi-

tated the amputation in the patient population. The patients in Wall's study underwent amputation because of neoplastic disease, whereas those in Katz & Melzack's had occlusive vascular disease or trauma.[171] It is interesting to note that Roth et al have reported recurrent phantom limb pain that progressively increased over an extended period of time instead of decreasing in two sarcoma patients. They surmised that the increased severity of the phantom pain was associated with the local recurrence of sarcoma in these patients.[172] These observations suggest that the presence of a neoplastic growth may alter the 'neuromatrix' or 'neurosignature' of the brain or neural pathway or activate pain pathways that differ from those involved in vascular occlusive disease.

Katz et al performed a study on the pattern of autotomy in rats after injury prior to neurectomy compared to no injury prior to neurectomy and found that the location of the injury affects the location along the limb that the rat will attack.[167]

TREATMENT

Treatment modalities are as varied and controversial as the etiology of phantom pain (Fig. 22.9). Moreover, most studies concerning the treatment of phantom pain used small groups (usually not more than five patients) with little or no follow-up analysis.[76] The reader is referred to Table 22.10 for a summary of results, sample size, and references to each treatment reviewed. More extensive follow-up studies are currently not available to evaluate the long-term results of these treatments. It is important to remember that some pain occurs in all patients after surgery and usually subsides. Stump pain is considerably different from phantom pain and a different approach to treatment must be taken. Treatment may be fashioned either to prevent the phantom pain completely or to alleviate an existing pain. It is the chronic phantom pain that is exceedingly difficult to treat. Mainly surgical and medical treatments will be discussed. Other modalities, such as biofeedback, although used in the treatment of phantom limb pain, are not discussed here, but are covered elsewhere in this text.

Surgical intervention

Surgical treatment is designed to interrupt the brain, spinal cord, and peripheral nerve intercon-

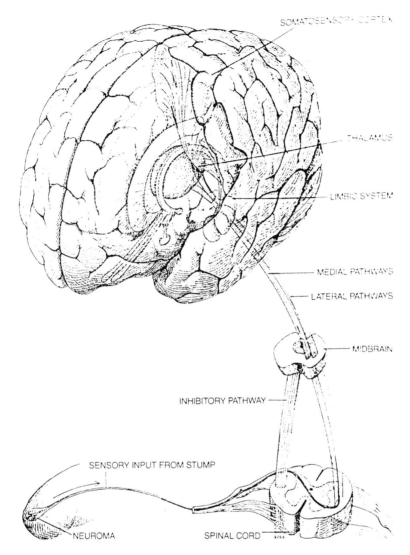

Fig. 22.8 Pathways of signals from the body to the brain are shown. After the loss of a limb, nerve cells in the denervated areas of the spinal cord and brain fire spontaneously at high levels and with abnormal bursting patterns.

nections leading to the cessation of pre-existing phantom limb pain. These interruptions can occur at various levels via cordotomy, rhizotomy, dorsal root entry zone (DREZ) lesions, or thalamotomy. The beneficial effects of anterolateral cordotomy diminish rapidly after 6 months.[179–181,208] These effects diminish because the spinal cord contains a network of interconnecting collateral fibers that eventually assume the same spinal functions of the severed major tracts.[182] Poor results have been achieved from posterior cordo-

tomy and rhizotomy, which consist of cutting the dorsal roots of the spinal cord.

The DREZ lesion procedure consists of destroying the entry zone area using a fine electrode (Fig. 22.10). The area of destruction extends from the dorsal surface of the spinal cord where the roots enter, to the depth of laminas V and VI.[183] These laminas consist of interneuronal synapses that transmit somatic and visceral sensory information. Consequently, the DREZ lesion has been shown to produce satisfactory analgesia

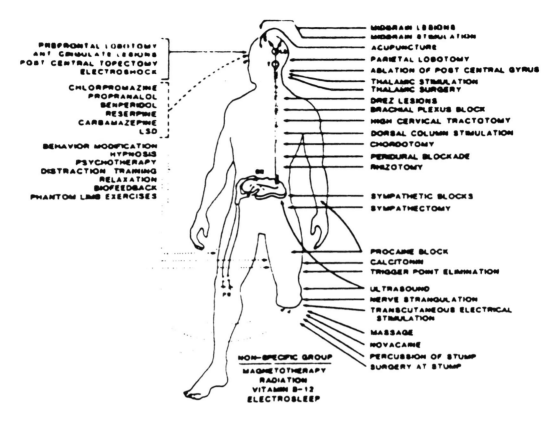

PREFRONTAL LOBOTOMY
ANT CINGULATE LESIONS
POST CENTRAL TOPECTOMY
ELECTROSHOCK

CHLORPROMAZINE
PROPRANALOL
BENPERIDOL
RESERPINE
CARBAMAZEPINE
LSD

BEHAVIOR MODIFICATION
HYPNOSIS
PSYCHOTHERAPY
DISTRACTION TRAINING
RELAXATION
BIOFEEDBACK
PHANTOM LIMB EXERCISES

MIDBRAIN LESIONS
MIDBRAIN STIMULATION
ACUPUNCTURE
PARIETAL LOBOTOMY
ABLATION OF POST CENTRAL GYRUS
THALAMIC STIMULATION
THALAMIC SURGERY
DREZ LESIONS
BRACHIAL PLEXUS BLOCK
HIGH CERVICAL TRACTOTOMY
DORSAL COLUMN STIMULATION
CHORDOTOMY
PERIDURAL BLOCKADE
RHIZOTOMY

SYMPATHETIC BLOCKS
SYMPATHECTOMY

PROCAINE BLOCK
CALCITONIN
TRIGGER POINT ELIMINATION

ULTRASOUND
NERVE STRANGULATION
TRANSCUTANEOUS ELECTRICAL STIMULATION
MASSAGE
NOVACAINE
PERCUSSION OF STUMP
SURGERY AT STUMP

NON-SPECIFIC GROUP
MAGNETOTHERAPY
RADIATION
VITAMIN B-12
ELECTROSLEEP

Fig. 22.9 Treatment modalities are as varied and controversial as the etiology of phantom pain (see text p. 390).

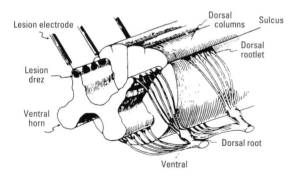

Fig. 22.10 The DREZ lesion procedure consists of destroying the entry zone area using a fine electrode, (see text on p. 391).

in about 65% of patients with phantom limb pain, but not for stump pain alone.[184] The DREZ lesion results are more promising for patients with traumatic amputation than with cancer or vascular insufficiency. Complications from this procedure include involuntary movements (treated with baclofen),[185] impotence, and urinary or rectal incontinence.

Surgery performed to remove neuromas at the stump or for resection have been largely unsuccessful in relieving phantom limb pain.

Dorsal column stimulation, where a stimulator is implanted around the dorsal column to stimulate nociceptive and inhibitory descending pathways, is based on Melzack & Wall's pain control theory where counterstimulation closes the pain gate.[182] However, this technique has not proven beneficial in the treatment of phantom pain (see Ch. 23).

Epidural blockade

If phantom limb pain is a 'memory' of pre-amputation pain or discomfort, then the use of epidural blockade prior to removal should eliminate pre-amputation pain and subsequently prevent phantom limb pain. Bach et al used lumbar epidural anesthesia to eliminate leg pain for 3 days before amputation.[170] Epidural anesthesia was then continued intraoperatively and postoperatively. All 11 patients who underwent this treatment experienced no phantom pain for 1 year after amputa-

Table 22.10 Phantom limb pain (PLP) treatments

Treatment	Description	Author(s)
Dorsal root entry	75% had 75% relief from PLP for 6 months (n = 8)	Nashold BS, Ostdahl RH (1979)[208]
Zone lesions (DREZ)	67% had good PLP relief for 6 months (n = 9)	Saris SC, Iacono RP, Nashold BS Jr (1988)[181]
Epidural anesthesia: 3 days before amputation, intraoperative, postoperative	Absence of PLP 1 year after amputation (n = 11)	Bach S, Noreng MF, Tjellden NU (1988)[170]
Subarachnoid fentanyl for diagnostic evaluation of relief followed by epidural opioid analgesia	Relief for 2 hours to 10 days after injection (n = 3)	Jacobson L, Chaba C (1989)[186] Jacobson L, Chaba C, Brody MC (1989)[187]
Spinal anesthesia plus IV subanesthetic doses of thiopental	Thiopental alleviates spinal anesthesia-induced PLP (n = 3)	Koyama K, Watanabe S, Tsuneto S, et al (1988)[189]
Spinal anesthesia plus calcitonin IV	Calcitonin alleviates spinal anesthesia-induced PLP (n = 1)	Fiddler DS, Hindman BJ (1991)[190]
Spinal anesthesia with bupivacaine and clonidine	Temporary relief of PLP for 3 days to 1 month (n = 2)	Gentili ME, Bonnet F (1993)[195]
Nerve sheath block during amputation and postoperatively	Absence of PLP 1 year after amputation (n = 11)	Fisher DS, Meller Y (1991)[196]
IV Infusion calcitonin	71% obtained pain relief for 2 years (n = 21)	Jaeger H, Maier C (1992)[197]
IV Infusion ketamine	One patient obtained relief for 6 months, 2 patients obtained relief but discontinued because of side effects (n = 3)	Stannard CF, Porter GE (1993)[198]
Oral opioids and anti-depressants	No opioid habituation in PLP patients in 22 months with over 50% pain relief (n = 5)	Urban BJ, Steinberger EK, et al (1986)[200]
Oral propanolol	Pain relief for 6 to 8 months (n = 2)	Marshland A, Weeks J, Atkinson R, et al (1982)[201]
Oral mexiletine Mexiletine plus clonidine patch	18 found some improvement while 11 needed clonidine in addition to the mexiletine (n = 31)	Davis RW (1993)[202]
Oral Fluoxetine	Patient was cured for 4 months (n = 1)	Power-Smith P, Turkington D (1993)[203]
TENS on contralateral leg	No PLP 6 months (n = 3)	Carabelli RA, Kellerman WC (1985)[205]
TENS bilateral auricular	Statistically decreases intensity of pain transiently (n = 11)	Katz J, Melzack R (1991)[206]

Note Duration of pain relief is quoted from articles and is usually not conclusive. Long-term studies need to be conducted in order to determine the true length of pain relief. 'n' means the number of subjects from PLP receiving the PLP. It does not include the control group or any group not suffering from PL.

tion. These results support Melzack's central theory of a neurosignature pattern forming as a result of learned body experiences because the memory of pain was 'permanently' blocked before the limb removal.

Spinal analgesia

Subarachnoid fentanyl can be used for diagnostic evaluation of phantom pain relief followed by epidural opioid analgesia.[186] This technique provided immediate relief from both phantom limb and stump pain, lasting from 2 hours in one patient to 9 days in another patient while a third had pain relief for at least 10 days after injection. A mild sense of warmth in the phantom limb was experienced by the three patients while pruritus was noted in one. Absence of supraspinal side effects such as drowsiness, lightheadedness, nau-

sea, and vomiting suggest that the opioid acts at the spinal cord level and does not migrate rostrally.[187]

Spinal anesthesia in amputees may cause the appearance or reappearance of phantom limb pain. Thus, patients with a history of phantom limb pain or amputated limb may not be suitable candidates for spinal anesthesia.[188] If spinal anesthesia must be used, two methods may be employed to decrease or abolish the phantom pain. One method involves intravenous administration of subanesthetic doses of thiopental concurrent with spinal anesthesia,[189] whereas the other employs calcitonin intravenously.[190]

Calcitonin has been theorized to work via central serotoninergic pathways independent of opiate receptors. Hence, calcitonin may act by increasing activity in descending pain inhibitory neural pathways, thereby reducing phantom pain.

Subarachnoid calcitonin has also been used successfully to treat intractable cancer pain.[191–194] Calcitonin can cause allergic reactions, hypocalcemia, neurotoxicity, and long-term tolerance. Although thiopental is more readily available, calcitonin may be cautiously used when the phantom pain is resistant to conventional therapy.[194]

Gentili & Bonnet also suggest that α_2-adrenergic agonists might be useful for the treatment of phantom limb pain. They report that two cases had their stumps revised and underwent spinal anesthesia with an association of bupivacaine and clonidine during the surgery. The result was temporary relief of phantom limb pain for 1 month in one patient and for 3 days in the other patient.[195]

Regional anesthesia

As a method to prevent phantom pain altogether, continuous postoperative regional analgesia by nerve sheath block during amputation has been suggested to provide both postoperative stump analgesia and a significant reduction in supplementary narcotic requirements. Fisher & Meller demonstrated the absence of phantom limb pain up to 1 year after surgery using this continuous femoral nerve blockade.[196]

Intravenous infusion

A double-blind, placebo-controlled study conducted by Jaeger & Maier on calcitonin in phantom limb treatment found that 1 and 2 years after the first calcitonin treatment, 62% still had more than 75% of phantom limb pain relief. After 1 week of the treatment, 90% had pain relief of more than 50%, 76% were pain free and 71% never again experienced phantom limb pain.[197] According to Jaeger & Maier, salmon calcitonin should be administered early for good results; the side effects are negligible and the treatment may be repeated.[197]

Stannard & Porter reported three case studies of successful phantom limb pain treatments with ketamine by IV infusion. Ketamine is a NMDA antagonist. It has been shown that NMDA antagonists can reduce certain plastic changes in the spinal cord and cortex and that NMDA receptors are involved in long-term potentiation of synaptic transmission in the hippocampus, which might be involved in memory. Side effects presumably occur because NMDA receptors are involved in the processing of sensory information in the brain resulting in confusion, delirium, vivid dreams, hallucination, and feelings of detachment from the body. Two out of the three patients in Stannard & Porter's study discontinued ketamine infusion because of side effects. The usefulness of ketamine as a phantom limb pain treatment awaits a randomized, double-blind clinical trial.[198]

Oral pharmacologic strategies

Long-term use of opioids in conjunction with anti-depressants has provided satisfactory relief from chronic phantom limb pain. Concerns surrounding opioid addiction have not been a problem when treating patients with chronic pain, especially caused by cancer.[199] However, terminal cancer patients usually have a shorter life expectancy than patients with phantom limb pain. Consequently, addiction symptoms may not have time to develop in cancer patients. Studies by Urban et al showed no signs of opioid habituation or addiction in phantom limb pain patients over a 22-month period.[200] Propanolol, a β-adrenergic antagonist has been cited by some sources as an effective treatment.[73,201]

Davis studied the effects of mexiletine in phantom limb treatment without a control sample. He found that out of 31 patients with phantom limb pain, 18 found mexiletine helpful while 11 needed mexiletine plus a clonidine TTS-1 patch. Others found that the side effect of persistent nausea precluded them from taking mexiletine at all. Mexiletine is an anti-arrhythmic drug which also is effective in decreasing activation potential duration and increasing the refractory period of WDR neurons with leaky sodium channels by blocking them.[202] Power-Smith & Turkington described a case in which fluoxetine (Prozac), a 5-hydroxytryptamine (5-HT) reuptake inhibitor completely cured a man's phantom limb pain after 8 weeks of treatment. The man had phantom limb pain for 5 years prior to treatment. It has long been shown that lowered 5-HT levels are implicated in the maintenance of chronic pain and from animal models, and that stimulation of 5-HT turnover inhibits nociception and increases the pain threshold.[203]

Feria et al conducted a study on the effects of selective neurotoxic lesions of lumbosacral serotonergic and noradrenergic systems on autotomy behavior in rats. They concluded that the pattern of rat autotomy can be affected by interfering with spinal cord serotonergic activity. They suggested that research should be conducted on the treatment of phantom limb pain by using drugs which activate or block spinal cord serotonergic receptor subtypes.[168]

Abbott & Young fed rats five times their normal requirements of tryptophan and raised the level of 5-HT and 5-hydroxy indoleacetic acid in the brain and spinal cord of these rats compared to controls. The effect of tryptophan supplementation on rat autotomy was studied and results show that dysethesia produced by denervation was not abolished. However, the intensity of autotomy by the rats on their own digits was reduced and tissue damage healed in most of the rats that were fed the extra tryptophan. It is suggested that increased 5-HT helped to reduce the intensity and duration of pain.[166]

Transcutaneous electrical nerve stimulation

TENS applied to the **contralateral leg** of an amputee is effective in decreasing the intensity of phantom limb pain and sensation.[204] Carabelli & Kellerman reported three cases in which TENS was applied to the contralateral leg that eliminated phantom limb pain.[205] TENS applied to the stump can exaggerate a fading phantom limb or revive a suppressed one. Thus, the phantom pain may result from a lack of inhibitory control exerted over the spinal cord. The effect of contralateral leg stimulation of spinal cord cells serving the phantom limb may facilitate inhibitory control and consequently decrease or eliminate the phantom limb pain.

TENS applied bilaterally behind the ears may also decrease the intensity of phantom pain.[204] A recent placebo controlled study conducted by Katz & Melzack on auricular TENS and its role in reducing phantom limb pain found a slight but statistically significant decrease in pain 10 minutes after stimulation. Phantom limb sensation intensity was decreased during the electrical stimulation. Katz & Melzack postulate that the relief brought about by this earlobe stimulation is transient but beneficial because it is easy enough for the patient to administer and helps build patient autonomy. A placebo-controlled study needs to be done to determine the long-term effectiveness of pain relief by this safe, non-invasive, drug-free and convenient method of treatment (see Ch 15).[206]

Other methods

Acupuncture has not only failed to eliminate phantom pain but actually exacerbates it. Consequently, Chong-cheng suggested that acupuncture should be used, not as a method of treatment but as a method in researching phantom pain pathways.[207]

SUMMARY

The treatment of chronic phantom pain is quite varied and controversial with the non-surgical methods being more successful than the surgical intervention.[80] The most promising methods in preventing phantom pain consist of epidural blockade before the operation to reduce pre-amputation pain or continuous postoperative regional anesthesia by nerve sheath blockade if the former is not feasible. The severity of the phantom pain should be assessed along with the reason for the amputation in order to plan an appropriate treatment. If mild, one should begin treatment with the less-invasive methods such as TENS and oral analgesics. As pain increases, subarachnoid fentanyl and epidural opioids, local anesthetics, or both may help to relieve the pain.[200]

Although not directly involved in the mechanism of phantom pain,[177] the psychological status of the patient is an important consideration. The patient should be reassured that this phenomenon is real. Finally, the patient should also be informed that complete relief of pain may not be obtainable but a reduction of pain is possible. As with any chronic pain process, the perceived pain intensity may be related to stress, anxiety, exhaustion, and depression.[80]

REFERENCES

1. Portenoy RK. Neuropathic pain. In: Portenoy RK, Kanner RM, eds. Pain management: Theory and practice. Philadelphia: FA Davis; 1996: 83–125.
2. Jänig W, Blumberg H, Boas RA, Campbell JM. The reflex sympathetic dystrophy syndrome: Consensus statement and general recommendations for diagnosis and clinical research. In: Bond MR, Charlton JE, Woolf CJ, eds. Pain research and clinical management, vol 4. Proceedings of the VIth World Congress on Pain. Amsterdam: Elsevier; 1991: 373–376.

3. Evans JA. Reflex sympathetic dystrophy. Surg Clin North Am 1946; 26: 780–790.

4. Winnie A. Reflex sympathetic dystrophy and causalgia: Diagnosis and management. In: Stanley TH, Ashburn MA, Fine PG, eds. Anesthesiology and pain management. Dordrecht: Kluwer Academic; 1991: 331–350.

5. McLeskey CH, Balestrieri FJ, Weeks DB. Sympathetic dystrophies. In: Warfield CA, ed. Principles and practice of pain management. New York: McGraw-Hill; 1993: 219–234.

6. Mailis A, Wade J. Profile of Caucasian women with possible genetic predisposition to reflex sympathetic dystrophy: a pilot study. Clin J Pain 1994; 10(3): 210–217.

7. Albert J, Ott H. Three brothers with algodystrophy of the hip. Ann Rheum Dis 1983; 42(4): 421–424.

8. Stanton-Hicks M, Jänig W, Hassenbusch S, et al. Reflex sympathetic dystrophy: Changing concepts and taxonomy. Pain 1995; 63: 127–133.

9. Stanton-Hicks M. Complex regional pain syndrome: A new name for reflex sympathetic dystrophy and causalgia. Curr Rev Pain 1996; 1: 34–40.

10. Roberts WJ. A hypothesis on the physiological basis for causalgia and related pains. Pain 1986; 24: 297–311.

11. Campbell JN, Meyer RA, Raja SN. Is nociceptor activation by α-1 adrenoreceptors the culprit in sympathetically maintained pain? APS J 1992; 1: 3–11.

12. Mitchell SW, Morehouse GR, Keene WW. Gunshot wounds and other injuries of nerves. Philadelphia: Lippincott; 1864: 164.

13. Doupe J, Cullen CH, Chance GQ. Post traumatic pain and the causalgia syndrome. J Neurol Neurosurg Psychiatr 1944; 7: 33–48.

14. Ochoa JL, Torebjork HE. Sensations evoked by intraneural microstimulation of single mechanoreceptor units innervating the human hand. J Physiol 1983; 342: 633–654.

15. Hooshmand H. Origins of RSD. In: Hooshmand H, ed. Chronic pain: Reflex sympathetic dystrophy. Prevention and management. Boca Raton: CRC Press; 1993.

16. Levine J, Taiwo Y. Inflammatory pain. In: Wall PD, Melzack R, eds. Textbook of pain. 3rd ed. Edinburgh: Churchill Livingstone; 1994: 45–56.

17. Livingstone WK. Pain mechanisms: A physiologic interpretation of causalgia and its related states. New York: Macmillan; 1944.

18. Melzack R, Wall PD. Pain mechanisms: a new theory. Science 1965; 150: 971–979.

19. Melzack R, Casey KL. Sensory, motivational and central determinants of pain. In: Kenshalo DR, ed. The skin senses. Springfield: Charles C Thomas; 1968.

20. Melzack R. Phantom limb pain: Implications for treatment of pathological pain. Anesthesiology 1971; 35: 409–419.

21. Bonica JJ. Causalgia and other reflex sympathetic dystrophies. In: Bonica J, Liebeskind J, Albe-Fessard D, et al, eds. Advances in pain research and therapy, vol. 3. New York: Raven Press; 1979: 141–166.

22. Payne R. Neuropathic pain syndromes, with special reference to causalgia and reflex sympathetic dystrophy. Clin J Pain 1986; 2: 59–73.

23. Helms CA, O'Brien ET, Katzberg RW. Segmental reflex sympathetic dystrophy syndrome. Radiology 1980; 135: 67–68.

24. Wilson PR. Sympathetically maintained pain: Diagnosis, measurement, and efficacy of treatment. In: Stanton-Hicks M, ed. Pain and the sympathetic nervous system. Norwell: Kluwer Academic; 1990: 91–123.

25. Sonneveld GJ, van der Meulen JC, Smith AR. Quantitative oxygen measurements before and after intravascular guanethidine blocks. J Hand Surg 1983; 8: 435–442.

26. Wesselmann U, Raja SN. Reflex sympathetic dystrophy and causalgia. Anesth Clin North Am 1997; 15(2): 407–427.

27. Arner S. Intravenous phentolamine test: Diagnostic and prognostic use in reflex sympathetic dystrophy. Pain 1991; 46: 17–22.

28. Raja SN, Treede RD, Davis KD, et al. Systemic alpha-adrenergic blockade with phentolamine: A diagnostic test for sympathetically maintained pain. Anesthesiology 1991; 74: 691–698.

29. Hannington-Kiff JG. Intravenous regional sympathetic block with guanethidine. Lancet 1974; 1: 1019–1029.

30. Wahren LK, Torebjörk E, Nystrom B. Quantitative sensory testing before and after regional guanethidine block in patients with neuralgia in the hands. Pain 1991; 46: 23–30.

31. Manchikanti L. Role of intravenous regional bretylium in reflex sympathetic dystrophy. Anesthesiology 1990; 73(3): 585–586.

32. Hana MH, Peat SJ. Ketanserin in reflex sympathetic dystrophy. A double-blind placebo controlled cross-over trial. Pain 1989; 38(2): 148–150.

33. Raja SN. Reflex sympathetic dystrophy: diagnosis and treatment. In: Comprehensive review of pain management. ASRA 1995; 119–130.

34. Rowlingson JC, Hamill RJ. Concomitant chronic pain syndromes. In: Rowlingson JC, Hamill RJ, eds. Handbook of critical care pain management. New York: McGraw-Hill; 1994: 543–554.

35. Rauck RL, Eisenach JC, Jackson K, Young LD, Southern J. Epidural clonidine treatment for refractory reflex sympathetic dystrophy. Anesthesiology 1993; 79(6): 1163–1169.

36. Gaumer D, Lennon RL, Wedel DJ. Axillary plexus block – proximal catheter technique for postoperative pain management. Anesthesiology 1987; 67(3A): A242.

37. Hooshmand H. Management of RSD. In: Hooshmand H, ed. Chronic pain: Reflex sympathetic dystrophy. Prevention and management. Boca Raton: CRC Press; 1993.

38. Wilkinson HA. Radio frequency percutaneous upper-thoracic sympathectomy: Technique and review of indications. N Engl J Med 1984; 311: 34–35.

39. Wilkinson HA. Percutaneous radiofrequency upper thoracic sympathectomy: A new technique. Neurosurgery 1984; 15: 811–814.

40. Wilkinson HA. Percutaneous radiofrequency upper thoracic sympathectomy. Neurosurgery 1996; 38(4): 715–725.

41. Shir Y, Cameron LB, Raja SN, Burke DL. The safety of intravenous phentolamine administration in patients with neuropathic pain. Anesth Analg 1993; 76950: 1008–1011.

42. Moore DC. Regional block. 4th ed. Springfield: Charles C Thomas; 1971: 211–218.

43. Stanton-Hicks MD. Blocks of the sympathetic nervous system. In: Stanton-Hicks M, ed. Pain and the sympathetic nervous system. Norwell: Kluwer Academic; 1990: 125–164.

44. Reid W, Warr JK, Gray TG. Phenol injection of the sympathetic chain. Br J Surg 1970; 57: 45.

45. Morros C, Cedo F. [Treatment with sympathetic intravenous block with reserpine in work-related reflex sympathetic dystrophy.] [Spanish] Revista Espanola de Anestesiologia y Reanimacion 1994; 41(5): 288–291.

46. Blanchard J, Ramamurthy S, Walsh N, Hoffman J, Schoenfeld L. Intravenous regional sympatholysis: a double-blind comparison of guanethidine, reserpine, and normal saline. J Pain Symptom Manage 1990; 5(60): 357–361.

47. Benzon HT, Chomka CM, Brunner EA. Treatment of reflex sympathetic dystrophy with regional intravenous reserpine. Anesth Analg 1980; 59(7): 500–502.

48. Rocco AG, Kaul AF, Reisman RM, Gallo JP, Lief PA. A comparison of regional intravenous guanethidine and reserpine in reflex sympathetic dystrophy. A controlled, randomized, double-blind crossover study. Clin J Pain 1989; 5(3): 205–209.

49. Chuinard RG, Dabezies EJ, Gould JS, Murphy GA. Matthews RE. Intravenous reserpine for treatment of reflex sympathetic dystrophy. South Med J 1981; 74(12): 1481–1484.

50. Duncan KH, Lewis RC Jr, Racz G, Nordyke MD. Treatment of upper extremity reflex sympathetic dystrophy with joint stiffness using sympatholytic Bier blocks and manipulation. Orthopedics 1988; 11(6): 883–886.

51. Jadad AR, Carroll D, Glynn CJ, McQuay HJ. Intravenous regional sympathetic blockade for pain relief in reflex sympathetic dystrophy: a systematic review and a randomized, double-blind crossover study. J Pain Symptom Manage 1995; 10(1): 13–20.

52. Hord AH, Rooks MD, Stephens BO, Rogers HG, Fleming LL. Intravenous regional bretylium and lidocaine for treatment of reflex sympathetic dystrophy: a randomized, double-blind study. Anesth Analg 1992; 74(6): 818–821.

53. Manchikanti L. Role of intravenous regional bretylium in reflex sympathetic dystrophy. Anesthesiology 1990; 73(3): 585–586.

54. Hanowell LH, Kanefield JK, Soriano SG 3d. A recommendation for reduced lidocaine dosage during intravenous regional bretylium treatment of reflex sympathetic dystrophy. Anesthesiology 1989; 71(5): 811–812.

55. Gargiulo RF. A method of facilitating intravenous regional bretylium. Anesthesiology 1988; 69(1): 147–148.

56. Ford SR, Forrest WH Jr, Eltherington L. The treatment of reflex sympathetic dystrophy with intravenous regional bretylium. Anesthesiology 1988; 68(1): 137–140.

57. Gschwind C, Fricker R, Lacher G, Jung M. Does peri-operative guanethidine prevent reflex sympathetic dystrophy? J Hand Surg (Br) 1995; 20(6): 773–775.

58. Ramamurthy S, Hoffman J. Intravenous regional guanethidine in the treatment of reflex sympathetic dystrophy/causalgia: a randomized, double-blind study. Guanethidine Study Group. Anesth Analg 1995; 81(4): 718–723.

59. Bonelli S, Conoscente F, Movilia PG, Restelli L, Francucci B, Grossi E. Regional intravenous guanethidine vs. stellate ganglion block in reflex sympathetic dystrophies: a randomized trial. Pain 1983; 16(3): 297–307.

60. Geertzen JH, de Bruijn H, de Bruijn-Kofman AT, Arendzen JH. Reflex sympathetic dystrophy: early treatment and psychological aspects. Arch Phys Med Rehabil 1994; 75(4): 442–446.

61. Arner S. Intravenous phentolamine test: diagnostic and prognostic use in reflex sympathetic dystrophy. Pain 1991; 46: 17–22.

62. Galer BS. Peak pain relief is delayed and duration of relief is extended following intravenous phentolamine infusion. Reg Anesth 1995; 20: 444.

63. Verdugo RJ, Ochoa JL. Sympathetically maintained pain. I. Phentolamine block questions the concept. Neurology 1994; 44(6): 1003–1010.

64. Verdugo RJ, Campero M, Ochoa JL. Phentolamine sympathetic block in painful

polyneuropathies. II. Further questioning of the concept of 'sympathetically maintained pain'. Neurology 1994; 44(6): 1010–1014.

65. Howng SL, Loh JK. Long term follow-up of upper dorsal sympathetic ganglionectomy for palmar hyperhydrosis: A scale of evaluation. Kaohsiung J Medical Sciences 1987; 3: 703–707.

66. Ghostine SY, Comair YG, Turner DM, Kassell NJ, Azar CG. Phenoxybenzamine in the treatment of causalgia. J Neurosurg 1984; 60: 1263–1268.

67. Abram SE, Lightfoot RW. Treatment of long-standing causalgia with prazosin. Reg Anesth 1981; 6: 79–81.

68. Prough DS, Mcleskey CH, Poehling GG, et al. Efficacy of oral nifedipine in the treatment of reflex sympathetic dystrophy. Anesthesiology 1985; 62: 796–799.

69. Davis KD, Treede RD, Raja SN, et al. Topical application of clonidine relieves hyperalgesia in patients with sympathetically maintained pain. Pain 1991; 47: 309–317.

70. Kirkpatrick AF, Desarai M. Transdermal clonidine: Treating reflex sympathetic dystrophy. (Letter) Reg Anesth 1993; 18: 140–141.

71. Simpson G. Propanolol for causalgia and Sudek's atrophy. JAMA 1974; 227:327.

72. Pleet AB, Tahmous AJ, Jennings JR. Causalgia: Treatment with propanolol. Neurol 1976; 26: 375.

73. Scadding JW, Wall PD, Parry CBW, Brook DM. Clinical trials of propanolol in postraumatic neuralgia. Pain 1982; 14: 283–292.

74. Broesta J, Roldan P, Gonzalez-Darder J, et al. Chronic epidural dorsal column stimulation in the treatment of causalgic pain. Applied Neurophysiol 1982; 45: 190–194.

75. Melzack R. Phantom limb. Sci Am 1992; 266(4): 120–126.

76. Sherman RA. Stump and phantom limb pain. Neurological Clinician 1989; 7: 249–264.

77. Jensen TS, Krebs B, Nielsen J, Rasmussen P. Immediate and long-term phantom limb pain in amputees: incidence, clinical characteristics and relationship to pre-amputation limb pain. Pain 1985; 21: 267–278.

78. Krebs B, Jensen TS, Kroner K, Nielsen J, Jorgenssen HS. Phantom limb phenomena in amputees 7 years after limb amputation. Pain 1984; Suppl 2: S85.

79. Melzack R. Central pain syndrome and theories of pain. In: Casey KL, ed. Pain and central nervous system disease. The central pain syndrome. New York: Raven Press; 1991; 59–64.

80. Sherman RA, Sherman CJ, Gall NG. A survey of current phantom limb pain treatment in the United States. Pain 1980; 8: 35–99.

81. Loeser J. Pain after amputation: Phantom limb pain. In: Bonica JJ, ed. The management of pain. 2nd ed. Philadelphia; Lea and Febiger; 1990.

82. Mitchell SW. Injuries of nerves and their consequences. Philadelphia: JB Lippincott; 1872; (reprint Dover Publications, NY 1926).

83. Heusner AP. Phantom genitalia. Trans Am Neurol Assoc 1950; 75: 128–184.

84. Ackerly W, Lhamon W, Fitts WT. Phantom breast. J Nerv Ment Dis 1955; 121: 177–178.

85. Bressler B, Cohen SI, Magnussen F. Bilateral breast phantom and breast phantom pain. J Nerv Men Dis 1955; 122: 315–320.

86. Weinstein S, Vetter RJ, Sersen EA. Phantom following breast amputation. Neuropsychologia 1970; 3: 185–197.

87. Hanowell ST, Kennedy SF. Phantom tongue pain and causalgia: Case presentation and treatment. Anesth Analg 1979; 58: 436–438.

88. Jamison K, Wellisch DK, Katz RL, Pasnau RO. Phantom breast syndrome. Arch Surg 1979; 114: 93–95.

89. Reisner H. Phantom sensations (phantom arm) in plexus paralysis. In: Siegfried J, Simmerman M, eds. Phantom and stump pain. Berlin: Springer; 1981; 62–65.

90. Postone N. Phantom limb pain. International Journal of Psychiatric Medicine 1987; 17: 57–70.

91. Nathanson M. Phantom limbs as reported by S. Weir Mitchell. Neurology 1988; 38: 504–505.

92. Mitchell SW. Phantom limb. The Lippincott Magazine 1871; 8: 563–569.

93. Jensen T, Rasmussen P. Phantom pain and related phenomena after amputation. In: Wall PD, Melzack R, eds. Textbook of pain. 2nd ed. Edinburgh: Churchill Livingstone; 1989: 508–521.

94. Sunderland S. Nerves and nerve injuries. 2nd ed. Edinburgh: Churchill Livingstone; 1978.

95. Pitres A. Etude sur les sensations illusiores des amputes. Ann Med Psychol (Paris) 1897; 8th series: 5–19.

96. Carlen PL, Wall PD, Nadvorna H, Steinbach T. Phantom limbs and related phenomena in recent traumatic amputation. Neurology 1978; 28: 211–217.

97. Cronholm B. Phantom limbs in amputees: Study of changes in integration of centripetal impulses with special reference to referred sensations. Acta Psychiatr Neurol Scand 1951; 72: 1–310. Supplement.

98. Solonen KA. The phantom phenomenon in amputated Finnish war veterans. Acta Orthopaed Scand 1962; 54: 7. Supplement.

99. Melzack R. Phantom limbs and the concept of a neuromatrix. Trends Neurosci 1990; 13: 88–92.

100. Katz J, Melzack R. Pain 'memories' in phantom

limbs: Review and clinical observations. Pain 1990; 43: 319–336.

101. Sliosberg A. Les algies des amutes. Paris; Masson; 1948.
102. Nathan PW. Pain traces left in the central nervous system. In: Keele CA, Smith R, eds. The assessment of pain in man and animals. Edinburgh; Churchill Livingstone; 1962; 129–134.
103. Wesolowshki JA, Lema MJ. 'Phantom limb pain.' Reg Anesth 1993; 18(2): 121–127.
104. Weiss A. The 'phantom limb.' Ann Int Med 1956; 44: 668–677.
105. Guerniot M. D'une hallucination du toucher (ou heterotropie subjective des extremities) particulière a certains amputes. J Physio Homme Animaux 1861; 4: 416.
106. Shukla GD, Sahu SC, Tripathi RP, Gupta DK. 'Phantom limb: A phenomenological study.' Br J Psych 1982; 141: 54–58. Abstract.
107. Henderson WR, Smyth GE. Phantom limbs. J Neurol Neurosurg Psych 1948; 11: 88–112.
108. Katz J. Psychophysiological contributions to phantom limbs. Can J Psych 1992; 37: 282–298.
109. Merzenich MM, Nelson RJ, Stryker MP, et al. Somatosensory cortical map changes following digit amputation in adult monkeys. J Comp Neurol 1984; 224: 591–605.
110. Haber WB. Effect of loss of limb on sensory functions. J Psychol 1955; 40: 115–123.
111. Teuber HL, Krieger HP, Bender M. Reorganization of sensory function in amputation stumps: Two-point discrimination. Fed Proc 1949; 8: 156.
112. Varma SK, Lal SK, Mukherjee A. A study of phantom experience in amputees. Indian J Med Sci 1972; 26: 185–188.
113. Morgenstern FS. The effects of sensory input and concentration on post-amputation phantom limb pain. J Neurol Neurosurg Psych 1964; 27: 58–65.
114. James W. The consciousness of lost limbs. Proceedings of the American Society for Physical Research 1887; (1): 249–258.
115. Haber WB. Observations on phantom limb phenomena. Arch Neurol Psych 1956; 75: 624–636.
116. Kallio KE. Phantom limb of forearm stump cleft by kineplastic surgery. Acta Chir Scand 1950; 99: 121–132.
117. Bors E. Phantom limbs of patients with spinal cord injury. Arch Neurol Psych 1951; 66: 610–631.
118. Bors E. Phantom limbs in patients with spinal cord injury. In: Harris P, ed. Spinal injuries. Proceedings of a symposium held in the Royal College of Surgeons of Edinburgh; 1963; 15–21.
119. Sweet W. Phantom sensations following intraspinal injury. Neurochirugie 1975; 18: 139–154.
120. Wynn Parry CB. Pain in avulsion lesions of the brachial plexus. Pain 1980; 9: 40–53.
121. Weiss SA, Fishman S. Extended and telescoped phantom limbs in unilateral amputees. J Abnorm Soc Psych 1963; 66: 489–497.
122. Riddoch G. Phantom limbs and body shape. Brain 1941; 64: 197–222.
123. Jensen TS, Krebs B, Nielsen J, Rasmussen P. Phantom limb, phantom pain, and stump pain in amputees during the first 6 months following limb amputation. Pain 1983; 17: 243–256.
124. Sherman R, Sherman C, Parker L. Chronic phantom and stump pain among American veterans: Results of a survey. Pain 1984; 18: 83–95.
125. Nystrom B, Hagbarth KE. Microelectrode recordings from transected nerves in amputees with phantom limb pain. Neurosci Lett 1981, 27: 211–216.
126. Fields HL. Pain. New York: McGraw-Hill; 1987.
127. Katz J. Psychophysical correlates of phantom limb experience. J Neurol Neurosurg Psych 1992; 55: 811–821.
128. Katz J. Psychophysiological contributions to phantom limbs. Comment in: Can J Psych 1993; 38(2): 151–153. Abstract.
129. Campbell JN, Raja SN, Meyer RA. Painful sequelae of nerve injury. In: Dubner R, Gebhart GF, Bond MR, eds. Proceedings of the 5th World Congress on Pain. Elsevier: Amsterdam, 1988; 135–143.
130. Delius W, Hagbarth KE, Hongell A, et al. Manoeuvres affecting sympathetic outflow in human skin nerves. Acta Physiol Scand 1972; 84: 177–186.
131. Hagbarth KE, Hallin RG, Hongell HE, et al. General characteristics of sympathetic activity in human skin nerves. Acta Physiol Scand 1972; 84: 164–176.
132. Parkes CM. Factors determining the persistence of phantom pain in the amputee. J Psychosom Res 1973; 17: 97–108.
133. Kolb LC. The painful phantom: psychology, physiology and treatment. Springfield: Charles C Thomas; 1954: 28–35.
134. Sherman RA, Gall N, Gormly J. Treatment of phantom limb pain with muscular relaxation training to disrupt the pain–anxiety–tension cycle. Pain 1979; 6: 47–55.
135. Arena JG, Sherman RA, Bruno GM, et al. The relationship between situational stress and phantom limb pain: cross-lagged correlational data from six month pain logs. J Psychosom Res 1990; 34: 71–77.
136. Merskey H. Psychiatry and chronic pain. Can J Psych 1989; 34(4): 329–336.
137. Sherman RA. Case reports of treatment of phantom limb pain with a combination of electromyo-

graphic biofeedback and verbal relaxation techniques. Biofeedback Self Regul, 1976; 1: 353.

138. Ribbers G, Mulder T, Rijken R. The phantom phenomenon: A critical review. Int J Rehabil Res 1989; 12: 175–186.

139. Melzack R. Phantom limb pain. Anesthesiology 1971; 35: 409–419.

140. Prevoznik SJ, Eckenhoff JE. Phantom sensations during spinal anesthesia. Anesthesiology 1964; 25: 767–770.

141. Davis RW. Phantom sensation, phantom pain and stump pain. Arch Phys Med Rehabil 1993; 74(1): 79–91.

142. Aanonsen LM, Lei S, Wilcox GL. Excitatory amino acid receptors and nociceptive neurotransmission in rat spinal cord. Pain 1990; 41: 309–321.

143. Pernow B. Substance P. Pharmacol Rev 1984; 35: 85–141.

144. Schneider SP, Perl ER. Selective excitation of neurons in the mammalian spinal dorsal horn. J Neurosci 1988; 8: 2062–2073.

145. Mayer ML, Westbrook GL. The physiology of excitatory amino acids in the vertebrate central nervous system. Prog Neurobiol 1987; 28: 197–276.

146. King AE, Thompson SWN, Urban L, et al. An intracellular analysis of amino acid induced excitations of deep dorsal horn neurones in the rat spinal cord slice. Neurosci Lett 1988; 89: 286–292.

147. Carlton SM, Westlund KN, Zhang DX, et al. Calcitonin gene-related peptide containing primary afferent fibers synapse on primate spinothalamic tract cells. Neurosci Lett 1990; 109: 76–81.

148. Lei SZ, Wilcox GL. Opioid and neurokinin activities of substance P fragments and their analogs. Eur J Pharmacol 1991; 87: 411–417.

149. Womack MD, Jessel TM. Substance P and the novel mammalian tachykinins: a diversity of receptors and cellular actins. Trends Neurosci 1988; 8: 43–45.

150. MacDermott AB, Mayer ML, Westbrook GL, et al. NMDA receptor activation increases cytoplasmic calcium concentration in cultured spinal cord neurons. Nature 1986; 321: 519–522.

151. Jorum E, Holm E, Lundberg LE, et al. Temporal summation in nociceptive systems. Pain 1990; (Suppl) 5: S314.

152. Collingridge GL, Singer W. Excitatory amino acid receptors and synaptic plasticity. Trends Pharmacol Sci 1990; 11: 290–296.

153. Dougherty P, Willis WD. Enhancement of spinothalamic neuron responses to chemical and mechanical stimuli following combined microiontophoretic application of NMDA and substance P. Pain 1991; 47: 85–93.

154. Dubner R. Neuronal plasticity and pain following peripheral tissue inflammation or nerve injury. In: Bond MR, Charlton JE, Woolf CJ, eds. Proceedings of the VIth World Congress on Pain. Amsterdam: Elsevier Science; 1991: 263–276.

155. Woolf CJ. Central mechanisms of acute pain. In: Bond MR, Charlton JE, Woolf CJ, eds. Proceedings of the VIth World Congress on Pain. Amsterdam: Elsevier Science; 1991: 25–34.

156. Wilcox GL. Excitatory neurotransmitters and pain. In: Bond MR, Charlton JE, Woolf CJ, eds. Proceedings of the VIth World Congress on Pain. Amsterdam: Elsevier Science; 1991: 97–117.

157. Thompson SWN, Woolf CJ. Primary afferent-evoked prolonged potentials in the spinal cord and their central summation: role of the NMDA receptor. In: Bond MR, Charlton JE, Woolf CJ, eds. Proceedings of the VIth World Congress on Pain. Amsterdam: Elsevier; 1991: 291–298.

158. Yoshimura M, Jessell TM. Primary afferent-evoked responses and slow potential generation in rat substantia gelatinosa neurones in vitro. J Neurophysiol 1989; 62: 96–108.

159. Herdegen T, Leah JD, Walker T, et al. Activated neurons in CNS pain pathways detected via early proto-oncogene products. Pain 1990: (Suppl) 5: S97.

160. Tolle TR, Castro-Lopoes JM, Evan G, et al. C-fos induction in the spinal cord following noxious stimulation: prevention by opiates but not by NMDA antagonists. In: Bond MR, Charlton JE, Woolf CJ, eds. Proceedings of the VIth World Congress on Pain. Amsterdam: Elsevier; 1991: 299–305.

161. Melzack R. Phantom limbs: Labat lecture. Reg Anesth 1989; 32: 285–287.

162. Yarnitsky D, Barron SA, Bental E. Disappearance of phantom pain after focal brain infarction. Pain 1988; 32: 285–287.

163. Tasker RAR, Choniere M, Libman SM, Melzack R. Analgesia produced by injection of lidocaine into the lateral hypothalamus. Pain 1987; 31: 237–248.

164. Vaccarino AL, Melzack R. Analgesia produced by injection of lidocaine into the anterior cingulum bundle of the rat. Pain 1989; 39: 213–219.

165. Vaccarino AL, Melzack R. The role of the cingulum bundle in self mutilation following peripheral neurectomy in the rat. Exp Neurol 1991; 111: 131–134.

166. Abbott FV, Young SN. The effect of tryptophan supplementation on autotomy induced by nerve lesion in rats. Pharmacol Biochem Behav 1991; 40(2): 301–304.

167. Katz J, Vaccarino AL, Coderre TJ, Melzack R. Injury prior to neurectomy alters the pattern of autotomy in rats. Behavioral evidence of central

neural plasticity. Comment in: Anesthesiology 1991; 75(5): 876–883.

168. Feria M, Sanchez A, Abad F, Abreu P. Effects of selective neurotoxic lesion of lumbosacral serotonergic and noradrenergic systems on autotomy behavior in rats. Pain 1992; 51(1): 101–109.

169. Melzack R, Loeser JD. Phantom body pain in paraplegics: Evidence for central pattern generating mechanism for pain. Pain 1978; 4: 195–210.

170. Bach S, Noreng MF, Tjellden NU. Phantom limb pain in amputees during the first 12 months following limb amputation, after preoperative lumbar blockade. Pain 1988; 33: 297–301.

171. Wall R, Novotny-Joseph P, MacNamara TE. Does preamputation pain influence phantom limb pain in cancer patients? South Med J 1985; 78: 34–36.

172. Roth YF, Sugarbaker PH, Weiss CM, Davidson DD. Increasing phantom limb pain as a symptom of cancer recurrence. Cancer 1984; 54: 373–375.

173. Scatena P. Phantom representations of congenitally absent limbs. Percept Mot Skills 1990; 70: 1227–1232.

174. Poeck K. Phantoms following amputation in early childhood and in congenital absence of limbs. Cortex 1964/1965; 1: 269–275.

175. McGrath PA, Hillier LM. Phantom limb sensations in adolescents: A case study to illustrate the utility of sensation and pain logs in pediatric clinical practice. J Pain Symptom Manage 1992; 7(1): 46–53.

176. Simmel ML. Phantom experiences following amputation in childhood. J Neurol Neurosurg Psych 1962; 25: 69–78.

177. Bruno GM, Sherman RA, Sherman CJ. Psychological factors influencing chronic phantom limb pain: An analysis of the literature. Pain 1987; 28: 285–295.

178. Kroner LC, Krebs B, Skov J, et al. Immediate and long-term phantom breast syndrome after mastectomy: Incidence, clinical characteristics and relationship to pre-mastectomy breast pain. Pain 1989; 36: 327–334.

179. Siegfried J, Cetinalp E. Neurosurgical treatment of phantom limb pain. In: Siegfried J, Simmerman M, eds. Phantom and stump pain. Berlin: Springer; 1981: 143–155.

180. White JC, Sweet WH. Pain and the neurosurgeon: A forty year experience. Springfield: Charles C Thomas; 1969: 68–86.

181. Saris SC, Iacono RP, Nashold BS Jr. Successful treatment of phantom pain with dorsal root entry zone coagulation. Applied Neurophysiology 1988; 51: 188–197.

182. Sherman RA. Published treatments of phantom limb pain. Am J Phys Med 1980; 59: 232–244.

183. Bonica JJ, Lindblon U, Iggo A. Surgical technique of DREZ coagulation. In: Advances in pain research and treatment. New York; Raven Press; 1981: 741–742.

184. Nashold BS, Ostdahl RH, Bullitt E, Friedman A, Brophy B. Dorsal root entry zone lesions: A new neurosurgical therapy for deafferentation pain. In: Bonica JJ, et al, eds. Advances in pain research and treatment. New York: Raven Press; 1983: 739–750.

185. Tourian A, Iacono R, Nashold B, Urban B, Sanders J. Involuntary movements of the lower extremity following dorsal root entry zone lesions in a man treated for phantom limb pain. Applied Neurological Physiology 1988; 51: 212–217.

186. Jacobson L, Chaba C. Prolonged relief of acute postamputation phantom limb pain with intrathecal fentanyl and epidural morphine. Anesthesiology 1989; 71: 984–985.

187. Jacobson L, Chaba C, Brody MC. Relief of persistent postamputation stump and phantom limb pain with intrathecal fentanyl. Pain 1989; 37: 317–322.

188. Mackenzie M. Phantom limb pain during spinal anesthesia: Recurrence in amputees. Anaesthesiology 1983; 38: 886–887.

189. Koyama K, Watanabe S, Tsuneto S, et al. Thiopental for phantom pain during spinal anesthesia. Anesthesiology 1988; 69: 589–600.

190. Fiddler DS, Hindman BJ. Intravenous calcitonin alleviates spinal anesthesia-induced phantom limb pain. Anesthesiology 1991; 74: 187–189.

191. Chrubasik J, Falke KL, Zindler M. Is calcitonin an analgesic agent? Pain 1986; 27: 273–276. Letter.

192. Shaw HL. Subarachnoid administration of calcitonin: A warning. Lancet 1982; 2: 390. Letter.

193. Eisenach JC. Demonstrating safety of subarachnoid calcitonin: Patients or animals? Anesth Analg 1988; 67: 298. Letter.

194. Candeletti S, Ferri S. Clinical use of subarachnoid neuropeptides: An experimental contribution. Anesth Analg 1989; 69: 416. Letter.

195. Gentili ME, Bonnet F. [Temporary relief from pain in the phantom limb after spinal anesthesia using a combination of bupivacaine and clonidine.] [French] Annales Francaises d Anesthesie et de Reanimation 1993; 12(3): 323–325.

196. Fisher A, Meller Y. Continuous postoperative regional analgesia by nerve sheath block for amputation surgery: A pilot study. Anesth Analg 1991; 72: 300–303.

197. Jaeger H, Maier C. Calcitonin in phantom limb pain: A double-blind study. Pain 1992; 48: 21–27.

198. Stannard CF, Porter GE. Ketamine hydrochloride in the treatment of phantom limb pain. Pain 1993; 54: 227–230.

199. Melzack R. The tragedy of needless pain. Sci Am 1990; 262: 27–33.

200. Urban BJ, France RD, Steinberger EK, Scott DL, Maltbie AA. Long-term use of narcotic/anti-depressant medication in the management of phantom limb pain. Pain 1986; 24(2): 191–196.

201. Marsland AR, Weekes JW, Atkinson RL, Leong MG. Phantom limb pain: a case for beta blockers? Pain 1982; 12(3): 295–297.

202. Davis RW. Successful treatment for phantom pain. Orthopedics 1993; 16(6): 691–695.

203. Power-Smith P, Turkington D. Fluoxetine in phantom limb pain. Br J Psych 1993; 163: 105–106.

204. Katz J, France C, Melzack R. An association between phantom limb sensations and stump skin conductance during transcutaneous electrical nerve stimulation. Pain 1989; 36: 367–377.

205. Carabelli RA, Kellerman WC. Phantom limb pain: relief by application of TENS to contralateral extremity. Arch Phys Med Rehabil 1985; 66(7): 466–467.

206. Katz J, Melzack R. Auricular transcutaneous electrical nerve stimulation (TENS) reduces phantom limb pain. J Pain Symptom Manage 1991; 6(2): 73–83.

207. Chong-cheng X. Acupuncture induced phantom limb pain and meridian phenomenon in acquired and congenital amputees. Chin Med J 1946; 99: 247–252.

208. Nashold BS, Ostdahl RH. Dorsal root entry zone lesions for pain relief. J Neurosurg 1979; 51: 59–69.

Invasive pain management for the trauma patient

Carol Harris, Miles Day and Gabor B Racz

Introduction

Management of the patient with chronic pain as a result of trauma
Sympathetic blockade
Radiofrequency thermocoagulation
Cryoneurolysis
Lysis of epidural adhesions

The Racz caudal catheter approach
Epiduroscopy
Spinal cord stimulation
Peripheral nerve stimulation
Implantable drug delivery systems

Summary

INTRODUCTION

Millions of accidental traumas occur annually and the majority of trauma patients experience persistent or recurrent pain requiring some form of medical or interventional treatment. Pain persisting beyond the normal recovery period can be considered chronic post-traumatic pain. For many patients, chronic pain is the most common reason for disability and non-productivity resulting in personal, social, psychological and economical hardship.

In the post-traumatic patient, the site of injury is an important factor for the development of chronic pain. Extremity injuries are prone to the development of Complex Regional Pain Syndrome I (CRPS I–reflex sympathetic dystrophy) or Complex Regional Pain Syndrome II (CRPS II–causalgia) (see Ch. 22).[1] The subsequent development of a sympathalgia can be expected in approximately 5% of trauma cases.[2] Burning, aching pain, initially localized and then spreading proximally, cold sensitivity, allodynia, as well as vasomotor and sudomotor disturbances characterize the clinical syndrome. As a result of a traumatic insult, the onset of changes occurs rapidly, often within days or weeks of the injury. Traumatic amputations can also be a source of

chronic pain. Post-amputation phantom sensations occur in nearly all amputees, with 5 to 72% developing phantom limb pain (see Ch. 22).[1]

Chronic pain differs from acute pain in many ways and as a result, therapeutic interventions often vary. In the acute setting, invasive treatments may be required for optimal performance of certain radiological or computed tomography studies and painful procedures such as closed reduction. In the trauma patient who experiences chronic pain that has failed conservative treatment, sympathetic blockade, radiofrequency, cryoneurolysis, spinal cord stimulation, implantable intrathecal pumps, Racz epidural catheters, and epiduroscopy are now frequently performed.

Many trauma patients who have developed chronic pain syndromes involving the peripheral and central nervous system, and have failed conservative treatments, can be successfully treated with radiofrequency thermocoagulation. Radiofrequency lesioning, a neurodestructive technique, is considered as an end-of-the-line treatment when conservative therapeutic procedures have failed. The physician should be highly trained and experienced in radiofrequency lesioning and appropriate fluoroscopic imaging and stimulation testing should be done. Paresthesias or motor paralysis occur very rarely.[8] The major advantage over other neurodestructive procedures is that the lesion is well controlled.

Cryoneurolysis and cryoanalgesia offer significant promise for the management of acute, postoperative and chronic intractable pain syndromes after a trauma injury.

Cryoanalgesia is a technique using extremely low temperatures by a cryosurgical probe to achieve pain relief by blocking peripheral nerves or destroying the nerve endings.[2] Percutaneous cryoprobe application has been used for many types of neural lesioning. Any nerve that can be isolated by percutaneous or direct vision cryoprobe can undergo cryoneurolysis.

Neuro-augmentation with spinal cord stimulation and peripheral nerve stimulation in the properly selected post-traumatic patients can provide significant pain relief. Spinal cord stimulation is appropriate for the treatment of various neuropathic pain syndromes. Spinal cord stimulation implantable techniques should be performed after patients have failed conservative therapy and are no longer surgical candidates. Peripheral nerve stimulation has been successfully used for the treatment of neurogenic pain secondary to peripheral nerve injuries. Stimulation effectively suppresses intractable pain of the upper extremities, lower extremities, and intercostal nerves.

Implantable pumps allow the delivery of opioid analgesics directly into the cerebrospinal fluid. Smaller opioid doses are delivered to the nociceptive fibers in the spinal cord, providing effective pain relief without necessarily causing systemic effects. Appropriate patient selection is crucial for optimal results to be achieved. Spinally administered narcotics are more appropriate for opioid-responsive nociceptive pain syndromes. In the post-traumatic patient, this technique can be used successfully for chronic pain that has not responded to more traditional therapies.

After traumatic injuries, hemorrhage into the epidural space can create adhesions that compress nerve roots. This can often be the cause of persistent pain in the back and lower extremities. The Racz, epidural, caudal catheter approach and epiduroscopy are two techniques commonly used for the placement of a local anesthetic and steroid solution directly into the area of adhesions.

MANAGEMENT OF THE PATIENT WITH CHRONIC PAIN AS A RESULT OF TRAUMA

Sympathetic blockade

Introduction

Trauma causes a state of vasoconstriction induced by either direct vascular injury or secondary to pain itself. Vasoconstriction produces nutrient imbalance, which interferes with cellular function. Sympathetic blockade decreases vascular resistance and improves skin and vascular graft flow. Earlier mobilization of the injured part preserves normal myofascial, pulmonary and gastrointestinal function. As a result, there is a reduction in postoperative morbidity and the development of post-traumatic pain syndromes.[1]

Sympathetically maintained pain (SMP) is a term commonly applied to post-traumatic pain conditions having both burning pain and allodynia. Sympathetic blockade relieves the pain of SMP. When treated early, repeated sympathetic blockade may eliminate the clinical findings. Vasomotor and sudomotor changes occur in some patients with phantom limb pain, therefore sympathetic interruption can be of some value in the treatment of these patients. There is some evidence that pretraumatic sympathectomy and pretraumatic epidural analgesia may prevent phantom limb pain following amputation.

Clinical applications

Sympathetic dystrophies affecting the upper extremity, head, neck, and chest can be managed using a cervicothoracic or stellate ganglion block. CRPS I or II is one of the prime indications. A typical patient usually requires multiple stellate ganglion blocks. Conditions such as traumatic injury or embolic occlusion of arteries, and post-amputation pain are additional indications for a stellate ganglion block[2] (Fig. 23.1) (see Ch. 22).

The upper thoracic sympathetic chain is an extension of the cervical sympathetic chain. Thoracic sympathectomy usually involves ablation of the sympathetic chain at the T2–T3 levels. These levels provide outflow to the upper extremity, especially the hand, and can be involved in sympathetically maintained upper extremity pain.[3] Test blocks should be performed with local anesthesia under fluoroscopic guidance prior to the radiofrequency procedure.

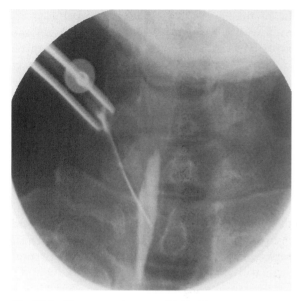

Fig. 23.1 Fluoroscopic spread of radio-opaque contrast dye at the C7 level, spreading toward C6 and T1 for a stellate ganglion block.

Lumbar sympathetic blocks are used extensively in the treatment of CRPS I and II for sympathetically maintained pain. The second and third lumbar ganglia provide the most complete denervation to the lower extremity because most of the fibers pass through these ganglia.[10] The pain relief is usually immediate and can be long-lasting. Other indications in the post-traumatic patient for lumbar sympathetic blocks include peripheral vascular insufficiency and deafferented pain syndromes such as phantom limb pain that has a component of sympathetically mediated pain.[2]

Radiofrequency thermocoagulation

Introduction

The first commercial radiofrequency generators became available in the 1950s and since that time, thermocoagulation techniques have been used successfully in making therapeutic lesions in the nervous system. Radiofrequency thermocoagulation is a neurodestructive procedure often used after a diagnostic blockade has provided some transient or temporary pain relief. The advantages of radiofrequency techniques versus other neurodestructive methods are:[4]

- Produce discrete therapeutic lesions

- Temperature control allows consistent lesioning from patient to patient without side effects of sticking, charring and the formation of gases
- Amenable to stimulation, impedence monitoring and recording, therefore it facilitates correct electrode placement
- Ability to utilize the same electrode cannula for different types of lesioning
- Safe, effective and simple to use
- There is a differential selection of pain fibers versus other neural fibers
- Lesioning can be done under local or sedative anesthesia
- There is rapid recovery after lesioning and a low incidence of morbidity and mortality with properly performed procedures
- Radiofrequency lesioning can be repeated after the neural pathways regenerate.

Concept of lesioning and monitoring

In radiofrequency lesioning, an insulated electrode needle with an uninsulated tip is placed into the nervous tissue via a circuit. The circuit consists of a radiofrequency generator as a voltage source, connected to grounding pads on the patient's body, allowing current to flow through the tissue between the generator and grounding pad. Heat lesioning is done at the tip of the radiofrequency electrode; therefore measuring and monitoring temperature at the tip of the electrode allows controlled lesioning.[4] At any given electrical current, thermal equilibrium is established in 60 seconds. (Cosman et al, 1983). In areas of high vascularity, greater time and power are needed to achieve thermal equilibrium since the blood tends to sink heat away from the surrounding tissue and produce an asymmetry in lesion shape. At our institution we use a lesioning time of 90 seconds at a constant 80°C for facet and lumbar sympathetic rhizotomy. A second lesioning at this temperature and duration is done after the curved, blunt tip electrode probe has been turned 180° to increase the area of lesioning. It has been shown that the most satisfactory method to control lesion size is that of maintaining a constant electrode tip temperature for a period of 1 to 2 minutes. (Cosman et al., 1983). Certain clinical conditions, such as dorsal root ganglionotomy and trigeminal ganglion radiofrequency, call for lower lesioning temperatures near 60 to 70°C because the highly myelinated A-β fibers survive better than the unmyelinated A-δ and C fibers. This allows preservation of tactile and motor innervation.

Although temperature monitoring is the primary parameter in radiofrequency success, it is mandatory that the system allows for stimulation at a wide range of frequencies, and ability to time the duration of the lesion, and to monitor the power, current, voltage, amperage and impedence to rule out malfunctions such as a short-circuit, system set-up failure, or a misplaced electrode tip.

Clinical applications of radiofrequency lesions in the trauma patient

Radiofrequency thermocoagulation has been used to ablate pain pathways for:

- Facet joint pain secondary to traumatic cervical, thoracic or lumbar spine injuries
- Sacroiliac joint pain
- Internally ruptured disc
- Pain from the lumbar spinal nerve
- Sympathetically maintained pain of the upper and lower extremities
- The treatment of post-traumatic headaches
- Facial trauma.

CRPS I (i.e. reflex sympathetic dystrophy) or CRPS II (i.e. causalgia), post-traumatic pain syndrome, circulatory insufficiency, phantom limb pain, or stump pain are all common indications for lumbar or thoracic sympathetic radiofrequency thermocoagulation. Sympathetic mediated pain of the upper extremity can be achieved with thoracic rhizotomy, while lumbar rhizotomy can treat lower extremity sympathetic mediated pain for patients who had previously responded to sympathectomy or sympathetic blocks.

Facet joint syndrome can occur as either acute or chronic pain after a trauma, especially with motor vehicle accidents. 50 to 67% of patients with chronic, low back pain can receive moderate-to-significant decrease in their pain after radiofrequency thermocoagulation. Radiographic findings may not reveal abnormalities. The patient may present with deep aching pain in the paravertebral region of the low back with somatic referred pain into the buttocks, posterior or lateral thigh, hip or knee. Hamstring pain and muscle spasm may be present. On physical exam, the patient may experience tenderness at the facet paravertebral joint and back pain with lumbosacral extension or lateral rotation. The pain only occasionally radiates

below the knee; when it does, it is usually associated with prolonged pathologic changes of the involved facet. A straight leg-raising test can be negative. Local anesthetic injection at the facet joint can assist in diagnosis.

A cervical facet syndrome may result from the sudden stop of a vehicle, athletic or occupational injuries, sleeping with a twisted neck, or a sudden jerk of the neck that results in overriding the superior on the inferior articular facet. Post-traumatic patients may present with symptoms of well-circumscribed pain overlying the cervical facet joints. They may also report pain in the neck and shoulder girth with associated chronic headaches and even ear pain. In addition, referred pain to the facial region may be seen. The patient frequently presents with decreased range of motion in the neck.

Radiofrequency techniques

The techniques involved in deinnervation of the lumbar facets are performed with the patient in a prone position on a fluoroscopy table. The patient is given small amounts of intravenous short-acting narcotic, but the patient should be awake enough to allow for motor and sensory stimulation testing for accurate electrode placement, and for communicating with the physician. Stimulation allows the physician to perform the procedure with a low incidence of morbidity.

Facet radiofrequency techniques

Using sterile techniques, the lumbar–sacral area is prepped and draped. A C-arm fluoroscopic machine is used to identify the correct radiofrequency target sites. Lidocaine is used for local skin infiltration at the target site. An angiocatheter, correctly fitted for the radiofrequency electrode, is inserted through the skin wheel in a parallel fashion to the X-ray beam. The superior and lateral aspect of the S1 foraminal opening is the first area lesioned. A small branch exits the superior lateral aspect of the S1 canal and extends in a superior fashion towards the base of the L5–S1 facet joint.

At the S1 level, the fluoroscopic unit is placed in a cranial fashion to correctly show the opening of the S1 foraminal canal. The cannula is passed parallel until it touches the periosteum at the superior lateral border of the S1 foramen. The second target zone includes the superior and medial junction of the sacral ala. A cannula is advanced until it touches the superior medial border of the sacral ala and after the periosteum has been contacted, the cannula is walked over the leading edge and advanced 2–3 mm in an anterior fashion.

The third, fourth and fifth target zones include the superior and medial aspects of the transverse process with the superior articulating process of its respective facet joint. Using an oblique fluoroscopic image, between 5 to 15°, the third, fourth, and fifth cannulas are placed until they touch the superior and medial aspect of the transverse process, or the point where the transverse process merges with the superior articulating facet (Fig. 23.2). The cannula is walked over the leading edge 2–3 mm in an anterior fashion to lie parallel to the nerve to be lesioned so that an entire lesion is created along the nerve. Frequent anteroposterior, lateral and oblique fluoroscopic views are taken to ensure correct needle placement and that it is not too close to the opening of the neuroforamina. Impedence monitoring is checked; the average impedence during facet rhizotomy is between 400–700 ohms. This is a good test for the integrity of the system.

Electrical stimulation is performed at 50 Hz.[4] Paresthesia to the back, paravertebral region or hip occurs when the medial branches are stimulated. Sensory stimulation should be noted at less than 1.0 volts at 50 Hz if the electrode is in correct alignment with the medial branch. Motor stimulation is performed at 2 Hz and lower extremity motor fasciculations should be absent at 3 volts stimulation.[4] After showing correct dissociation between motor and sensory stimulation, it is assumed that the cannulas are in correct position. 1–2 cc of a local anesthetic and steroid solution is injected through each cannula and a 30-second delay is allowed to occur. Thermal lesioning at each level is performed at 80°C for 90 seconds. The curved tip is then turned 180° for a second lesioning at 80°C for 90 seconds.

After the lesions are completed, the cannulas are removed and a sterile bandage is placed at each puncture site. Complications from lumbar facet rhizotomy include transient lower extremity numbness and weakness, dyesthesia, pain in the paravertebral region and upper buttock which is thought to be secondary to spasm of the quadratus lumborum muscle.

Thoracic facet joint pain can also be treated with radiofrequency rhizotomy. The technical aspects are quite similar to lumbar facet rhizotomy. The targets points are the superior–medial aspects of the transverse processes. The fluoroscopic camera is angled in a cranial or caudal manner to show separation of the transverse process from its associated rib. A less oblique view is needed as compared to the lumbar region. The risks in the thoracic region are similar to the lumbar region. The primary risk in the thoracic region includes a small risk of pneumothorax. The vascular supply of the thoracic cord has less collateral flow than other regions. Vascular injury during the course of this or any other procedure could have serious consequences, such as cord ischemia.

Cervical facet deinnervation is safe and effective and can be done after a diagnostic injection of the cervical facet joints. The posterior primary ramus of the cervical facet wraps around in a posterior fashion and sends branches along the waist of the cervical facet column (Fig. 23.3). These branches supply joints above and below the level from which they are derived; therefore lesioning should be performed at multiple levels to properly deinnervate a specific facet segment.

To deinnervate the facet joints at C2–3, C3–4, C4–5, and C5–6, the patient is placed in the supine position. For the lower facets, the patient is placed in a prone position and a similar approach to the lumbar facet deinnervation is taken.[4] The facets are palpated and a line is drawn with a

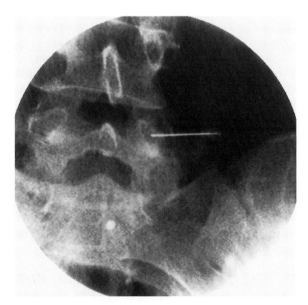

Fig. 23.2 Posteroanterior radiograph of the lumbar spine, showing needle placement for the posterior primary medial branch at L4.

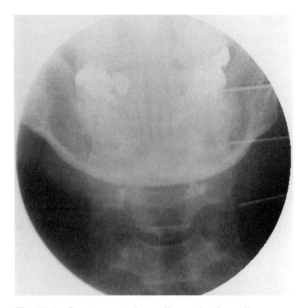

Fig. 23.3 Posteroanterior radiograph of needle placement for cervical facet deinnervation at the left C3, C4 and C5. The posterior primary ramus sends branches along the waist of the cervical facet column.

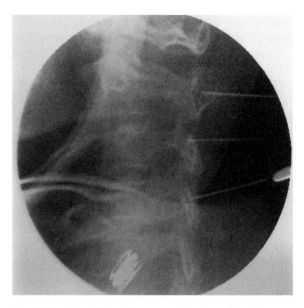

Fig. 23.4 30° oblique fluoroscopic view, showing needle placement at the respective C2, C3, C4 cervical facet pedicle or 'bead'.

marker from the mastoid process caudal over the palpable cervical transverse process. The neck is then prepped in a sterile fashion. After adequate sedation, a 5 cm RFTC needle with a 5 mm curved, blunt active tip is used for lesioning. An oblique fluoroscopic view is used to advance the cannula from an area posterior to the spine to an anterior fashion, achieving alignment with the waist of the facet joint column. An oblique imaging view allows correct needle placement at the respective bead of the cervical facet (Fig. 23.4).

Stimulation is performed at each level after the cannulas are in position, in a manner similar to lumbar radiofrequency thermocoagulation. Stimulation at 50 Hz should be felt in the neck and shoulder region at 1.0 volts or less. Absence of upper extremity motor fasciculations should be noted with 2 volts at 2 Hz stimulation. After proper stimulation, a local anesthetic and steroid solution is passed through each cannula to anesthetize the lesion site. Lesioning is then performed at 80°C for 90 seconds.

Most patients show good relief from cervical facet rhizotomy, but some can develop minor dyesthesia and patchy numbness. Painful hypersensitivity of the neck and shoulders can occur. Lesions of C2–3 facet joint can also produce short-term symptoms of vertigo. These complica-

tions usually resolve within 2 to 4 weeks after the procedure.

Radiofrequency thermocoagulation of the sympathetic chain

The lumbar sympathetic radiofrequency technique is performed with the patient in the prone position. The C-arm is rotated in an oblique view, at the chosen vertebral body, so that spinous process lay over the zygapophyseal joint on the opposite side, usually at 25–30°.[7] A 15 cm Radionics, 5 or 10 mm curved, blunt tip RFTC needle is placed 6–8 cm lateral to the midline at the second, third or fourth lumbar vertebrae. Skin entry is made inferior to the transverse process so that the probe can pass under the transverse process but over the exiting nerve root.

Once the probe has reached the psoas muscle, a lateral fluoroscopic image is used to avoid advancement anterior to the vertebral body. The sympathetic chain lies just anterior to the psoas muscle; lesions should be placed when the probe tip penetrates the psoas. Lateral fluoroscopic image will reveal the spread of a contrast dye in a thin ribbon superiorly and inferiorly (Fig. 23.5). The anteroposterior view will show the contrast spreading in a vacuolated appearance along the lateral border of the vertebral column and should not show muscle striations.

The patient's response to electrical stimulation at 50 Hz and at 2 Hz is noted. Contraction of skeletal muscles signify that the needle is too close to a somatic nerve root and injury to the nerve may result if a lesion is made. If electrical stimulation causes pain referred to the inner aspect of the thigh, the needle should be repositioned or lesioning may result in postsympathetic neuralgia. A local anesthetic and steroid are injected prior to lesioning to produce analgesia and decrease the incidence of postsympatholytic neuralgia. Electrocoagulation of the area is performed at 80°C for 90 seconds. The curved tip is then turned 180° for a second lesioning at 80°C for 90 seconds.

To perform radiofrequency thermocoagulation of the upper thoracic sympathetic chain, one must have knowledge of the precise location of the sympathetic ganglionic chain in relation to radiological landmarks, i.e. ventral surface of the vertebral body and disc interspaces.[6]

The patient is placed in the prone position with a C-arm fluoroscope in position. Skin wheals are raised with local anesthetics on the side to be lesioned overlying the T1–T2 and T2–T3 intercostal spaces. A 10 cm curved, blunt tip RFTC probe is placed under fluoroscopic guidance to the ventral surface of the vertebral body, near the center of the vertebral body[5] (Fig. 23.6). It is important that the cannulae be kept medial to the costal angle so as to prevent puncture of the lung (Fig. 23.7)

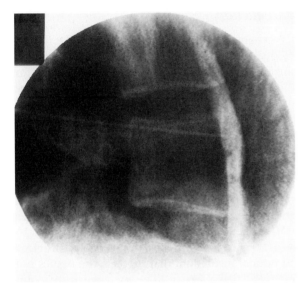

Fig. 23.5   Lateral fluoroscopic imaging, showing spread of a radio-opaque contrast dye in a thin ribbon superiorly and inferiorly from the anterior border of the L3 vertebral body.

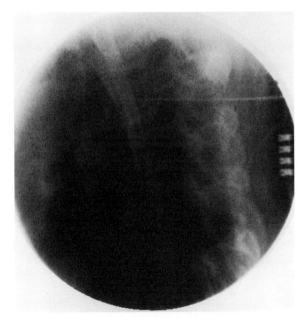

Fig. 23.6   Lateral fluoroscopic imaging, showing needle placement near the center of the vertebral body for a T2 thoracic radiofrequency thermocoagulation.

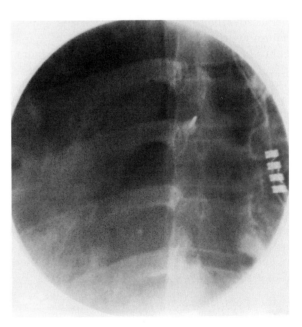

Fig. 23.7   Placement of a radiofrequency thermocoagulation needle in the 30° oblique view medial to the costal angle of the vertebral body to prevent lung puncture.

Electrical stimulation is carried out to minimize the risk of painful intercostal nerve damage. Lesioning is performed at 80°C for 90 seconds. The curved tip needle is turned 180° for a second lesioning at 80°C for 90 seconds. A rapid rewarming and vasodilatation of the affected upper extremity should be observed immediately after the procedure, and pain relief should quickly follow. Horner's syndrome, bradycardia, intercostal neuralgia, and pneumothorax are the primary complications from the upper thoracic technique.

Discussion

The most commonly used procedures for the post-traumatic patient with chronic pain include neurodestruction of the facet joint at the cervical, thoracic, and lumbar region and radiofrequency lesioning of the sympathetic chain for sympathetic maintained pain of the upper and lower extremities. Radiofrequency lesioning has also been performed for sacroiliac joint pain, lumbar discogenic pain by lesioning of the ramus communicans nerve, treating pain from the thoracic, lumbar and sacral spinal nerves with radiofrequency of the dorsal root ganglionotomy, stellate ganglion lesioning for sympathetically maintained pain of the upper extremity, and sphenopalatine and trigeminal ganglion lesioning for pain from facial trauma.

Pulsed radiofrequency in Europe has gained enormous popularity in the treatment of spinal pain and within the next year, pulsed radiofrequency should be available for use in the USA. Sluijter states that this technique involves a discontinuous-pulsed application of radiofrequency. The generator output can be kept equal to the level which is normally used for making radiofrequency heat lesions, with a correspondingly 'normal' strength of the electrical field. The inactive phase allows for the elimination of heat, which has been produced during the active phase. Initial studies of dorsal root ganglia procedures for spinal pain have indicated that pulsed radiofrequency has a far better effect than continuous radiofrequency with a low generator output. Pulsed radiofrequency has the following advantages:

- It is a non-destructive method.
- It is suitable for use in the treatment of neuropathic pain.
- It is not followed by neuritis-like reactions.
- It is suitable to use for procedures in peripheral nerves such as suprascapular nerves.

- It is a painless procedure since the frequency of RF (500 000 Hz) is far outside the physiological range and since the minimal rise in tip temperature is non-painful.

Cryoneurolysis

Introduction

Cryotherapy was first introduced by Dr Irvine Cooper in 1961. The first clinical application of this technique was in the field of neurosurgery for the treatment of Parkinsonism. The cryoprobe works on the principle of the Joule–Thompson effect (Fig. 23.8). It is composed of an inner tube, an outer tube, and a working tip. When a high-pressure gas, such as nitrous oxide, is allowed to expand in the probe tip, there is a rapid fall in temperature, causing a cooling to –60°C. The currently manufactured cryoprobes have insulation around them, but using a standard intravenous (IV) catheter (12 and 14 gauge catheters for 14 and 16 gauge cryoprobes, respectively) provides additional insulation, that protects the tissues not intended to be frozen. The mechanism of cold-

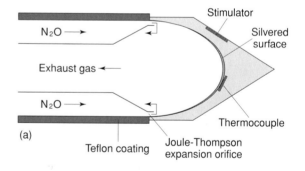

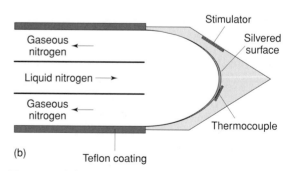

Fig. 23.8 (A) Diagrammatic cross-section of gas-expansion (Joule–Thompson). (B) Liquid nitrogen cryoprobe tips. (From Raj P, ed. Pain medicine, a comprehensive review. Mosby)

induced nerve injury is still unknown. Many explanations have been suggested, including hypertonicity of intracellular and extracellular fluids, physical destruction by larger cellular ice crystals, minimal cell volume, damage to proteins, membrane rupture caused by rapid water loss, ischemic necrosis, and the production of autoantibodies.[9] A cryolesion is reversible and has not been associated with neuritis and the formation of neuromas. The extent of cell destruction by a cryolesion will be dependent on several factors, but the rate of freezing and thawing and the temperature attained by the tissue in proximity to the cryoprobe are the most important. The repeated freeze–thaw cycles greatly enhanced the size of the cryolesion. It is critical for a minimum length of 4 mm of the nerve to reach a temperature of $-20°C$ or below in order to stop nerve conduction.

Indications

Indications for percutaneous cryoneurolysis in the trauma patient include:

- Post-thoracotomy pain syndrome
- Intercostal neuralgia
- Low back pain
- Facial pain
- Postsurgical neuralgia
- Painful neuromas
- Cervical and lumbar facet syndromes
- Pain from the interspinous ligaments.

Numerous cutaneous nerve branches are responsive to cryodenervation, such as:

- The infrapatellar branch of the saphenous nerve after blunt injury to the tibial plateau or following knee replacement
- The deep and superficial peroneal and intermediate dorsal cutaneous nerves after an injury to the foot or ankle
- The superior gluteal branch of the sciatic nerve following a lifting injury of the low back and hip
- Supraorbital nerve neuralgia at the supraorbital notch caused by deceleration against an automobile windshield. Commonly confused with migraines and frontal sinusitis, the pain of supraorbital neuralgia often manifests as a throbbing frontal headache. This neuralgia often worsens with time, most likely secondary to scar formation around the nerve
- Infraorbital nerve of the trigeminal nerve can develop in an irritative neuropathy at the infraorbital foramen, secondary to blunt trauma or fracture of the zygoma with entrapment of the nerve in the bony callus. Commonly confused with maxillary sinusitis, the pain of infraorbital neuralgia most often manifests as pain exacerbated by smiling and laughter
- Posterior auricular neuralgia is often seen after blunt injury to the mastoid – common in abused women in whom the left side is more often involved because of the preponderance of right-handedness in humans. The clinical presentation consists of ear pain and tenderness. Cryolesioning of this nerve can be done at the posterior border of the sternocleidomastoid muscle, superficial and immediately posterior to the mastoid.

Technique

Percutaneous cryoblations are performed after a diagnostic anesthetic block of the nerve to be lysed has provided adequate results. A 14 or 16 gauge cryoprobe is placed, through a 12 or 14 gauge IV angiocatheter respectively, as close as possible to the nerve to be lysed. It is critical for a minimum of 4 mm of the nerve to reach a temperature of $-20°C$ in order to stop nerve conduction.[9] Fluoroscopy can be used to check for correct probe placement prior to lesioning. Nerve stimulation in the cryoprobe can be used after proper probe placement. If any motor component is seen, the probe is repositioned to prevent freezing of motor nerves. Sensory stimulation is performed to specifically reproduce the patient's pain in the desired area of lesioning.

Cryolesioning is performed from 1.0 to 1.5 minutes. The nitrous oxide gas-expansion probe reaches a temperature of -60 to $-70°C$ at the tip with maximum freezing occurring at 1.5 minutes. The freeze–thaw–refreeze technique is used to expand the freeze zone. After the 1.5-minute freeze cycle has been completed, the probe is thawed for 20 to 30 seconds without removing the probe; a second 1.5-minute freezing is performed. Multiple sites of freezing are frequently done, but the probe must thoroughly thaw before removing it from one area to another.

Complications of cryotherapy

Cryoneurolysis is not a benign procedure and some complications do exist for the use of the percutaneous probe. A significant leakage of refrigerant can cause freezing along the shaft of the cryoprobe and subsequent freezing of structures other than those intended. The most common problem is frostbite of the skin at the entry site, which can be prevented by an introducer sheath. Motor damage can occur with cryoneurolysis of motor nerve, but the patient usually recovers.

Conclusion

Cryoneurolysis is a safe and effective method that lacks the formation of neuromas and has a low incidence of neuritis. Therapeutic effectiveness cannot be predicted and pain can last from 3 to 1000 days[9] (mean pain relief duration, 60 days).

Lysis of epidural adhesions

Introduction

Epidural adhesions are commonly caused by hemorrhage into the epidural space following surgical intervention of the spine and the healing that subsequently occurs. Inflammation and nerve root compression by adhesions are the mechanisms of persistent pain in patients after a laminectomy, ruptured disc, or vertebral body fracture. Epidural adhesions may also contribute to the pain of failed facet joint syndrome. The use of epidural catheters and epiduroscopy makes the treatment lesion-specific, because the injectable solution is placed into the actual area of the adhesions.

The Racz caudal catheter approach

Previously described techniques for epiduroscopy and lysis of adhesions involved placement of a single needle without fluoroscopic guidance into the epidural space. The Racz approach to epidural lysis of adhesions places a catheter into the actual area of the adhesions. Fluid injected into the epidural space takes the path of least resistance and frequently bypasses the area of adhesion formation. Increasing the volume of injectate does not break up the adhesions, because the extra solution simply bypasses the scarred area and may potentially cause spinal cord compression. The epidural catheter placement makes treatment lesion-specific.[10]

Indications

Indications for the epidural lysis of adhesions in the trauma patient include:[10]

- Failed back surgery syndrome
- Radiculopathy of the upper/lower extremities
- Disc disruption
- Traumatic vertebral body compression fracture
- Facet pain
- Epidural scarring from trauma or meningitis
- Pain unresponsive to spinal cord stimulation
- Pain unresponsive to spinal opioid
- Occipital neuralgia.

Technique

The sacral hiatus is the preferred site of entry to the epidural space for low back pain and lower extremity radiculopathy. This entry site is chosen because:

1. there is less likely subdural placement
2. solutions placed in the lumbar epidural space take the path of least resistance and may not reach the area of adhesions or
3. it may be difficult or impossible to pass a lumbar catheter caudally into the area of scarring.

The patient is placed in a prone position on the fluoroscopy table and the sacral area is prepped and draped in a sterile fashion. The sacral cornu and sacral hiatus are palpated. The entry point through the skin is in the gluteal fold opposite the affected side, approximately 1–2 cm lateral and

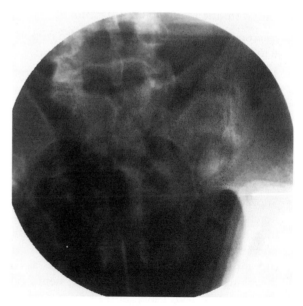

Fig. 23.9 In the posteroanterior view, note the epidural needle placement in the sacral hiatus at the S3 foramina with the needle tip toward the affected side.

2 cm inferior to the sacral hiatus. A 16 gauge epidural needle (preferably an R-K needle) is passed through the entry point and into the sacral hiatus. The needle is advanced to the S3 foramina. Lateral fluoroscopic view confirms that the needle is within the bony canal and an anteroposterior view should verify that the needle tip is toward the affected side (Fig. 23.9).

After negative aspiration for cerebrospinal fluid (CSF) and blood, 10 mL of Omnipaque 240 dye is injected under fluoroscopy. A Christmas tree pattern of dye is seen under fluoroscopy as the dye spreads within the bony canal along the perineural structures. Epidural adhesions prevent the spread of contrast medium in this characteristic pattern, preventing outlining of the involved nerve roots. A Racz Tun-L-Kath is passed through the needle into the adhesions (Figs 23.10 and 23.11). After negative apiration for CSF or heme, 5–10 mL of contrast dye is injected through the catheter. It should be seen spreading into the area of the previous filling defect.

Hyaluronidase (Wydase) 1500 units, mixed in 10 mL of preservative-free saline, is used as a spreading factor to increase the spread of medications within the epidural space as well as into the adhesions. After negative aspiration, a 3 mL test dose of a local anesthetic and steroid solution is given (at our institution we commonly use 0.25% bupivacaine or 0.2% ropivacaine with 40 mg aristocort). After negative evidence of subarachnoid, subdural or intrathecal spread, an additional 7 mL of the steroid and local anesthetic solution are given.

Usually in the recovery room and 30 minutes after the second local anesthetic and steroid injection, without evidence of intrathecal or subdural block, 10 mL of 10% saline is infused over 30 minutes.

Hypertonic saline has a mild, reversible local anesthetic effect and reduces edema of scarred or inflamed nerve roots. Injection of hypertonic saline into the epidural space is painful unless preceded by local anesthetic. The catheter is flushed at the end of the hypertonic saline infusion with 2–3 mL of normal saline to prevent catheter occlusion. The catheter is left in place for a total of 3 days, and is re-injected on days 2 and 3 with 10 mL of a local anesthetic solution without steroid. This is followed by an infusion of hypertonic saline. The catheter is removed after the third injection. The patient is discharged home with an oral cephalosporin antibiotic for 5 to 7 additional days.

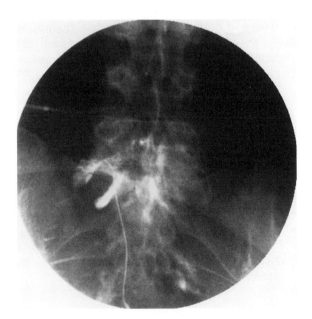

Fig. 23.10 A Racz Tun-L-Kath placed anteriorly at the L5 foraminal level in the area of adhesions. Note the dye spreading into the area of previous filling defect outlining the L4 and L5 nerve roots.

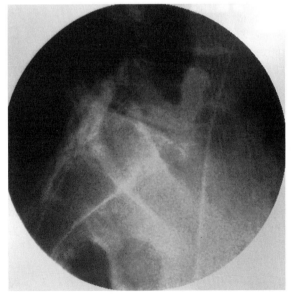

Fig. 23.11 Lateral fluoroscopic view, showing the Racz epidural catheter in the ventral epidural space at the mid-L5 level.

The technique for lysis of epidural adhesions in the cervical, thoracic and lumbar spine is modified. The patient is placed in the lateral position on the fluoroscopy table. In the cervical and thoracic area, the paramedian approach provides easier access to the epidural space. The C7–T1 or T1–T2 interspaces provide the easiest point of entry for cervical catheter placement. Fluoroscopy in the anteroposterior and lateral views confirm correct needle placement. A Racz Tun-L-Kath epidural catheter is passed toward the filling defect until the catheter enters the area of adhesions. After negative aspiration for CSF or heme, 6 mL of saline with Wydase, 6 mL of the local anesthetic and steroid solution and 6 mL of hypertonic saline are injected in the cervical epidural; in the lumbar epidural space 10 mL of saline with Wydase, 10 mL of the local anesthetic and steroid, and 10 mL of hypertonic saline are injected.

Complications

Potential complications of epidural lysis of adhesions include infection, subarachnoid or subdural injection of local anesthetic or hypertonic saline, bowel or bladder dysfunction, paralysis, spinal cord compression with rapid injection, catheter shearing, and sensitivity to hyaluronidase.

Conclusion

Epidural lysis of adhesions is considered after other conservative treatments have failed such as rest, narcotics and non-narcotics, muscle relaxants, epidural steroid injections, and physical therapy. Prevention of surgical intervention in post-traumatic patients suffering from herniated disc, radiculopathies, compression fractures and facet joint pain is possible with the lysis of adhesion technique.

The technique is lesion-specific and allows placement of the medication directly into the area of adhesion through a soft-tip catheter. The steroid, local anesthetic and hypertonic saline solution reach the inflamed nerve root to open up the perineural space. As a result of the procedure, there is a reduction in inflammation at the nerve root and pain relief is provided.

Epiduroscopy

Epiduroscopy can be used in the trauma patient to allow direct visualization of the epidural space. It is an excellent diagnostic and therapeutic invasive technique used for accurate placement of a local anesthetic and steroid solution into the epidural space. For over 60 years, clinicians have been working with various types of endoscopes. In 1931, Michael Burman, an orthopedic surgeon from New York Hospital for Joint Diseases performed a direct visualization of the spinal canal.[11] In 1937, a neurosurgeon, J. Lawrence Pool, attempted to assess lumbar–sciatic syndrome by examining anesthetized patients with a myeloscope. He was able to identify neuritis, herniated nucleus pulposus, hypertrophied ligamentum flavum, neoplasms, varicose vessels and arachnoid adhesions.[11] The lack of photographic equipment, rigid metal scopes, illuminating lighting, myelography, computerized tomography and magnetic resonance imaging delayed the development of epiduroscopy. Unlike the Racz caudal catheter technique for lysis of adhesion, epiduroscopy provides a three-dimensional, color view of the adhesion and adjacent anatomy. This provides an advantage over the two-dimensional, black-and-white fluoroscopic projections or epidurograms.

Indications

Saberski and Kitahata considered non-surgical candidates with persistent radiculopathy.[13] The patients had not responded to physical therapy or two to three caudal epidural injections. Pseudoradiculopathy such as pain from myofascial or biomechanical nature was ruled out.

Contraindications

Epiduroscopy should be avoided in patients with:

- Infection
- Coagulopathy
- Raised intracranial pressure
- Central nervous system space-occupying lesions
- Cerebrovascular disease
- Patients with pre-existing bladder and bowel dysfunction as a complication of sacral nerve injury.

Technique

The caudal approach to the epidural space is preferred over the paramedian approach by many clinicians because there is a straight entry into the epidural space, which allows easier steering of the fiberoptic scope.

The patient is placed in a prone position. The sacral hiatus is identified by palpating the sacral cornua. A midline position is confirmed with posteroanterior fluoroscopy. After skin infiltration with a local anesthetic, a 17 gauge Tuohy needle is inserted into the sacral hiatus. Correct needle placement in the sacral canal is confirmed with lateral fluoroscopic views. A non-ionic contrast, 5–15 mL, outlines nerve roots and scar adhesions. Under posteroanterior fluoroscopy, a flexible guidewire is threaded cephalad through the Tuohy needle. After placement of the wire, the Tuohy needle is removed. A small incision with a No. 11 scalpel is made to widen the canal aperture for easier passage of the introducer sheath and dilator. The dilator is then removed, leaving the introducer sheath. The side arm of the introducer sheath is flushed with 5–10 mL of normal saline. The fiberoptic cable is placed through the steering handle. The steering handle and cable are then passed through the introducer. The camera and video recorder are started, and the steering handle containing the fiberoptic is advanced into the caudal epidural space to the area of concern (Fig. 23.12). The epidural space is distended by sustained pressure of normal saline either from a syringe or a pressurized bag to 50–75 mmHg. Pressure is sustained for 3 minutes at a time and then reduced to resting pressure for at least 1 minute, to prevent compromises in perfusion. In general, the amount of fluid injected is approximately 60 mL per procedure.

Complications

Significant pain at the procedure site is a potential complication of epiduroscopy. The pain can be severe enough to require intravenous opioid medication and an increased level of care with overnight hospitalization. Saberski et al report that

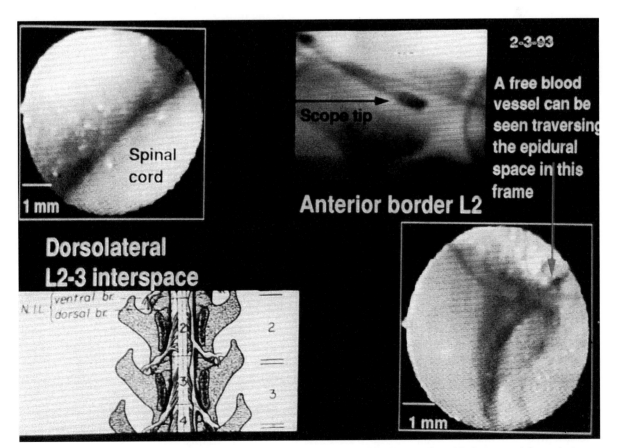

Fig. 23.12 Visualization of the epidural space using epiduroscopy. The fiberoptic cable is steered through the epidural space to the area of concern.

another possible complication of this technique is the generation of significant epidural pressures that could affect local perfusion. Epidural endoscopy when performed correctly does not appear to affect bowel, bladder or neurologic function.[12]

Spinal cord stimulation

Introduction

Spinal cord stimulation for the treatment of intractable pain was introduced in 1967 by Shealy et al in response to Melzack and Wall's gate control theory. The gate control theory of pain describes an ability to suppress transmission of pain signals in small diameter fibers (A-δ and C) by activation of large diameter, non-noxious fibers (A-β).[14] Many other theories have been proposed to explain the pain-relieving effects of spinal cord stimulation. These theories include inhibiting transmission of the spinothalamic tract, activation of supraspinal mechanisms, activation sympathetic blocking mechanisms, and neurochemical alterations in the central nervous system.

In general, spinal cord stimulation is rarely used as a first-line treatment and should be reserved for patients with chronic, intractable pain. It is imperative that post-traumatic patients suffering from chronic pain undergo a complete multidisciplinary evaluation prior to implantation. An accurate diagnosis must be established and a psychological evaluation must be performed. Failure of previous, less-invasive treatment modalities should be documented. The patient must lack drug-seeking behavior, there should not be any unresolved compensation or litigation issues, and a successful, trial spinal cord stimulation should have been performed prior to implantation of a permanent spinal cord stimulator. With trial stimulation, the patient should have noted at least a 50% reduction of pain, increased function and decreased or stable medication usage.

Indications

In the post-traumatic patient, spinal cord stimulation can be successfully used for the treatment of various pain conditions. Common indications include:[16]

- Sympathetically mediated pain
  — CRPS I (RSD)
  — CRPS II (causalgia)

- Arachnoiditis or epidural fibrosis
- Intercostal neuralgia
- Peripheral neuropathy
- Phantom limb pain
- Postamputation stump pain
- Nerve root avulsion
- Spinal cord injury
- Failed back surgery syndrome
- Radicular pain.

Contraindications

Contraindications for permanent placement of a spinal cord stimulator include:

- Failure of trial spinal cord stimulation
- Patient refusal to implantation
- Patient is adverse to electrical stimulation
- A coagulopathy at time of implantation
- Localized or disseminated infection
- Physician's lack of experience or training
- Patient with a demand cardiac pacemaker
- Patient needing a magnetic resonance imaging in the future
- Untreated drug dependency
- Undocumented cause of pain.

Technique for implantation

There are several protocols for implantation of a spinal cord stimulator. At our institution, we conduct a trial stimulation using a percutaneous non-tunneled lead in the operating room using fluoroscopy and under sterile conditions. The patient is discharged home on the morning of the following postoperative day with a course of oral antibiotics. The exteriorized lead is connected to a stimulator box and the patient is instructed on its usage. The patient is informed that the stimulator paresthesia should cover the area of pain. After 5 days of trial stimulation, the patient returns to clinic to have the percutaneous lead removed. We do not implant the entire system at the time of trial because: the patient is under intraoperative sedation which may ease some of the patient's pain, the patient is not participating in any routine activities during this time, and changes in body position may alter pain generators, therefore the patient may not be able to evaluate his/her pain in the most exaggerated form during placement in the operating room.

Available leads for trial and permanent implantation of spinal cord stimulators include the Quad

3487, the Quad plus 3488 and 3516 Dual. The Quad plus lead provides a longer length and larger area of stimulation and is frequently used for bilateral stimulation and for more difficult areas such as the back (Fig. 23.13).

After a successful trial stimulation the patient returns in 2 to 3 weeks for permanent lead placement in the operating room under sterile conditions. Prophylactic antibiotics are administered prior to the procedure. Our patients are routinely placed in the lateral decubitus position, although many physicians prefer the prone position. The entry level varies according to pain distribution. The usual entry level for lower extremity and hip pain is at T12–L1.

A 15 gauge Medtronic epidural needle is placed under fluoroscopic guidance, using the loss-of-resistance technique, into the epidural space. The stimulating electrode is placed under fluoroscopic guidance through the needle into the dorsal epidural compartment. Final lead position depends on elicitation of stimulation paresthesias over the painful region. The lead is anchored to the supraspinous ligament and tunneled to an upper abdominal or buttock subcutaneous pocket for connection to an implantable pulse generator (IPG). Prior to wound closure the system is activated and the integrity is checked. Once the

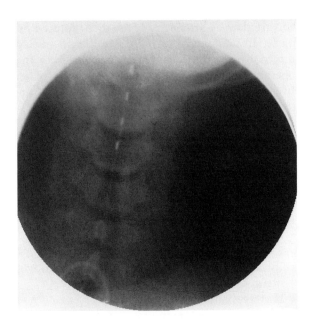

Fig. 23.13   A Quad plus spinal cord stimulator electrode from C2–C4 in the midline for bilateral upper extremity stimulation.

patient has demonstrated the capability of operating the system, the patient is discharged home on oral antibiotics within 24 to 48 hours and is instructed to return to the clinic in 1 week for wound examination.

Complications

Side effects or complications with spinal cord stimulation can occur intraoperatively or postoperatively. Intraoperative complications can include:

- Uncooperative, overly sedated patients may have difficulty determining whether the induced paresthesia is covering painful areas or providing pain relief
- Inability to position leads properly
- Inability to access the epidural space
- Difficulty overlapping stimulation-produced paresthesia with the patient's pain pattern
- Inadvertent dural puncture
- Nerve root injury.

Postoperative complications related to surgical technique include:

- Postoperative bleeding or hematoma
- Wound dehiscence
- Pocket infection
- Pocket seroma
- CSF hygroma
- Epidural abscess or meningitis
- Post-dural puncture headache
- Spinal cord compression by an epidural hematoma.

Specific complications related to the spinal cord stimulator include:

- Lead migration
- Lead fracture
- Lead disconnection
- Pulse generator battery failure
- Lack of effective stimulation
- Erosion of electrode or generator through the skin.

Conclusion

Prior to placement of a permanent spinal cord stimulator, the patient must meet certain criteria and should have undergone a successful trial stimulation period. Spinal cord stimulation implantable techniques should be performed after the patient has failed conservative therapy and is no longer a surgical candidate. Spinal cord stimulation is more appropriate for the treatment of various neuropathic pain syndromes.

Peripheral nerve stimulation

Introduction

Peripheral nerve stimulation (PNS) has been used since 1965. The scientific basis for the use of PNS as pain therapy is based on Melzack and Wall's spinal gate control theory. Peripheral nerve stimulation produces a low-threshold afferent activation that reduces pain by activating local inhibitory circuits within the dorsal horn of the spinal cord. The inhibitory effect then diminishes nociceptive transmission through the spinal cord. Another proposed mechanism is that the PNS produces a nondecipherable code, thereby 'jamming' sensory input to the central nervous system.[16]

Pain reduction with a trial of transcutaneous electrical nerve stimulation (TENS) or with local anesthetic nerve block is often used as a screening procedure for PNS. Other selection criteria for PNS placement include: chronic intractable pain, recalcitrant to other therapies, no psychological contraindications, and objective evidence of pathology.

Indications

In the post-traumatic patient, the best results from peripheral nerve stimulation are obtained in patients who have pain in the distribution of a single traumatized peripheral nerve. Clinical indications for peripheral nerve stimulation include:

- CRPS I and II
- Plexus avulsion
- Operative trauma
- Entrapment neuropathies
- Injection injuries.

Technique

Under general anesthesia, a peripheral nerve stimulator placement is performed by a surgeon. The first step of the procedure involves implantation of the stimulating electrode, followed by a trial period of 3 days. The nerve is exposed after dissecting down to the neurovascular bundle and an electrode is placed proximal to the injury, along the side of or underneath the nerve. The nerves

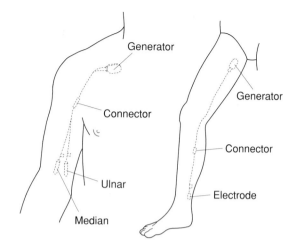

Fig. 23.14   Implantation sites for generator and stimulation electrode: (A) ulnar or median nerve; (B) tibialis nerve. (From Raj P, ed. Pain medicine, a comprehensive review. Mosby)

commonly used for PNS are the median, ulnar, radial, common peroneal, sciatic and posterior tibial nerves. A flap of fascial tissue from intermuscular septum is folded over the electrode to prevent direct contact of the electrode with the nerve. Scar formation caused by direct contact between the nerve and the cuff can lead to nerve constriction. The electrode is then sutured in place. If adequate pain relief is obtained during the trial period, the patient is taken back to the operating room for permanent placement of an Itrel (Medtronic) programmable stimulating battery pack (Fig. 23.14).

Complications

Potential complications can include:

- Infection
- Bleeding
- Poor pain relief
- Lead fracture
- Intraoperative and postoperative lead movement
- Battery malfunction
- Transmitter malfunction
- Scarring between nerve and electrode
- Interference with cardiac pacemakers
- Fluid shorting electrical connections

- Tissue damage when PNS equipment transmits output of radiofrequency devices, such as electrocautery and radiofrequency lesioning, to electrode contacts.

Implantable drug delivery systems

Introduction

Opiate receptors and endogenous opioid peptides in the central nervous system were discovered in the early 1970s. By 1979, the first controlled study of analgesic affects of intrathecal morphine was reported, and since that time there has been widespread use of intraspinal opioids for pain relief. Intraspinal opiates act at the substantia gelatinosa of the dorsal horn of the spinal cord to produce analgesia. This has led to the clinical use of intraspinal opiates for the treatment of malignant pain and for the control of chronic, non-malignant pain. In patients who have not responded to more traditional pain therapies, the administration of intrathecal narcotics can successfully alleviate pain and improve the quality of life.

Indications

Opioid-responsive nociceptive pain is described as 'dull, aching, sharp, or throbbing pain'. Nociceptive pain is responsive to opioid therapies administered orally, parenterally, or spinally. Examples of nociceptive pain include post-surgical pain and pains of trauma. Indications for placement of an implantable intrathecal pump include:

- Conservative therapies have failed
- Surgical intervention is not indicated
- A successful trial has been performed.

Other issues to consider prior to implantation include the presence of infection or sepsis, anticoagulation status, behavioral and psychological abnormalities, the cost of the delivery system, needles, and supplies, no untreated drug habits, and life expectancy.

Technique

Prior to placement of a permanent, implantable drug delivery system, a pre-implantation trial must be performed to determine whether or not the patient receives adequate pain relief by a spinal drug. At our institution we perform a 3-day trial, typically using 0.5 mg intrathecal morphine on the first day, a placebo on the second day, and 1.0 mg intrathecal morphine on the third day. We proceed with the implantation of a drug delivery system if the patient receives greater than 50% pain relief of pre-injection intensity, with a duration of at least twice the half-life of the agent, 8 to 12 hours for morphine with either of the intrathecal morphine trial doses and no severe opioid side effects. The patient should not demonstrate pain relief with the placebo. Failure to provide pain relief during a pre-implantation trial with the opioid may occur secondary to: the drug not placed correctly into the subarachnoid space, psychological reasons, opioid tolerance, incorrect dose of drug, or the patient's pain is not susceptible to spinal opioids such as seen in deafferentation pain.

After a successful trial has been performed, the patient is taken to the operating room for permanent placement of an intrathecal catheter and an implantable programmable infusion pump. The patient is placed in a lateral position for catheter placement to allow both the posterior incision and tunneling of the catheter to the anterior wall. A spinal anesthetic is administered for the procedure. The lumbosacral region is prepped and draped in a sterile fashion. The desired interspace is identified fluoroscopically, usually at L1–L2. Using a paramedian approach, a 15 gauge R-K epidural needle is inserted and advanced with fluoroscopic direction until a free-flow of CSF is obtained. Needle tip position is confirmed in the anteroposterior, lateral and oblique fluoroscopic views with needle advancement. Fluoroscopic confirmation of correct needle placement is obtained by injecting Omnipaque 240 contrast with spread along the subarachnoid space with a fluoroscopic image consistent with a myelogram. There should be no obstruction to rostral spread of the contrast dye.

The radio-opaque intrathecal catheter is then passed through the needle into the subarachnoid space and advanced cephalad to the spinal target, which is determined by the dermatome of origin of the patient's pain (Fig. 23.15). At our institution, the tip of the catheter is placed at T10. Aspiration of the catheter should produce a clear fluid consistent with CSF. An incision is made around the needle and carried down to the supraspinous fascial plane. A pursestring 2–0 silk suture is placed into the supraspinous fascia

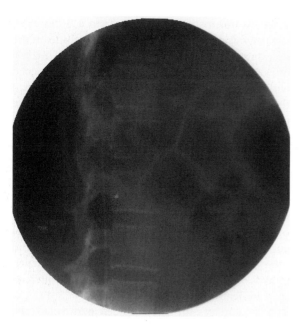

Fig. 23.15 Lateral fluoroscopic view of a radio-opaque intrathecal catheter in the subarachnoid space for a Medtronic synchromed pump placement.

around the epidural needle. The needle is then withdrawn under fluoroscopic direction, ensuring correct catheter placement. A silastic anchor is placed around the catheter and sutured to the supraspinous fascia. The catheter is clipped to prevent loss of CSF. At this point, the pump is prepared, primed, and filled for placement. An incision for the pump pocket is made in the right lower quadrant of the abdomen. The pump catheter is then subcutaneously tunneled from the pump pocket to the back wound. It is essential to ascertain free flow of CSF and prevent obstruction to flow. The back wound and pump pocket are irrigated with an antibiotic irrigation and closed in a two-layer closure.

Complications

- Side effects to the spinal opioids
  — Pruritus
  — Urinary retention
  — Early and late respiratory depression
  — Nausea and vomiting
  — Hypotension
  — Somnolence
- Infection
- Bleeding

- Epidural hematoma
- Post-dural puncture headaches
- Pump battery depletion
- Pharmacologic overdoses
- Development of tolerance
- Catheter dislocation, rupture, kinking, obstruction and migration
- Subcutaneous seroma
  — CSF hygromas
  — Spinal cord injury.

Conclusion

Implantable drug-delivery systems with intraspinal narcotics have dramatically influenced the way chronic pain is managed. Intraspinal opioids should be used after conservative therapies have failed and further surgical intervention is not indicated. Intraspinal opioids should be used as a last resort and should be used only in the context of clearly defined opioid responsiveness.

SUMMARY

Some patients suffer from chronic pain after traumatic injuries, while other patients with similar injuries avoid chronic suffering. The site of injury is important in the development of chronic pain, whereas extremity injuries are prone to the development of CRPS I and II. CRPS can be expected in approximately 5% of trauma patients. Few chronic pain patients benefit from neural blockade in comparison to acute post-traumatic pain patients, therefore other methods of treatment should be considered. Invasive pain management procedures for the treatment of chronic pain are now commonly employed. For patients to be considered for invasive pain procedures, the patient should have failed conservative treatments, lack psychological or behavioral abnormalities, lack drug addiction, lack contraindications to the procedure and should have passed a successful trial.

REFERENCES

1. Hartrick C. Pain due to trauma including sports injuries. In: Raj P, ed. Practical management of pain. 2nd ed. Mosby–Yearbook; 1992.
2. Subhash J. Nerve blocks. In: Warfield C, ed. Principles and practice of pain management. New York: McGraw-Hill.

3. Campbell J. Complex regional pain syndrome and the sympathetic nervous system. Baltimore: Department of Neurosurgery, Johns Hopkins University School of Medicine.

4. Kline MT. Stereotactic radiofrequency lesions as part of the management of pain. St Lucie Press; 1996.

5. Wilkinson HA. Percutaneous radiofrequency upper thoracic sympathectomy: A new technique. Neurosurgery 15(6): 811–813.

6. Yarzebski JL, Wilkinson HA. T2 and T3 sympathetic ganglia in the adult human: A cadaver and clinical-radiographic study and its clinical application. Neurosurgery 1987; 21(3): 339–341.

7. Rocco A. Radiofrequency lumbar sympatholysis: The evolution of a technique for managing sympathetically maintained pain. Reg Anesth 1995; 20(1): 3–12.

8. Noe C, Racz G. Radiofrequency. In: Raj P, ed. Pain medicine, a comprehensive review. Mosby.

9. Arthur J, Racz G. Cryolysis. In: Raj P, ed. Pain medicine, a comprehensive review. Mosby.

10. Racz G, Heavner J, Diede J. Lysis of epidural adhesions: Utilizing the epidural approach. In: Waldman, Winnie AP, eds. Interventional pain management. Philadelphia: WB Saunders; 1996.

11. Saberski L, Brull S. Spinal and epidural endoscopy: A historical review. Yale J Biol Med 1995; 68: 7–15.

12. Saberski L, Gerena F. Safety of epidural endoscopy. Reg Anesth Pain Med 1998; 23(3): 324–325.

13. Saberski L, Kitahata L. Review of the clinical basis and protocol for epidural endoscopy. Conn Med 1996; Feb: 71–73.

14. Krames E. Neuroaugmentation. Mechanisms of action of spinal cord stimulation. In: Waldman, Winnie AP, eds. Interventional pain management. Philadelphia: WB Saunders; 1996.

15. Heavner J, Racz G, Diede J. Peripheral nerve stimulation: Current concepts. In: Waldman, Winnie AP, eds. Interventional pain management. Philadelphia: WB Saunders; 1996.

16. Bedder M. Spinal cord stimulation and intractable pain: Patient selection. In: Waldman, Winnie AP, eds. Interventional pain management. Philadelphia: WB Saunders; 1996.

17. Krames E. Spinal administration of opioids for nonmalignant pain syndromes: A U.S. experience. In: Waldman, Winnie AP, eds. Interventional pain management. Philadelphia: WB Saunders; 1996.

Index

Note: Page numbers in *italics* refer to illustrations and tables

Abbreviated injury scale 19
ABC phenomenon *373*
Abdominal trauma 176–177
Accident prevention 24–25
Acetaminophen (paracetamol) 64
Acetic acid derivatives 64
Acid–base balance 96
α_1-acid glycoprotein 222
Acidosis 133
  and propofol 144
Acromegaly 95
ACTH (adrenocorticotropic
    hormone) 48
Activated partial thromboplastin
    time 98, 201
Active range of motion (ARDM)
    149–150
  see also Contractures
Activities of daily living, in
    spasticity 153
Acupuncture 4, 259
Acute/chronic trauma patients
    62–63
Acute compartment syndrome
    156–157
  events in *156*
Acute post-traumatic pain
    management 59–60
Acute renal failure 96–97
  causes of *97*
Acyclovir 291–292
Addison's disease 96
Adhesions, epidermal, lysis of 412
Adrenal suppression 96
Adson's maneuver 157
Adult respiratory distress syndrome
    (ARDS) 92
Advanced trauma life support 23
A fibers 302
A-delta fibers 29–33, 140, 258,
    316
Age
  of children 266
  and death, causes (USA) *9*
  and patient-controlled analgesia
    (PCA) 167
Airbags, in cars 24–25

Airway management, emergency
    133
Alanine aminotransferase 93
Alarms 110
Alcoholism 94
  see also Ethanol
Aldosterone *48*
Alfentanil 123–124, 192
  for dressings *173*
Algogenic agents *31*, 32
Alkaline phosphatase 93
Allen test 157
Allergy, and patient-controlled
    analgesia (PCA) 167
Allodynia 39–41, 68
α_1-receptor blockers 383
Alprazolam 68
'Alternative' medicine 260
Ambulance helicopters 110, 113
Ambulation aids, in spasticity *152*
American Society of
    Anesthesiologists (ASA)
    guidelines, non-operating
    non-anesthesia *126*
AMH receptors 30
Amino amide local anesthetics
    74–75
Amitriptyline 66
  plus perphenazine 67
Amphotericin B 96
Analgesia
  enteral 111–114
  epidural *see* Epidural analgesia
  goals of 137–139
  in the intensive care unit
    140–142
  parenteral 111–114
  pre-emptive 52
  provision of 23–24
  sedation technique and 125
  systemic 59–60
  see also Pain control; Patient-
    controlled analgesia
'Analgesia' vs. 'anesthesia' 114
Anesthesia
  historical aspects 4–5
  in the operating room 24

Anesthesiologists 21–24
  Advanced Trauma Life Support
    23
  analgesia provision by 23–24
  in-hospital care 22–23
    trauma resuscitation and 23
  in the operating room 24
  post-operative critical care 24
  pre-hospital care 22–23
  pre-operative critical care 24
  team leaders for 23
  and transfer of patients 24
  and trauma resuscitation 22
Angiotensin-converting enzyme
    (ACE) 91
Ankle block 117, 122
Ankle-foot orthosis 151–152
  Klenzak *152*
  thermoplastic molded *152*
Anthranilic acid derivatives 65
Antibiotics 291–292
Anticoagulated patients 97–101
Anticoagulation therapy 178,
    201–202
Anticonvulsants 67–68
Antidepressants 65–67
  guidelines for using 66–67
  see also Tricyclic antidepressants
Antidiuretic hormone (ADH) *see*
    Vasopressin
Anti-emetics 173
Antihistamines 68–69
Antimalarials 291–292
$\alpha 1$-Antitrypsin deficiency 94
Anxiety, and patient information
    254
Anxiolytics 68
Aortic stenosis 91, 360
Arachidonic acid 31, 63–64
  see also Prostaglandins
Arachnoiditis 416
Arachnoid mater 179
Aristocort 413
Army surgeons *see* War
Arrow Single-shot needle *215*
Aspartate 34
Aspartate aminotransferase 93

Aspirin 64
  see also Non-steroidal anti-
    inflammatory drugs
    (NSAIDs)
Assaults see Homicide
Atelectasis 132
Atenolol 91
Atherosclerotic cardiovascular
    disease 86–91
Atracurium 353–354
Avicena 4
Axillary approach, to brachial
    plexus 268
Axillary brachial plexus block 359
Axillary nerve 158
Axillary nerve block 117
Axillary perivascular brachial plexus
    block 213

Babinski index 151
Backache 200
Baclofen, intrathecal 153
Bacteremia 101–102
Bacterial infection 132, 178, 200,
    217, 359
  and propofol 144
  and regional anesthesia
    101–102
Balanin 34
Barbiturates 5, 143
Battlefield analgesia 164
'B'-bevel needles, for children
    267–268
Bed sores 153–154
Behavior 254–255
Behavior reinforcement, for burns
    308
Behavioral techniques, 308
Beliefs 254
Benzodiazepine 68, 114, 123–125,
    142–143, 145–146, 291,
    305–306, 345–346
  for burns 305–306
Betadine 181
Bible, and trauma 4
Bicarbonate ion, and local
    anesthesia 73
Bier's block 121, 381–383
Bilirubin 93
Biofeedback techniques 257–258,
    300
Bispectral index 140
Blood coagulation 97–98
  see also Anticoagulated patients
Blood, maternal, in pregnancy 290
Blood pressure monitoring 111

Bolus dosing, in patient-controlled
    analgesia (PCA) 166
Bone density 377
Botulinum toxin type A 160
Brachial plexus block 117, 122,
    268
  anatomy of 212–213
  axillary perivascular 213, 359
  infraclavicular 217–218, 358–359
  interscalene 220–222, 357–358
  musculocutaneous 213–217
  subclavian perivascular 218–219
Bracing 155
Bradykinin 31
Brain see CNS
Brain function, 132
  and nociception 33
  see also CNS; Spinal cord
Breastfeeding 293
  and antibiotics 291
Brena-Chapman clusters 62
Bretylium 382–383
'Buddy-buddy' injections 164
'Bullet-tipped' needle 216
Bupivacaine 69–77, 188–190, 198,
    217, 221–223, 227–228, 232,
    243–245, 248, 281, 283, 323,
    324, 326–328, 331, 334, 354,
    356–357, 359
  and breastfeeding 293
  in children 267
  efficacy 176
  maximum dose of 117
  plus 2–chloroprocaine 73
  in pregnancy 290
  vs. ropivacaine 296
  see also Local anesthetics
Buprenorphine 112
Burns 40, 127, 301–308
  and benzodiazepines 305–306
  and butorphenol 305
  depth classification of 302
  and diazepam 305
  and enflurane 307
  and fentanyl 305
  inhalational agents and 306–307
  ketamine and 306
  lorazepam and 305
  management of 303–308
  methoxyflurane and 307
  and midazolam 305–306
  and morphine 304
  and nalbuphine 305
  nitrous oxide and 306–307
  non-steroidal anti-inflammatory
    drugs (NSAIDs) and 306
  and opioids 304

pain experience of 301
pain mechanisms in 301–302
patient-controlled analgesia
    (PCA) for 304–305
  in pregnancy 288
  stages of 303
  types of 302–303
Burst vertebral fractures 154–155
Buspirone 68
Butorphanol 305

Caffeine 199
Calcitonin gene-related protein
    (CGRP) 31, 34
Calcium-channel blockers 383
Calcium ions 189
Canes, in spasticity 152
Cannon's phenomenon 373
Cannulae see Catheterization
Carbamazepine 68
Carbocaine 74
Carbon dioxide 111, 141
  retention, in the CNS 347
Cardiac risk index (ACP) 87
Cardiac risk, in surgery 87–91
  and surgical procedure 89
Cardiovascular disease 86–92
Cardiovascular system 50, 197
  and inhalational anesthesia
    144–145
  and opioids 141
  in pregnancy 288–289
  see also Heart
Carpal tunnel syndrome (CTS)
    157–158
  associated disorders 157–158
Cars see Motor vehicle accidents
    (MVAs)
Catecholamines 132–133
  see also Epinephrine (adrenaline)
Catheterization
  of children 282–283
  for epidurals 183
Catheters, for epidurals 183
  and musculocutaneous nerve
    block 213–217
Cauda equina syndrome 200
Caudal anesthesia 281–282
Caudal block 279–283
  continuous 282
Caudal epidural techniques
    185–187
  in children 188
Causalgia see Complex regional
    pain syndrome II
Cellulitis 102

Central hypersensitization 49–50
Central nerve blocks 122, 329
    see also Spinal cord
Cephalin 99
Cephalosporins 291–292
Cerebral blood flow 339–340
Cerebral vasodilatation, and
        ketamine 143
Cerebrospinal fluid (CSF) 179,
        183, 187, 419–420
Cervical epidural techniques
        184–185
    at C6–C7 186
Cervical facet rhizotomy 408
Cervical facet syndrome 406–407
Cervical spine instability 325
C fibers 29–33, 40–41, 140, 258,
        301–302, 316
    spinal cord 33
Chakra balancing 260
Chassignac's tubercle 271
Chayan technique 230–231
Chemoreceptor trigger zone 173
    see also Nausea; Vomiting
Chest percussive therapy 138
Chest wall anatomy 311–314
Children
    caudal epidurals 196
    continuous caudal/epidural
        catheterization 282–283
    epidurals for 187–188
    regional anesthesia for, in trauma
        265–286
Chinese medicine 3–4
Chloramphenicol 291–292
Chlordiazepoxide 291
2–Chloroprocaine 69–77
    in children 267
    plus bupivacaine 73
Chloroquine 291–292
Cholestasis 95
Cholecystokinin 34–35
Choline magnesium trisalicylate 64
Chronic compartment syndrome
        156–157
    events in 156
Chronic obstructive pulmonary
        disease (COPD) 8, 9, 92–93,
        360
    and death 9
Chronic pain 369–402
    management of 61–62
Chronic post-traumatic pain 58–59
Chronic renal insufficiency 97
Cirrhosis 94–95
Citanest 68
Clonidine 148, 193–194, 248, 383

CNS 339–349
    delirium and 145
    ketamine 143
    local anesthetic toxicity 77
    pathology of 177–178
    and phantom pain 388–390
    in pregnancy 290
    see also Brain; Spinal cord
Coagulation defects, in regional
        anesthesia 132–133, 178
Coagulation tests 99
Coagulopathy 97–101
Cocaine 74
Codeine 63
Cognition, and pain control
        255–256
Cognitive intervention, in burns
        therapy 307–308
    see also entries under Behavior
Cold hyperalgesia 40
Cold therapy 259
Collagen 159
Coma 340–341
    and the Glasgow Coma Scale 341
Compartment syndrome 156–157
Common peroneal nerve block 279
Complex regional pain syndrome
        39, 370–384, 403–406, 411,
        418
    α1–blockers and 383
    β-blockers and 383–384
    acute 'hyperemic' phase of 374
    'atrophic' phase of 375
    Bier's block and 381–383
    bone scan and 377
    calcium channel blockers and 383
    central α2–agonists and 383
    central processes of 373–374
    classification of 371
    contact thermography and 376
    criteria for 371
    diagnosis of 375
    diagnostic sympathetic block 377
    digital plethysmography 376
    dystrophic 'ischemia' phase of
        374–375
    epidural sympathetic block and
        380
    guanethidine blockade and 378
    infrared thermography 376
    local anesthetic sympathetic
        ganglion block and 377
    management of 378
    neurostimulatory techniques for
        384
    oscillometry and 376
    pathogenesis 372

percutaneous sympatholytic
        techniques 379–380
    peripheral nerve blocks and 380
    peripheral processes and 372–373
    phentolamine administration for
        380–381
    phenotlamine infusions 377–378
    Q-SART sweat reponse test
        376–377
    radiofrequency percutaneous
        sympatholysis 380
    radiographic bone density 377
    skin blood flow measurements
        376
    skin conductance response 377
    skin temperature measurements
        376
    stellate ganglion block 379
    surgical management of 383
    sweating 376–377
    sympathetic block 379
    sympathetic ganglion block
        379–380
    sympathetically independent pain
        372
    syndrome I (reflex sympathetic
        dystrophy) 38–39, 58, 59,
        133, 370–384, 403–406,
        411, 418
    definition of 371–372
    syndrome II (causalgia) 38–39,
        370–384, 403–406, 411, 418
    definition of 372
    taxonomy 371
    transcutaneous electrical nerve
        stimulation (TENS) 384
    transcutaneous oxygen
        monitoring 376
Compression vertebral fractures
        154–155
Computerized tomography 198
Conscious sedation 125
    see also Sedation
Congenital disorders see Teratology
Contact thermography 376
Continuous analgesia/sedative
        therapy, i.v. 145–146
Continuous brachial plexus needle
        215
Continuous epidurals 194–199
Continuous passive motion 150
    see also Contractures
Continuous peripheral nerve blocks
        209–238
    rationale for 210–211
Contiplex Continuous Brachial
        Plexus Anesthesia Tray 216

Cordotomy 153
Coronary artery disease prediction 89
Coronary revascularization 87–91
Corticotropin-releasing hormone (CRH) 48
Cortisol 48, 132
Contractures 149–150
Costoclavicular space 157
Costs, and trauma care 17–18
Coumadin 98
C-polymodal nociceptors 30, 373
Crawford needle 214, 282
Critical care 24
    post-operative 24
    pre-operative 24
'Cross-talk' theory 373
CRPS I see Complex regional pain syndrome I
CRPS II see Complex regional pain syndrome II
Crutches, in spasticity 152
Cryolesioning 411
Cryoneurolysis 410–411
    intercostal 330
Cryoprobe 410, 411
Cryotherapy 411
Cubital tunnel syndrome 188
Cutaneous blood flow 376
Cutaneous sensations 385
Cutaneous stimulation 356
Cyclobenzapine 69
Cyclooxygenase 64
    pathways 63–64
Cyclooxygenase 2 inhibitors (COX 2 inhibitors) 65
Cyclosporine 95
Cytokines 31
Cytomegalovirus 94

Dalens sciatic nerve block 273–274
Dantrolene 145
Death
    in the UK 9, 10
    in the USA 8, 10
    worldwide statistics 11
Deaths, trimodal distribution of 21
Decerebrate rigidity 151
Decorticate rigidity 151
Decubitus ulcers 153–154
    grading system for 153, 154
    prevention of 153–154
    treatment of 154
Deep-heating devices 260
Deep sedation 125
    see also Sedations

Deep venous thrombosis 317–318
Delayed diagnosis 120
Delirium 145
Demand dose, patient-controlled analgesia (PCA) 166
Deoxyhemoglobin 111
Dextran 100
Diabetes mellitus 95
Diaphragmatic/abdominal breathing 255
Diaphragmatic paresis 219
    hemi- 221
Diaphragmatic rupture 315
Diathermy 260
Diazepam 58, 68, 123, 142, 146, 291, 305, 345
    see also Benzodiazepines
Diclofenac 64–65
Differentiated pain management, in emergency room 128
Diflunisal 64
Digital nerve blocks 121
Digital plethysmography 376
Diphenhydramine 168
Disc disruption 412
Disseminated intravascular coagulopathy (DIC) 98
Distal upper extremity blocks 272
Distraction techniques, and burns 307–308
Domestic violence, in pregnancy 288
Dorsal root entry zone (DREZ) 391–392
Dorsal root ganglion 32, 38
Dosage intervals, in patient-controlled analgesia (PCA) 166
Drapes 134
Dressing changes 173
Dressing devices 153
Drowning, in River Thames 4–5
Drug abusers 202
Drug delivery, implantable systems 418–420
Dupuytren's disease 382
Dura mater 179
Dysfibrinogenemias 99
Dynorphin 34

Earlobe stimulation, and TENS 395
Eating utensils 153
'Ebb' phase 47, 49
Ebers Papyrus 3–4
ECG (electrocardiography) 111

see also Cardiovascular system; Heart
Education of patients 254
EEG (electroencephalography) 139–140
    see also CNS, Spinal cord
Egyptian Civilization 3–4
Eicosanoids 63–64
    see also Prostaglandins
Electric current, and needles 354–355
Electrical stimulation, radiofrequency techniques 405–410
Electrocution 288
    in pregnancy 288
Electrolyte disorders 96–97
Emergency medical service (EMS) 22–24, 109–118
    pain management and 119–129
Emergency room pain management 121–127
    drug administration and 122–125
    for fractures 127
    for head injuries 127
    monitoring in 126
    nerve blocks for 121–122
    safety of 126
    shock and 127
    techniques in 125
    thermal injuries in 127
Emergency visits, hospital, USA 17
EMLA cream 266, 272
Endocrine disorders 95–96
Endogenous opioids 34
Endorphins 34, 48
End-tidal carbon dioxide 111
Enflurane 144–145, 307
Enkephalins 34
Enlightenment, the 4
Enoxaparin sodium 100, 201
Enthesitis 159
Entonox 115
Entrapment neuropathies 418
Enzymes, liver 93
Ephaptic transmission theory 373
Ephedrine 135
Epidemiology of trauma 6–18
Epidural adhesions 412
Epidural analgesia 132–133, 240–244, 247–8, 322–325, 354
    advantages of 196
    alfentanil 192, 194, 321
    contraindications 177–178
    disadvantages of 196

effects and complications 196–199
after extremity trauma 177
fentanyl 191, *194–195, 196*, 243, 247, 321, 324, 334
and the gastrointestinal system 197
hydromorphone 176, 190–191, 194, 195, 321, 323, 324, 334
in local anesthesia 188–189
morphine 176, 190, *194–195, 196*, 243, 247–9, 312, 321, 323, 324
opioids 177, 189–193, *194, 195*, 245, 248, 320, 321–322
pediatric 187–188
in pregnancy trauma patient surgery 293–294
respiratory depression and 196
sufentanil 191, *194, 195*
technique see Epidural blocks
urinary retention and 197
see also Lumbar epidural analgesia; Thoracic epidural analgesia
Epidural blocks 240, 244, 247, 279–283, 324–325
after abdominal/pelvic trauma 176–177, 320–326
caudal 185–186
cervical 184–185
in children 187–188, 282–283
circulatory effects of 197
continuous protocols 194–196, 243, 320, 323–324
and the gut 197
infusions see Infusions
local toxicity 198
lumbar 180–184, 241
mechanism 179–180
neurologic sequelae 197–198
opioids see Opioids
patient-controlled (PCEA) 177, 195, 324–325
vs. peripheral nerve block *211*
and phantom pain 392–393
respiratory complications with 196
technique 178, 179–180
thoracic 176, 184, *197*, 198, 240–241, 247, 248, 324–325
and urinary retention 197
see Epidural analgesia
Epidural scarring 412
Epidural space 179

Epidural sympathetic block 380
Epiduroscopy 414
Epinepherine (adrenaline) 48, 135, 232
and caudal anesthesia 281
and distal upper extremity blocks, in children 272
with local anesthetics *72, 117*, 121, 189
Epstein-Barr virus 94
Equipment, for emergency airway management 133
Ergonomics 158
Erythromycin 291–292
Erythropoietin 97
Ester local anesthetics 74
Ethambutol 291–292
Ethanol (alcohol) 16, 24, 134–135, 326
abuse of 326
see also Alcoholism
liver and 94
Etidocaine 69–77
see also Local anesthetics
Etodolac 65
Etomidate 143
Evoked potentials 139–140
Excitatory amino acids 34, 387–388
Exercises 155
Exsanguination, in intravenous regional anesthesia 272–273
Exteroceptive sensation 385
'Extracath' technique 214, 226
Extremity trauma 177

Faces pain scale 139
Facet joint pain 406, 407, 410
Facet joint syndrome 406–410
cervical 406–408, 411
lumbar 411
Facial pain 411
Failed back surgery syndrome 412, 416
Falls 14
in pregnancy *288*
Fascia iliaca block 276–277
vs. 'three-in-one' block 277
Fatty liver 94
Femoral nerve 223–225
Femoral nerve block 116–117, 122, 275–276, 363–365
indications for 116
technique of 116–117
Femoral nerve entrapment 158–159
Fenoprofen 65

Fentanyl 112, 123, 141, 191, *194–6*, 243, 247–248, 281, 283, 305, 321, 324–326, 329, 334, 346
Fetus see Pregnancy, and trauma
Fibrin 99
Fibrinogen 99
Fibrinolysis 50
Finances, of trauma care 17–18
Fingers
and nerve block 121–122
splints for 150
Firearms 15, 25
and pregnancy *288*
First-degree burns 302–303
First pain 30
Flail chest 314–315
Flexion—distraction fractures 154–155
'Flow phase' 47
Flow Sheets, in patient-controlled analgesia (PCA) 168, *170*
Flumazenil 346
Fluphenazine 66
Flurbiprofen 65
Fluoroscopy *404*, 405, *408, 409, 413*, 419, *420*
Foot drop 159
Fourth-degree burns *302*, 303
Fractures 127
hip 359–360, 362
vertebral 154–155
types of *154*
Functional residual capacity, and thoracic trauma *315*
Fungal infections, and propofol 144
see also Amphotericin B

GABA (γ-aminobutyric acid) receptors 33, 142, 143
Galen 4
Gastrointestinal system 51, 132
and epidural analgesia 197
and opioids 142
in pregnancy 290
Gate theory (Melzack & Wall) pain theory 253–254, 258, 374
General anesthesia, for heart disease 91–92
Geography, and trauma statistics 6–18
Gilbert's disease 93–94
Glasgow Coma Scale 19, 111, 341
Glomerular filtration rate (GFR) 97
Glucagon *48*, 142

Glucocorticoid equivalents, for drugs 96
Glucocorticoids 48
Glucose metabolism 132–133
Glutamate 34, 189
γ-Glutamyl transpeptidase 93
Glycine 34–35
'Golden Hour' 21, 23
Goiter 95–96
Graves' disease 95
Greek Civilization 4
Growth hormone 48
Guanethidine 381–382
  blocks with 378
Guardini sciatic nerve block 274
Guns see Firearms

Haloperidol 348
Halothane 144, 245, 281
Hand, and nerve block 121–122
Hand splints 150
Hand, trauma, children 272
'Hanging drop' technique 185, 242
Head see CNS
Headaches, and spinal anesthesia 103
  see also Post-dural puncture headache
Head injuries 127, 132, 339–349
  algorithm for treatment 342
  see also Brain; CNS
Heart 50, 132
  and inhalational anesthesia 144–145
  and local anesthetic toxicity 77
  and opioids 141
  in pregnancy 288–289
  see also Cardiovascular system
Heat injuries see Burns
Heat therapy 259–260
Helicopters 110, 113
Hemothorax 314
Heparin 98, 99, 201–202
  low-molecular-weight (LMWH) 100–101, 201–202
Heparin-antithrombin III complex 99
Hepatic disease 93–95
Hepatitis 94
Hepatotoxicity, with halothane 144
Herniation 155
Hip fractures 359–364
  femoral nerve block 363
  lateral femoral cutaneous nerve block 363

lumbar plexus block 360–362
obturator nerve block 363–364
Histamine 31, 68–69
History, of trauma anesthesia 3–6
HIV 8, 102
  deaths and 9
Homer (Iliad) 4
Homocide 14–15
Horner's syndrome 132, 219, 222, 352, 353, 357
Hospitals, and trauma
  in-hospital resuscitation 23
  pre-hospital care 22–23
  working conditions and 110
Humane Society 4
Hyalouronidase 413
Hydrogen ions 31
Hydromorphone 63, 190–191, 324–326, 329
Hydroxychloroquine 291–292
Hydroxyzine 68–69
Hyperabduction syndrome 157
Hyperalgesia 38–41, 302
Hypercoagulability 51
Hyperflexion injuries 155
Hyperglycemia 95, 133
Hypertension, CNS see Intracranial pressure (ICP)
Hyperthyroidism 95–96
Hypertonic saline 413
Hypertonic states 151
Hypesthesia 40
Hypnotics 124, 143, 256
  for burns 308
  imagery 256
  suggestions 256
  see also Etomidate; Sedation
Hypoglycemia, and teratogenicity 291
Hypotension 57–58, 134, 143, 199–200
Hypothalamic–pituitary–adrenal axis 48
Hypothalamus 48
Hypothyroidism 95–96
Hypovolemia 57–58, 113, 135, 143, 178
Hypoxemia 132
Hypoxia, and patient-controlled analgesia (PCA) 172

Ibuprofen 65
ICU see Intensive care units
Iliacus muscle 224
Imagery 256
Immune system 51

Implantable drug-delivery systems 419–420
Indomethacin 64
Infection see Bacterial infection
Infiltration
  of local anesthetics 121, 353
  and thoracic trauma 326
Inflammation, and myofascial pain 159
  see also Non-steroidal anti-inflammatory drugs (NSAIDs)
Infraclavicular brachial plexus block 217–218, 358–359
Infrared thermography 376
Infusion 176–177, 190–191, 193, 199, 202
  alfentanil 192, 194, 321
  bupivacaine 188–189, 196, 198, 243, 244, 247, 249, 323, 324, 326–328, 33–332, 334
  continuous epidural 194–196, 243, 430, 323–324
  fentanyl 191, 194–195, 196, 243, 247, 321, 324, 334
  hydromorphone 176, 190–191, 194, 195, 321, 323, 324, 334
  lidocaine 188, 241, 244
  lumbar epidural 241, 243, 247–248
  local anesthetic 188–189, 241, 247, 248
  morphine 176, 190, 194–195, 196, 243, 247–9, 312, 321, 323, 324
  opioids 177, 189–193, 194, 195, 245, 248, 320, 321–322
  ropivacaine 189
  sufentanil 191, 194, 195
  thoracic epidural 240–243, 247
Inguinal ligament 224
Inguinal paravascular lumbar plexus block 226–228
Inhalational anesthetics 115–116, 144, 306–307
In-hospital vs. pre-hospital working conditions 110
Injection injuries 418
'Injury' see Trauma
Injury Severity Scale 19, 20
Injury site, and chronic post-traumatic pain 58–59
Insulated needles 354–355
  see also Sheathed needles
Insulin 132–133

Intensive care units (ICUs)
    137–147
    muscle relaxants and 348
    see also Emergency medical
        service (EMS)
Intercostal nerve block 241–244,
    248, 326–327
Intercostal nerve cryoneurolysis
    330
Intercostal neuralgia 418
Intercostal space 241, 242,
    313–314
Interleukins 31
International Classification of
    Disease (ICD-9) 6–7
International death rates 11
International Normalized Ratio
    (INR) 99
International trauma statistics
    6–18
Interpleural (intrapleural) analgesia
    242, 244, 245, 248–249,
    327–328
Interscalene-directed brachial
        plexus block 122, 220–222,
        270, 357–358
Interspinous ligament 178
    pain from 411
'Intracath' techique 214, 226
Intracompartmental tissue pressure
    156–157
Intracranial pressure (ICP) 178,
        339–342
    and carbon dioxide retention
        347
    monitoring 342–343
Intramuscular analgesia 353
Intramuscular injections 163
    method of 165
Intrapleural analgesia see
    Interpleural analgesia
Intravascular injections 267
Intravascular volume 360
Intravenous analgesia 353
    and thoracic trauma 245, 249
Intravenous PCA see Patient-
    controlled analgesia (PCA)
Intravenous regional anesthesia
        272–273, 353–354
    in children 272–273
    see also Bier's block
Intubation 340–341
    analgesia for 341
Invasive blood pressure 111
Ionization, of local anesthetics 71
Islam 4
Isoflurane 144–145

Jewett hyperextension
        (thoracolumbosacral
        (TLSO)) orthosis 155
Joint pain 36
Joule-Thompson effect 410–411

Kaolin 99
Ketamine 57–58, 60, 113–114,
        123, 143, 306
    and phantom limb pain 394
    side effects of 114, 123, 143
Ketoacidosis 95
Ketoprofen 65
Ketorolac 60, 65, 140
Kidneys 96–97
Kinesthetic sensations 385
Kleishauer–Betke test 290
Klenzak foot—ankle orthosis 152
Knee nerve blocks 278
Knife wounds 15
    and pregnancy 288

Laminas, spinal cord 32–33
Laryngeal block 219, 222
Laryngeal mask airway 266
Lateral femoral cutaneous nerve
        block 278
    thigh 363
'Late death', after trauma 21
    UK vs. USA rates 21
Levorphanol 63
Lidocaine (lignocaine) 69–77, 74,
        188, 232, 382–383
    in children 267, 272–273
    headaches and 103
    maximum doses of 117
    seizures with 272
    see also Local anesthetics,
        Infusion
Ligamentum flavum 178
Lipophilicity, of opioids 189
Lipoxygenase 63–64
Lissauer's tract 32
Literature, and trauma 3–6
Liver
    disease 93
    and halothane 144
Livingston's reverberatory circuit
        theory 373–374
Loading dose, in patient-controlled
        analgesia (PCA) 166
Local anesthetics 69–77, 116–117,
        241–242, 247–248, 267,
        291, 324, 328, 329
    amino acid 74

bicarbonation 73
    for brachial plexus block, in
        children 268
    and breastfeeding 293
    bupivacaine infusion 188–189,
        196, 198, 243, 244, 247,
        249, 323, 324, 326–328,
        33–332, 334
    carbonation and 73
    cardiovascular system and 77
    chemical properties of 70
    children, in trauma 267
    chiral forms of 71
    clinical profile of 75
    combinations of 73
    CNS toxicity of 77
    concentration of 72
    contrivous epidural 194–196,
        243, 430, 323–324
duration of action 71
    emergency room use of 121–122
    plus epinephrine 72, 117, 189
    equipotency of 70
    ester 74
    infusion see Infusion, see under
        names of drugs
    injection site and 72–73
    ionization of 71
    lidocaine infusion 188, 241,
        244
    lipid solubility of 70
    local tissue toxicity 76
    minimum concentration
        (MLAC) 188
    onset time 73
    physical properties of 70
    in pregnancy 73
        trauma patient surgery and
            295–296
    protein binding 70–71
    reaction to, differential diagnosis
        61
    ropivacaine infusion 189
    sodium ions and 72
    sympathetic ganglion block 377
    systemic toxicity 76
    temperature and 73
    toxicity of 76, 198, 200
        and chirality 71
    vasconstrictor agents and 72
        and epinephrine 72, 117, 189
    volume of 72
Lockout intervals, in patient-
        controlled analgesia 166
Longitudinal ligaments 179
Lorazepam 142, 306
    as Ativan 345

'Loss of resistance' method 181, 242
Lovenox 100, 201
Lower extremity blocks, in children 273–274
  via sciatic nerve 273–274
    anterior approach to 274
    lateral approach to 274
    posterior approach to 273–274
Lower extremity continuous plexus blocks 223–233
Low back pain 411
Low-molecular-weight heparin (LMWH) 100–101, 201–202
Lumbar epidural techniques 180–184, 241
  complications with 197, 198
  lateral decubitus position for 180–181
  see also Epidural analgesia; Epidural blocks; Thoracic epidural analgesia; Thoracic blocks; Thoracic epidural blocks
Lumbar epidural opioids 241, 243, 247–248, 321
  see also Epidural analgesia; Infusions; Opioids
Lumbar intrathecal opioids 248, 323
  see also Epidural analgesia; Infusions; Opioids
Lumbar nerve root entrapment 158
Lumbar plexus 223–225, 275
Lumbar plexus block 277, 360–362
Lumbar plexus, perivascular approach to see 'Three-in-one' block
Lumbar puncture, complications of 103
Lumbosacral plexus block 229–230
Lumbosacral spinal anesthesia 187
Lungs 132, 340–341
  intrapleural (intrapleural) analgesia 242, 248–249, 314–316
  in pregnancy 290
  and thoracic trauma 314–316
  see also Chronic obstructive pulmonary disease (COPD); Pulmonary disease
Lympho-adrenal axis 48
Lysis of adhesions, epidural 412

Magnesium ions 189, 290
Major nerve blocks 122

Major Trauma Outcome Study 20
Malleolus, and ankle block 117
Manipulation 259
Marcaine 74, see Bupivacaine
Massage 259
Maternal trauma see Pregnancy, and trauma
McGill Pain Questionnaire 301
Mean arterial pressure, and head injuries 340
Mechanical allodynia 39–41
Meclofenamate 65
Median nerve block, in children 272
Mefenamic acid 65
Melzack and Wall pain theory 253–254, 258, 374, 416, 418
  phantom limb pain 380–390, 403, 416
Meningitis 101–102
Mental acuity, for patient-controlled analgesia (PCA) 167, 173
Mental function 132
  see also entries under Behavior
Meperidine 63, 141
Mepivacaine 69–77, 223, 232
  in children 267
  see also Local anesthetics
Methadone 63, 146, 202
Methionine synthase 144
Methotrexate 94
Methotrimeprazine 67
Methoxyflurane 307
N-Methyl-D-aspartate (NMDA) receptors 34, 189
  phantom limb pain and 394
Metronidazole 291–292
Microwave diathermy 260
Midazolam 124, 125, 142, 146, 305–306, 346
  see also Benzodiazepines
Midline approaches, to epidurals
  lumbar 180–181
  thoracic 184
Midline spinal anesthesia 187
Minnesota Multiphase Personality Inventory 59
Minor nerve blocks 121–122
Missed diagnosis 120
Mitral regurgitation 91
Mitral stenosis 91
Monoradiculopathy 200
Morphine 63, 67, 69, 112, 123, 141, 249, 281, 294–295, 304
  for burns 304
  as elixir 329

infusion 176, 190, 194–195, 196, 243, 247–249, 312, 321, 323, 324
  for neurologic injuries 346
  and respiratory depression 190
  for thoracic trauma 243, 320–321, 324–326, 331, 332, 334
  see also Epidural analgesia
Morphine 6–glucuronide 141
Morphine sulfate (MS-Contin) 329, 346
  see also Opioids
Motion see Range of motion (ROM)
Motor vehicle accidents (MVAs) 5–6, 10–14
  in pregnancy 288
  prevention 24–25
MRI 198
Multiple dressing changes 173
Murder see Homocide
Muscle relaxants 68–69, 348
  ideal, qualities of 348
  intubation and 340–341
Muscle sensory receptor classification 36
Muscular pain 36
Musculocutaneous nerve block 213–217
Musculoskeletal system, in pregnancy 290
Music 134, 307
MVAs see Motor vehicle accidents
Myelinated sensory fibers 36
Myofascial pain 159
Myotendinitis 159
Myxedema 96

Nabumentone 65
Nalbuphine 63, 112, 305
Naloxone 124, 142, 168, 283
  see also Opioids
Naphthyl-alkanones 65
Naproxen 65
Narcotics see Opioids
National trauma statistics 6–18
Nausea 173, 192, 200
Needles 211–212
  for caudal block 279
  insertion, in epidurals 181–184, 186
  insulated 354–355, see Sheathed needles
  selection of 267
  and thoracic trauma 323

Nerve blocks *see under specific anatomical locations*

Nerve entrapment syndromes 157–159

Nerve growth factor 31

Nerve root avulsion 416

Nerve stimulators 266–267, 354–356

Neural damage 268

Neurokinin A 189

Neuroleptic malignant syndrome 145

Neuroleptics 67, 145
  guidelines for using 67

'Neuromatrix', CNS, and phantom limb pain 388–390

Neuroma 411
  formation *38*

'Neuromodule', CNS, and phantom limb pain 388–390

Neuromuscular blockers, and intensive care units 138–139

Neuropathic pain 38

Neuropathy, entrapment 418

'Neurosignature', CNS, and phantom limb pain 388–390

New Injury Severity Scale 19

Nifedipine 383

Nitrogen, liquid 410–411

Nitrous oxide 5, 124, 144, 306–307
  contraindications for *124*
  oxygen and 115–116
  side effects of *124*

Nociceptor subtypes *30*

Nociception 29–35
  ascending sensory pathways 35
  central sensory neurochemistry 33–35
  CNS anatomy of 32–33
  descending inhibitory pathways 35
  peripheral neuroanatomy 29–32
  peripheral neurochemistry 31–32
  and thoracic trauma 316–318
    central facilitation 316
    neuroendocrine responses 317
    peripheral sensitization 316
    sympathoadrenal activation 316–317

Nociceptive information flow 33

Non-fatal injuries 16–17

Non-steroidal anti-inflammatory drugs (NSAIDs) 64–65, 113, 123, 140, 158, 249, 306, 322, 353
  for burns 306
  mechanism of action 63–64

Norepinephrine (noradrenaline) 31, *48*, 141
  see also Epinephrine (adrenaline)

5'-Nucleotidase 93

Nutrition 132

Observer Assessment of Alertness/Sedation Scale 139

Obturator nerve block 363–364

Occipital neuralgia 412

Octanol:buffer coefficients *190*

Oddi, sphincter of 142

Omnipaque 413, 419

Operating-room pain management *131–136*

Opiates *see* Opioids

Opioids 31–32, 59–60, 62–63, 111–113, 123–124, 140–141, 291, 346, 394
  administration routes 111, *112*
  for burns 304, *305*
  and caudal anesthesia 281
  classification of 111–112
  epidurals 189–193
  equivalent epidural doses *192*
  and the gut 142
  and the heart 141
  implantable drug-delivery systems 419, 420
  infusion 177, 189–193, *194*, *195*, 245, 248, 320, 321–322
  lumbar epidurals 247–248
  octanol-buffer coefficients *190*
  in pregnant trauma patient surgery 295–296
  receptors 33–34
  relative potencies of *63*
  and respiratory depression 124, 141
  side effects of 63, 141–142
    epidurals 192–193
    and thoracic trauma 323–326
  tolerance to 124
  see also Fentanyl; Hydromorphine; Morphine; Patient-controlled analgesia (PCA); Thoracic epidural analgesia

Oral techniques 329

Order Sheets, in patient-controlled analgesia (PCA) 168, *169*

Orthopedic trauma 351–368
  analgesia for 353–354
  brachial plexus blocks for 357–359
  femoral nerve block 364–366
  hip fractures 359–364

nerve blocks 354–355
  sciatic nerve block 364–366
  skin stimulation 356

Oscillometry 376

Oxicam derivatives 65

Oxycodone *63*, 329

Oxycontin 329

Oxygenation 111, 132

Oxygen, transcutaneous 376

Oxyhemoglobin 111

Pain
  by acute injury 56–58
    and hypotension 57–58
    hypovolemia 57–58
  assessment 111, 120–121
  cardiovascular responses 50
  central hypersensitization 49–50
  classification of 35–36
  clinical effects of 48–49
  ebb-flow phases 49
  gastrointestinal complications 51
  hematological consequences 51
  hypothalamic-pituitary-adrenal axis 48
  immune consequences of 51
  joint pain and 36
  location-based management of 109–160
    see also under specific anatomical locations
  lympho-adrenal axis and 48
  management of 56–57
    principles of 56–57
    rationale for 56
  mechanisms of 29–45
  muscular 36
  neuropathic 38
  perioperative management, and trauma 163–261
  psychological factors 59
    see also entries under Behavior
  pulmonary dysfunction 50–51
  referred 37
    see also Phantom limb pain
  and rehabilitation 149–160
  somatic 35–36
  and specific trauma patient populations 265–421
  subtypes of 35
  sympathomedullary adrenal axis 48
  and trauma, interface 3–106
  unresponsive to spinal cord stimulation 412
  unresponsive to spinal opioid 412

Pain (*continued*)
visceral 36
'wind up' 49–50
Pain consultants 260
Pain control 253–260
acupuncture 259
behavioral strategies 254–255
beliefs 254
biofeedback techniques 257–258
breathing 255
cognitive approaches to 255–256
energy-based approaches to 260
hypnosis and 256
imagery and 250
information and 254
manipulation 259
massage 259
mobilization techniques 259
psychotherapy 257
Qigong technique for 260
Reiki technique for 260
social support 254
TENS (transcutaneous electrical
nerve stimulation) 258–259
tense-release exercises 255
therapeutic cold 259
therapeutic heat 259–260
traction for 259
ultrasound for 260
undermedicating 254
underreporting 254
Pancreatitis, with propofol 144
Paracelsus 4
Paracetamol *see* Acetaminophen
Paramedian approaches, to
epidurals 183–184
lumbar 183
thoracic 184
Paramedian spinal anesthesia 187
Paramedic 22–23, 109–111
Paraproteinemias 99
Paraquat 16
Parascalene block, brachial plexus
271
Paratendinitis 159
Paravertebral block 328–329
Partial thromboplastin time 99
Passive range of motion (PROM)
149–150
see also Contractures
Patient-controlled analgesia (PCA)
60, 145, 163–174, 242, 254,
322, 353
advantages of 165
age and 167
allergy and 167
basal infusion rate for 166–167

bolus 166
for burns 304–305
in children *167*
confusion and 173
contraindications for 167
demand dose 166
disadvantages of 165
epidurals (PCEA) *see* Patient-
controlled epidural analgesia
and entries under Epidural
Flow Sheets 168, *170*
hypoxia and 172
ideal qualities for 168–171
loading dose of 166
lockout interval (dosage interval)
166
mental acuity 167
nausea 173
Order Sheets 168, *169*
paradigm for 164–165
patient selection 167
pump manufacturers 173–174
respiratory depression 172
side effects of 171
social history 167
starting dose 168
technology for 168
terminology for 166
thoracic block and 242
thoracic trauma and 173, 322
total hourly dose and 167
trauma and 173, 322
urinary retention and 173
vomiting and 173
Patient-controlled epidural
analgesia (PCEA) 177, 188,
195, 244, 324–325
Patroclus 4
Pectoralis minor syndrome 157
Pediatric lower extremity blocks
273–279
Pediatric techniques 187–188
Pedatric upper extremity blocks
268–272
Pelvic fractures 366
Pelvic trauma 176–177
Pelvis, blood supply to *367*
Penicillin 291–292
Pentazocine *63*
Percutaneous cryoneurolysis
410–411
Peripheral nerve blocks 103,
209–233, 354–355, 380
axillary perivascular brachial
plexus block 213
brachial plexus 212–213
clinical considerations 222–223

infraclavicular brachial plexus
block 217–218
interscalene brachial plexus block
220–222
musculocutaneous nerve block
213–217
rationale for 210–211
sheathed needles for 211–212
stimulators for 211–212, *see*
Insulated needles
subclavian perivascular brachial
plexus block 218–219
Peripheral nerve stimulation
211–212, 418–419
phantom limb pain and 386–387
Peripheral neuropathy 416
Peripheral regional anesthesia, in
pregnant trauma patient
surgery 294
Peroneal nerve block 279
Peroneal nerve entrapment 159
Perphenazine 67
Persistent pain *see* Chronic post-
traumatic pain
pH, of local anesthetics 71–72
Phantom limb pain 133, 384–395,
416
acupuncture for 395
central (supraspinal) 388–390
clinical characteristics of 385
clonidine for 394
concept of 385
definition of 385
epidural blocks for 392–393
fluoxetine for 394
history of 384
intravenous infusions 394
mexiletine 394
opioids for 394
pathogenesis of 385–390
pathophysiology of 385–390
peripheral nerves in 386–387
propranolol for 394
regional anesthesia for 394
spinal analgesia 393–394
spinal anesthesia for 393–394
spinal nerves 387–388
surgical intervention in 390–392
telescoping in 385
transcutaneous electrical nerve
stimulation (TENS) 395
treatment of 390–395
tryptophan and 395
'Phantom limb sensation' 385
Phenoxybenzamine 383
Phentolamine 383
Phentolamine block 380–381

Phentolamine infusion test 377–378
Phenylbutazone 65
Pheochromocytoma 95
Philosophy, and trauma 3–6
Pinprick hyperalgesia 40
Plantar reflex 151
Plexus avulsion 418
Pliny the Elder 4
Pneumothorax 134, 219
Popliteal fossa sciatic nerve block
    278
Post-amputation stump pain 385,
    403, 416
Post-dural puncture headaches 103,
    187, 198–199
Post-surgical neuralgia 411
Post-thoracotomy pain syndrome
    411
Post-traumatic chronic pain test 59
    acute pain 59–60
    chronic pain 58–59
Post-traumatic stress disorder 59
Power spectral analysis 139–140
Prazosin 383
Pre-emptive analgesia 52
Pregnancy, and trauma 287–299
    algorithm for evaluation 289
    anesthetic issues in 290, 292–296
        epidurals 294
        peripheral regional 294
        spinal 293–294
    antibiotics for 291–292
    cardiovascular changes in
        288–289
    central nervous system changes
        290
    epidural anesthesia for 294
    fatty liver in 94
    FDA classification of pain
        medication 292
    gastrointestinal changes 290
    hematological considerations 290
    injuries in 288
    and local anesthesia 73, 291
    musculoskeletal changes in 290
    opioids for 291
    perioperative pain management
        294–295
    peripheral/regional anesthesia
        techniques 294
    physiology of 288
    postoperative regional techniques
        295–296
    pulmonary issues in 290
    ropivacaine 296
    sedatives for 291
    spinal anesthesia for 293–294

teratology of 290–291
Pre-hospital induction, of
    anesthesia 114–115
Pre-hospital vs. in-hospital working
    conditions 110
Pre-hospital monitoring 110–111
    qualities of 110
Pre-hospital working conditions
    109–110
Preoperative cardiac assessment
    algorithm 90
Pressure-relieving cushions
    153–154
Pressure ulcers 153–154
Prilocaine 69–77
    see also Local anesthetics
Primary hyperalgesia 39–41
Procaine 69–77
    see also Local anesthetics
Progesterone, and local anesthesia
    73
Propionic acid derivatives 65
Propiocaine 74
Propofol 124, 144, 146, 266,
    346–347
    and the CNS 347–348
    and head injuries 347–348
    side effects of 144
Propranolol 383–384
Propriomelanocortin 48
Prostaglandin synthetase see
    Cyclooxygenase
Prostaglandins 31, 63–64, 140
Prothrombin time 98–99, 201
Pruritus 192
Psoas compartment block 230–231
Psoas major 224
Psychology, and pain 59
Psychotherapy 257
    see also entries under Behavior
Pulmonary aspiration 132
Pulmonary disease 92–93
    see also Chronic obstructive
        pulmonary disease (COPD)
Pulmonary dysfunction 50–51
Pulmonary embolism 92–93
Pulmonary function tests 92
Pulse oximetry 111, 135
Pump manufacturers 173–174
Pumps, for patient-controlled
    analgesia (PCA) 165
Pupillary constriction 132
Pyrazolone derivatives 65

Qigong technique 260
Q-START (sweat test) 376–377

Quad plus spinal cord stimulator
    416–417
Quadratus lumborum 224

Racz caudal catheter 404, 412
Racz epidural catheter 404, 412
Racz Tun-L-Kath 413, 413, 414
Radial nerve block, in children 272
Radial nerve entrapment 158
Radicular pain 416
Radiculopathy 412
Radiofrequency lesioning 153
Radiofrequency percutaneous
    sympatholysis 380
Radiofrequency techniques
    406–409
    facet 406–408
    sympathetic chain 408–410
Radiofrequency thermocoagulation
    405–410
    see also Sedation
Radiograph 406
Ramsey sedation scale 139, 146
    see also entries under Sedation
Range of motion (ROM) 149–150
    and compartment syndrome 156
    see also Contractures
Ranitidine 290
Reappraisal technique, in burns
    307–308
    information techniques in 308
Referred pain 37
    see also Phantom limb pain
Reflex sympathetic dystrophy
    definition of 370
    see also Complex regional pain
        syndrome I
Regional anesthesia 60–61, 307
    advantages of 102, 131, 132–133,
        352
    and bacterial infections 101–102
    and burns 307
    and cardiovascular function
        91–92, 132
    and cerebral function 132
    in coagulation disorders 99–100
    contraindications 103, 133
    in the emergency room 121–122
    equipment for 133
    in the field 116
    gastrointestinal 132
    musculoskeletal function and 133
    neuroendocrine function and
        132–133
    operative intervention 131–136
    and pediatric trauma 265–286

Regional anesthesia (*continued*)
  for phantom limb pain 394
  potential problems with 134–135
  in pregnancy 294–296
    contraindications and *293*
  respiratory function and 132
  risks of 102–103, 353
    of peripheral nerve block 103
    of spinal anesthesia 103
  see also Analgesia; Epidural
      anesthesia; Epidural blocks;
      Local anesthetics; Opioids;
      Thoracic analgesia; Thoracic
      blocks *and under specific
      location and specific block*
Rehabilitation centers 149–160
Reiki technique 260
Relaxation imagery 256
Relaxation techniques, for burns
    308
Remifentanil 141–142
  side effects of 142
Renaissance, the 4
Renal disorders 96–97
Reptilase 99
Reptilase test 98
Reptilase time 98
Reserpine 381
  see also Neuroleptics
Respiration 255
  in fractured hip 360
  and thoracic injury 314–316
Respiratory depression 124, 141,
    190, 192–193, 196,
    239–240, 325–326
  and patient-controlled analgesia
      (PCA) 172
  and propofol 144
Respiratory function 132
  emergencies, equipment for *133*
Resuscitation 22–23, 339–340
Retropulsed fragmentation 155
Revised Trauma Score 19–20
Rexed classification 32
RFTC needle 408, *409*
Rh-negative, maternal 290
Rheumatoid arthritis 97
Rhizotomy 153
Rifampin 291–292
Rigidity 151
  decerebrate 151
  decorticate 151
Ritodrine 290
Road accidents *see* Motor vehicle
    accidents (MVAs)
Roman Civilization 4
Ropivacaine 69–77, 189, 281, 296

  vs. bupivacaine *296*
  in pregnancy 290
  see also Local anesthetics
Rosenblatt technique 213–214
Royal Society (London) 4

Sacrum, needle trajectory, caudal
    epidurals *186*
Salicylates 64
  see also Non-steroidal anti-
      inflammatory drugs
      (NSAIDs)
Salsalate 64
Scalene triangle 157
Scalp block 343–345
Scarring, epidural 412
Sciatic nerve 273–274
Sciatic nerve block 228–229, 273,
    364–366
  anterior approach to 274, 365
  lateral approach to 274
  popliteal fossa *278*
  supine approach 365–366
Scoring systems, trauma 18–20
  *see also under specific systems by
      name*
Seatbelts, in cars 24–25
  see also Motor vehicle accidents
      (MVAs)
Secondary hyperalgesia 40
Second-degree burns 302–303
Second pain 30
Sedation 124, 125, 134, 137–146,
    291, 344–348
  assessment of 139
  conscious 125
  deep 125
  Ramsay scale for *346*
Sedative hypnotics 68
Selander technique 213
Self-hypnosis 256, *257*
'Self' injections 164
Sensitization 39–41
  central 50
  nociception 30
Sensorcaine 74
Sensory fibers, classification of *30*
Sentient neural hub 388
Serotonin (5–hydroxytryptamine,
    5–HT) 31
'Sheathed' needles 211–212, *see*
    Insulated needles
Shock 127
  see also Trauma
Short-wave diathermy 260
'Shrimp' position 180

Single-shot dosing 188, *194*
Sitting position, for lumbar
    epidurals 180–181
Skin conductance 377
Skin, and muscle sensory receptors
    36–38
Skin sores 153–154
Skin stimulation 357
Skin temperature 376
Skin, trans-, electrical stimulation
    see Transcutaneous electrical
      nerve stimulation (TENS)
'SMA-6' electrolytes 96
Social history, and patient-
    controlled analgesia (PCA)
    167
Social support 254
Sodium ions 189
Sodium pentobarbital 5
Somatic pain 35–36
Somatostatin 31–32, *34*
Spasticity 150–153
  stepped care approach to *151*
Spinal anesthesia 103, 187
  backache 200
  'failed' 200
  hypotension and 199–200
  nausea and 200
  neurological sequelae of 200
  for phantom pain 393–394
  in pregnant trauma patient
      surgery 293–294
  'total' 200
  vomiting and 200
  vs. peripheral nerve block *211*
Spinal cord 32–35, 387–388
Spinal cord injury 416
Spinal cord ischemia 200
Spinal cord stimulation 156–157,
    416
Spinal injuries 354
Spinal nerves, and phantom pain
    287–288
Spiritual healing 260
Splints 150
Sport-related injuries 58–59
Statistical sources, on trauma 6–18
Stellate ganglion block 379
Steroids 404, 408, 413, 414
'STP' 5
Stress 48–49
  endocrine response to 48–49
  metabolic response to 49
  prevention of 51
Stretching 150
'Stump pain' 385
Subarachnoid analgesia 354

Subarachnoid hemorrhage 200
Subarachnoid injection, accidental 198
Subarachnoid space 179
Subclavian perivascular brachial plexus block 218–219
Substance abuse 202
    see also Alcoholism; Ethanol
Substance P 31, 34, 189
Sudomotor axon reflex test (Q-SART) 376–377
Sufentanil 191
Suicide 15–16
    in pregnancy 288
Sulindac 64–65
Sumatriptan 199
'Super added phantom sensation' 385
Superficial skin stimulation 356
Supraclavicular blocks 117
Supraclavicular-directed brachial plexus block 122
Supraspinous ligament 178
Surface area, body, and burns 303
Surgery, and chronic pain 59
Survival, probability of (Ps) 20
Sweating, measurement of 376–377
Sympathetic block 404–406
'Sympathetic-efferent/somatic-afferent' mechanism 386–387
Sympathetic ganglion block 379–380
Sympathetically independent pain 372
Sympathetically maintained pain 372
Sympathectomy, drug-induced 383–384
Sympatholytic blocks 379–383
    intravenous 379–380
    percutaneous 379–380
Sympathomedullary-adrenal axis 48
Systemic lupus erythematosus (SLE) 97
Systemic toxic reactions 267
Systemic vascular resistance 91

'Telescoping' 385
Temporal summation 30–31
Tendon-muscle junction inflammation 159
Tense-release exercises 255
Teratology 290–291
    see also Pregnancy, and trauma
Terazocin 383

Terbutaline 290
Tetracaine 69–77
    in children 267
    see also Local anesthetics
Tetracycline 291–292
Thalamus 33
Thermal hyperanalgesia 40
Thermal injuries see Burns
Thermal lesioning see Thermocoagulation
Thermocoagulation, radiofrequency 405–406
Thermography 376
Thermoplastic molded ankle-foot arthrosis 152
Third-degree burns 302, 303
Thoracic blocks 180–184, 198, 239–250, 326–328
    epidural analgesia see Thoracic epidural analgesia
    epidural blocks see Thoracic epidural blocks
    intercostal nerve blocks 241–244, 248, 326–327
    intrapleural analgesia 242, 244, 245, 248–249, 327–328
    intravenous analgesia 245, 249, 353
    lumbar epidural block 180–184, 197, 198, 241
        and opioids 247–248
    lumbar intrathecal opioids 248
    patient-controlled analgesia (PCA) for 242
Thoracic epidural adrenergic agonists 248
Thoracic epidural analgesia 184, 240, 242–244, 247, 324–325
    continuous infusions 194–196, 243, 320, 323–324
    local anesthetics 248
    opioids see Opioids
    techniques 184
    see also Thoracic epidural blocks, see Infusions
Thoracic epidural blocks 176, 184, 240–241, 247, 322–323
    complications of 197, 198
    local anesthetics and 188–189, 196, 247, 248
    opioids see Opioids
Thoracic facet joint pain 407
Thoracic outlet syndrome 157
Thoracic paravertebral block 328, 329
Thoracic trauma 176, 246, 314–316

associated disorders 246
comparative treatment modalities 330–332
    optimal 332, 334
isolated 246
neuroaxial analgesia 323–324
neuroendocrine responses 317
on-demand analgesia 320–322
patient-controlled analgesia (PCA) 173, 322
phases in 318–320
    acute 319
    chronic 320
    emergent 319
    rehabilitation 319–320
pre-existing illness and 246
respiratory depression and 325–326
Thoracolumbosacral orthosis 155
Thoracotomy, locoregional analgesia 249
Thorax, anatomy of 312–314
'Three-in-one' block 122, 225, 226–228, 275
    in children 276–277
    vs. fascia iliaca blocks 277
Thrombin time 98, 99
Thromboembolism 132
Thromboprophylaxis 100–101, 201–202
    see also Low-molecular-weight heparin (LMWH)
Thrombus formation 51
Thyroid disease 95–96
Thyroid hormones 96
Tinel's sign 38
Tocolytics 290
Toes, and nerve block 121–122
Tometin 65
Tourniquets, for intravenous regional anesthesia 272–273
Traction 259
Tramadol 123, 173, 193–194, 329
Transcutaneous electrical nerve stimulation (TENS) 258–259, 330, 384, 395
Transcutaneous oxygen 376
Transport, of trauma patients 24, 109–118
'Trapped nerves' see Nerve entrapment syndromes
Trauma
    anesthesia 3–6
    anesthesiologists and 21–22
    care, costs of 17–18
    by country, fatalities 8
    courses on 23

Trauma (*continued*)
  death after, and time 21
  ebb phase in 49
  epidemiology of 6–7
  extremities, and continuous
      peripheral nerve block
      209–238
  flow phase in 49
  historical aspects on 3–6
  hormones released in major 48
  international statistics on 7–10
  intensive pain management
      403–421
  multiple-site 134
  and neurological injuries
      339–349
  orthopedic injuries 351–368
  outcome from 18–20
  and pain, interface of 3–106
  pediatric 265–286
  perioperative pain management
      in 163–261
  in pregnancy 287–299
    see also Pregnancy, and trauma
  pre-hospital care 22–23
  prevention of 24–25
  regional anesthesia in 85–106
  resuscitation 23
  specific types of 10
      and pain 265–421
  survival chain in *25*
  thoracic 311–338
      block 239–251
      management strategies 246
  transfer, of patients 24, 109–118
Trauma scoring systems 18–20
  Abbreviated Injury Scale 19
  Glasgow Coma Scale 19
  Injury Severity Score 19
  New Injury Severity Score 19
  Revised Trauma Score 19–20
Trauma team leaders 23
Trauma trimodal death distribution
      21
Tricyclic antidepressants 35, 65–66

Triage Index 19–20
Trigger points 159
TRISS (Trauma Score-Injury
      Severity Score) 20
Turbulence, in complex regional
      pain syndrome *373*
Twitch response 355
  fine tune mode in 355
  search mode 355

UK, deaths, causes of *9, 10*
  see also Trauma, epidemiology
Ulcers *see* Pressure ulcers
Ulnar nerve block, in children 272
Ulnar nerve entrapment 158
Ultrasound 120, 260
Uncooperative patients 178
Unmyelinated sensory fibers 36
Upper abdominal trauma 311–338
Upper extremity blocks, in children
      268–273
  brachial plexus 268–271
  distal 272
Upper extremity continuous plexus
      blocks 212–223, 359
Upper motor neurons, injury to
      150–152
Uremia 97
Urinary retention 192, 197
USA
  deaths, causes of *8*
      and age *9*
  emergency hospital visits 17
  YPLL concept 10
  see also Trauma, epidemiology
Utensils, for eating *153*

Valvular heart disease 91
Vasoactive intestinal peptide *34*
Vasopressin (antidiuretic hormone,
      ADH) *48*
Venflon catheter 213
Ventilation–perfusion (V/Q) 50–51

Verapamil 95
Vertebral body compression 412
Vertebral column 178–179
  lateral view of *179*
Vertebral fractures 154–155
Viral hepatitis 94
Visceral pain 36–38
Viscerosomatic neurons 37
Visual Analog Scale (VAS) 111,
      121, 247–249, 308
Vitamin K 99
Vomiting 173, 192, 200
Von Willebrand's disease 99

Walkers, in spasticity *152*
War 5–6, 384
Warfarin 100
Weiss needle 182
'Werther effect' 16
Wheelchairs *152*
Whiplash injuries 159
Wide-dynamic range neurons
      (WDR) 33, 40, 41, 316,
      373
Wilson's disease 94
Wind-up concept 49–50
Winnie's technique 277–278
Worldwide trauma statistics 6–18
Wright maneuver 157
Wrist blocks 121–122
Wrist splints 150
Writing aides 153
Wydase 413, 414

Xylocaine 74
  see also Local anesthetics, *see also*
      Lidocaine

Years of potential life lost (YPLL)
      concept 10
  in the USA *10*
  see also Trauma, epidemiology